HOLT

Lifetime HEALTH

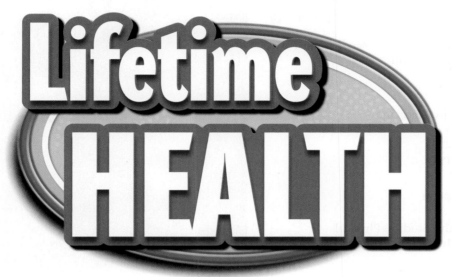

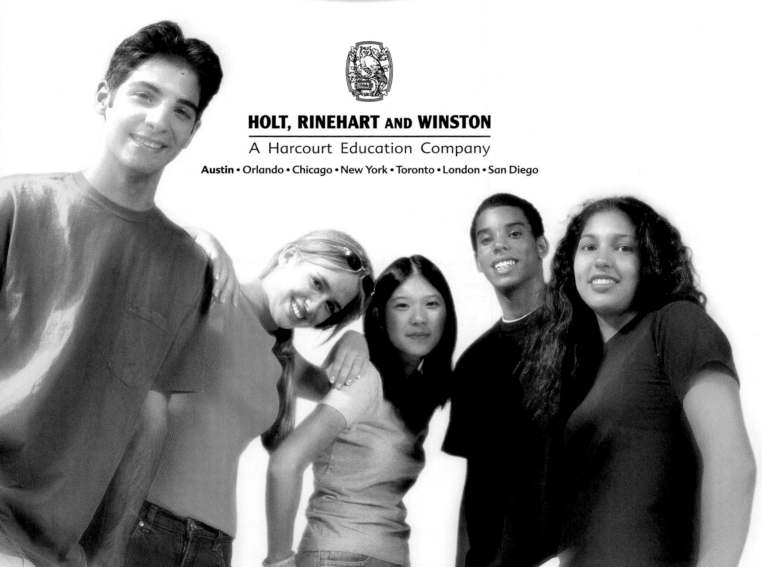

HOLT, RINEHART AND WINSTON

A Harcourt Education Company

Austin • Orlando • Chicago • New York • Toronto • London • San Diego

AUTHORS

David P. Friedman, Ph.D.
Professor, Department of Physiology & Pharmacology
Deputy Associate Dean for Research
Wake Forest University School of Medicine
Winston-Salem, North Carolina

Curtis C. Stine, M.D.
Professor
Department of Family Medicine
    and Rural Health
College of Medicine
Florida State University
Tallahassee, Florida

Shannon Whalen, Ph.D.
Assistant Professor
Department of Health Studies, Physical
    Education and Human Performance
Adelphi University
Garden City, New York

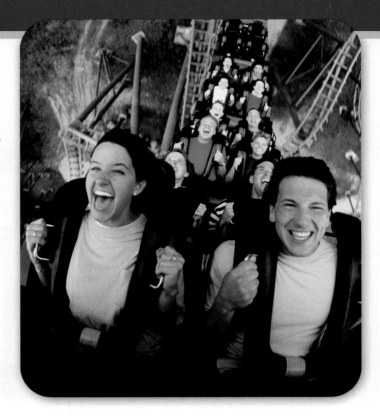

Acknowledgments

CONTRIBUTING AUTHORS

Mary B. Grosvenor, M.S., R.D.
Science and Health Writer
Delta, Colorado

Shahla Khan, Ph.D.
Adjunct Professor
Department of Health Science
University of North Florida
Jacksonville, Florida

Mitchell Leslie
Science and Health Writer
Albuquerque, New Mexico

Josh R. Mann, M.D., M.P.H.
Clinical Assistant Professor
Department of Family and
    Preventive Medicine
University of South Carolina
Columbia, South Carolina

Joe S. McIlhaney, Jr., M.D.
President
The Medical Institute for Sexual
    Health
Austin, Texas

Margaret Meeker, M.D., F.A.A.P.
Pediatrician
Traverse City, Michigan

Jane A. Petrillo, Ed.D.
Assistant Professor
Department of Health, Physical
    Education, and Sport Science
Kennesaw State University
Kennesaw, Georgia

Lori A. Smolin, Ph.D.
Department of Nutritional
    Sciences
University of Connecticut
Storrs, Connecticut

Robert Wilson III
Chairman
Department of Health and
    Physical Education
Morehouse College
Atlanta, Georgia

Kathleen Young, Ph.D.
Research Scientist
Center of Health Promotion and
    Disease Prevention
University of New Mexico
Albuquerque, New Mexico

CONTRIBUTING WRITERS

Sandra Alters, Ph.D.
Science and Health Writer
Montreal, Canada

Daniel H. Franck, Ph.D.
Science and Health Writer
Spencertown, New York

Linda K. Gaul, Ph.D.
Epidemiologist
Texas Department of Health
Austin, Texas

Rosemary E. Previte
Science and Health Writer
Lexington, Massachusetts

Inclusion Specialist

Ellen McPeek Glisan
Special Needs Consultant
San Antonio, Texas

Teacher Edition Development

Sandra Alters, Ph.D.
Science and Health Writer
Montreal, Canada

Linda K. Gaul, Ph.D.
Epidemiologist
Texas Department of Health
Austin, Texas

**Marilyn Massey-Stokes, Ed.D.,
C.H.E.S.**
Associate Professor
Health, Exercise, and Sport
    Sciences
Texas Tech University
Lubbock, Texas

Su Nottingham
*Health and Life Management
    Teacher*
Waterford Mott High School
Waterford, Michigan

Jane A. Petrillo, Ed.D.
Assistant Professor
Department of Health, Physical
    Education, and Sport Science
Kennesaw State University
Kennesaw, Georgia

Debbie Rummel
Health Teacher
Antioch Community High School
Antioch, Illinois

Wendy Schiff, M.S.
Adjunct Lecturer
St. Louis Community College—
    Meramec
St. Louis, Missouri

Joan A. Solorio
Special Education Director
Austin Independent School
    District
Austin, Texas

Kathleen Young, Ph.D.
Research Scientist
Center of Health Promotion and
    Disease Prevention
University of New Mexico
Albuquerque, New Mexico

(continued on p. 684)

CONTENTS *In Brief*

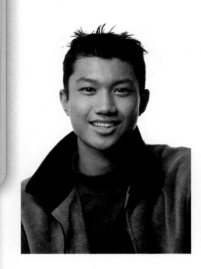

UNIT 1 Health and Your Wellness

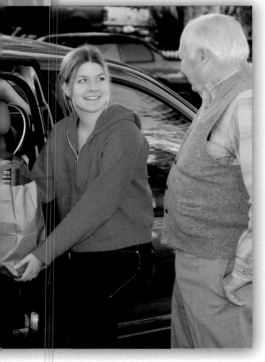

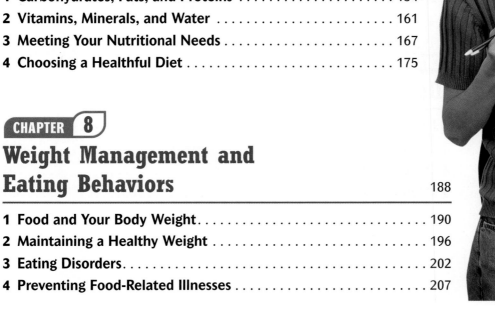

UNIT 3 Drugs

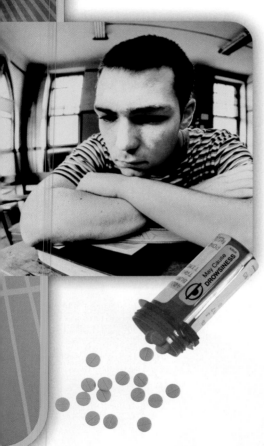

UNIT 4 Diseases and Disorders

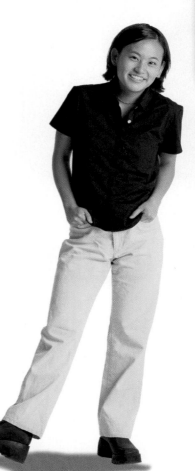

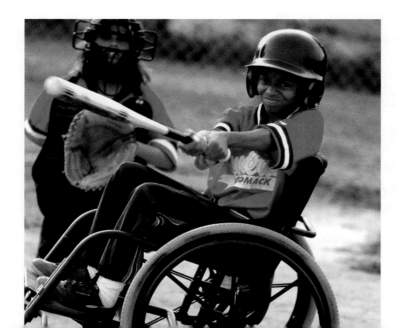

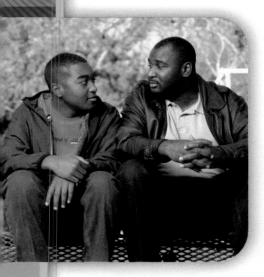

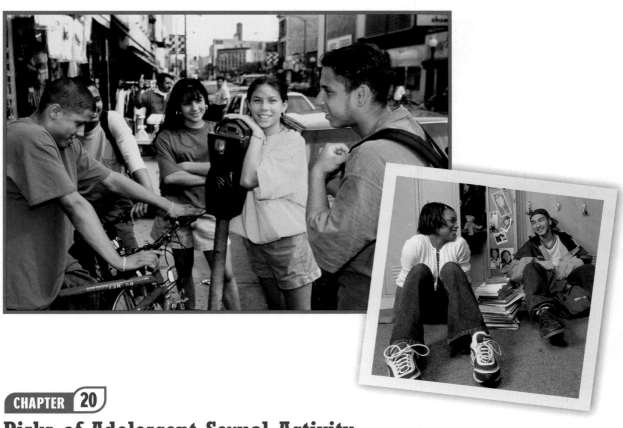

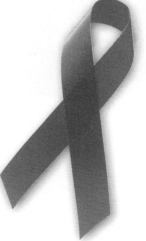

HEALTH Handbook

EXPRESS Lessons

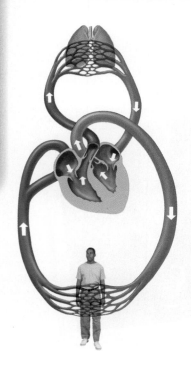

How Your Body Works

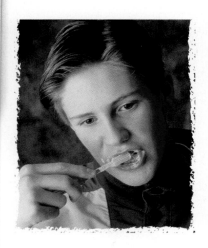

What You Need to Know About...

First Aid and Safety

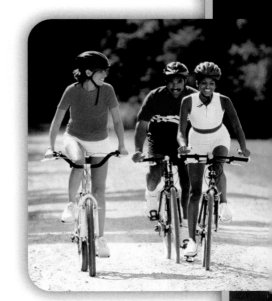

LIFE SKILLS *QUICK REVIEW*

REFERENCE Guide

FEATURES

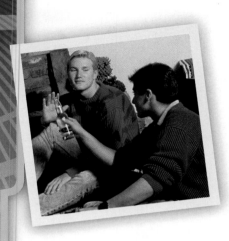
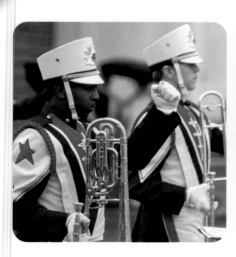

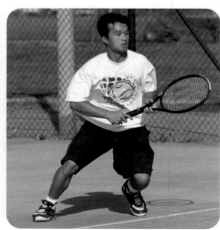

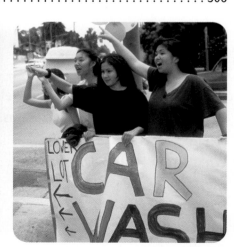

Analyzing DATA

Interpret health data, and draw accurate conclusions.

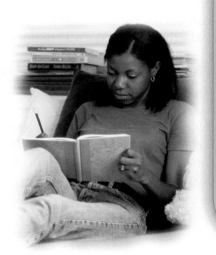

real life Activity

Use these hands-on activities to practice what you've learned.

YOUR Health YOUR World

Analyze the influence of media, technology, and culture on your health.

HOW TO USE YOUR TEXTBOOK

Your Road Map for Success with *Lifetime Health*

Read the Objectives

Objectives tell you what you'll need to know.

STUDY TIP Reread the objectives when studying for a test to be sure you know the material.

Study the Key Terms

Key Terms are listed for each section. Learn the definitions of these terms because you will most likely be tested on them. Use the glossary to locate any definition quickly.

STUDY TIP If you don't understand a definition, reread the page where the term is introduced. The surrounding text should help make the definition easier to understand.

Take Notes and Get Organized

Keep a health notebook so that you are ready to take notes when your teacher reviews the material in class. Keep your assignments in this notebook so that you can review them when studying for the chapter test.

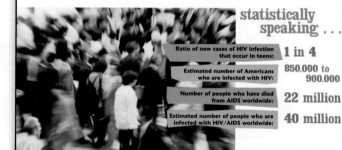

SECTION 1

HIV and AIDS Today

OBJECTIVES

Distinguish between an HIV infection and AIDS.
Name the three areas in the world that have the greatest number of people living with HIV/AIDS.
Compare the number of people in the United States living with HIV infection to the number of people in the United States living with AIDS.
Summarize why teens are one of the fastest-growing groups infected with HIV.

KEY TERMS

human immunodeficiency virus (HIV) the virus that primarily infects cells of the immune system and that causes AIDS
acquired immune deficiency syndrome (AIDS) the disease that is caused by HIV infection, which weakens the immune system
pandemic a disease that spreads quickly through human populations all over the world

Every day, about 110 Americans are infected with HIV. Three million people died from AIDS in 2000. Currently, there is no cure for AIDS. Do you know how to help fight against the spread of HIV and AIDS?

What Are HIV and AIDS?

HIV and AIDS are different. **Human immunodeficiency virus (HIV)** is the virus that primarily infects cells of the immune system and that causes AIDS. **Acquired immune deficiency syndrome (AIDS)** is the disease that is caused by HIV infection, which weakens the immune system.

HIV infection is an infection in which HIV has entered the blood and is multiplying in a person's body cells. HIV specifically infects cells of the immune system. HIV eventually destroys the body's ability to fight off infection. After someone is infected with HIV, the virus

statistically speaking . . .

Ratio of new cases of HIV infection that occur in teens:	1 in 4
Estimated number of Americans who are infected with HIV:	850,000 to 900,000
Number of people who have died from AIDS worldwide:	22 million
Estimated number of people who are infected with HIV/AIDS worldwide:	40 million

Be Resourceful, Use the Web

*HEALTH LINKS*sm

Internet Connect boxes in your textbook take you to resources that you can use for health projects, reports, and research papers. Go to **scilinks.org/health,** and type in the HealthLinks code to get information on a topic.

Visit go.hrw.com
Find worksheets, articles from *Current Health,* and other materials that go with your textbook at **go.hrw.com.** Click on the textbook icon and the table of contents to see all of the resources for each chapter.

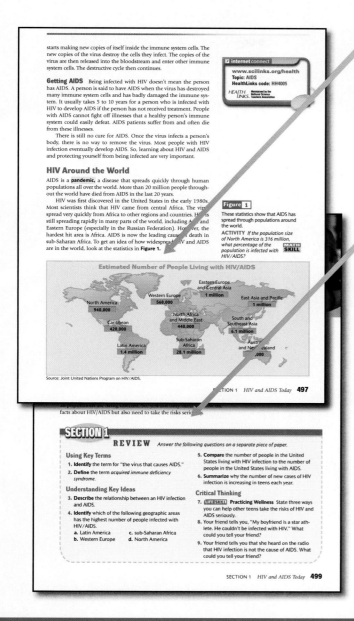

starts making new copies of itself inside the immune system cells. The new copies of the virus destroy the cells they infect. The copies of the virus are then released into the bloodstream and enter other immune system cells. The destructive cycle then continues.

Getting AIDS Being infected with HIV doesn't mean the person has AIDS. A person is said to have AIDS when the virus has destroyed many immune system cells and has badly damaged the immune system. It usually takes 5 to 10 years for a person who is infected with HIV to develop AIDS if the person has not received treatment. People with AIDS cannot fight off illnesses that a healthy person's immune system could easily defeat. AIDS patients suffer from and often die from these illnesses.

There is still no cure for AIDS. Once the virus infects a person's body, there is no way to remove the virus. Most people with HIV infection eventually develop AIDS. So, learning about HIV and AIDS and protecting yourself from being infected are very important.

HIV Around the World

AIDS is a **pandemic**, a disease that spreads quickly through human populations all over the world. More than 20 million people throughout the world have died from AIDS in the last 20 years.

HIV was first discovered in the United States in the early 1980s. Most scientists think that HIV came from central Africa. The virus spread very quickly from Africa to other regions and countries. HIV is still spreading rapidly in many parts of the world, including Asia and Eastern Europe (especially in the Russian Federation). However, the hardest hit area is Africa. AIDS is now the leading cause of death in sub-Saharan Africa. To get an idea of how widespread HIV and AIDS are in the world, look at the statistics in **Figure 1**.

internet connect
www.scilinks.org/health
Topic: AIDS
HealthLinks code: HH4005
HEALTH LINKS. Maintained by the National Science Teachers Association

Figure 1
These statistics show that AIDS has spread through populations around the world.

ACTIVITY *If the population size of North America is 316 million, what percentage of the population is infected with HIV/AIDS?* **MATH SKILL**

Estimated Number of People Living with HIV/AIDS

Eastern Europe and Central Asia
1 million

Western Europe
560,000

North America
940,000

East Asia and Pacific
1 million

Caribbean
420,000

North Africa and Middle East
440,000

South and Southeast Asia
6.1 million

Latin America
1.4 million

Sub-Saharan Africa
28.1 million

Austra and New Zealand
,000

Source: Joint United Nations Program on HIV/AIDS.

SECTION 1 *HIV and AIDS Today* **497**

facts about HIV/AIDS but also need to take the risks seriously.

SECTION 1

REVIEW *Answer the following questions on a separate piece of paper.*

Using Key Terms

1. **Identify** the term for "the virus that causes AIDS."

2. **Define** the term *acquired immune deficiency syndrome.*

Understanding Key Ideas

3. **Describe** the relationship between an HIV infection and AIDS.

4. **Identify** which of the following geographic areas has the highest number of people infected with HIV/AIDS.
   a. Latin America   c. sub-Saharan Africa
   b. Western Europe   d. North America

5. **Compare** the number of people in the United States living with HIV infection to the number of people in the United States living with AIDS.

6. **Summarize** why the number of new cases of HIV infection is increasing in teens each year.

Critical Thinking

7. **LIFE SKILL** **Practicing Wellness** State three ways you can help other teens take the risks of HIV and AIDS seriously.

8. Your friend tells you, "My boyfriend is a star athlete. He couldn't be infected with HIV." What could you tell your friend?

9. Your friend tells you that she heard on the radio that HIV infection is not the cause of AIDS. What could you tell your friend?

SECTION 1 *HIV and AIDS Today* **499**

Use the Illustrations and Photos

Art shows complex ideas and processes. Learn to analyze the art so that you better understand the material you read in the text.

Tables and graphs display important information in an organized way to help you see relationships.

A picture is worth a thousand words. Look at the photographs to see relevant examples of health concepts you are reading about.

Answer the Section Reviews

Section Reviews test your knowledge of the main points of the section. Critical Thinking items challenge you to think about the material in greater depth and to find connections that you infer from the text.

STUDY TIP When you can't answer a question, reread the section. The answer is usually there.

Do Your Homework

Your teacher will assign Study Guide worksheets to help you understand and remember the material in the chapter.

STUDY TIP Answering the items in the Chapter Review will prepare you for the chapter test. Don't try to answer the questions without reading the text and reviewing your class notes. A little preparation up front will make your homework assignments a lot easier.

Visit Holt Online Learning
If your teacher gives you a special password to log onto the Holt Online Learning site, you'll find your complete textbook on the Web. In addition, you'll find some great learning tools and practice quizzes. You'll be able to see how well you know the material from your textbook.

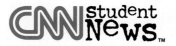

Visit CNN Student News
You'll find up-to-date events in health and fitness at **www.cnnstudentnews.com**.

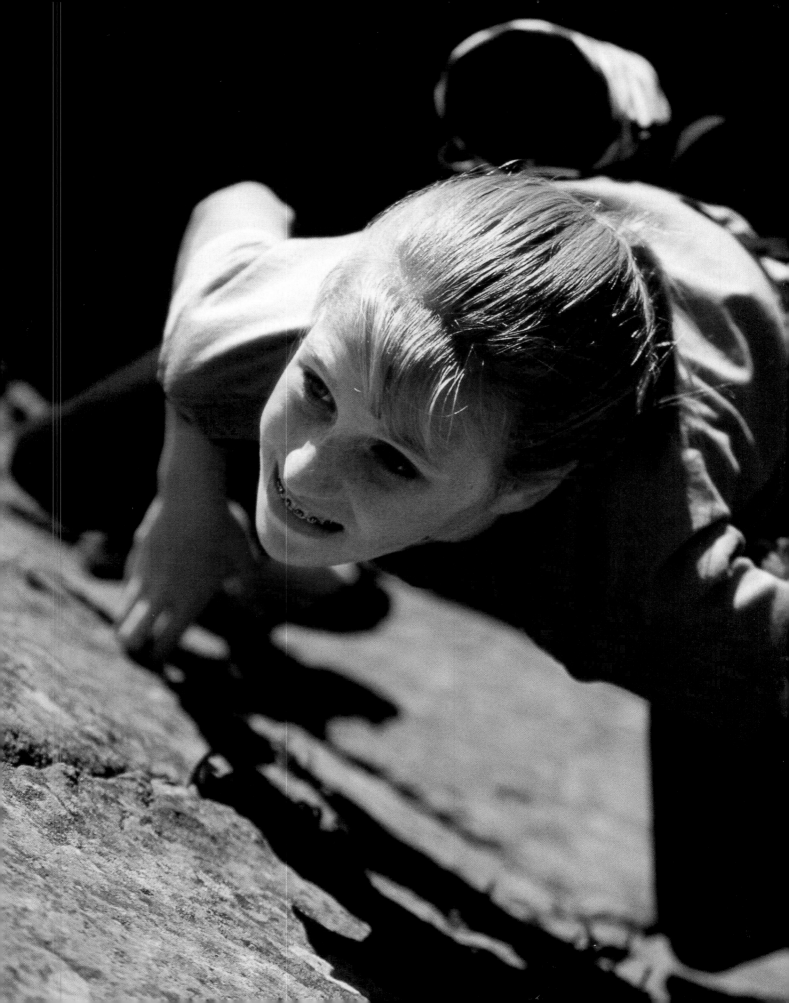

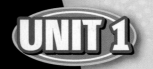

UNIT 1

Health and Your Wellness

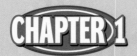

CHAPTER 1

Leading a Healthy Life

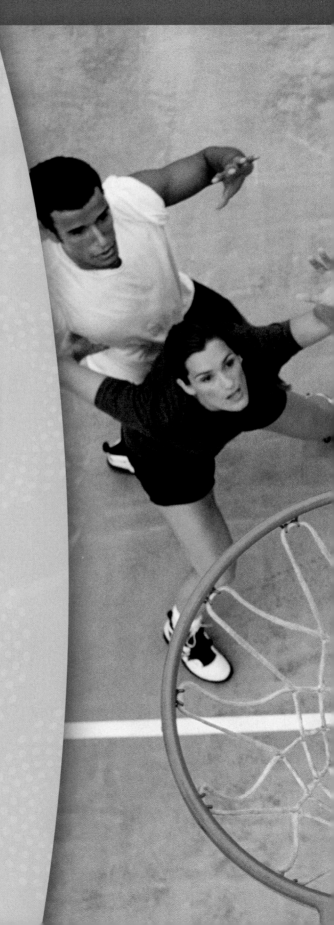

What's Your Health IQ?

KNOWLEDGE

Which of the statements below are true, and which are false? Check your answers on p. 642.

1. Most deaths are caused by our behaviors.

2. If you have a history of heart disease in your family, there is nothing you can do about your risk for heart disease.

3. The leading cause of death in teens is motor vehicle accidents.

4. Smoking is the single leading preventable cause of death in the United States.

5. Eating at least five servings of fruits and vegetables a day can lower your chances of suffering from cancer or heart disease.

6. If you are not physically sick, then you are healthy.

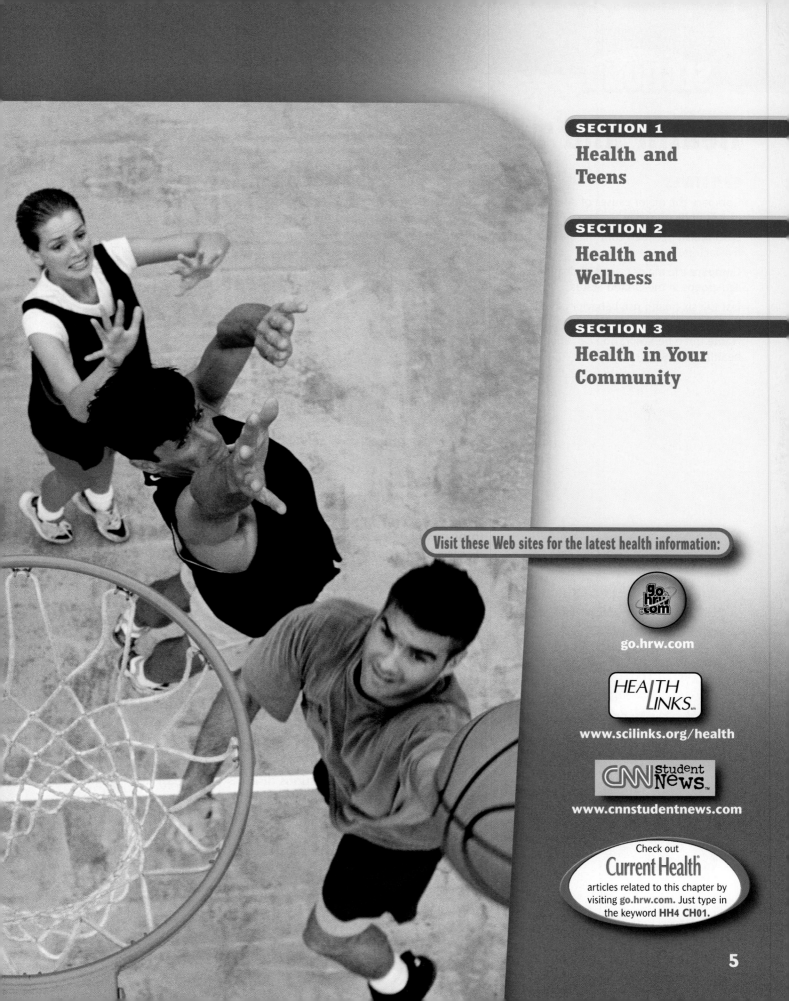

Visit these Web sites for the latest health information:

go.hrw.com

HEALTH LINKS℠

www.scilinks.org/health

CNN student News™

www.cnnstudentnews.com

Check out **Current Health** articles related to this chapter by visiting **go.hrw.com.** Just type in the keyword **HH4 CH01.**

Health and Teens

OBJECTIVES

Compare the major causes of death in the past with the major causes of death today.

Distinguish between controllable risk factors and uncontrollable risk factors.

Compare the major causes of death for teens with those for other age groups in the United States.

List the six health risk behaviors that lead to health problems in teens.

Name three behaviors you can adopt now to improve your health. **LIFE SKILL**

Y ou have the power to protect yourself from the dangers that threaten your health. The first step to protecting yourself is learning what these dangers are and what you can do to prevent them.

Health Today

What does being healthy mean to you? Focus on the first thing you think of when you read the word *healthy*. Did you think of not having diseases? being physically fit? eating right? Many people think that being healthy simply means not being sick. In the past, this was true.

Health in the Past: Infectious Diseases   In the 1800s and early 1900s, the leading causes of death in the United States were *infectious diseases*—diseases caused by pathogens, such as bacteria. Infectious diseases can be passed from one person to another. Examples of infectious diseases include polio, tuberculosis, pneumonia, and influenza (the flu). Infectious diseases were a constant threat. That is why people thought of being healthy as being free from disease!

Health Today: Lifestyle Diseases   Over the years, medical advances, better living conditions, and a focus on preventative medicine have helped bring infectious diseases of the past under control. As a result, most of the diseases that were common 50 to 100 years ago can now be prevented or cured. Today, most health problems in the United States are related to the way we live, or our lifestyle. **Lifestyle diseases** are diseases caused partly by unhealthy behaviors and partly by other factors. They are diseases influenced by the choices you make that affect your health. Examples of diseases that can be influenced by lifestyle are some types of diabetes, some types of heart disease, and some types of cancer.

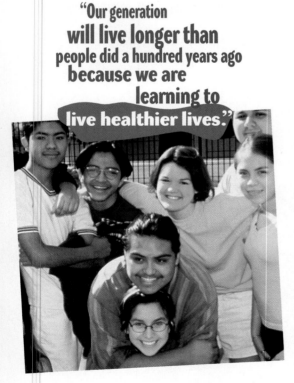

"Our generation **will live longer than** people did a hundred years ago **because we are** learning to **live healthier lives.**"

Table 1 **Controllable Risk Factors for Heart Disease**

Controllable factor	Behavior		
	Bad	Better	Best
Physical activity	▶ watching TV very often	▶ walking the stairs instead of taking elevator	▶ playing a team sport three times a week
Smoking	▶ smoking every day	▶ smoking every so often	▶ quit smoking or not smoking
Weight	▶ weighing 20 percent more than recommended body weight	▶ weighing 10 percent to 20 percent more than recommended body weight	▶ weighing recommended body weight
Diet	▶ eating fast food every day	▶ eating junk food several times a week	▶ eating healthful, nutritious meals

Health Risk Factors

All health problems have risk factors. A **risk factor** is anything that increases the likelihood of injury, disease, or other health problems. For example, the risk factors for heart disease include a history of heart disease in your family, a high-fat diet, stress, being overweight, smoking, and lack of exercise. All of these factors increase a person's chance of developing heart disease. Notice that some of the risk factors can be controlled by your behavior, while others cannot.

Controllable Risk Factors *Controllable risk factors* are risk factors that you can do something about. They can be controlled by your behavior. For example, what can you do to decrease your risk of developing heart disease? As shown in **Table 1,** you can exercise regularly, avoid smoking, manage a healthy weight, and eat healthful, nutritious meals.

Uncontrollable Risk Factors Unfortunately, not all health risk factors are controllable. The ones that can't be changed are called *uncontrollable risk factors*. Examples of uncontrollable risk factors for heart disease are age, race, gender, and heredity. For example, the older a person is, the more likely he or she is to develop heart disease. African Americans are more likely to have high blood pressure, which can lead to heart disease, than European Americans are. Men are more likely to develop heart disease than women are.

You can't make yourself younger or change your race or gender. However, by focusing on controllable risk factors, which you can change through your behavior, you can protect your health.

Uncontrollable Risk Factors

▶ **Age**
▶ **Race**
▶ **Gender**
▶ **Heredity**

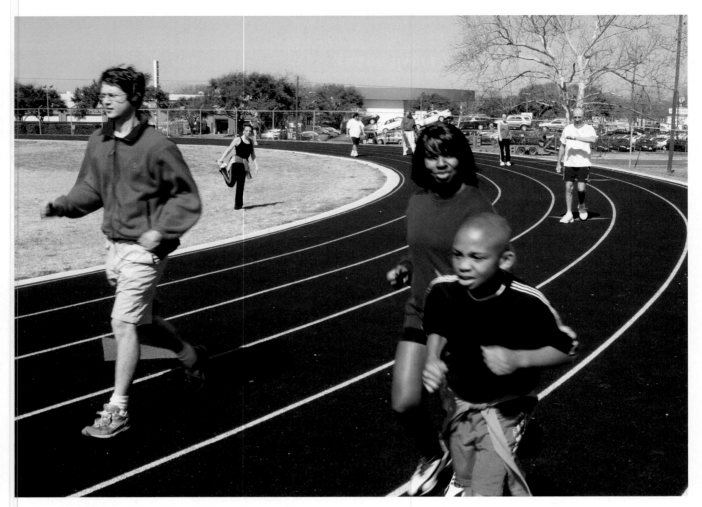

Everyone, no matter what age, can do things to take control of his or her health.

Risk Factors and Your Health

You can't control the uncontrollable risk factors. However, you can protect your health by focusing on controllable risk factors, which you can change through your behavior. What behaviors can you focus on at this point in your life? First, you should know the leading causes of death for people your age in the United States:

▶ motor vehicle accidents
▶ homicide
▶ suicide
▶ other accidents

These four causes of death make up almost three-fourths of all teen deaths. For children and infants, motor vehicle accidents are also the No. 1 cause of death.

Your health behaviors affect not only your health today but also your future health. Thus, you should be aware of the leading causes of death for other age groups. For example, the leading cause of death for adults between 19 and 65 years of age is cancer. The leading cause of death for adults over 65 years of age is heart disease.

The next section describes the health behaviors that most affect you and other teens. By learning these risk behaviors, you can take control in improving your health today and in the future.

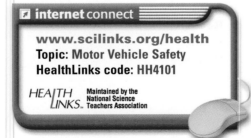

☐ internet connect

www.scilinks.org/health
Topic: Motor Vehicle Safety
HealthLinks code: HH4101

HEA/TH LINKS. Maintained by the National Science Teachers Association

Analyzing DATA

Health Today

1 Each slice of the pie represents the percentage of deaths among *teens* that are a result of the cause indicated.

2 Each slice of the pie represents the percentage of deaths for *all ages* that are a result of the cause indicated.

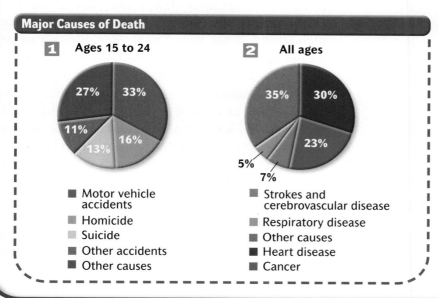

Major Causes of Death

1 Ages 15 to 24

27% 33% 11% 13% 16%

- ■ Motor vehicle accidents
- ■ Homicide
- ■ Suicide
- ■ Other accidents
- ■ Other causes

2 All ages

35% 30% 5% 7% 23%

- ■ Strokes and cerebrovascular disease
- ■ Respiratory disease
- ■ Other causes
- ■ Heart disease
- ■ Cancer

Your Turn

1. What is the No. 1 cause of death for your age group?

2. What percentage of deaths for all ages are caused by heart disease and cancer? **MATH SKILL**

3. Using one or both pie charts, list at least four causes of death that are affected by health risk behaviors.

4. **CRITICAL THINKING** Describe what you can do to protect yourself from each of the causes of death that you listed in item 3.

Source: Centers for Disease Control and Prevention.

Six Health Risk Behaviors

There are six types of risk behaviors that cause the most serious health problems.

1. **Sedentary lifestyle** Not taking part in physical activity on a regular basis is referred to as being **sedentary.** Those who have sedentary lifestyles, even if they are not overweight, raise their risk of certain diseases such as heart disease and diabetes.

2. **Alcohol and other drug use** Alcohol abuse can cause liver disease, certain types of cancer, heart disease, and brain damage. Alcohol and drug use are also major factors in car accidents, physical fights, depression, suicide, and mental disorders. Alcohol and drug use are also factors in the spread of *sexually transmitted diseases* (STDs). These are diseases that are spread through sexual activity. An example of a sexually transmitted disease is acquired immune deficiency syndrome (AIDS), caused by the human immunodeficiency virus (HIV).

3. **Sexual activity** Sexual activity outside of a committed relationship, such as marriage, puts people at risk for health problems. These health problems include HIV infection, other sexually transmitted diseases, and unplanned pregnancy.

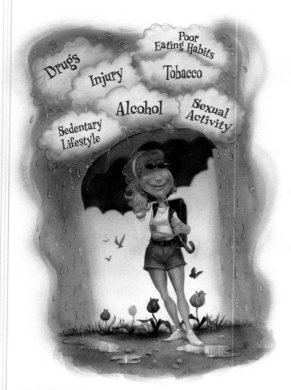

Figure 1

You have the power to protect yourself from the six types of risk behaviors.

ACTIVITY *What risk behaviors do you think are the most common at your school?*

4. **Behaviors that cause injuries** As mentioned, the four major causes of death for teenagers are motor vehicle accidents, other accidents, homicide, and suicide. For example, a risk behavior that can lead to homicide is carrying a weapon. Not using a seat belt is a risk behavior that can lead to death in a motor vehicle accident.

5. **Tobacco use** Smoking is the single leading preventable cause of death in the United States. Smoking is a controllable risk factor for heart disease, cancer, and respiratory disease. These are three of the leading causes of death for all age groups. The choice to smoke often takes place in high school, if not before then. Smoking as a teenager greatly increases your risk for the three leading causes of death.

6. **Poor eating habits** Your eating habits can either increase or lower your chances of developing many diseases. Eating at least five servings of fruits and vegetables a day can lower your chances of suffering from cancer or heart disease. On the other hand, eating foods that are high in fat and weighing more than your recommended weight puts you at risk for heart disease, cancer, and stroke.

The choices you make can either raise your risk for certain health concerns or lower your risk. Learning about the risk behaviors summarized in **Figure 1** will help you make better choices to protect yourself.

SECTION 1

REVIEW   *Answer the following questions on a separate piece of paper.*

Using Key Terms

1. **Identify** the term for "a disease caused partly by unhealthy behaviors and partly by other factors."

2. **Identify** the term for "not taking part in physical activity on a regular basis."

Understanding Key Ideas

3. **State** the type of disease that causes most deaths in the United States today.

4. **List** three examples of uncontrollable risk factors.

5. **Identify** which of the following is *not* a controllable risk factor.
   a. exercise   **c.** age
   b. diet   **d.** weight

6. **Compare** the leading causes of death for teens with those of all ages.

7. **State** the six risk behaviors that lead to health problems in teens.

8. **Identify** the risk behavior that leads to the most deaths in teens.

9. **Identify** the risk behavior that is the leading preventable cause of death in the United States.

Critical Thinking

10. **LIFE SKILL** **Practicing Wellness** List three of your behaviors that you can change to improve your health.

11. **LIFE SKILL** **Practicing Wellness** Use Table 1 to give another example of a "best" behavior you can do for the controllable factor physical activity.

Health and Wellness

OBJECTIVES

Describe each of the six components of health.

State the importance of striving for optimal health.

Describe four influences on wellness.

Describe three ways to take charge of your wellness.

Name two ways you can improve two components of your health. **LIFE SKILL**

KEY TERMS

health the state of well-being in which all of the components of health—physical, emotional, social, mental, spiritual, and environmental—are in balance

value a strong belief or ideal

wellness the achievement of a person's best in all six components of health

health literacy knowledge of health information needed to make good choices about your health

ris was in good physical shape. Abel couldn't remember the last time he had to stay home because he had a cold. Do you think Iris and Abel are healthy?

Six Components of Health

Being healthy is much more than being physically fit and free from disease. **Health** is the state of well-being in which all of the components of health—physical, emotional, social, mental, spiritual, and environmental—are in balance. To be truly healthy, you must take care of all six components. The six components are described in more detail below.

Physical Health Abel used to think that being physically healthy meant being strong and muscular like an Olympic athlete. Being in good physical shape is part of physical health. However, you don't have to be an athlete or even good at sports to be physically healthy. *Physical health* refers to the way your body functions. Physical health includes eating right, getting regular exercise, and being at your recommended body weight. Physical health is also about avoiding drugs and alcohol. Finally, physical health means being free of disease and sickness.

Emotional Health *Emotional health* is expressing your emotions in a positive, nondestructive way. Everyone experiences unpleasant feelings at one time or another. Emotionally healthy people can cope with unpleasant emotions and not get overwhelmed by them. For example, when Abel feels down, he knows he can go to his best friend or his family for support. Are you aware of how you feel and to whom you can go for support?

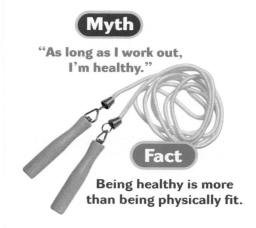

Myth

"As long as I work out, I'm healthy."

Fact

Being healthy is more than being physically fit.

Six Components of Health

Physical Health
▶ eats a well-balanced, diet
▶ exercises regularly
▶ avoids tobacco, alcohol, and drugs
▶ is free of disease

Mental Health
▶ has high self-esteem
▶ enjoys trying new things
▶ is free of mental illness

Emotional Health
▶ expresses emotions constructively
▶ asks for help when sad

Spiritual Health
▶ has a sense of purpose in life
▶ follows morals and values
▶ feels a unity with other human beings

Social Health
▶ respects others
▶ has supportive relationships
▶ expresses needs to others

Environmental Health
▶ has access to clean air and water
▶ has a clean and uncrowded living space
▶ recycles used paper, glass products, and aluminum

Figure 2

To be healthy, a person must attend to all six components of health.

ACTIVITY *Which component of your health do you think needs the most improvement?*

Social Health   Social health does not mean being the most popular kid in school. A person who is popular can be socially unhealthy! *Social health* is the quality of your relationships with friends, family, teachers, and others you are in contact with. As listed in **Figure 2,** a person who is socially healthy respects others. A socially healthy person also stays clear of those who do not treat him or her with respect and tolerance. For example, Abel gets together with his friends each week. However, he avoids his neighbor who bullies him. He is also learning to better work out disagreements with his parents.

Mental Health   Your mental health can be strongly influenced by your emotional health. *Mental health* is the ability to recognize reality and cope with the demands of daily life. Sometimes people who have gone through intensely troubling times develop mental illnesses. An example of a mental illness is a phobia. A phobia is an irrational and excessive fear of something, such as a fear of heights. But mental health is about more than not having mental illness. Mental health is also having high self-esteem. Having high self-esteem is feeling comfortable and happy about yourself. For example, Iris is now trying out for the drama club. She had been hesitant to try out because none of her friends liked acting, but she decided to try out anyway.

Spiritual Health *Spiritual health* is maintaining harmonious relationships with other living things and having spiritual direction and purpose. Spiritual health means different things to different people. For some people, spiritual health is defined by the practice of religion. For others, it is understanding their purpose in life.

Spiritual health also includes living according to one's ethics, morals, and values. A **value** is a strong belief or ideal. Being spiritually healthy may mean you live in harmony with your environment. It may also mean that you are at peace with yourself and those around you. For example, Iris says she feels most valuable and united with others when she helps out at her city's homeless shelter.

Environmental Health The environment is made up of the living and nonliving things in your world. The environment includes air, water, and land. Your environment is your surroundings—where you live, work, or play. *Environmental health* is keeping your air and water clean, your food safe, and the land around you enjoyable and safe. Iris started a recycling program for her family when she realized the importance of her environmental health to her well-being.

Wellness: Striving for Optimal Health

As you may have noticed, many of the components of health can be affected by the other components. If one component of health is weak, it can affect a person's overall health. This is why being healthy is defined as the balance of all the components of health. **Wellness** is the achievement of a person's best in all six components of health.

It would be unrealistic to think that a person could achieve complete wellness all of the time. Think of striving for wellness in the same way you think of always striving to have a good day. Do you always have a really good day or a really bad day? Most of your days are most likely somewhere in between. That is how the wellness continuum works, too.

The wellness continuum represents the idea that a person is neither completely healthy nor completely unhealthy. Think of the wellness continuum as resembling the scale on a bellringer, commonly seen at amusement parks. As shown in **Figure 3,** at the top of the scale is optimal health, and at the bottom of the scale is illness and death. The harder you strive to hit the hammer on the pedal, the higher the ball goes on the scale. For most of us, the ball reaches somewhere in the middle of the scale.

People who can cope with their emotions, have healthy relationships, and make smart decisions probably fall near the optimal wellness side of the continuum. On the other hand, people who eat poorly, engage in health risk behaviors, never exercise, and are unhappy probably fall closer to the illness side. Where you fall on the continuum can change on a yearly, monthly, and even daily basis. Fortunately, you have the power to change your behaviors to move closer to optimal health.

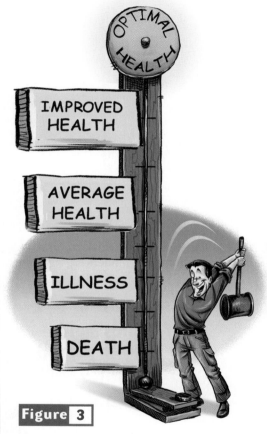

Figure 3

The wellness continuum shows that wellness is about always striving for optimal health, even though most people are never completely healthy.

Influences on Your Wellness

As you strive for optimal health, it's important to recognize that there are many factors that influence your health.

Hereditary Influences   Your health can be influenced by your *heredity*—the traits you inherit from your parents. For example, if several members of your family have developed diabetes, you may be at risk for diabetes. However, if you have a hereditary disease in your family, it doesn't mean you will definitely develop that disease. By focusing on controllable risk factors, you can decrease your risk for hereditary diseases.

Social Influences   Your health is also influenced by the relationships you have with other people. For example, if your friends convince you to go to a party where alcohol is available, your friends are influencing your health in a negative way. If your parents or grandparents deal with anger by talking out their problems instead of yelling and fighting, you will be more likely to talk out your problems. Your parents are influencing your health in a positive way.

Cultural Influences   *Culture* is the values, beliefs, and practices shared by people that have a common background. Your culture can strongly influence your health. For example, some Asian cultures eat a lot of vegetables and seafood in their diet. This cultural influence is thought to be one of the reasons people from some Asian cultures have a lower risk of heart disease. What cultural influences do you think influence your health?

Many factors influence your health, including hereditary, social, cultural, and environmental influences.

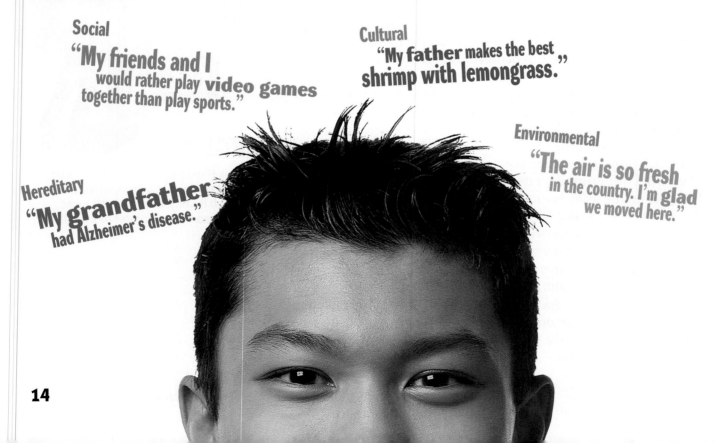

Social
"My friends and I would rather play **video games** together than play sports."

Cultural
"My **father** makes the best shrimp with lemongrass."

Environmental
"The air is so fresh in the country. I'm glad we moved here."

Hereditary
"My grandfather had Alzheimer's disease."

Environmental Influences Your surroundings, the area where you live, and all the things you have contact with are part of your environment. Pollutants, safety regulations, and the availability and use of medical care are aspects of your environment that affect your health. The government enforces air- and water-quality regulations to keep your environment free from pollutants. The government also maintains safety regulations, such as traffic laws, to keep you safe.

Taking Charge of Your Wellness

Three ways you can take charge of your health are through your knowledge, through your lifestyle, and through your attitude.

Knowledge An important way to improve your health is through your knowledge. **Health literacy** is the knowledge of health information needed to make good choices about your health. Studying health in school will certainly increase your health literacy. However, it's important to keep up with current health issues. Your parents, teachers, healthcare providers, and library are great resources for health information. They can also lead you to other resources for health information.

Lifestyle One of the most important ways to improve your health is to make behavioral changes in your lifestyle. Putting your knowledge into action is a sure way to take charge of your wellness.

Unfortunately, most people don't always behave in a way that shows they know what is healthy. For example, most smokers know that smoking cigarettes can lead to lung cancer, but they still smoke. **Table 2** shows some examples of consequences that can happen when health behavior doesn't follow health knowledge. Some ways you can put your health knowledge into action are to exercise regularly, always wear a seat belt, and eat healthy and nutritious foods.

Table 2 Health Knowledge Versus Health Behavior		
Health knowledge *knowing the consequences of your behavior on your health*	**Health behavior** *taking action that affects your health, either negatively or positively*	**Consequences** *facing the effect of your behavior on your health*
Example 1		
▶ Steven knows that eating junk food can make him overweight and may lead to heart disease later in life.	▶ Steven eats candy bars and chips and drinks soda almost every day.	▶ Steven starts putting on weight which increases his risk for diabetes and heart disease.
Example 2		▶ Karen does poorly on her exams, gets sick, and misses the junior prom.
▶ Karen knows she needs enough sleep to stay healthy.	▶ Karen doesn't plan her studying well and stays up late all week cramming for final exams.	

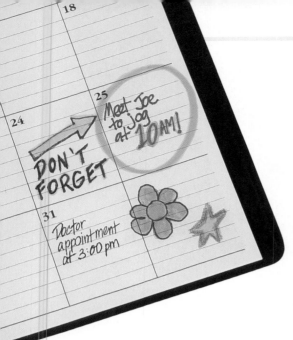

Attitude A person's way of thinking, or attitude, greatly affects that person's health. By changing your attitude, you can act in ways that work to make you a healthier person. For example, you could try to change your attitude toward stress. You can try to relax and stop letting the "little things" bother you. If you can keep stress from affecting you, you will find that you feel better mentally and physically. You can also try to change your attitude about anger. Don't get so worked up about things you can't control!

Your attitude can also help you make the best of a bad situation. People who have suffered through a long-term illness have benefited by having a positive attitude. People with positive attitudes are more hopeful and will strive harder to overcome illness. Having a positive attitude can be critical when overcoming an illness.

Perhaps the most important attitude you can change is the way you feel about yourself. To achieve wellness, you have to feel good about yourself, or have positive self-esteem. *Self-esteem* is a person's confidence, pride, and self-respect. You can be free from disease, be physically active, have a healthy diet, and have many supportive relationships. However, if you don't feel good about yourself, you will never be truly healthy. Eventually, low self-esteem can affect your health and actually make you physically ill. As a result, it is important to build a healthy self-esteem.

Taking charge of your wellness will help you lead a healthy life. Leading a healthy life is about balancing the six components of health. Getting the best out of each component of health has a lot to do with the choices you make and the actions you take. The good news is that you have the power to make the right choices and live life to its fullest!

> "Health knowledge is useless without positive health behavior. You must put what you know into action for it to work!"

SECTION 2

REVIEW   *Answer the following questions on a separate piece of paper.*

Using Key Terms

1. **Define** the term *health*.

2. **Identify** the term for "a strong belief or ideal."

3. **Define** the term *wellness*.

4. **Identify** the term for "knowledge of health information needed to make good choices about your health."

Understanding Key Ideas

5. **Describe** each of the six components of health.

6. **Identify** the health component that involves working on the quality of your relationships with others.
   - **a.** mental health
   - **b.** social health
   - **c.** emotional health
   - **d.** environmental health

7. **Describe** the importance of striving for wellness.

8. **Discuss** each of the four influences on your wellness.

9. **Describe** how your attitude can help you take charge of your health.

Critical Thinking

10. **LIFE SKILL** **Practicing Wellness** State two ways you can improve two components of your health.

11. **Describe** how your family members influence and promote health in your family.

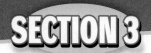

SECTION 3

Health in Your Community

OBJECTIVES

Describe four ways society addresses health problems.

List three ways you can promote an issue to improve the health of others. **LIFE SKILL**

KEY TERMS

public health the practice of protecting and improving the health of people in a community

advocate to speak or argue in favor of something

public service announcement (PSA) a message created to educate people about an issue

Three years ago, Maureen's mother was so sick from diabetes that she had to be hospitalized. Thanks to new developments in medicine, she's feeling better than she has in years. Maureen's mother is now more free to do the things she loves.

Four Ways Society Addresses Health Problems

Everyone has the responsibility of taking care of his or her health. However, many health problems need to be tackled by the cooperation and experience of many people. **Public health** is the practice of protecting and improving the health of people in a community.

Our community is able to promote and protect the health of people in many ways. Four ways in which our community addresses health problems are through medical advances, technology, public policy, and education.

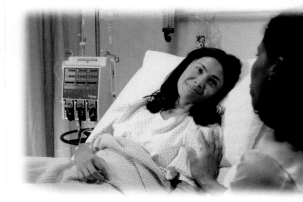

Medical advances and technology have saved lives and helped people recover from many diseases.

1. **Medical advances** Conducting medical research is one way our society addresses health concerns. One medical advancement that came about through medical research was the development of the insulin pump.

   The implanted insulin pump is being developed for people with a certain type of diabetes. *Diabetes* is a serious disease in which the body is not able to obtain glucose (better known as *sugar*) from the blood. Diabetes kills tens of thousands of people every year in the United States. People who live with diabetes must constantly manage the levels of glucose in their bloodstream. To do so, diabetics must monitor their diet, exercise regularly, and, in many cases, receive daily insulin shots.

   The surgically implanted insulin pump is being developed to replace the need for daily insulin shots. A microchip embedded in the pump makes monitoring and controling blood-sugar levels possible. If a diabetic's blood-sugar level is low, the pump will release insulin. With the insulin pump, the diabetic will no longer need daily insulin shots and can easily manage blood-sugar levels.

 HEALTH Handbook For more information about public health, see the Express Lesson on p. 552 of this text.

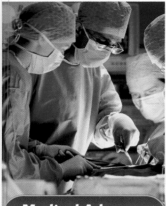
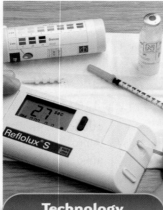
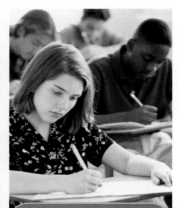
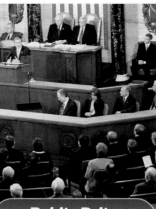

Medical Advances
Doctors are developing insulin pumps that can be surgically implanted to make managing blood-sugar levels easier.

Technology
Glucose meters indicate blood-sugar levels for diabetics.

Public Policy
Congress passes laws that provide funds for research on diseases such as diabetes.

Education
School health classes teach students how to decrease their risk of developing diabetes.

Figure 4

Society has worked in many ways to address health problems such as diabetes.

ACTIVITY *Can you think of how another health problem has been addressed for one of these four ways?*

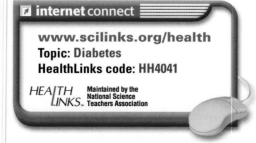

internet connect

www.scilinks.org/health
Topic: Diabetes
HealthLinks code: HH4041

HEALTH LINKS. Maintained by the National Science Teachers Association

2. **Technology** Another way in which our society works to solve health problems is through technology. Through the use of computers, lasers, and other revolutionary technologies, new and better products have been made to help people lead healthier lives.

   One example of a product made through the use of technology is the glucose meter, such as the one shown in **Figure 4.** The glucose meter was designed to let diabetics know their blood-sugar level by requiring only a very small amount of blood. The glucose meter makes monitoring blood-sugar levels easier.

3. **Public policy** Governmental policies and regulations can also help to address health problems. Tobacco regulation is one way that laws can help prevent disease. Examples of these laws are placing taxes on cigarettes, enforcing an age limit to buy tobacco products, and limiting how tobacco companies can advertise. These laws are aimed at trying to keep people from smoking. Smoking can cause diseases such as lung cancer.

   Congress can also pass laws that provide tax dollars for research on diseases. This money helps fund the development of products such as the glucose meter. The money also helps advance medical research, such as surgically implanting insulin pumps.

4. **Education** Health education has been a key factor in the prevention of disease and illness in this country. For example, most states require that students take some form of health class. Health teachers teach students about the benefits of exercising and eating nutritious foods. Health teachers also discuss the risks of smoking, drinking, and behaving violently.

   In addition, many community agencies provide health education. For example, the American Diabetes Association teaches the public about diabetes and ways to prevent it.

What You Can Do

Many people have improved the health of others by speaking out and promoting health issues. To speak out or argue in favor of something is to **advocate.** You may know of people in your community who work tirelessly to promote health issues. Maybe they help take hot meals to elderly people in their homes. Or perhaps they organize rallies to promote certain health issues. Others may work in a health field.

You Can Be an Advocate!   Although few people devote their lives to being advocates, we all have the potential to better our own wellness as well as the wellness of others. For example, you could volunteer at a local health clinic or public agency. You could become involved at school in addressing health issues important to teens. You could serve as an example to others by practicing your best health behaviors. You can even be an advocate by training for a career in a health field!

HEALTH Handbook For more information about health careers, see the Reference Guide on p. 632 of this text.

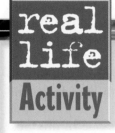

real life Activity

SPEAK OUT!

LIFE SKILL
Communicating Effectively

Materials

✔ magazines
✔ scissors
✔ colored paper
✔ poster board
✔ glue
✔ markers

Procedure

1. **Choose** a health issue in your school or community that you would like to address by supporting others in making positive health choices.

2. **Think** about the message you want to communicate and the audience you want to receive your message.

3. **Cut** out magazine pictures that can help you express your health message.

4. **Use** magazine pictures, colored paper, poster board, glue and markers to create a poster that expresses your message.

Conclusions

1. **Summarizing Results** What was the main health message of your poster?

2. **Evaluating Information** What technique or style did you use to make your health message stand out?

3. **Predicting Outcomes** How do you think the audience you want to send your message to will respond to your poster?

4. **CRITICAL THINKING** Using other methods, such as the Internet or a video camera, how would you communicate your health message differently?

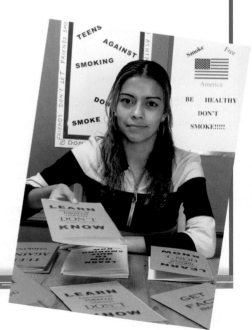

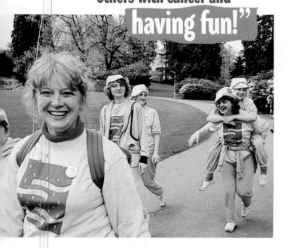

"Our mother survived cancer. Now, we're helping others with cancer and having fun!"

Getting Your Point Across One way to reach many people about health issues is through a public service announcement. A **public service announcement (PSA)** is a message created to educate people about an issue. Most PSAs are in the form of a commercial that you hear on the radio or on television. You can also create a PSA in other forms. For example, you can publish an essay in the school newspaper. You could also create posters and post them around your school.

There are several things you should think about when choosing the way to communicate your message:

▶ **Make sure you have the most current and accurate information.** Be sure to research your topic. Ask a family member or teacher about an organization that specializes in your topic. Your parents can also help you find information on the Internet.

▶ **Know your audience.** To whom are you trying to send your message? How do you think your audience will respond to your message? Some issues bring up strong feelings and opinions in people. The success of your message can depend on how sensitive you are to these feelings and opinions.

For example, how would you get your best friend to stop smoking? How would she react if you told her that she should quit because her clothes smell and her breath stinks? Your comments likely wouldn't convince her to quit. However, what would happen if you recommended a technique that would make it easier for her to quit? You could offer to buy her favorite CD as she reaches a specific goal. You could also suggest that her doctor may have some advice about how to quit smoking. In this way, you are using your health knowledge and showing your friend that you care about her.

Advocating for your health and others' health is one of the most important things you can do in your life. Being well informed about your health, knowing how you feel about yourself, and making an effort to maintain a healthy lifestyle are the foundations for your and others' wellness.

SECTION 3

REVIEW *Answer the following questions on a separate piece of paper.*

Using Key Terms

1. **Define** the term *public health*.

2. **Identify** the term for "a message created to educate people about an issue."

Understanding Key Ideas

3. **List** four ways society addresses health issues.

4. **Identify** the way in which society teaches others to live healthy lives.
   - **a.** medical advances
   - **b.** education
   - **c.** technology
   - **d.** public policy

5. **Identify** which of the following areas addresses community health through governmental decisions.
   - **a.** public policy
   - **b.** medical advances
   - **c.** technology
   - **d.** education

Critical Thinking

6. **LIFE SKILL** **Communicating Effectively** Describe why good communication skills are important for advocating a health issue.

7. **LIFE SKILL** **Practicing Wellness** List three ways you can communicate a health issue to your community.

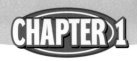

CHAPTER 1

Highlights

Key Terms

SECTION 1

lifestyle disease (6)
risk factor (7)
sedentary (9)

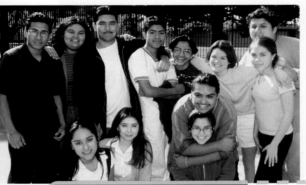

SECTION 2

health (11)
value (13)
wellness (13)
health literacy (15)

SECTION 3

public health (17)
advocate (19)
public service
announcement (PSA) (20)

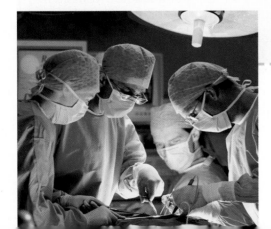

The Big Picture

✔ In the past, deaths were caused mainly by infectious diseases. Today, most health problems are related to the way we live, or our lifestyle.

✔ All health problems have risk factors. You have the power to change controllable risk factors.

✔ The major cause of death for adults over the age of 65 is heart disease. The major cause of death for adults between 19 and 65 years of age is cancer. The major causes of death for teens are motor vehicle accidents, homicide, suicide, and other accidents. The major cause of death for children and infants is motor vehicle accidents.

✔ The six types of behavior that lead to health problems for teens are sedentary lifestyle, alcohol and drug use, sexual activity, behaviors that result in unintentional and intentional injuries, tobacco use, and poor eating habits.

✔ Health is the state of well-being in which all of the components of health—physical, emotional, social, mental, spiritual, and environmental—are in balance.

✔ Wellness is the achievement of your best in all of the components of health.

✔ The four influences on your wellness are hereditary, social, cultural, and environmental influences.

✔ You can take charge of your wellness through your lifestyle, through your attitude, and through your knowledge.

✔ Society addresses health problems in four ways: medical advances, technology, public policy, and education.

✔ Everyone has the power to try to improve the wellness of others.

✔ Public service announcements are an effective way to advocate for a health issue.

✔ Communication skills are very important when you advocate for a health issue.

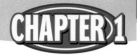

Review

Using Key Terms

advocate (19)
health (11)
health literacy (15)
lifestyle disease (6)
public health (17)
public service announcement (PSA) (20)

risk factor (7)
sedentary (9)
value (13)
wellness (13)

1. For each definition below, choose the key term that best matches the definition.
   a. the practice of protecting and improving the health of people in a community
   b. a message created to educate people about an issue
   c. the achievement of a person's best in all six components of health
   d. a strong belief or ideal
   e. not taking part in physical activity on a regular basis
   f. anything that increases the likelihood of injury, disease, or other health problem
   g. knowledge of health information needed to make good choices about your health

2. Explain the relationship between the key terms in each of the following pairs.
   a. *health* and *lifestlyle disease*
   b. *advocate* and *public service announcement*

Understanding Key Ideas
Section 1

3. How have the causes of health problems changed from the past to today?

4. Heart disease is an example of which type of disease: infectious or lifestyle?

5. Which of the following is a controllable risk factor?
   a. race
   b. age
   c. gender
   d. exercise

6. Which of the following is *not* a common cause of death for your age group?
   a. heart disease
   b. motor vehicle accidents
   c. suicide
   d. homicide

7. Describe how a sedentary lifestyle can lead to health problems.

8. Driving without a seat belt is an example of which of the six health risk behaviors?

9. Describe how the risk behavior tobacco use can lead to health problems.

10. **CRITICAL THINKING** What are some behaviors you can practice now that will improve your chances of living a long, healthy life?

Section 2

11. Which component of health involves avoiding drugs and alcohol?

12. The ability to cope with the demands of daily life is part of which component of health?

13. Describe how you can reach higher levels on the wellness continuum.

14. Give an example for how each of the following factors influences your wellness.
    a. heredity
    b. culture
    c. society
    d. the environment

15. Describe how you can take charge of your wellness through your attitude. **LIFE SKILL**

16. **CRITICAL THINKING** Describe how you can use health knowledge to improve the physical component of your health.

Section 3

17. Which of the following is *not* an example of how society addresses health problems?
    a. education
    b. public policy
    c. smoking
    d. medical advances

18. Explain why it's important to know your audience when you advocate for better health.

19. Why is it important to have the most current and accurate information when you advocate for a health issue?

20. **CRITICAL THINKING** Describe how technology has improved your health and the health of others in the world.

Understanding Graphics

Study the figure below to answer the questions that follow.

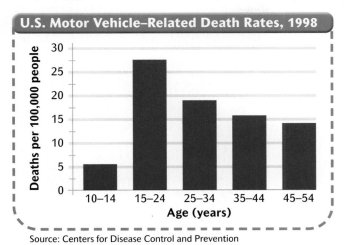

U.S. Motor Vehicle–Related Death Rates, 1998

Deaths per 100,000 people / Age (years)

Source: Centers for Disease Control and Prevention

21. What is the motor vehicle death rate for your age group?

22. Which age group has the highest motor vehicle death rate?

23. CRITICAL THINKING Why do you think the age group that you answered in item 22 has the highest motor vehicle death rate?

Activities

24. Health and Your Community Interview a person over the age of 70 to find out what health problems were most common during his or her teenage years. Prepare a one-page report comparing what you learned in the interview with what you learned in this chapter about health problems facing teens today. **WRITING SKILL**

25. Health and You For 1 week, keep a diary of everything that influences your wellness. Separate the influences into four categories: hereditary, social, cultural, and environmental. **WRITING SKILL**

26. Health and Your Community Collect newspaper or magazine pictures that show healthful behaviors and harmful behaviors. Glue these pictures on a poster board. Show your poster to the class, and discuss how advertisements can influence your health choices.

Action Plan

27. LIFE SKILL Practicing Wellness Create a personal health plan that improves or promotes each of the six components of health.

Standardized Test Prep

Read the passage below, and then answer the questions that follow. **READING SKILL** **WRITING SKILL**

Kent knows that there are many benefits to exercising regularly. He knows that regular exercise makes him feel as if he has more energy. He also knows that it will help him maintain his weight. However, Kent can't remember the last time he exercised. Kent prefers to play video games after school. After he gets bored playing video games, he usually watches some TV. When Kent put his jeans on this morning, he noticed they were tight. Today, he was feeling too <u>lethargic</u> to pay attention in math class. Kent couldn't understand why he was so tired if he slept 9 hours last night. He felt that he was getting sick.

28. In this passage, the word *lethargic* means
   A hungry.
   B excited.
   C lacking in energy.
   D bored.

29. What can you infer from reading this passage?
   E Kent's health behavior does not reflect his health knowledge.
   F Kent has an infectious disease that is making him sick.
   G Kent needs more sleep each night.
   H none of the above

30. Explain what may happen to Kent's energy level if Kent starts exercising at least three times a week.

31. Write a paragraph describing how Kent can change his daily routine to find more time to exercise.

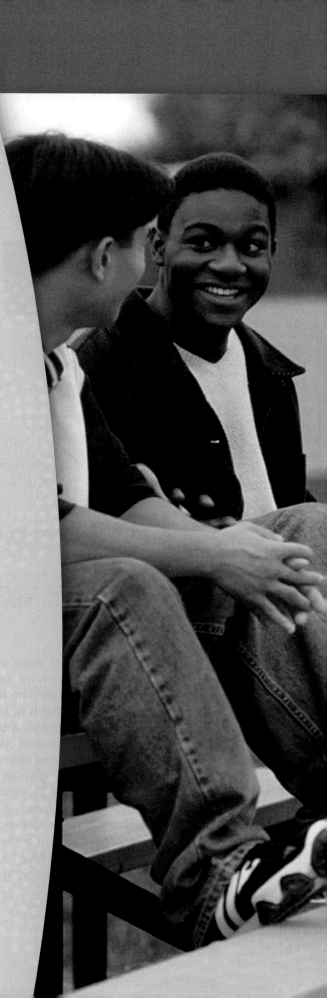

CHAPTER 2

Skills for a Healthy Life

What's Your Health IQ?

BEHAVIOR

Indicate how frequently you engage in each of the following behaviors (1 = never; 2 = occasionally; 3 = most of the time; 4 = all of the time). Total your points, and then turn to p. 642.

1. I review all of my choices before I make a decision.

2. I think about the outcome for each possible choice.

3. I make decisions that support my beliefs.

4. I think about the decisions I make afterward so that I can learn from them.

5. I stop to think about who might be affected by the decisions I make.

6. I usually ask for advice when I have a tough decision to make.

7. If I make a bad decision, I try to correct any problem my decision caused.

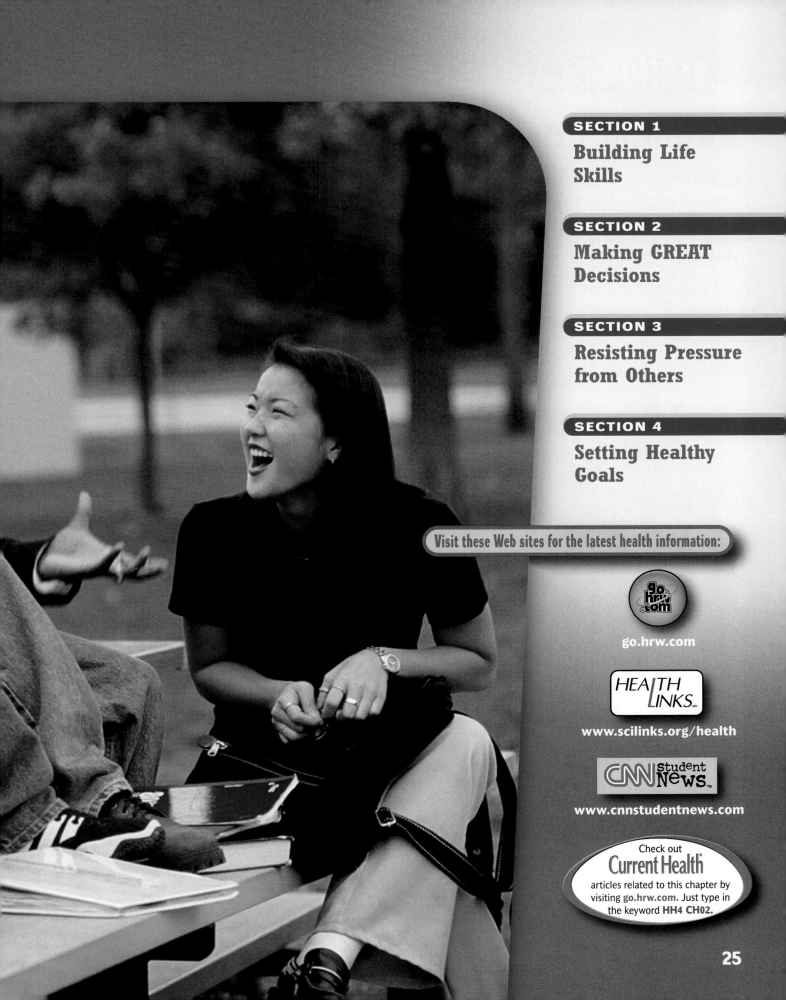

Visit these Web sites for the latest health information:

go.hrw.com

go.hrw.com

HEALTH LINKS.

www.scilinks.org/health

CNN student News.

www.cnnstudentnews.com

Check out
Current Health
articles related to this chapter by visiting **go.hrw.com**. Just type in the keyword **HH4 CH02.**

Building Life Skills

OBJECTIVES

State the importance of practicing life skills for lifelong wellness.

List 10 life skills that you need for a healthy life.

Predict how you can use each of the 10 life skills in your daily life.
LIFE SKILL

KEY TERMS

life skill a tool for building a healthy life

coping dealing with problems and troubles in an effective way

consumer a person who buys products or services

media all public forms of communication, such as TV, radio, newspaper, the Internet, and advertisements

resource something that you can use to help achieve a goal

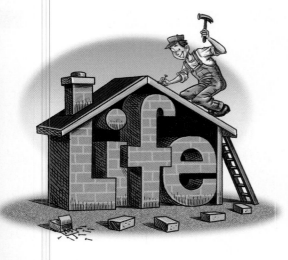

Just like you need skills to build a house, you also need skills to build a happy, healthy life.

Amin has been so frustrated. He argues with his dad every day. His allergies are driving him crazy, and he doesn't know which medicine to buy. What's worse is that the class bully has been following him around school. Amin knows things need to get better, but he isn't sure where to begin.

What Are Life Skills?

Like Amin, everybody wants to enjoy the benefits of a healthy life. We all want to be free from sickness. We want to feel good about who we are. However, having a healthy life doesn't come without effort.

Just like you need skills to build a house, you need skills to build a happy, healthy life. Building a house is not an easy task. A lot of hard work is required, and you need the right tools, such as a hammer, nails, and wood. You need tools for building a healthy life, too. These tools for building a healthy life are called **life skills.**

Life skills will help you improve the six components of health: physical, emotional, social, mental, spiritual, and environmental. For example, one life skill can improve your social component of health by teaching you how to communicate more effectively. Another life skill can help your emotional health by suggesting ways to deal with difficult times, such as the death of a family member.

Some life skills can affect all components of your health. For example, one life skill provides suggestions for making good decisions. From the foods you choose to the friends you choose, the decisions you make can affect every component of your health.

Learning to use life skills will boost your wellness throughout your lifetime. However, using life skills takes practice. Just as an experienced builder makes a better house, you can practice life skills to build a healthier life!

Ten Life Skills

Figure 1 lists 10 life skills that can help you lead a healthy life. You will find these life skills throughout this textbook. The life skills are identified by this icon: **LIFE SKILL**

1. **LIFE SKILL** **Assessing Your Health** How healthy are you? How do you know if you are doing the right thing for your health? This life skill will help you evaluate your health. It will also help you to evaluate how your actions and behaviors affect your health. This will enable you to find out what you need to do to improve your health!

2. **LIFE SKILL** **Communicating Effectively** Have you ever had trouble dealing with a classmate or your parents? Have you ever struggled for the right word to say how you feel? This life skill will teach you good communication skills, which include knowing how to listen and speak effectively. These skills will help improve your relationships with your family, friends, classmates, teachers, and other adults.

3. **LIFE SKILL** **Practicing Wellness** This life skill will show you how to practice healthy behaviors daily so that you can have good lifelong health. Examples of healthy behaviors you may practice are getting enough sleep, choosing nutritious foods, and avoiding risky behaviors.

4. **LIFE SKILL** **Coping** Dealing with troubles or problems in an effective way is referred to as **coping.** This life skill will help you deal with difficult times and situations and with emotions such as anger, depression, and loss of a loved one.

5. **LIFE SKILL** **Being a Wise Consumer** A **consumer** is a person who buys products (such as food, CDs, or clothing) or services (such as

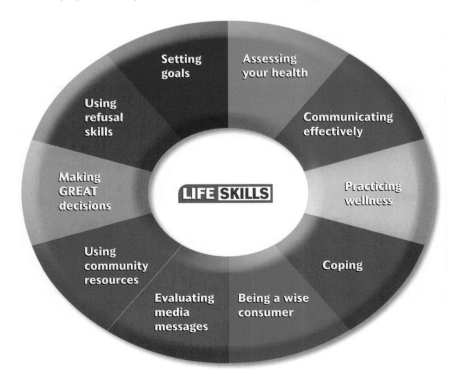

Figure 1

Practicing these 10 life skills will help you lead a healthy life.

Setting goals

Assessing your health

Using refusal skills

Communicating effectively

Making GREAT decisions

LIFE SKILLS

Practicing wellness

Using community resources

Coping

Evaluating media messages

Being a wise consumer

medical care or auto repair). Therefore, you are a consumer! This life skill will help you make good decisions when buying health products and services. It will show you how to decide what is appropriate for your health.

6. **LIFE SKILL** **Evaluating Media Messages** Public forms of communication, such as TV, radio, movies, newspaper, the Internet, and advertisements are referred to as the **media.** The media have a significant influence on what you learn about the world. This life skill will give you the tools to analyze media messages. Knowing how to analyze media messages will help you make better decisions about your health.

7. **LIFE SKILL** **Using Community Resources** A **resource** is something that you can use to help achieve a goal. For example, health clinics, libraries, and government agencies are all community resources. Every community has a wealth of services that provide help for all six components of health. This life skill will help you find these services and will describe how they can assist you.

The following three life skills will be described in more detail in the next three sections of this chapter.

8. **LIFE SKILL** **Making GREAT Decisions** Everyone wants to make the right decisions for themselves. This life skill will provide you with steps to help you do just that. Section 2 of this chapter will discuss these steps in more detail.

9. **LIFE SKILL** **Using Refusal Skills** This life skill will provide you with different ways you can say "no" to something you do not want to do. Section 3 of this chapter will describe refusal skills in more detail.

10. **LIFE SKILL** **Setting Goals** This life skill will provide you with tips to help you reach your goals. Section 4 of this chapter will discuss these tips on setting goals in more detail.

> The average number of advertisements a person sees in 1 day is 3,000.

SECTION 1

REVIEW
Answer the following questions on a separate piece of paper.

Using Key Terms

1. **Define** the term *coping.*

2. **Identify** the term for "a person who buys products and services."

3. **Identify** the term for "something that you can use to help achieve a goal."

Understanding Key Ideas

4. **Summarize** the importance of practicing life skills for lifelong wellness.

5. **Name** the life skill that teaches you good listening skills.

6. **Identify** the life skill that helps you make good decisions when buying health products or services.
   a. Coping
   b. Practicing Wellness
   c. Assessing Your Health
   d. Being a Wise Consumer

7. **Name** the life skill that will help you say no to something you don't want to do.

Critical Thinking

8. **LIFE SKILL** **Practicing Wellness** Choose three life skills. Then, describe how you can apply each of these life skills in your life.

Making GREAT Decisions

OBJECTIVES

Describe the importance of making decisions.

Summarize what you should do if you make a wrong decision.

Apply the Making GREAT Decisions model to make a decision. **LIFE SKILL**

Describe a time when you worked with someone else to make a decision. **LIFE SKILL**

KEY TERMS

consequence a result of your actions and decisions

collaborate to work together with one or more people

O n her way to school, Sina was daydreaming about Marty, the cute senior she met yesterday. To her surprise, he pulled up in his car with his friends. Marty and his friends were planning to skip school and wanted her to come along. Sina froze as she quickly tried to decide what she should do.

Importance of Making Decisions

How many decisions have you made today? You've probably made more decisions than you even realize. Every day, people make decisions about what clothes to wear, what to eat, what channel to watch on TV, and whether to press the snooze button on the alarm clock again. These decisions often happen on the spur of the moment. You may even make these decisions without even thinking about them.

Making snap decisions without really thinking about them is alright for the easy things. But if you make impulsive decisions all of the time, you may run into some negative consequences. **Consequences** are the results of your actions and decisions. Sexually transmitted diseases, pregnancy, tobacco and alcohol addiction, overdoses, and car accidents are examples of negative consequences that many teens have faced because they made fast decisions.

Making decisions is important because you are responsible for the consequences of your decisions. The decisions you make not only affect your health but also can affect the health of others. For example, choosing to drink and drive not only puts the driver in danger but also puts everyone on the road in danger.

Your decisions can also promote the health of your family and the health of your community. For example, you can start a recycling project with your family. You can also start a neighborhood watch program in your community.

Deciding not to take part in risky behavior will protect you from negative consequences.

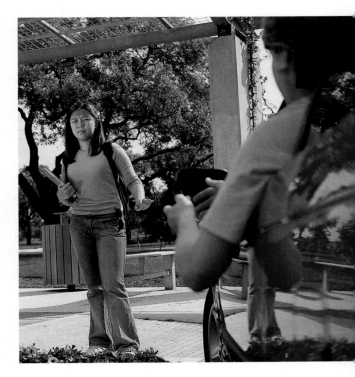

Figure 2

The Making GREAT Decisions model will help you make great decisions.

ACTIVITY *Use the steps of the Making GREAT Decisions model for a decision you need to make today.*

Using the Making GREAT Decisions Model

How many times have you made a decision that you regretted later? This is where the life skill for making GREAT decisions can help you by providing a decision-making model. The Making GREAT Decisions model is useful because it requires you to think about the choices and the consequences before making a decision. If you learn how to use the decision-making model, you are more likely to make decisions that have positive consequences.

The steps of the Making GREAT Decisions model are listed in **Figure 2.** Notice that each step uses the first letter of the word *great*. Let's use the model for the decision Sina was facing at the beginning of this section. Recall that Sina has just been asked to skip school with Marty.

GIVE Thought to the Problem If Sina doesn't stop to think about the decision, she might do something she regrets. Therefore, Sina pauses before giving Marty an impulsive answer.

REVIEW Your Choices At first glance, you might say that Sina has two choices. One choice is skip school and get into the car with Marty. Another choice is to tell Marty, "No, thanks," and keep walking to school. Are those two choices the only ones that Sina has? Can you think of any others? Why is Sina tempted to skip school with Marty in the first place? She probably likes him. Maybe she can suggest that they get together at another time.

EVALUATE the Consequences of Each Choice In this step, Sina weighs the pros and cons of each possible choice. If Sina skips school, she could get caught and could be suspended from school. If her parents found out, she would be grounded. These consequences would be the short-term consequences.

Sina could also face long-term consequences. These consequences would affect her years from now. Sina thinks that she spotted a six-pack of beer in the back seat. What would happen if she were in the car and they were arrested? She could have an arrest on her record. Or they could get into an accident!

What if Sina follows her second choice—not to get into the car with Marty but to keep walking to school? If she makes this decision, she will not face any serious consequences. But she will miss a chance to be with Marty.

What if she follows her third choice—to turn down Marty's offer but to suggest that they get together another time? Sina won't get into trouble for skipping school. Also, she won't risk getting into a car with people who drink and drive. Wait a minute. If Marty drinks and drives and skips school now, is he likely to do so again? If Sina gets together with Marty, might she find herself in this situation in the future?

ASSESS and Choose the Best Choice   During this step, Sina makes her choice. She decides which choice best reflects her values. You may recall that a value is a strong belief or ideal. For example, honesty is one of Sina's values. Values have a big effect on your decision making. If you make a decision that goes against your values, you will feel bad about the decision later. Respecting your values is respecting yourself.

Sina chose not to skip school with Marty. She also did not offer to get together with him later. Lying to her teachers and parents about her whereabouts went against her values. She would face too many negative consequences for skipping school. Going straight to school was a lot less stressful. Sina politely told Marty, "No, thanks."

THINK It Over Afterward   Sina thought about her decision. She was glad she didn't have to lie to her parents. She was also glad that she didn't have to worry about getting in trouble.

Making GREAT Decisions Together

You will likely face situations in which you are not sure what the right decision is. These decisions generally affect your life and health significantly. For this reason, you may feel more pressured to make the right decision. When you have to make difficult decisions, seeking advice from your friends, teachers, and parents can be very helpful. They might see a positive or negative consequence that you didn't. They can also support you when you need to make an unpopular decision.

Sometimes, we don't realize how our decisions affect others. For example, if you decide to baby-sit when you feel sick, you might pass the sickness on to the baby. These are the decisions about which you probably would want to ask for advice.

For some decisions, you may need more than just advice. Many decisions require you to collaborate with others. To **collaborate** is to work together with one or more people. For example, working on a science project with your classmate requires you to collaborate. Some collaborations are more serious. For example, you discover your friend has been talking about suicide. You need to collaborate with your parents to find out how to help your friend. No matter how serious the situation is, learning to work with others helps you find the right solution.

As you get older you will find that skills in collaborative decision making will be very useful. You will use these skills to make decisions with co-workers at your current or future jobs. You will also use collaborative decision making skills with the family you will form. Learning these skills now will help you make better decisions in the future.

Collaborating with parents can help you make GREAT decisions.

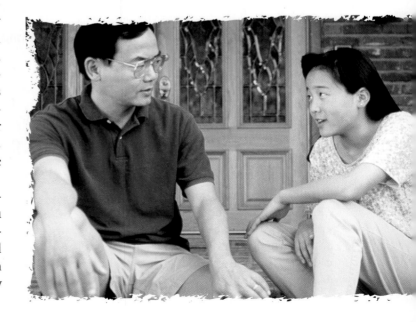

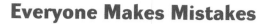

Everyone Makes Mistakes

What happens if you find you made a poor decision? It is possible, even likely—even after practicing your decision-making skills! Sometimes, the consequences of wrong decisions are embarrassing or humiliating. Everybody has had that kind of experience. Sometimes, however, wrong decisions can be dangerous to you and to the people around you. These kinds of decisions need to be dealt with as soon as possible.

Stop, Think, and Go   If you made a poor decision, you can use the Stop, Think, and Go process to correct the problem. The Stop, Think, and Go process uses the following steps:

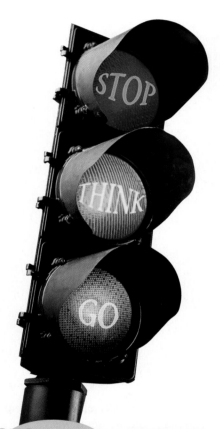

▶ **STOP** First, stop and admit that you made a poor decision. When you admit that you made a wrong decision, you take responsibility for what you've done.

▶ **THINK** Then, think about to whom you can talk about the problem. Usually, a parent, teacher, school counselor, or close friend can help you. Tell whomever you choose about your decision and its consequences. Discuss ways to correct the situation.

▶ **GO** Finally, go and do your best to correct the situation. Maybe you simply need to leave the situation you are in. You may have to tell someone about an unsafe situation. You may have to apologize to someone you hurt. In any case, you have had the opportunity to learn from your mistake.

Admitting that you have made the wrong decision is not always easy. You might risk getting in trouble with your parents or teachers. You might make your friends angry. In the long run, though, you'll feel better. You will know that you adhered to your values and tried to do the right thing.

SECTION 2

REVIEW   *Answer the following questions on a separate piece of paper.*

Using Key Terms

1. **Identify** the term for "a result of your actions and decisions."

2. **Define** the term *collaborate*.

Understanding Key Ideas

3. **Describe** the importance of making decisions.

4. **Identify** the step that is *not* a part of the Making GREAT Decisions model.
   a. Review your choices.
   b. Assess and choose the best choice.
   c. Think it over afterward.
   d. Think quickly.

5. **Summarize** why it is important to think about decisions you make afterward.

6. **Describe** what you can do if you make a wrong decision.

Critical Thinking

7. **LIFE SKILL** **Making GREAT Decisions** Apply the Making GREAT Decisions model to a situation in which you need to make a decision.

8. **LIFE SKILL** **Making GREAT Decisions** Describe a time when you worked effectively with someone else to make a decision.

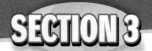

Resisting Pressure from Others

OBJECTIVES

State the people and groups that influence our behavior.

Identify three types of direct pressure.

Identify three types of indirect pressure.

State an example of each of the 12 types of refusal skills.

Apply one of the refusal skills to a pressure in your life. **LIFE SKILL**

" ere, take this! Don't say anything or I'll say it was your idea!" Maiyen's friend Jeff stuffed candy that he was planning to steal into Maiyen's pocket. At that moment, Maiyen's uncle came out from behind the store counter. "Maiyen! How's your dad?"

Who Influences You?

What style of clothes do you wear? What kind of hairstyle do you have? Your behaviors and decisions are often influenced by many people. For example, your friends can influence you through peer pressure. **Peer pressure** is a feeling that you should do something because that is what your friends want. Your family can also influence your behaviors and decisions. Even the media (movies, TV, books, magazines, newspapers, the Internet, and radio) influence the decisions you make every day. These influences can be positive or negative.

Positive Influences Having positive role models and being influenced to improve yourself can be good. For example, let's say that your closest friends are joining the track team. You decide to join the team, too, to spend more time with your friends. Running around the track improves your physical health, doesn't it?

Negative Influences On the other hand, being pressured to do something that you don't want to do is not healthy. For example, Maiyen is being pressured to steal from her uncle's store. The consequences of negative pressure can be serious. Some pressures can be life threatening. Examples of pressures that can threaten your life include smoking, drinking alcohol, and using drugs. These pressures often come from your own friends.

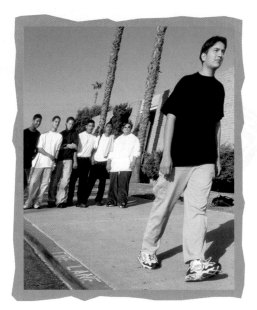

Everybody has felt some type of pressure from his or her friends at one time or another.

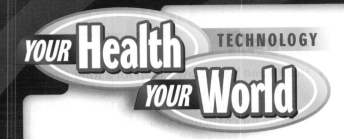

Self-Diagnosis and the Internet

More and more people are using the Internet to diagnose their medical conditions. This Internet research has some benefits but has a lot of serious drawbacks, too.

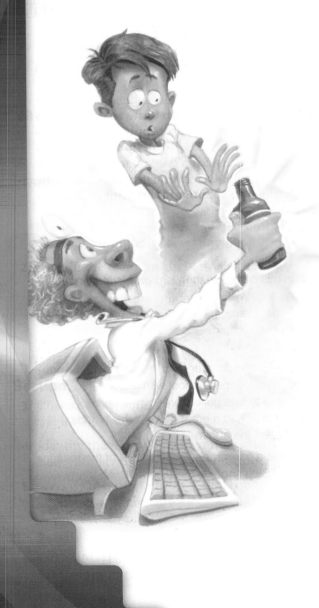

Self-diagnosis is our personal evaluation of our own health issues. We usually use self-diagnosis, for example, when we are coming down with a cold, when we have the flu, or when we have a rash from poison ivy. In the past, if a condition were more complex or more dangerous, people went to a doctor for a professional diagnosis. Most people still do, but today many people are turning to the Internet to find the answers to their medical questions.

Web Sites Often Have Inaccurate Information

One health issue that many people go to the Internet to understand is skin cancer. Doctors at the University of Michigan wanted to find out if Internet sites that provide information on skin cancer were accurate. What they found was quite alarming. Their study revealed that most sites contained incomplete information and that one in eight contained wrong information. It is important to remember that many Web sites lack accurate information about prevention, diagnosis, and treatment.

Some Sites Are Not What They Claim To Be

Unfortunately, some sites contain areas of self-diagnosis simply to sell you a worthless product. Many unscrupulous Internet merchants are simply seeking to make a lot of money in a hurry. If someone sells you a bracelet to cure a rash, it does more harm than only costing you money. If you buy the bracelet, you may be using a useless trinket to ignore a serious condition. Such bogus sites often spring up on the Internet and then disappear just as quickly. Other sites mean well but offer cures that have not been fully tested. The people behind these sites may have your best interest at heart, but their sites may not have the objectivity of a carefully trained doctor.

How Can the Internet Help?

The Internet has many sites that offer self-diagnosis charts, tests, and evaluations. For example, if you have a skin problem, you can go to a site, answer a few questions, and arrive at a medical conclusion. In many cases, such Internet sites can help you understand your problem. By comparing your symptoms with those listed on a site, you may figure out what is wrong.

As good as Web self-diagnosis may be, it is also filled with dangers. Self-diagnosis on the Web

▶ is not a substitute for a doctor's professional evaluation

▶ may be based on information that is inaccurate or false

▶ is often conducted on sites that want to sell you something or that contain highly questionable health practices

Your Doctor Knows

A doctor has been trained to look carefully for all of the evidence of a disease or disorder. In addition, your doctor is less likely to make a mistake than you are while you are sitting and worrying in front of a computer. For example, suppose that moving the left side of your face became difficult and you couldn't blink your left eye. If you looked up the symptoms on a computer, you might think you had Bell's Palsy, an annoying disruption of your facial nerves. According to the Internet, your problem will go away on its own. Your doctor, however, may ask you if you had a recent rash, had joint pain, or had been hiking. Your doctor knows that nerve problems in the face can be a symptom of something else. He or she will evaluate all of your symptoms and might diagnose Lyme disease and take appropriate steps. Your self-diagnosis would have prevented you from getting the antibiotics needed to combat Lyme disease.

Wise Use of the Web

The Internet can help you see the seriousness of a symptom or can provide additional information. For example, if you have already seen a doctor, you can

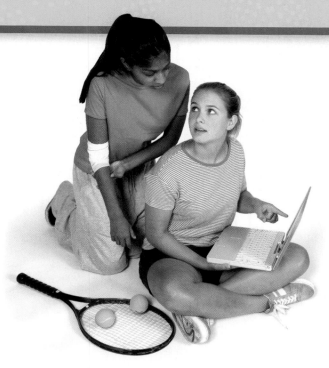

read more about your diagnosis and can educate yourself. In addition, you can use the Internet to gather information in private. But the Internet is only one tool to support your health. Use it wisely in addition to consulting health professionals.

YOUR TURN

1. **Summarizing Information** What are three dangers of using Internet sites for self-diagnosis of health issues?

2. **Applying Information** How has Internet technology changed self-diagnosis from the way people diagnosed themselves in the past?

3. **CRITICAL THINKING** How can you determine if a Web site contains medically accepted information?

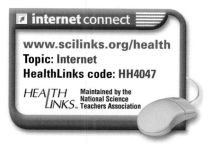

internet connect

www.scilinks.org/health
Topic: Internet
HealthLinks code: HH4047

HEALTH LINKS. Maintained by the National Science Teachers Association

Self-Esteem and Mental Health

What's Your Health IQ?

BEHAVIOR

Indicate how frequently you engage in each of the following behaviors (1 = never; 2 = occasionally; 3 = most of the time; 4 = all of the time). Total your points, and then turn to p. 642.

1. I praise myself when I do a good job.

2. I do what I know is right, even if others use pressure to try to stop me from doing the right thing.

3. I am confident enough to try new things, even if I might fail at them.

4. I ask people for help if I need it.

5. I like to volunteer to help others when I can.

6. I concentrate on my strengths and work to improve my weaknesses.

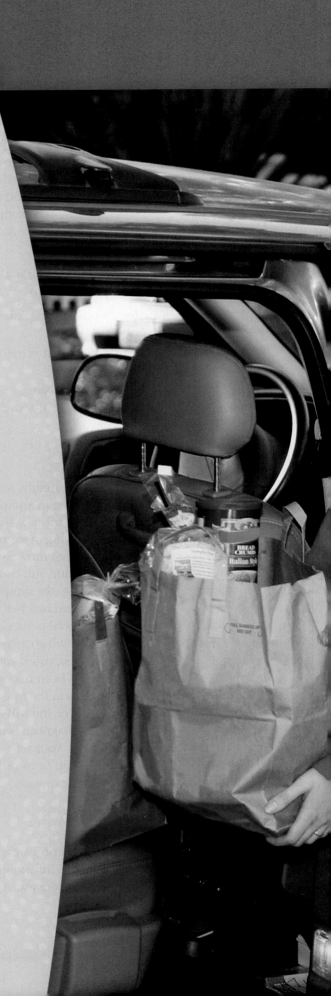

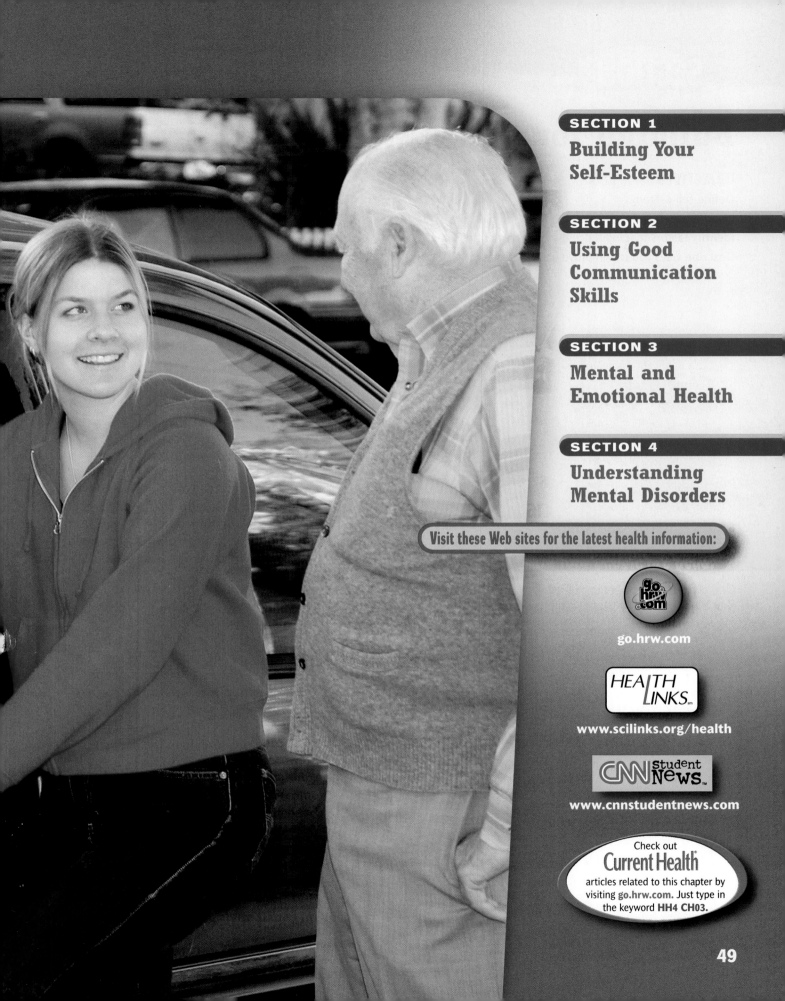

Visit these Web sites for the latest health information:

go.hrw.com

HEALTH LINKSsm

www.scilinks.org/health

CNN student News™

www.cnnstudentnews.com

Check out **Current Health** articles related to this chapter by visiting go.hrw.com. Just type in the keyword **HH4 CH03.**

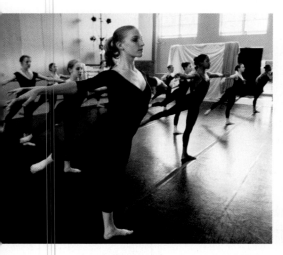

Building Your Self-Esteem

OBJECTIVES

Define self-esteem.

List the benefits of high self-esteem.

Identify factors that influence the development of self-esteem.

Describe ways you can improve your self-esteem. **LIFE SKILL**

KEY TERMS

self-esteem a measure of how much you value, respect, and feel confident about yourself

self-concept a measure of how you view yourself

integrity the characteristic of doing what you know is right

One characteristic of high self-esteem is not being afraid to try new things.

Leyla started taking ballet 3 months ago. She doesn't dance as well as the rest of the class. The other dancers have been practicing ballet much longer than Leyla has. However, Leyla loves every minute of rehearsal. She can't wait to perform on stage.

What Is Self-Esteem?

Self-esteem is a measure of how much you value, respect, and feel confident about yourself. How you feel about yourself affects everything you do. It affects how you communicate with people and what decisions you make about your health. For example, if you feel good about yourself, you can more easily talk with people and share your feelings. However, if you don't feel good about yourself, you might not have the confidence to use your refusal skills or to avoid disrespectful people.

Benefits of High Self-Esteem   Below are a list of the benefits people who have high self-esteem experience.

▶ **Increased respect** People with high self-esteem respect themselves by taking care of themselves. They will not do anything to harm themselves, such as smoking or abusing drugs and alcohol. They don't criticize or put themselves down. Furthermore, they exercise, eat right, and get plenty of rest.

People with high self-esteem respect their values and beliefs. They are less likely to let others pressure them to take part in risky behavior. Nor will they pressure others to take part in harmful behavior.

▶ **Increased ability to reach goals** If you have confidence in yourself, you are more likely to set realistic goals and stick with the goals you set for yourself until you reach those goals. The longer you stick with a goal and the harder you try, the better the chance you have at reaching it. Because people with high self-esteem are more likely to reach their goals, they are more likely to challenge themselves to set higher goals and accomplish more.

- **Increased willingness to try** People with high self-esteem have the will to try new things and don't get discouraged easily. For example, Leyla had the courage to try something new—ballet dancing. More important, when she found out she wasn't as good as the others, she didn't give up. Instead, she kept trying her best. She did it for herself, not for competition.
- **Increased feelings of value** People with high self-esteem feel like they are a valuable part of their family, school, and community. They are more likely to ask for help when they need it. They are also more likely to volunteer in their communities because they know they have the power to help others.

Risks of Low Self-Esteem People with low self-esteem share many characteristics as listed in **Figure 1.** For example, people with low self-esteem are more vulnerable to peer pressure. As a result, they are more likely to make unhealthy decisions, such as smoking.

People with low self-esteem may not be respectful to themselves or others. Those who do not feel good about themselves will often put themselves down. They are also more critical of others.

Low self-esteem is also harmful to one's mental health. People with low self-esteem are at risk for depression and suicide. Low self-esteem is also linked to eating disorders, running away, and violence.

People with low self-esteem do not have to experience the risks of low self-esteem. Everyone has the power to choose healthy behaviors that show respect for others and themselves.

Figure 1

You can't tell if someone has high self-esteem or low self-esteem just by looking at him or her.

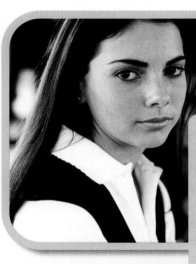

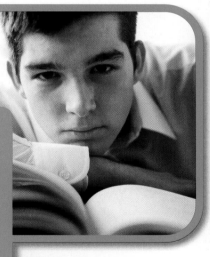

High Self-Esteem
- Speaks up for self
- Respects self and others
- Has confidence
- Tries new things
- Feels valuable to society
- Adjusts to change
- Feels optimistic
- Makes decisions based on values

Low Self-Esteem
- Feels insecure
- Disrespects self and others
- Vulnerable to peer pressure
- Doesn't feel valuable
- Feels depressed
- Fears failure
- Uses drugs and alcohol
- Feels pessimistic
- Behaves destructively

Ten Tips for Building Self-Esteem

▶ Volunteer at a soup kitchen or other community service.

▶ Make a list of your strengths.

▶ Speak positively about yourself and others.

▶ Take care of your physical health.

▶ Reward yourself when you do well.

▶ Try something new.

▶ Choose friends who support you and your positive choices.

▶ Set a goal to improve a weakness.

▶ Cheer yourself through hard times.

▶ Have fun.

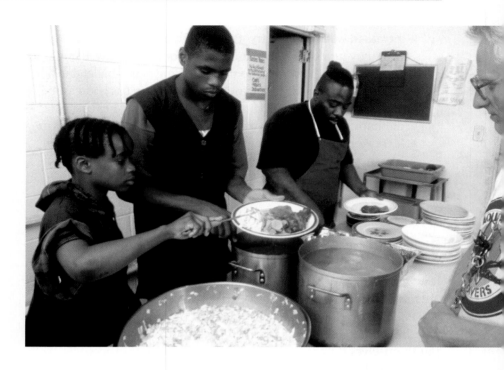

The Development of Self-Esteem

Self-esteem begins to develop the day you are born. Across your entire life, your level of self-esteem can vary. At one time, it may be high, and at a different time or in a different situation, it may be low.

Self-Concept   A measure of how one views oneself is **self-concept.** For example, if you think of yourself as a valuable and likeable person, you have a positive self-concept. If you have a positive self-concept, you have high self-esteem. However, if you don't think of yourself as very likeable or valuable, you probably have a negative self-concept and therefore, have low self-esteem.

Interpreting Messages From Others   How you interpret messages about yourself has a lot to do with how you view yourself. These messages come from family, friends, teachers, neighbors, and even strangers. The messages can be positive, such as "You are fun to be around." Messages can also be negative, such as "You always complain about everything." These messages shape what you think about yourself. How you think about yourself shapes your self-esteem.

Some negative messages can serve as good advice. Good advice on how to improve yourself is called *constructive criticism.* For example, if you have not been getting along well with your parents, your brother might recommend that you try being more cooperative with your parents.

Other negative messages can be hurtful. But your self-esteem doesn't have to suffer. Remember that self-esteem is how you feel about yourself, not how others feel about you or what others say about you. Only you have the power to control your self-esteem.

Improving Your Self-Esteem

Everyone can work at improving his or her self-esteem. You can improve your self-esteem by using positive self-talk, acting with integrity, choosing supportive friends, and accepting yourself.

Use Positive Self-Talk   You learned that the messages you receive from others influence your self-esteem. The same is true for the messages *you* send to yourself. The things you say to yourself strongly influence your self-esteem.

We are constantly talking to ourselves, whether we realize it or not. You may say or think things like, "My painting really looks neat!" or "I'm too stupid for this class." The things you say about yourself can make you feel good, or they can make you feel not so good.

To practice treating yourself well, you can use a technique called *self-talk*. Self-talk is a way of coaching yourself about your own self-worth. Go ahead and talk to yourself. Tell yourself you can do what you set out to do when you set realistic goals and ask for help. Tell yourself that you are a valuable person.

real life Activity

SELL YOURSELF

LIFE SKILL
Practicing Wellness

Materials

✔ poster board
✔ magazines
✔ markers
✔ scissors
✔ paste

Procedure

1. **Think** about why you are a wonderful person.
2. **List** five reasons why you are wonderful on your poster board.
3. **Think** of different techniques advertisers use to sell their products. Use these techniques in your own advertisement to express why you are fabulous.
4. **Cut** out magazine clippings to help express the five reasons you are great.

Conclusions

1. **Summarizing Results** What are the five reasons you are great?
2. **Evaluating Information** What technique or style did you use to make yourself stand out?
3. **Analyzing Methods** Describe why this activity may have been hard for you or easy for you.
4. **CRITICAL THINKING** List at least five additional reasons that you are special.

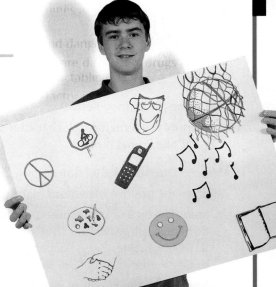

Act with Integrity The characteristic of doing what one knows is right is **integrity.** For example, your integrity prompts you to be honest and return the extra $10 the cashier mistakenly gave you, even if your friends want you to spend it on a movie with them.

When you have integrity, you respect others, yourself, and your values. You don't let people pressure you to go against what is right and important to you. People who have low self-esteem may be unsure of themselves and can be swayed to do something they don't feel right about. On the other hand, people who have high self-esteem recognize when they need to stand up for their beliefs to continue to respect themselves.

Choose Supportive Friends It is easier for you to treat yourself well if the people you know also speak well of you. Avoid critical or disrespectful people. Maintain friendships with people who acknowledge your strengths and support you in your goals and values.

Accept Yourself People who have high self-esteem do not think they are perfect. They know they are not perfect. People who have high self-esteem accept who they are. They see all their imperfections and still think of themselves as valuable.

People who accept themselves celebrate their strengths and concentrate on what they do well. They also strive to improve weaknesses by setting short-term goals. However, if they can't change a weakness, they let it go. For example, if you're not as tall as you would like to be, wishing and hoping won't make you taller. However, dwelling on your height may lower your self-esteem.

Once you accept yourself, you'll find that others will accept you, too. If you project a confident attitude, others will sense—and respect you for—your confidence. You will then feel better about yourself!

> ....
> **Until you accept who you are, you will never be happy with what you have.**
> ....

SECTION 1

REVIEW   *Answer the following questions on a separate piece of paper.*

Using Key Terms

1. **Define** the term *self-esteem*.

2. **Identify** the term for "the characteristic of doing what one knows is right."

Understanding Key Ideas

3. **State** the positive benefits of high self-esteem.

4. **Identify** which of the following is *not* a characteristic of high self-esteem.
   a. feels valuable
   b. pessimistic
   c. confidence
   d. self-respect

5. **Summarize** the effects of low self-esteem.

6. **Identify** factors that influence the development of self-esteem.

7. **Identify** which of the following is *not* a way to improve your self-esteem.
   a. using positive self-talk
   b. accepting yourself
   c. acting with integrity
   d. denying your faults

Critical Thinking

8. **Describe** how respecting yourself and respecting your values can improve your self-esteem.

9. **LIFE SKILL** **Practicing Wellness** Describe three ways you can improve your self-esteem.

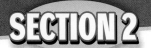

Using Good Communication Skills

OBJECTIVES

Summarize why good communication is important.

Differentiate between passive, assertive, and aggressive communication styles.

Name five characteristics of good listening skills.

List three examples of body language.

List five ways to improve your speaking skills. **LIFE SKILL**

KEY TERMS

passive not offering opposition when challenged or pressured

aggressive hostile and unfriendly in the way one expresses oneself

assertive direct and respectful in the way one expresses oneself

empathy the ability to understand another person's feelings, behaviors, and attitudes

Rina was planning to have some friends over for her birthday. But her friends have been acting strange. They whisper when they think she isn't looking. They pretend not to see her when she walks down the hall. No one will even return her phone calls.

Good Communication Is Important

Communication is a process through which two or more people exchange information. One person sends the message, and one or more people receive it. However, if the message is not properly sent or is unclear, misunderstandings can arise.

Preventing Misunderstandings Rina's situation shows how easy it is to miscommunicate. Rina was receiving messages that made her feel unwanted. What she found out later was almost the opposite. Rina's friends were being secretive because they were planning a surprise for her birthday. Fortunately, her situation had a positive outcome; she was pleasantly surprised. However, miscommunication can have some negative effects such as arguments and hurt feelings.

Building Healthy Relationships Communication is important for building caring and satisfying relationships with your family, friends, co-workers, and society. How you communicate with others affects how people relate to you. For example, if you are mean or insult others, they probably won't want to be around you. However, if you let people know how important they are to you, they will be more likely to treat you the way you want to be treated.

Expressing Yourself Good communication skills are also important for letting others know what you need and want. These skills also help you to express how you feel. Just think how difficult life would be if you couldn't tell someone that you needed help.

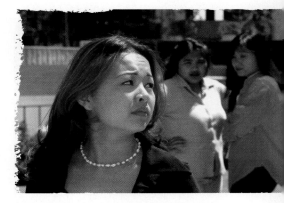

Miscommunication can result in hurt feelings.

Communication Styles

There are three communication styles: passive, aggressive, and assertive. The following descriptions compare these three communication styles.

Passive A person who has a communication style that is **passive** does not offer opposition when challenged or pressured. Such a person tends to go along with what other people want and does not protest or resist when challenged. For example, let's say your brother borrowed your shirt and tore it. If you had a passive response, you would give your brother the silent treatment and then just throw your shirt away.

Aggressive To be hostile and unfriendly in the way one expresses oneself is to be **aggressive.** For example, an aggressive response in the same situation with your brother would be to tell him, "You are such a jerk! Let's see how you feel when I ruin your things!" Aggressive communication is not effective and usually leads to a bigger conflict.

Assertive The third and most healthy communication style is the assertive style. To be **assertive** is to express oneself in a direct, respectful way. For example, you could say to your brother, "My favorite shirt is ruined. I spent a lot of money on this shirt. I would like you to replace it." With this response, you calmly expressed to your brother how his action affected you. This response was also respectful to your brother, which is an important part of being assertive.

Using the assertive communication style might not be easy when someone has done something that really upsets you. However, practicing can help you improve. **Table 1** lists more examples of passive, aggressive, and assertive communication responses. See if you can think of some examples of your own.

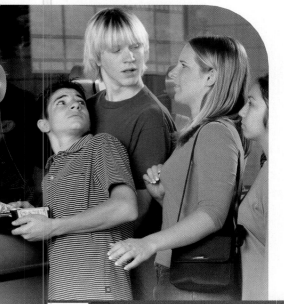

Use assertive communication if someone is disrespectful to you, such as cutting in front of you in line.

Table 1 Communication Styles

Situation	Passive response	Aggressive response	Assertive response
Someone cuts in front of you in line.	You don't say anything.	"Well, you must think you're special!"	"Excuse me, but I believe I'm next in line."
Your best friend tells someone else one of your secrets.	You don't say anything, but you vow never to tell her another secret.	"I hate you! I'm never going to trust you again!"	"It hurt me to find out you told my secret to someone else. Please don't repeat my secrets again."
Your boss asks you to work late for the third night in a row.	You agree but feel worried about finishing your homework tonight.	"You are so inconsiderate! I quit!"	"Sorry, I can't work tonight. I have a lot of homework do."

Speaking Skills

Think about the way you communicate. Are there any areas that you would like to improve? Have you ever been at a loss for words? Have you ever been frustrated because you can't get someone to understand you? Everyone has felt that way before. There are many skills you can learn to help you communicate better.

One of the main ways we communicate is verbally. *Verbal* communication refers to the specific words and tones that we use when we speak. Because most of us can speak, we frequently use speech to communicate.

You may ask yourself, what could I possibly need to learn about talking, something I've been doing almost my whole life? It is true that you have a lot of practice with this type of communication. However, learning effective speaking skills can be helpful when you need to give a speech in class. Effective speaking skills also can give you the confidence to discuss sensitive issues with your parents, such as sexual activity or marraige.

Voice Volume   How loud or soft you are speaking is called *voice volume*. If someone increases how loud he or she says something, what does that increase in voice volume generally mean? You don't even have to know what the person is saying to know that he or she may be mad. What does it mean if someone lowers the volume of communication to a whisper? That person may be either trying to tell you a secret or trying not to get caught talking to you in class! Be aware of the voice volume you use when speaking with others.

Tone and Pitch   Tone of voice and pitch refer to the *inflections* or emphasis in your voice when you speak. Tone and pitch convey the attitude you are trying to express.

For example, if your older sister says, "What are you doing?" the tone and pitch of her voice tell you that she is asking you a question. But if she says, "WHAT are you doing!" you know she is angry. If she says, "What ARE you doing?" she sounds arrogant. She could also say, "What are you DOING?" and sound very upset. See if you can say, "What are you doing?" and sound questioning, angry, arrogant, and upset. Can you think of any other tones and pitches that you could use with the same phrase?

"I" Messages and "You" Messages   A good technique for communicating assertively is to use "I" messages. An "I" message is a way of talking that explains how you feel while remaining firm, calm, and polite. Sometimes, when people are mad or upset, they say things that seem like they are blaming another person. This type of statement is called a "you" message. "You" messages sound like the following: "You did this" or "You are so selfish." It is very easy to get in a fight when "you" messages are being sent. An "I" message, on the other hand, is a tool that allows you to express your feelings without blaming another person.

WHAT are you doing?

What **ARE** you doing?

What are you **DOING?**

When using "I" messages, say how you feel and why you feel that way. For example, suppose you put your bag on the front seat of the bus to save it while you run to get something. When you come back, someone has moved your bag and taken your seat. To use an "I" message, you could say, "I'm upset that you moved my bag and took my seat. I want to sit there because my stop is the first stop."

Let's say your sister is playing music so loud that you can't study for your history test. You could use "I" messages to tell her, "I can't study for my test because the music is so loud. Please turn it down."

Empathy The ability to understand another person's feelings, behaviors, and attitudes is called **empathy.** Showing empathy can be an effective way to communicate. For example, let's say you ask your neighbor if you can borrow his bike. He tells you he needs it for his job delivering newspapers. If you respond by telling him he can deliver newspapers later, that would not show empathy. Your neighbor would probably respond, "Go take a hike." However, if you responded by asking to borrow the bike when he's done, he might be more likely to lend it to you.

LIFE SKILL Activity

Communicating Effectively

Say What?

Practicing "I" messages will help you communicate more effectively. Try role-playing a situation in which "I" messages would be helpful.

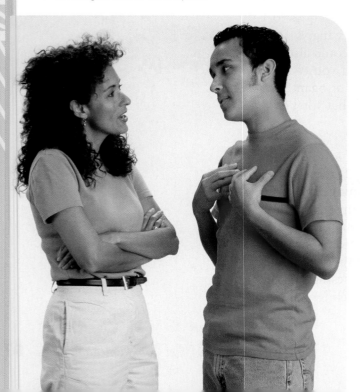

1. Decide who will be the "parent" and who will be the "teen."

2. Decide on a situation in which you need to talk to your parent about something that upset you, such as chores or going out with friends.

3. First, use "you" messages to talk to the "parent."

4. Now, try "I" messages to tell the "parent" how you feel.

5. Switch roles with your partner, and repeat steps 4 and 5.

LIFE SKILL **Communicating Effectively**

1. When you were the "parent," describe how you felt when the "teen" was using "you" messages.

2. Now, describe how you felt when the "teen" used "I" messages. Which form of communication do you think would be most effective? Explain your answer.

Listening Skills

Have you ever spent a lot of energy explaining how you felt to someone but found out that the person wasn't paying attention? How did the situation make you feel? What did it do to your self-esteem?

Communication includes not only sending messages but also receiving messages, or listening. It makes people feel good when they know you are listening and that you really care about what they are saying. Two important ways to show you are listening are to use active listening and to paraphrase. **Figure 2** lists more suggestions for being a good listener.

Active Listening *Active listening* means letting the speaker know you are listening and clarifying anything that is confusing. You can do so by asking the speaker questions and by using expressions such as

▶ "I guess you must have felt . . . "
▶ "Tell me about . . . "
▶ "Hmmm."
▶ "Really?"
▶ "Uh-huh."

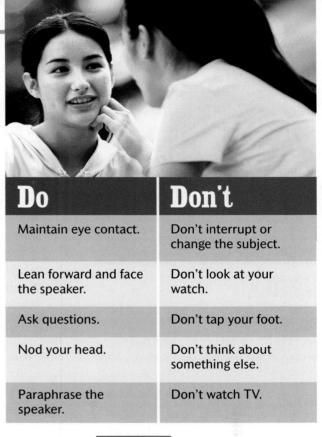

Do	Don't
Maintain eye contact.	Don't interrupt or change the subject.
Lean forward and face the speaker.	Don't look at your watch.
Ask questions.	Don't tap your foot.
Nod your head.	Don't think about something else.
Paraphrase the speaker.	Don't watch TV.

Figure 2

Maintaining eye contact is a good way to show that you are listening. Here are some more tips to show that you are listening.

To practice active listening, give the speaker your full attention. Giving your full attention means you should not think about what you are going to say next. Try to identify the main concepts and ideas that are being communicated. Provide feedback to the speaker, but wait until the speaker is finished before you start talking.

Paraphrasing *Paraphrasing* is using your own words to restate what someone else said. You may have heard teachers use this term when telling you how to write a research paper. When writing a paper, you paraphrase other authors to show the teacher that you understood what you read. In a conversation, you paraphrase to show the other person that you understand what he or she is saying.

Here is an example of paraphrasing. Your friend spends 10 minutes telling you how unhappy he is because his parents are divorced, and you say, "The divorce really is making you unhappy, isn't it?" Paraphrasing allows you to show the person that you care about what he or she is saying. Paraphrasing may seem like restating the obvious, but you would be amazed how sometimes you hear something differently from what the speaker means. Paraphrasing helps you to accurately understand the speaker.

Paraphrasing can also be used if you don't understand what someone is saying. For example, imagine your health teacher is talking about the fat content in food. If you were paraphrasing, you might say, "So, what you are saying is that white-meat chicken has less fat than dark-meat chicken does?" Then, the teacher could either agree or try to explain the topic in a different way.

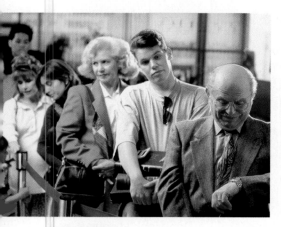

Figure 3

Body language can tell a lot about how a person is feeling.

ACTIVITY *What are the first three people in line feeling? How can you tell?*

Body Language

Earlier, you learned that one way to communicate is to speak. However, you can communicate without saying a word. You reveal a lot about how you feel through facial expressions, gestures, and posture. This nonverbal communication is called *body language*. Below are some examples of body language. See if you can guess what each one may be communicating.

▶ opening your eyes wide
▶ scratching your head
▶ opening your mouth wide
▶ snarling
▶ scrunching your eyebrows in a V shape
▶ standing up straight and tall
▶ winking

Can you think of any other examples of body language? Try some body language of your own. Act excited. Go on—do it. What did you do? You probably smiled, looked alert, and clapped your hands. Now, act bored. You probably slumped your shoulders and drooped your face. If someone was watching you, he or she would have been able to tell how you were feeling even though you didn't say a word. What do you think the people in **Figure 3** are feeling?

Misunderstandings often occur when our body language says one thing but our mouths say another. Think back to the example of Rina and her friends. What made her suspicious of her friends? What type of body language was she receiving from them? Usually, when body language is giving a message that is different from what you are saying, people tend to believe the body language message. Therefore, paying attention to the messages you are sending nonverbally is important. Also, you can learn a lot about what others are feeling by watching their body language.

SECTION 2

REVIEW *Answer the following questions on a separate piece of paper.*

Using Key Terms

1. **Identify** the term for "direct and respectful in the way one expresses oneself."

2. **Define** the term *empathy*.

Understanding Key Ideas

3. **Describe** why good communication is important.

4. **Identify** the communication style that is most likely to lead to conflict.

5. **List** five characteristics of good listening skills.

6. **Identify** which of the following behaviors is *not* an example of a good listening skill.
   a. watching TV   c. paraphrasing
   b. facing the speaker   d. leaning forward

7. **Identify** which of the following behaviors is *not* an example of body language.
   a. winking   c. snarling
   b. raising your voice   d. clapping hands

Critical Thinking

8. **LIFE SKILL** **Communicating Effectively** List five ways you can improve your speaking skills.

Mental and Emotional Health

OBJECTIVES

Describe characteristics of positive mental health.

Compare the stages of Maslow's hierarchy of needs.

Describe how you can learn to express emotions in positive ways.

Identify the limitations of defense mechanisms.

Describe three positive strategies for managing your emotions. **LIFE SKILL**

KEY TERMS

mental health the state of mental well-being in which one can cope with the demands of daily life

self-actualization the achievement of the best that a person can be

emotion the feeling that is produced in response to life experiences

defense mechanism an unconscious behavior used to avoid experiencing unpleasant emotions

L ast night, John's girlfriend broke up with him. He layed in bed feeling sad for hours before he fell asleep. The next morning, he still felt sad. He wanted to try to make himself feel better, so he decided to talk to a friend about his sadness.

Mental Health

Mental health is the state of mental well-being in which one can cope with the demands of daily life. Good mental health means having high self-esteem and being able to develop healthy, intimate relationships. Having high self-esteem, handling daily frustrations, and building relationships depend on your ability to express and manage your emotions in positive ways. Therefore, to be mentally healthy, you also must be emotionally healthy.

People who are mentally and emotionally healthy have the following characteristics:

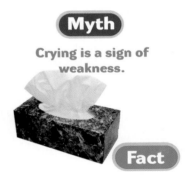

Myth

Crying is a sign of weakness.

Fact

Holding your emotions in can be destructive to your health.

▶ **A sense of control** Mentally healthy people have a sense of control and take charge of their lives. Because they feel in control, they also take responsibility for their behavior. They are less likely to blame others for situations they may face.

▶ **Ability to endure failures and frustrations** Mentally healthy people are more likely to persist through setbacks because they understand that frustrations are part of learning.

▶ **Ability to see events positively** Mentally healthy people are optimistic and see the challenges of life as opportunities.

▶ **Ability to express emotions in a healthy way** Mentally healthy people do not hold in emotions or deny how they feel. They express their emotions in healthy ways and talk with friends when they need support.

For example, when John was feeling sad he decided to talk with a friend. He did not deny his emotions or express them destructively. John has characteristics of someone who has good mental health.

Maslow's Hierarchy of Needs

Having good mental health has benefits. For example, mentally and emotionally healthy people are more likely to reach self-actualization. **Self-actualization** is the achievement of the best that a person can be. People who have achieved self-actualization have reached their potential and feel that they have received the most out of life.

Abraham Maslow, a *psychologist*, a person who studies emotions and behaviors, believed that everyone has a basic drive to reach self-actualization. Maslow stated that to reach self-actualization, a person has to first achieve some very basic needs. He listed these needs and called the list the *hierarchy of needs*, which is shown in **Figure 4.**

According to Maslow, the first needs a person must meet are the basic physical needs of the body, such as the need for food, water, sleep, and exercise. Once these needs are met, the next need is safety. This need includes the needs for shelter and protection from danger. After the need for safety is achieved, the person is free to strive for social needs, such as love, acceptance, and friendship. Once social needs are met, the person can focus on achieving esteem. Esteem is met through self-respect and the achievement of goals. Finally, after all of the other needs are met, the person could reach self-actualization.

Figure 4

Everyone has basic needs he or she strives to meet in order to get the most out of life.

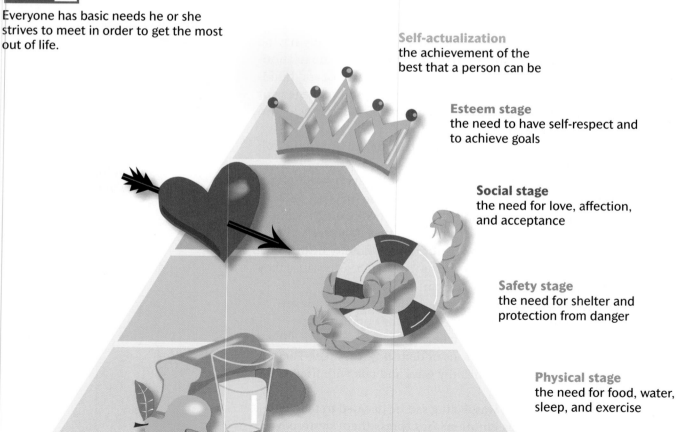

Self-actualization
the achievement of the best that a person can be

Esteem stage
the need to have self-respect and to achieve goals

Social stage
the need for love, affection, and acceptance

Safety stage
the need for shelter and protection from danger

Physical stage
the need for food, water, sleep, and exercise

Most people work on more than one stage at a time. Even people who have reached self-actualization may have to struggle with hardships that threaten their basic needs throughout their lives. Basic needs such as love and safety may not be met all of the time. However, you can still strive for the higher stages. Some ways you can work toward self-actualization in your teen years are by building healthy relationships, setting goals, and working toward achieving those goals.

Expressing Emotions

An **emotion** is the feeling that is produced in response to life experiences. Emotions aren't categorized as good or bad. However, the expression of emotions can have positive or negative effects. For example, pretend you can't study for your test because your family is making a lot of noise. Feeling frustrated is normal. But if you run around the house tearing at your hair and screaming, you probably won't get a positive response from your family.

Whether the emotion is anger, sadness, or joy, expressing it in a positive way is important. Denying an emotion will not make it go away. Instead, the emotion can build up inside of you and be expressed in a negative way. Learning to express and manage emotions in healthy ways are key to mental and emotional health and to self-actualization.

Learning to Express Emotions
How you decide to express your emotions is based in large part on how others around you express their emotions. For example, your family might deal with anger by yelling and throwing things. It is likely you would learn to deal with your anger in the same way.

You can learn to express your emotions more constructively regardless of how others around you express their emotions. To relearn how to express an emotion, practice expressing the emotion in a positive way. For example, role-play with a friend a situation in which you lost your temper with someone. This time, use the speaking skills you learned earlier to calmly tell that person what made you upset. Practicing will help you positively express your emotions naturally.

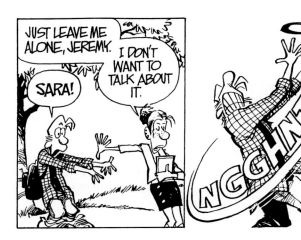
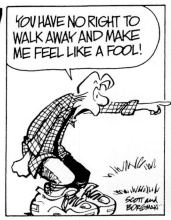
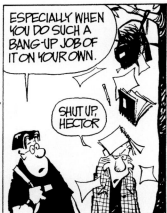

ZITS reprinted with special permission of King Features Syndicate, Inc.

Managing Emotions

Emotions can be overwhelming, especially during your teenage years. Understanding and recognizing the emotions you feel can be challenging.

It is especially difficult if you are feeling more than one emotion at a time. For example, should you go up and talk to that cute, new student? Or should you run and hide in the bathroom? Trying to deal with so many emotions can be frustrating. The following are suggestions to help you manage your emotions.

1. **Talk it out.** One way you can make sense of what you are feeling is by talking with someone you trust. For example, John made plans to talk with his friend after his girlfriend broke up with him. Just talking about a problem can help you manage your emotions.

2. **Blow off steam.** When emotions become bottled up inside of you, releasing that energy in some positive way often helps. Activities such as exercising, building something, or playing a sport are positive ways to let off steam.

3. **Be creative.** You can also release emotions in creative ways. Some people write or draw when they are troubled. Some people enjoy singing, playing a musical instrument, or painting. All of these activities help release tension.

Some emotions are more difficult to manage than other emotions. These emotions deserve special attention and are discussed in more detail below.

Anger Often, anger results from frustration or helplessness. For example, the computer crashes and causes you to lose the report that is due next class. You may want to grab the computer and smash it on the floor. That response will definitely not get your report back. In fact, that response may get you into a lot of trouble. Understanding that there was nothing you could do and letting things like this go will release a lot of tension.

Anger can *always* be dealt with in an appropriate manner. A person may make you angry, but that person doesn't make you hit him or her. You and only *you* are responsible for how you express your emotions.

The first step in keeping your anger from getting out of your control is learning to recognize when you feel angry. If you can recognize quickly when you start to become angry, you can more easily control your anger. When you get angry, do you clench your fists? Does your heart beat faster? When you feel the anger coming on, stop. Count to 10, take a deep breath, and calm down before you react. You may want to walk away and think about how best to deal with the situation. You may want to talk with someone or jog a few blocks while you think.

Once you feel in control of your anger, you may want to talk with the person who made you upset. This can help resolve your feelings. Be sure to use the "I" messages you learned earlier.

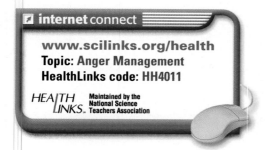

internet connect

www.scilinks.org/health
Topic: Anger Management
HealthLinks code: HH4011

HEALTH LINKS. Maintained by the National Science Teachers Association

Yelling at others when you are angry may make you feel better but it may cause more problems later.

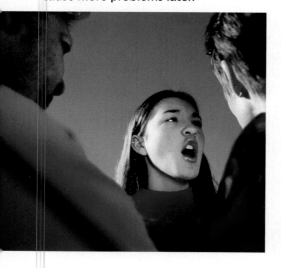

Fear Fear may not be a pleasant emotion, but it can be a helpful one. For example, our sense of fear is what helps protect us from danger. You jump out of the way of a speeding car because you fear getting run over.

Speeding cars are good things to fear. However, many people fear things that are not harmful. The fear may even get in the way of your normal life. For example, the fear of speaking in front of class can prevent you from giving a good speech.

To get over a fear, you can use self-talk. Instead of thinking about being scared, tell yourself that you have nothing to be afraid of. Another way to manage your fear is through controlled exposure to the fearful situation. For example, if you are afraid of speaking in front of a large group of people, you can start by speaking in front of one person. You can then work your way up to speaking in front of a large group.

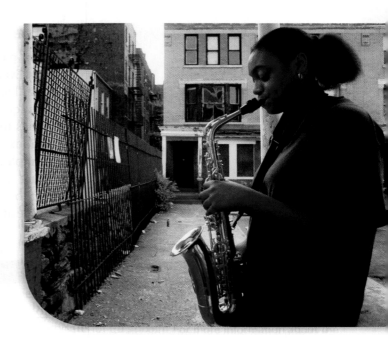

Guilt Guilt is another emotion that may not be pleasant but can serve a purpose. It alerts you that you are behaving in a way that goes against your values. Guilt can keep you true to yourself.

The best way to deal with guilty feelings is to do your best to right the wrong. If someone was hurt, apologize. If you stole something from a store, return it. Making amends lifts the weight of guilt off your shoulders because you are taking responsibility for your behavior. You'll feel much better in the long run.

Jealousy Jealousy is often caused by a fear that something you own or love will be lost. For example, if John's ex-girlfriend starts to date another person, John may feel jealous. A twinge of jealousy now and then is natural. However, if jealousy is not controlled, it can make you bitter and ruin your relationships.

If your girlfriend's or boyfriend's flirting has been bothering you, try talking about it with your boyfriend or girlfriend. However, remember that dating someone doesn't mean you own the person. If you don't trust your partner, you should examine your relationship and why you feel distrustful.

Loneliness Loneliness is an emotion that makes you feel isolated from others—not physically isolated, but emotionally isolated. You can be in a room of people, but if you don't feel close to any of them or feel rejected, you can still feel lonely. On the other hand, you can be by yourself and not feel lonely at all. In fact, being able to enjoy time by yourself is a sign of positive mental health.

A good way to manage loneliness is to join a group or club. You could also do volunteer work or start a job. Don't wait for people to approach you. You'll never be able to make close friends unless you go out and meet people.

Tips for Managing Emotions

▶ **Sing, or play a musical instrument.**

▶ **Write down how you feel.**

▶ **Talk to a friend.**

▶ **Exercise, or play a sport.**

▶ **Let go of what you can't control.**

▶ **Draw or paint a picture.**

Understanding Mental Disorders

OBJECTIVES

Describe what mental disorders are.

List seven signs of a mental disorder.

Summarize causes of mental disorders.

Identify community resources available for mental health problems.

KEY TERMS

mental disorder an illness that affects a person's thoughts, emotions, and behaviors

symptom a change that a person notices in his or her body or mind and that is caused by a disease or disorder.

depression a sadness and hopelessness that keeps a person from carrying out everyday activities

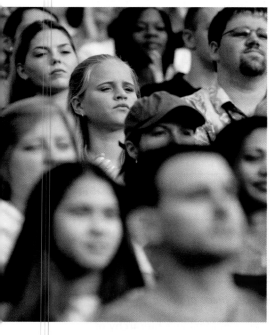

Anyone can be affected by a mental disorder.

I t is just after noon, and Lisa is still in bed. She doesn't see any point in getting up. She doesn't want to do anything. She has felt this way for days. She doesn't even want to be around her friends. She feels that anything she does is useless.

What Are Mental Disorders?

In the last section, you learned that mental health is being able to meet the daily challenges of life, having high self-esteem, and developing healthy relationships. Sometimes, however, people are not mentally healthy. They may suffer from a mental disorder. A **mental disorder** is an illness that affects a person's thoughts, emotions, and behaviors. Those who suffer from a mental disorder may not be able to have fun. They may not feel good about themselves or may have a difficult time developing intimate relationships. They may have difficulty dealing with everyday routines. Many homeless people suffer from a mental disorder.

Lisa is an example of someone experiencing a mental disorder. She feels hopeless and doesn't have the energy to do regular activities or build relationships.

Mental Disorders Are Often Misunderstood Unfortunately, many people who have a mental disorder don't get help because they don't understand mental disorders. Some people are afraid of mental disorders or the people who have the disorders. Identifying and understanding different kinds of mental disorders can help prevent the fear associated with the disorder. Most of these mental disorders are treatable.

To understand mental disorders, you need to learn about their symptoms. A **symptom** is a change that a person notices in his or her body or mind and that is caused by a disease or disorder. For example, Lisa's symptoms were hopelessness and low energy.

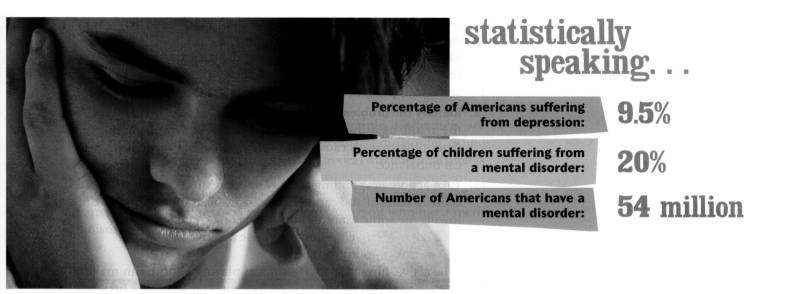

statistically speaking. . .

Percentage of Americans suffering from depression:	9.5%
Percentage of children suffering from a mental disorder:	20%
Number of Americans that have a mental disorder:	54 million

Types of Mental Disorders

There are many types of mental disorders, and they have a variety of symptoms. If you experience any of the symptoms listed below, talk to a trusted adult. However, only licensed professionals can diagnose a mental disorder.

- ▶ too much or too little sleep
- ▶ feeling of extreme sadness
- ▶ unexplained mood changes
- ▶ drug or alcohol abuse
- ▶ inability to concentrate
- ▶ extreme anxiety or irrational fear
- ▶ personality changes
- ▶ false perceptions of reality

Several disorders are common and require some additional description. These disorders are depression, attention-deficit/hyperactivity disorder, and anxiety disorders.

Depression   Everyone feels sad or down at times. However, sadness and hopelessness that keep a person from carrying out everyday activities is called **depression.** Depression, also known as major depressive disorder, is a serious disorder that if left untreated can lead a person to consider suicide. Some of the symptoms of depression are listed below.

- ▶ lack of energy
- ▶ withdrawal from people
- ▶ loss of appetite or overeating
- ▶ too much or too little sleep
- ▶ feelings of helplessness and hopelessness

Experiencing one or more of these symptoms from time to time is not uncommon. However, if you experience several of these symptoms for several days, you should seek professional help.

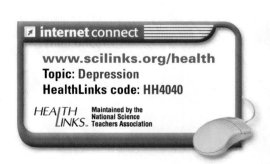

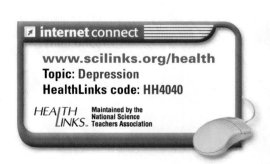**internet** connect

www.scilinks.org/health
Topic: Depression
HealthLinks code: HH4040

HEALTH LINKS Maintained by the National Science Teachers Association

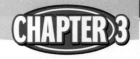

CHAPTER 3

Review

Using Key Terms

aggressive (56)	**mental health** (61)
assertive (56)	**mental disorder** (68)
defense mechanism (66)	**passive** (56)
emotion (63)	**self-actualization** (62)
empathy (58)	**self-concept** (52)
integrity (54)	**self-esteem** (50)
depression (69)	**symptom** (68)

1. For each definition below, choose the key term that best matches the definition.
  a. the ability to understand another person's feelings, behaviors, and attitudes
  b. the achievement of the best that a person can be
  c. a change that a person notices in his or her body or mind and that is caused by a disease or disorder
  d. the characteristic of doing what one knows is right
  e. not offering opposition when challenged or acted upon
  f. an illness that affects a person's thoughts, emotions, and behaviors
  g. a sadness and hopelessness that keeps a person from carrying out everyday activities
  h. an unconscious behavior used to avoid experiencing unpleasant emotions

2. Explain the relationship between the key terms in each of the following pairs.
  a. *aggressive* and *assertive*
  b. *self-concept* and *self-esteem*
  c. *emotion* and *mental health*

Understanding Key Ideas

Section 1

3. Describe how you can show respect for yourself.

4. List the benefits of high self-esteem.

5. Describe how self-esteem develops.

6. Explain how accepting yourself can improve your self-esteem.

Section 2

7. Which of the following is *not* a reason why communication is important?
  a. builds healthy relationships
  b. leads to unclear messages
  c. lets you express yourself
  d. prevents misunderstandings

8. Which of the following statements is *not* an example of assertive communication?
  a. I don't want to talk to you ever again!
  b. I have to go because I'm running late.
  c. Don't yell at me.
  d. I don't want to see that movie.

9. Describe how to be an active listener.

10. List three examples of body language.

11. **CRITICAL THINKING** Describe a situation in which you can use "I" messages. **LIFE SKILL**

Section 3

12. Describe characteristics of positive mental and emotional health.

13. State the stage of Maslow's hierarchy of needs that requires food.

14. How can you learn to express your emotions in a positive way?

15. Which defense mechanism is being used when someone refuses to accept reality?

16. **CRITICAL THINKING** Describe a positive strategy for managing your anger. **LIFE SKILL**

Section 4

17. List three characteristics of mental disorders.

18. Which of the following symptoms is *not* a sign of depression?
  a. lack of energy   **c.** high self-esteem
  b. loss of appetite   **d.** too much sleep

19. Give two examples of disorders that can be treated with medication.

20. **CRITICAL THINKING** List two mental disorders that could be caused by a traumatic experience.

Interpreting Graphics

Study the figure below to answer the questions that follow.

Assertive Communication

Situation	Response
1. Your boyfriend/girl-friend tells you to stop wearing a certain shirt	**1.** _____ _____ _____
2. Your mother throws out your favorite torn jeans.	**2.** You calmly but firmly tell your mother not to throw out your things.
3. Your little sister borrows your tennis racket without asking.	**3.** You yell at your sister and then take her stuff so she can see what it feels like.

21. Which response in the table is an assertive response?

22. Which response in the table is an aggressive response?

23. **CRITICAL THINKING** Fill in an assertive response for the first situation.

Activities

24. Health and You Optimism helps a person reach his or her goals or overcome hard times. Think of a situation that you will face this week and that you have been worried about. Now, write a detailed description of how you want that situation to turn out. **WRITING SKILL**

25. Health and Your Community Ask each classmate to write down one nice thing about each other student in the class. Have your classmates give their anonymous lists to you. Organize the comments according to student names. Hand back the nice comments to the students so that they can read the nice things written about them!

26. Health and You Identify a person you admire for their community involvement. Compare this person's characteristics with characteristics you already possess or hope to acquire. **WRITING SKILL**

Action Plan

27. **LIFE SKILL** **Communicating Effectively** Use the communication skills you learned in this chapter to create a step-by-step action plan to improve communication in one of your relationships.

Standardized Test Prep

Read the passage below, and then answer the questions that follow. **READING SKILL** **WRITING SKILL**

Rina's birthday party on Saturday night was a big hit. Everyone had fun except Jessica and Tessa, who had an argument. Jessica became <u>agitated</u> when Tessa broke Jessica's necklace. Tessa was trying it on when it caught on her watch and the clasp snapped. Jessica called Tessa an idiot and yelled, "Don't ever touch my things again!" Tessa was so offended that she told Jessica she didn't want to be friends with her anymore. Jessica left the party early. Tessa stayed, but she was very quiet and withdrawn.

28. In this passage, the word *agitated* means means
  A worried.
  B angry.
  C jealous.
  D curious.

29. What can you infer from reading this passage?
  E Tessa knows how to manage her anger.
  F Rina will never have another party again.
  G Both Jessica and Tessa were hurt by the argument.
  H none of the above

30. Write a paragraph describing how the situation would have turned out more positively if Jessica and Tessa used the communication skills listed in this chapter.

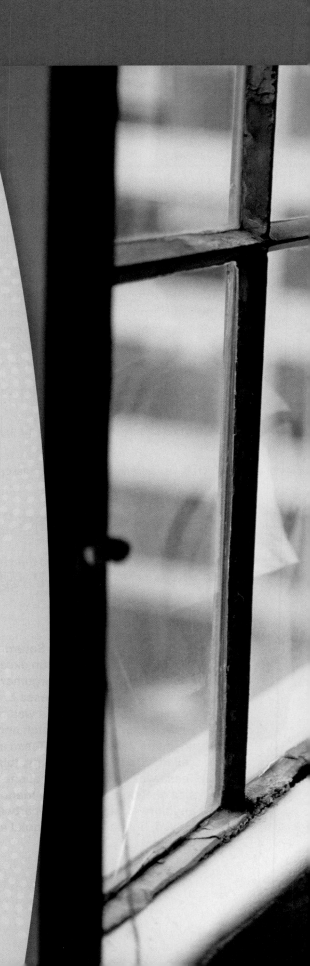

CHAPTER 4

Managing Stress and Coping with Loss

What's Your Health IQ?
BEHAVIOR

Indicate how frequently you engage in each of the following behaviors (1 = never; 2 = occasionally; 3 = most of the time; 4 = all of the time). Total your points, and then turn to p. 642.

1. I exercise and eat well.

2. I make time in my schedule to do the things that I really enjoy.

3. I ask for support from family and friends when I feel too much stress.

4. I have an optimistic view of changes in my life.

5. I do the most important projects I want to accomplish first.

6. I say no if my boss repeatedly asks me to work late on a school night.

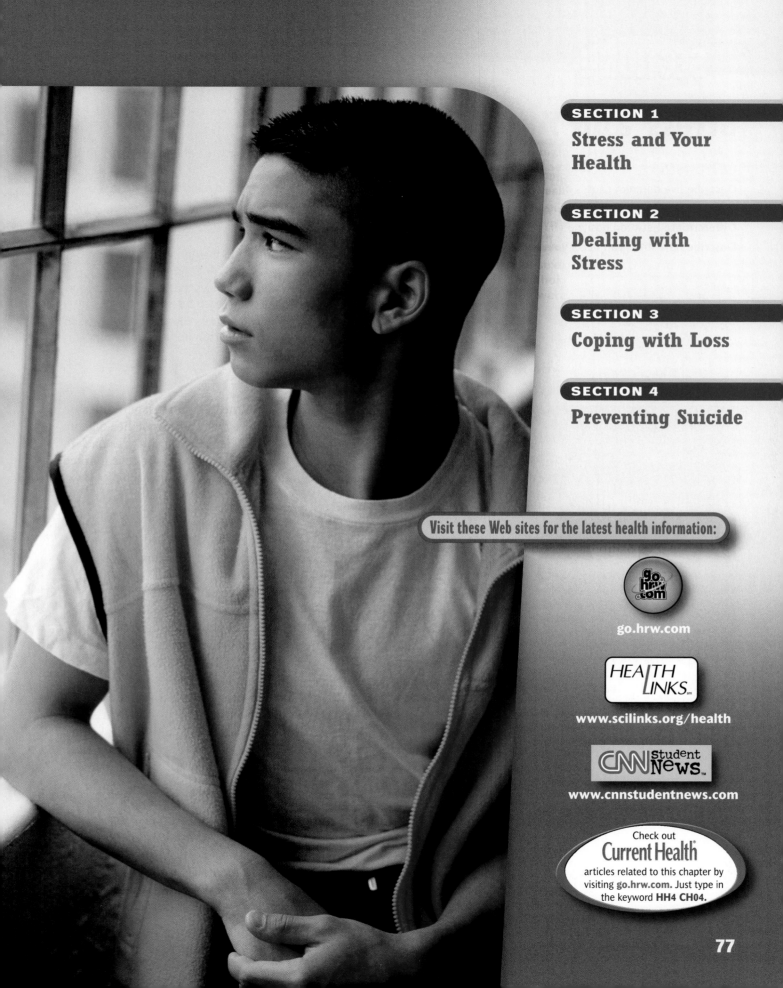

SECTION 1
Stress and Your Health

SECTION 2
Dealing with Stress

SECTION 3
Coping with Loss

SECTION 4
Preventing Suicide

Visit these Web sites for the latest health information:

go.hrw.com

www.scilinks.org/health

www.cnnstudentnews.com

Check out **Current Health** articles related to this chapter by visiting go.hrw.com. Just type in the keyword **HH4 CH04.**

Stress and Your Health

OBJECTIVES

Describe five different causes of stress.
Describe the body's physical response to stress.
Differentiate between positive and negative stress.
Describe how stress can make you sick. **LIFE SKILL**

KEY TERMS

stress the body's and mind's response to a demand

stressor any situation that puts a demand on the body or mind

epinephrine one of the hormones that are released by the body in times of stress

eustress a positive stress that energizes a person and helps a person reach a goal

distress a negative stress that can make a person sick or can keep a person from reaching a goal

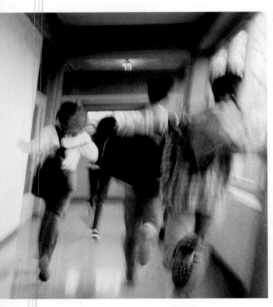

Many people experience stress because they take on too many responsibilities or don't manage time well.

It's 1:05 P.M. Paula is running down the hall and is late for algebra class. Halfway to class, she realizes that she forgot her algebra homework in her locker. She'll get a detention if she goes back to get it and is late to class again. When she gets to class, she is marked late. Paula's head begins to pound with an intense headache.

What Causes Stress?

Do you ever feel stressed? **Stress** is the body's and mind's response to a demand. You may not even be aware that you are under stress until you get a headache, as Paula did.

Stress can be caused by many different situations or events. For example, going out on a date can cause stress and so can taking a test or watching a football game. Stress is caused by stressors. A **stressor** is any situation that puts a demand on the body or mind. There are several different types of stressors.

Environmental Stressors Environmental stressors are conditions or events in your physical environment that cause you stress. For example, pollution, poverty, crowding, noise, and natural disasters are things in your environment that can cause you stress.

Biological Stressors Some stressors are biological. These are conditions that make it difficult for your body to take part in daily activities. For example, having an illness, a disability, or an injury are biological stressors.

Thinking Stressors Any type of mental challenge can cause stress. A good example of this is taking a test. Paula's algebra homework is probably a stressor for her.

Behavioral Stressors Unhealthy behavior, such as not getting enough sleep or exercise, can lead to stress. Using tobacco, alcohol, or drugs also puts stress on your body. Paula was experiencing behavioral stress because she didn't manage her time well.

Life Change Stressors Any major life change, whether positive or negative, can be a cause of stress. For example, death of a loved one, getting married, and other personal events can cause stress. The teen years are a time when you experience many changes and, thus, stress. **Table 1** lists some common life changes that can lead to stress.

ACTIVITY *To measure how much your life has changed, add up the life change units below for the changes that you experienced in the past year. Compare your score with the scale below.*

Table 1 Life Changes That Can Lead to Stress			
Life event	**Life change units**	**Life event**	**Life change units**
Experiencing the death of a parent	▶ 119	Having more arguments with parents	▶ 51
Experiencing the death of a brother or sister	▶ 102	Getting married	▶ 50
Going through your parents' divorce	▶ 98	Failing a grade in school	▶ 42
Having a serious illness	▶ 77	Seeing an increase in arguments between parents	▶ 40
Having a parent go to jail	▶ 75	Beginning or ending school	▶ 38
Experiencing the death of a close friend	▶ 70	Breaking up with a boyfriend or girlfriend	▶ 37
Being pregnant	▶ 66	Making an outstanding achievment	▶ 36
Getting a new job	▶ 62	Moving to a new school district	▶ 35
Gaining a new family member	▶ 57	Being suspended from school	▶ 29
Experiencing a significant change in family's financial status	▶ 56	Having trouble with a teacher	▶ 28
Experiencing the serious illness of a parent	▶ 56	Change in sleeping habits	▶ 26
Being excluded from a social circle	▶ 53	Going on vacation	▶ 25
		Getting a traffic ticket	▶ 22

Your Life Change Score: If your score is less than 100, your life has changed little. If your score is between 100 and 200, you have experienced moderate change. If your score is more than 200, your life has changed significantly.

Adapted from Mark A. Miller and Richard H. Rahe, "Life Changes Scaling for the 1990s," *Journal of Psychosomatic Research* 43 (1997).

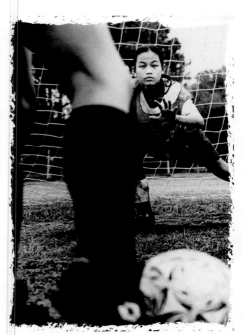

The physical changes in response to stress prepare the body to run away or stay and fight.

HEALTH Handbook For more information about the endocrine system, see the Express Lesson on p. 545.

Physical Response to Stress

Imagine that you are riding your bike and you suddenly find yourself in the path of a fast-moving car. You feel a sudden burst of energy that allows you to get out of the way of the car. Now imagine that you are a goalie in a soccer game. The ball has been kicked by an opposing team player and it's headed straight to the goal. Your heart starts to beat faster as you jump for the ball and make the block.

In both of these situations, your body responded to a stressful situation, but in a different way. When the car was in the path of your bike, the response was to move away, or "take flight." When the soccer ball was coming to the goal, the response was to confront the situation, or "fight." The physical changes that prepare your body to respond quickly and appropriately to stressors is called the *fight-or-flight response.*

The Fight-or-Flight Response During the fight-or-flight response, your body provides you with the energy, reflexes, and strength you may need to respond to the stressor. As part of the fight-or-flight response, your body releases epinephrine. **Epinephrine** (EP uh NEF rin), formally called *adrenaline*, is one of the hormones that are released by the body in times of stress. Epinephrine prepares the body for quick action by triggering the changes listed below.

▶ Your breathing speeds up, which helps get more oxygen throughout your body.
▶ Your heart beats faster, which increases the flow of blood to carry more oxygen to your muscles.
▶ Your muscles tense up, which prepares you to move quickly.
▶ The pupils of your eyes get wider, which allows extra light for more sensitive vision.
▶ Your digestion stops, since this is an unnecessary activity during an emergency.
▶ Blood sugar increases to provide more fuel for fighting or running.

Emotional and Behavioral Response to Stress

The way you respond to a stress emotionally and behaviorally depends on whether you consider the stress to be positive or negative, as shown in **Figure 1.**

Positive Stress Let's say you have to give a speech in front of your class. If you choose to consider this in a positive way, this type of stress can motivate you to do your best. Positive stress can help you respond well in a stressful situation. A positive stress that energizes one and helps one reach a goal is called **eustress.** Eustress will make you feel alert and lively. You will appear confident and in control.

A person who presents speeches when experiencing eustress often attracts and holds the attention of the audience. The words roll off the speaker's tongue. One point flows into the others, and the speaker rarely forgets what to say next.

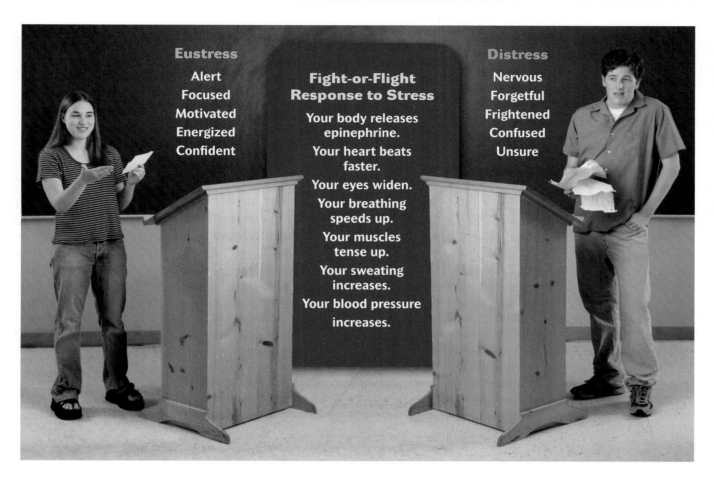

Eustress
Alert
Focused
Motivated
Energized
Confident

Fight-or-Flight Response to Stress
Your body releases epinephrine.
Your heart beats faster.
Your eyes widen.
Your breathing speeds up.
Your muscles tense up.
Your sweating increases.
Your blood pressure increases.

Distress
Nervous
Forgetful
Frightened
Confused
Unsure

Negative Stress If you choose to consider giving a speech to be a negative stress, you may experience distress. **Distress** is negative stress that can make a person sick or keep a person from reaching a goal. Distress can keep you from doing your best, no matter how capable you are.

People who attempt to give a speech while experiencing distress may forget the points they want to make. They may have practiced the speech for days, but when they stand up in front of a room full of people, they lose their concentration. Their words don't flow well. Their voice may sound too soft and shaky, revealing a lack of confidence. The audience may become bored or confused.

Try to Make Stress Positive Obviously, it is better to approach stressful situations as positive and not negative. However, it is not always easy to control your response to a stressor. One way you can help yourself experience eustress is to be optimistic about dealing with a stressor. Instead of thinking, I can't do this, think, What can I do to accomplish this? Concentrate only on what you can control in the situation. Let go of what you cannot control. Do what you can to build confidence that you can succeed in the situation. If you set your mind to it and prepare to meet the challenge, you will find yourself approaching situations in a positive way!

Figure 1

Everybody experiences the same physical responses to stress—the fight-or-flight response. But each person's emotional and behavioral response differs depending on whether he or she views the stress as positive (eustress) or negative (distress).

ACTIVITY *Which student do you think has a better chance at winning the debate? Explain your answer.*

Stress-Related Diseases and Disorders

▶ **Tension headache**
▶ **Cold and flu**
▶ **Asthma**
▶ **Migraine headache**
▶ **Backache**
▶ **Temporomandibular joint dysfunction (TMJ)**
▶ **Heart disease**
▶ **Stroke**
▶ **High blood pressure**
▶ **Chronic fatigue**
▶ **Ulcer**
▶ **Anxiety disorder**
▶ **Insomnia**
▶ **Depression**

Long-Term Stress Can Make You Sick

If your body experiences stress continuously over a long period of time, you increase your risk for a wide range of stress-related diseases. For example, stress causes the muscles in your neck and head to tense, which can cause headaches. Long-term stress can cause changes in your body that can lead to a heart attack. Long-term stress can also weaken your immune system, the system of your body that defends against infections. As a result, you are more likely to suffer from infections, such as colds.

The *general adaptation syndrome* is a model that describes the relationship between stress and disease. Learning the stages will help you understand how stress can affect your health. There are three stages in the model:

1. **Alarm stage** In the alarm stage, the body and mind become alert. This stage includes the events brought on by the flight-or-flight response. All of your body's efforts go into responding to the demand. A person in this stage may experience headaches, stomachaches, difficulty sleeping, and anxiety.

2. **Resistance stage** If the stress continues, your body becomes more resistant to disease and injury than normal. You can cope with added stress, but only for a limited time.

3. **Exhaustion stage** In this stage, your body cannot take the resistance to the stressor any longer, especially if several stressors occur in a row. You become exhausted, not in the normal sense like after a long, busy day, but in a more serious way. Organs such as your heart may suffer, and your immune system can no longer fight illness.

By learning to manage stress, you can protect yourself from many illnesses and can enjoy a healthier life.

SECTION 1

REVIEW *Answer the following questions on a separate piece of paper.*

Using Key Terms

1. **Compare** the terms *stress* and *stressor*.
2. **Identify** the term for "a positive stress that energizes a person and helps a person reach a goal."

Understanding Key Ideas

3. **List** five different causes of stress.
4. **Identify** which of the following is *not* a part of the fight-or-flight response.
   a. heart rate speeds up   c. muscles tense
   b. increased sweating   d. digestion occurs

5. **Identify** a hormone that is released during the fight-or-flight response.
6. **Compare** positive and negative stress.
7. **LIFE SKILL** **Assessing Your Health** Using the stages of the general adaptation syndrome, describe how stress can make you sick.

Critical Thinking

8. **LIFE SKILL** **Practicing Wellness** Describe how two stressors led you to experience eustress.
9. What do you think would be the consequences of not having a fight-or-flight response?

Dealing with Stress

OBJECTIVES

Describe how you can take care of yourself to avoid stress-related illnesses.

Describe two relaxation techniques.

List eight skills or resources for building resiliency.

Evaluate the effect of a positive attitude on stress reduction.

List three ways that you can manage your time more efficiently. **LIFE SKILL**

KEY TERMS

resiliency the ability to recover from illness, hardship, and other stressors

asset a skill or resource that can help a person reach a goal

prioritize to arrange items in order of importance

Anthony has a final exam tomorrow. He told his friend Ricardo that he couldn't help him fix his bike because he needed to study for a couple of hours. It's now 10 P.M. Anthony has studied for 3 hours and is now listening to music to relax. He plans to go to bed when the CD finishes so that he can get a good night's sleep.

Take Care of Yourself

Stressful events will occur throughout your life. At this time, you may be experiencing stressors such as tests and peer pressure. When you get older, your stressors may be managing money or raising children. Whatever stressors you experience, learning to manage them will help you remain healthy throughout your life.

In the last section, you learned how your body responds to stress. If stress continues over time, stress-related illnesses can develop. People who are in better physical health are more likely than others to resist developing an illness. An important way to defend yourself from stress-related illness is to take care of yourself! Exercising regularly, getting enough rest, and eating right will help you prevent some of the negative consequences of stress.

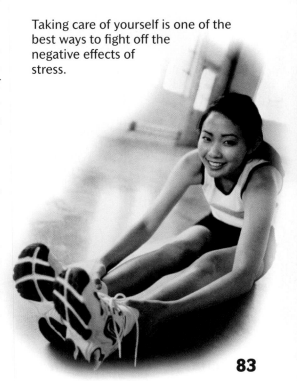

Taking care of yourself is one of the best ways to fight off the negative effects of stress.

Exercise Regularly Exercise will not only keep you physically fit, but it will also relieve tension. *Tension* is a physical effect of stress marked by straining of muscles. During the fight-or-flight response, the body is tensed and ready for a great amount of physical activity. However, many stressors, such as taking a test, don't require much physical activity. Keeping the body in a heightened state of alertness when you don't need to run or fight stresses your heart, muscles, and immune system. Health problems such as tension headaches and heart disease can result from such long-term stress. Exercise can relieve this tension in a healthy way.

Get Enough Rest You should get at least 9 hours of sleep every night. Not getting enough sleep can lead to exhaustion, which can cause illness. Also, if you haven't slept enough, you are less alert and less capable of dealing with a stressor. For example, Anthony knows that if he has a good night's sleep, his mind will be prepared and alert for the exam.

Eat Right Eating nutritious foods gives you the vitamins, minerals, and energy you need to deal with everyday demands. You need vitamins and minerals for your immune system to function properly. The better shape your immune system is in, the better it can defend you from stress related illnesses.

Learn to Relax

During the response to stress, you build up a lot of tension. At the same time, energy is pulled away from body systems that need the energy to fight sickness. Using relaxation techniques can help you relieve tension and reserve energy for fighting illness. The following are a couple of relaxation techniques you can try.

Breathing Exercises One relaxation technique is deep breathing. It requires completely filling the lungs with air instead of taking shallow breaths. Deep breathing brings more oxygen to all parts of your body. More oxygen helps muscles and organs function more effectively. More oxygen also helps keep your brain alert and focused. Deep breathing also produces a calming effect that helps relax you. When you practice deep breathing, your heart rate slows down and your blood pressure drops.

To practice deep breathing, find a comfortable place to sit. Close your eyes, and concentrate only on your breathing. Inhale slowly until your lungs cannot hold any more air. Then, exhale slowly. Repeat this process for at least 15 minutes.

Tension-Releasing Exercises When you are under stress, it's common to hold the tension in your muscles. You may not even notice the tension in your muscles until they start to ache.

To release tension, start by tensing the muscles in one part of your body, such as your shoulders. Notice how it feels to have those muscles tensed. Now, relax those muscles. Notice how those muscles feel relaxed. You can then move to another muscle group and repeat the tensing and relaxing until your entire body is relaxed.

Deep breathing and tension-releasing exercises are only two ways for you to relax. You can put your body at ease in many other ways. For example, Anthony relaxes by listening to music. Someone else may relax by reading a book. You may already have your own special technique. Keep in mind that although relaxation techniques can help you manage the symptoms of stress, this should not stop you from dealing with the stressor directly.

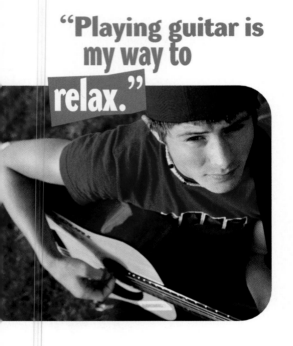

"Playing guitar is my way to relax."

Table 2	Eight Assets for Building Resiliency	
Asset	**Description**	**Example**
Support	▶ having family, friends, and others to help you	▶ You talk to the school counselor about a problem.
Empowerment	▶ feeling as if you are a valuable member of your community and family	▶ You volunteer to start a drug-free campaign at school.
Boundaries	▶ having a clear set of rules and consequences for school, family, and relationships	▶ You know that if another teen bullies you at school, a teacher will speak with that teen.
Productive use of time	▶ choosing creative and productive activities	▶ You join a school club instead of playing video games after school.
Commitment to learning	▶ understanding the value of schoolwork	▶ You spend time every day working on homework assignments.
Positive values	▶ having values that include caring, integrity, honesty, self-responsibility, equality, and justice	▶ You support a friend who tells the truth even though doing so may get him or her in trouble.
Social skills	▶ communicating effectively, respecting others, and avoiding peer pressure	▶ You talk out a disagreement instead of yelling.
Positive identity	▶ having high self-esteem, having a sense of control, and feeling as if you have a purpose	▶ You use positive self-talk to prepare yourself for a speech.

Source: Adapted from Benson, Peter L., Ph.D., Espeland, Pamela, and Galbraith, Judy, M. A., *What Teens Need to Succeed*.

ACTIVITY *Provide an additional example of how you can strengthen each asset.*

Build Resiliency

The ability to recover from illness, hardship, and other stressors is called **resiliency.** Resilient people continue to be optimistic when life gets tough. They seem to struggle less and succeed more. They accomplish difficult tasks and make other people ask, "How did they do that?"

Many resilient people get their strength from their assets. An **asset** is a skill or resource that can help you reach a goal. For example, support is an asset. Having people to support you can get you through some hard times. You don't have to have a big family or be popular to have a strong support system. Resilient people build strong support systems by asking for help. They ask for support from their family, friends, teachers, school counselors, neighbors, community leaders, and religious leaders.

You have the power to strengthen these assets. **Table 2** lists eight assets and provides examples of how each asset can work for you. For example, if you want to strengthen the asset entitled "positive identity," you can use the skills such as positive self-talk to improve your self-esteem. The stronger you make your assets, the stronger you will feel, and the healthier you will be.

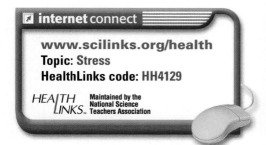

internet connect

www.scilinks.org/health
Topic: Stress
HealthLinks code: HH4129

HEALTH LINKS. Maintained by the National Science Teachers Association

Change Your Attitude

You have control over the number of stressors in your life. Because stress is caused by how you perceive a new or potentially threatening situation, you can choose to see the situation as a challenge instead of as a problem. Having a positive attitude about the outcome of potentially stressful events can eliminate a lot of stress. If you approach the situation with a positive attitude, you won't feel as nervous. If you don't feel so nervous, a positive consequence is more likely to happen.

Use Positive Self-Talk Say or think positive things to yourself. For example, let's say you are invited to go on a date to go see a movie. You are nervous about the date because you really like the person that invited you on the date. You can think to yourself, I must be fun and desirable if this person wants to go out with me. You can also predict a realistic, positive outcome. You can imagine that you and your date have a great time and make plans to meet again.

LIFE SKILL
Activity

Coping

Positive Attitude

Approaching the stressors in your life with a positive attitude will not only help you produce additional positive effects, but it will also relieve a lot of tension. How can you have a positive attitude about the stressors in your life?

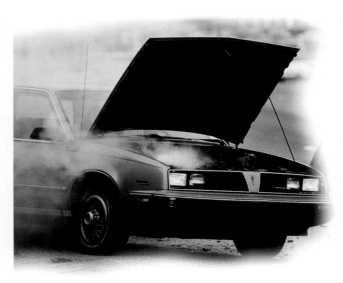

1 List five stressors. If you would like to, you can list your own stressors.

2 Describe how you could have a positive emotional response to each stressor.

3 Describe how you could have a positive physical response to each stressor.

4 Describe a positive outcome to each stressor.

LIFE SKILL Practicing Wellness

1. Predict how this activity will affect your actual responses to these stressors.

2. Describe how you felt when you finished step 4. Did you see the stressors more optimistically?

Be Confident About Yourself The better you feel about yourself, the more positive your perception of a situation will be. The more positive your perception is, the more positive your response and the consequences will be! To build your self-confidence, you can remember similar challenges you have met successfully.

Don't Worry About Things Out of Your Control Accept the things you can't change, and then make the best out of the situation. Put your energy only into things you can control.

Manage Your Time

One of the most common stressors that people experience is the feeling of not having enough time. Many people feel overwhelmed by the pace of their lives. However, by organizing your time, you can feel in control of your life. Having a sense of control will minimize the effects of stress.

Many of us get into trouble when we take on more things to do than we have time for. Helene is overwhelmed because today she has to go to swim practice, study for a French test, do her history homework, go to dance rehearsal, cover the late shift at work, and help prepare dinner.

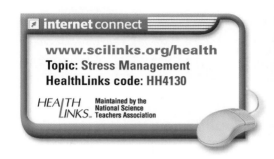

internet connect

www.scilinks.org/health
Topic: Stress Management
HealthLinks code: HH4130

HEALTH LINKS Maintained by the National Science Teachers Association

List and Prioritize Your Projects The first step in managing your time is to make a list of your projects and to prioritize your goals. To **prioritize** is to arrange items in order of importance. You may not be able to do everything on your list. However, if you put the most important items first, you can be sure to get them done. Prioritizing also helps you decide which activities can be eliminated.

Helene organized her priorities as follows: (1) French test, (2) swim practice, and (3) history homework. Helene was able to eliminate three activities. She didn't have to prepare dinner because she traded nights with her sister. She arranged to have a co-worker cover her shift at work. Finally, she went to dance practice as a way to relieve stress through exercise and having fun.

Know and Set Your Limits One major reason that some people have hectic schedules is that they don't know their limits when they commit to projects. For example, Helene has taken on much more than she can handle. Signing up for dance, swimming, and a part-time job is too much for anybody. If Helene does not drop some of her responsibilities, her health will begin to suffer.

Helene can also manage her time by learning to say no. Helene shouldn't have promised her boss that she would work. Some people have a hard time saying no. They are afraid people will think that they don't care. However, saying no sometimes is a healthy way of taking care of yourself.

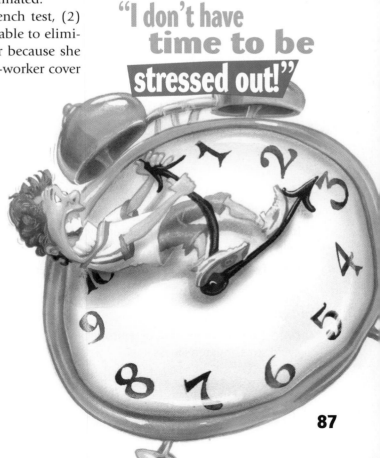

"I don't have time to be stressed out!"

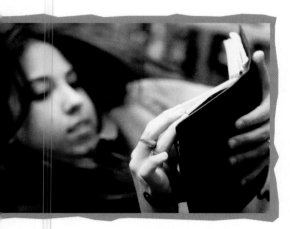

Make a Schedule Once you have prioritized your projects and have decided what you can accomplish, you can make a schedule. Some people use calendars or planners to keep track of their schedule. But all you really need is a pen and a notebook. The following points will help you make your schedule.

▶ **Enter your priorities first.** When setting aside time for projects, start with the projects at the top of your list to make sure that you give them the time needed. Schedule your most difficult tasks for the hours when you are most productive. Consider scheduling your least favorite tasks first.

▶ **Be realistic.** Set realistic goals. Don't cram your day with more activities than you can possibly do. Make sure you plan enough time for each activity. Break up long-term goals into short-term goals. For example, if you have a big research paper to turn in, break the paper down into manageable parts. Schedule one day to gather your references, a second day to write the outline of your paper, and so on. Your steady progress will motivate you to continue.

▶ **Prepare for problems.** Life is never perfect. Therefore, it helps to think about possible problems ahead of time. You may want to give yourself a little more time in your schedule, just in case.

▶ **Make time to relax.** Don't forget to fit in time to have fun or to do the things you really enjoy. Remember that relaxing is important to your health.

▶ **Do it.** Stop thinking about what you have to do and just do it. Sometimes you can get overwhelmed by just thinking of all of the things you have to do. Tackle each task one at a time.

If you practice the stress management techniques you learned in this chapter, you can begin to control the stress in your life. Not only will you protect your health, you will have more time to enjoy your life!

Five Tips for Managing Your Time

1 Prioritize your goals.

2 Learn to say no.

3 Keep a schedule.

4 Don't overload yourself.

5 Plan for fun activities.

SECTION 2

REVIEW *Answer the following questions on a separate piece of paper.*

Using Key Terms

1. **Define** the term *resiliency*.

2. **Identify** the term for "a skill or resource that can help a person reach a goal."

3. **Identify** the term for "to arrange items in order of importance."

Understanding Key Ideas

4. **Describe** how taking care of yourself can help you avoid stress-related illness.

5. **Describe** two techniques you can use to relax.

6. **Name** eight assets for building resiliency.

7. **Describe** how a positive attitude can change your response to stress.

8. **LIFE SKILL** Practicing Wellness Describe three ways to manage your time more efficiently.

Critical Thinking

9. Why do you think the phrase "burned out" is used to describe a person who has been under a lot of stress?

Coping with Loss

OBJECTIVES

Describe the effects of loss.

Name the stages of the grieving process.

Describe how funerals, wakes, and memorial services help people cope with the loss of a loved one.

Propose three ways you can cope with the loss of a loved one. **LIFE SKILL**

> **KEY TERMS**
>
> **grieve** to express deep sadness because of a loss
>
> **wake** a ceremony to view or watch over the deceased person before the funeral
>
> **funeral** a ceremony in which a deceased person is buried or cremated
>
> **memorial service** a ceremony to remember the deceased person

Fidencia cannot imagine life without Ben. She can't believe her parents are making her move away from him. She was so angry with them that she wanted to scream. Today is the day that they move. She feels as if she is losing a part of herself.

Effects of Loss

There are many forms of loss. Some examples of loss are the death of a family member, the divorce of one's parents, the death of a pet, a breakup with a boyfriend or girlfriend, and a move away from your home.

All forms of loss can cause you to experience a range of emotions, from sadness to anger to numbness. These feelings are normal and common reactions to loss. You may not be prepared for how intense your emotions may be or how suddenly your moods may change. You may even begin to doubt your mental stability. It is important to know that these feelings are healthy and normal and will help you cope with your loss. However, if the feelings don't pass over time, you should seek the help of a parent or trusted adult.

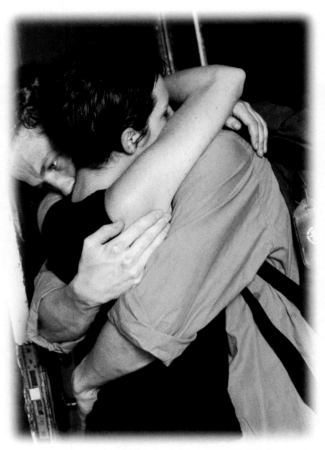

Moving away from someone you care deeply for is an example of a loss that can cause stress.

Loss Can Cause Stress When you experience loss, you can feel the physical and emotional effects of stress. For example, after a loss, you may develop tension headaches or an increase in blood pressure. You may also feel irritable and confused. Just like other stressors, the stress caused by a loss needs to be managed or it can lead to a stress-related illness. The tension-relieving skills that you learned in the last section can keep you healthy. The last thing you need through a trying time is to have a sickness weigh you down.

The Grieving Process

To express deep sadness because of a loss is to **grieve.** Allowing yourself to grieve is important because grieving helps you heal from the pain of a loss.

When grieving, you may feel agitated or angry. You may find concentrating, eating, or sleeping difficult. You might even feel guilty. For example, you may wish you had told a loved one that died how you felt about him or her. This period of unpredictable emotions may turn to short periods of sadness, silence, and withdrawal from family and friends. During this time, you may be prone to sudden outbursts of tears that are triggered by reminders and memories of this person. Over time, the pain, sadness, and depression will start to lessen. You will begin to see your life in a more positive light again.

This journey to recovery is called the *grieving process.* There are five stages of the grieving process. Not everyone goes through all of the stages or goes through the stages in the same order. However, understanding these stages and the importance of expressing feelings of grief will help you recover from a loss.

Stages of Grief

▶ **DENIAL**
"This can't be happening to me!"

▶ **ANGER**
"Why me? It's not fair."

▶ **BARGAINING**
"I'd do anything to have him back."

▶ **DEPRESSION**
"There is no hope. I'm so sad. I just want to be alone."

▶ **ACCEPTANCE**
"It's going to be OK."

The Five Stages of the Grieving Process Although you may never completely overcome the feelings of loss, the grieving process can help you accept the loss. Try to move forward through the stages. If you feel stuck in a stage, ask your parents or a trusted adult for help.

1. **Denial** The first reaction you may face when dealing with a loss is denial. In denial, the person refuses to believe the loss occurred. Denial can act as a buffer to give you a chance to think about the news. However, you must eventually reach the other stages in order to heal.

2. **Anger** Experiencing anger or even rage is normal when you face a loss. You may even try to blame yourself or others for the loss. Be careful about accusing others, and use anger management skills.

3. **Bargaining** Bargaining is the final attempt at avoiding what is true. For example, some people make promises to change if the person or thing they lost is returned to them.

4. **Depression** Sadness is a natural and important emotion to express when you experience loss. However, if feeling very sad keeps you from daily activities for more than a few days, ask a parent or a trusted adult for help.

5. **Acceptance** During this stage, you begin to learn how to live with a loss. The loss continues to be painful, yet you know you will get through it and that life will go on.

Funerals, Wakes, and Memorial Services

Different types of ceremonies may take place after the death of a loved one. These ceremonies honor the person who has passed away. They also help the family and friends of the loved one to get through the grieving process. Different cultures and religions have different ceremonies for handling grief. However, most people use some form of service to help them grieve.

A **wake** is a ceremony that is held to allow family and friends to view or watch over the deceased person before the funeral. Viewing the body of the deceased can help family and friends accept the death. A wake also gives family members and friends an opportunity to come together and to support each other emotionally. For example, in Ireland, the wake is commonly held in the home of the deceased's family.

A **funeral** is a ceremony in which a deceased person is buried or cremated. To *cremate* means to burn the body by intense heat. During a funeral, the death is formally acknowledged. The funeral honors the deceased and offers family and friends the opportunity to pay tribute to the loved one.

A **memorial service** is a ceremony to remember the deceased person. A memorial service provides the same opportunity to mourn the loss of a loved one that funerals and wakes do. However, memorial services can take place long after the death of the loved one. These services may also present a memorial or structure, such as the Vietnam War Memorial, to remember and honor the deceased.

The Vietnam Veterans Memorial Wall is dedicated to honoring those who died in the Vietnam War. Visiting the memorial has helped many people cope with the loss of a loved one who died in the war.

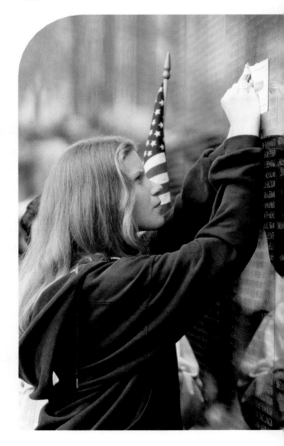

You have mixed feelings about seeing Nate at school this morning. He has just lost his brother, and you want to show your support. However, you and your friends feel awkward. You are not sure how to relate to Nate after his tragic loss.

Write on a separate piece of paper how you might give your friend Nate support. Remember to use the decision-making steps.

Give thought to the problem.

Review your choices.

Evaluate the consequences of each choice.

Assess and choose the best choice.

Think it over afterward.

Help for Dealing with a Loss

There are several things you can do to help yourself as you cope with a loss.

▶ Get plenty of rest and relaxation, but try to stick to any routines you kept before the loss.

▶ Share memories and thoughts about the deceased.

▶ Express your feelings by crying or by writing in a journal.

▶ If the loss was unintentional, do not blame yourself or others. Blaming only creates a way of avoiding the truth about the loss.

Helping Others   Sometimes people feel uncomfortable in the presence of a person who has experienced a loss. Small, kind actions such as the touch of a hand on a shoulder is a powerful way to show your support. There are other ways you can help a friend cope with a loss.

▶ Show your support through simple actions, such as offering to run errands or cook a meal.

▶ Let the person know that you are there for him or her, and allow the person to talk about his or her thoughts and feelings.

▶ Tell the person that you have faith that he or she is strong and will learn to live with this loss.

▶ If the person seems depressed, avoids family and friends, or doesn't seem to be making any progress, tell a trusted adult.

Your support can help your friend accept his or her loss. He or she will appreciate your help.

SECTION 3

REVIEW   *Answer the following questions on a separate piece of paper.*

Using Key Terms

1. **Define** the term *grieve*.

2. **Identify** the term for "a ceremony to view or watch over the deceased person before the funeral."

3. **Identify** the term for "a ceremony to remember the deceased person."

Understanding Key Ideas

4. **Describe** the effects of loss.

5. **Identify** which of the following is *not* a stage of the grieving process.
   a. death
   b. acceptance
   c. bargaining
   d. anger

6. **Identify** in which of the following stages you might say, "Why me?"
   a. acceptance
   b. bargaining
   c. anger
   d. depression

7. **Compare** how funerals, wakes, and memorial services help people grieve.

8. **LIFE SKILL Coping** Describe three ways that you can help someone cope with a loss.

Critical Thinking

9. Why should a person not be afraid to show emotion, such as crying, when faced with a loss?

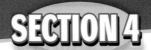

Preventing Suicide

OBJECTIVES

List four facts about suicide.

Describe why teens should be concerned about suicide.

State seven warning signs of suicidal behavior.

Describe steps that you can take to help a friend who has talked about suicide. **LIFE SKILL**

Kim had six types of pills in a variety of colors in front of her. She didn't know what half of them were for. It didn't matter. Nothing mattered. Or did it? Kim decided to make one last phone call.

Facts About Suicide

Suicide is the act of intentionally taking one's own life. It is shocking to think that someone would want to die. The truth is that most people who attempt suicide don't really want to die. They feel helpless about how to end their emotional pain. However, suicide is never the solution. There are other ways to deal with emotional suffering. Asking someone for help is the first step in making yourself feel better.

Suicide is an uncomfortable topic for many people. Because so many people avoid the subject, many myths about it have arisen. Knowing the following truths about suicide can put an end to the myths and can help prevent suicide.

▶ Many people who have considered suicide considered it only for a brief period in their life.

▶ Most people who have attempted suicide and failed are usually grateful to be alive.

▶ Suicide does not happen without warning. People who have attempted suicide often asked for help in an indirect way. All talk of suicide should be taken seriously.

▶ The use of drugs or alcohol can put people at risk of acting on suicidal thoughts because their judgment is impaired.

Suicide is a serious issue for all teens. Any talk or mention of suicide by a friend should not be taken lightly. If you think a friend is in trouble, talk with your friend. More important, tell a parent or trusted adult about your friend's intentions right away.

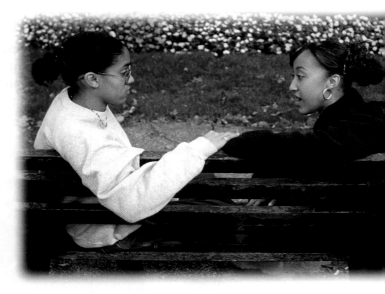

Talking to someone is one of the best things you can do when you feel hopeless or sad.

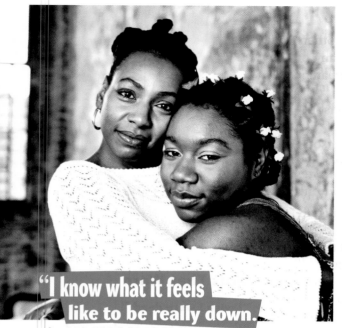

"I know what it feels like to be really down. I'm glad I talked with someone."

Giving and Getting Help

When you or someone you know is thinking of suicide, do not ignore the problem. Thoughts of suicide are a cry for help. You should act immediately by talking with a friend, parent, or trusted adult. The following are things that you can do if a friend has talked about suicide.

▶ **Take all talk of suicide seriously.** If your friend mentions suicide, tell a trusted adult even if you think your friend is joking.

▶ **Tell your friend that suicide is not the answer.** Emphasize to your friend that suicide is not the answer to temporary problems. Remind your friend of all the things that would be missed if he or she were no longer alive. Suggest that your friend talk to a trusted adult.

▶ **Change negative thoughts into positive thoughts.** Help your friend use positive self-talk to look at things with a different perspective.

▶ **Don't keep a secret.** Do not agree to keep a secret if your friend asks you not to tell anyone that he or she is thinking of suicide. This is a serious situation that requires the help of a trusted adult.

Anyone who is suicidal needs professional help and cannot fix the problem by himself or herself. It is very important that you get help for a friend who is suicidal. Likewise, if you are feeling depressed, don't delay asking a trusted adult for help.

Most cities have a variety of health organizations that offer services to people in need. Some of these services are free. A parent or guardian can help you find the right organization. The important thing is to tell someone and to get the help that you or your friend needs.

SECTION 4

REVIEW   *Answer the following questions on a separate piece of paper.*

Using Key Terms

1. **Define** the term *suicide*.

Understanding Key Ideas

2. **Name** four facts about suicide.

3. **Describe** why suicide is an especially serious problem for teens.

4. **Identify** the number that suicide ranks as the cause of death in teens.
   - **a.** first
   - **b.** third
   - **c.** fifth
   - **d.** ninth

5. **State** seven warning signs that someone may be thinking about committing suicide.

6. **Describe** how positive self-talk can help a person who is thinking of suicide.

7. **LIFE SKILL** **Practicing Wellness** Describe four things that you can do if your friend is thinking about suicide.

Critical Thinking

8. **LIFE SKILL** **Practicing Wellness** Describe how you can protect yourself from the risks of suicide during the teen years.

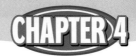

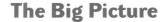

Highlights

Key Terms

The Big Picture

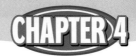

Key Terms

SECTION 1

stress (78)
stressor (78)
epinephrine (80)
eustress (80)
distress (81)

The Big Picture

✔ Stress is your body's and mind's response to a demand. Anything you perceive as threatening can cause stress.

✔ The fight-or-flight response is your body's physical response to help you deal with a stressor.

✔ Eustress is positive stress and can motivate and energize a person to reach a goal. Distress is negative stress and can make a person sick or keep a person from reaching a goal.

✔ If your body is under stress for a long period of time, you may become exhausted and may develop a stress-related illness.

SECTION 2

resiliency (85)
asset (85)
prioritize (87)

✔ Eating right, exercising regularly, and getting enough rest will keep you healthy so that your body can avoid stress-related illnesses.

✔ You can learn to relax by practicing deep breathing exercises and tension-releasing exercises.

✔ Assets are skills or resources that can help a person build resiliency against stressors.

✔ Having a positive attitude about a potentially threatening situation can help relieve stress.

✔ You can manage your time more effectively by listing your projects in order of priority, knowing your limits, and making a schedule.

SECTION 3

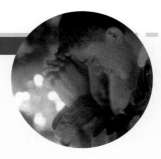

grieve (90)
wake (91)
funeral (91)
memorial service (91)

✔ Loss may cause the same emotional and physical effects that characterize stress.

✔ The stages of the grieving process are denial, anger, bargaining, depression, and acceptance.

✔ Funerals, wakes, and memorial services can help you accept the loss of a loved one and receive emotional support from family and friends.

✔ Sharing memories of the deceased and listening to your friend are a couple of ways you can help a friend cope with a loss.

SECTION 4

suicide (93)

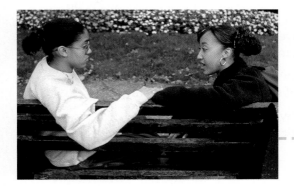

✔ Learning the facts about suicide can prevent the development of myths about suicide and can help prevent suicide.

✔ Teens should be concerned about suicide because it is the fifth leading cause of death in people between the ages of 15 and 24.

✔ Giving away personal things, feeling hopeless, and sleeping too much are a few of the warning signs for suicide.

✔ Taking all talk of suicide seriously, suggesting that your friend talk to a trusted adult, and not keeping any talk of suicide secret are a few ways you can help a friend who may be considering suicide.

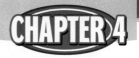

Review

Using Key Terms

asset (85)

distress (81)

epinephrine (80)

eustress (80)

funeral (91)

grieve (90)

memorial service (91)

prioritize (87)

resiliency (85)

stress (78)

stressor (78)

suicide (93)

wake (91)

1. For each definition below, choose the key term that best matches the definition.
   a. any situation that puts a demand on the body or mind
   b. the ability to recover from illness, hardship, and other stressors
   c. to arrange items in order of importance
   d. a ceremony in which a deceased person is buried or cremated
   e. a skill or resource that helps a person reach a goal
   f. the act of intentionally taking one's own life
   g. to express deep sadness because of a loss
   h. the body's and mind's response to a demand made upon it
   i. one of the hormones that are released by the body in times of stress

2. Explain the relationship between the key terms in each of the following pairs.
   a. *wake* and *memorial service*
   b. *distress* and *eustress*

Understanding Key Ideas

Section 1

3. What is the difference between a biological stressor and an environmental stressor?

4. Describe how the fight-or-flight response can help you respond to a threatening situation.

5. Which of the following does *not* describe someone in distress?
   a. confused
   b. unsure
   c. nervous
   d. motivated

6. In which stage of the general adaptation syndrome are you most likely to get sick from response to stress?

Section 2

7. Explain how exercise can help you deal with stress.

8. Explain how breathing deeply can help you deal with stress.

9. Which of the following is *not* an asset for building resiliency?
   a. occasional exercise
   b. support
   c. positive values
   d. empowerment

10. Explain how self-talk can help you deal with a stressor.

11. Which of the following is *not* a helpful suggestion for making a schedule? **LIFE SKILL**
    a. Be realistic.
    b. Make time to relax.
    c. Order your activities randomly.
    d. Prepare for problems.

12. **CRITICAL THINKING** Use the tips you learned in the chapter to make a schedule for yourself for today.

Section 3

13. Describe how loss can cause stress.

14. List the stages of the grieving process.

15. Describe three ceremonies that honor a loved one who has passed away.

16. Describe why you should not blame others for a loss if the loss was an accident. **LIFE SKILL**

Section 4

17. Explain why it is important to know the facts about suicide.

18. Which of the following does *not* describe a behavior that can lead teens to react quickly on thoughts of suicide?
    a. impulsive
    b. highly emotional
    c. silent
    d. focused on today

19. Explain why giving away personal things might be a sign of someone considering suicide.

20. Explain why it is important not to ignore a friend's talk about suicide. **LIFE SKILL**

Interpreting Graphics

Study the figure below to answer the questions that follow.

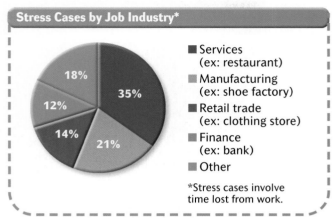

Stress Cases by Job Industry*

- 18%
- 12%
- 14%
- 21%
- 35%

■ Services
(ex: restaurant)
■ Manufacturing
(ex: shoe factory)
■ Retail trade
(ex: clothing store)
■ Finance
(ex: bank)
■ Other

*Stress cases involve time lost from work.

Source: U.S. Department of Labor Bureau of Statistics.

21. Which job industry accounts for the highest percent of stress cases?

22. What is the total percent of stress cases for the services and manufacturing job industries?

23. **CRITICAL THINKING** What types of stress cases do you think workers experience in the job industries listed?

Activities

24. **Health and You** Using the time management skills you learned in this chapter, develop a schedule for the next 7 days.

25. **Health and Your Community** Research and write a two-page report on the ways that people in the United States cope with loss. **WRITING SKILL**

26. **Health and You** Describe the grieving process as it relates to a loss you have experienced or a loss you could have experienced.

27. **Health and Your Community** Create a list of family members and friends you can turn to for help if you or a person you know is considering suicide.

Action Plan

28. **LIFE SKILL** **Practicing Wellness** Use the stress management techniques—taking care of yourself, building resiliency, changing your attitude, and managing your time—to create a stress management program. Follow the program for 1 week. Keep track of your stress management activities and how these activities affect your stress level.

Standardized Test Prep

Read the passage below, and then answer the questions that follow. **READING SKILL** **WRITING SKILL**

As Cindy hung up the phone, she thought about Hallie's comments. Cindy didn't understand why Hallie was so <u>adamant</u> about not going to her sister's funeral. Cindy tried to talk Hallie into going to the funeral. She told Hallie that the funeral might be uncomfortable but that she would be happy later if she went. However, Hallie's last words to Cindy were "I love my sister, but I hate funerals. My parents will be so angry with me, but I just can't imagine sitting through a funeral." Cindy sat in silence, thinking. She wanted to help and comfort her friend, but didn't know how.

29. In this passage, the word *adamant* means
    A negative.
    B not clear.
    C not giving in.
    D hopeful.

30. What can you infer from reading this passage?
    E Hallie is sad and confused.
    F Cindy will be going to the funeral.
    G Cindy's sister died.
    H all of the above

31. Write a paragraph that describes ways that Cindy could help Hallie with her loss.

32. Write a paragraph that describes why it may help Hallie through the grieving process if she goes to her sister's funeral.

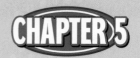

Preventing Violence and Abuse

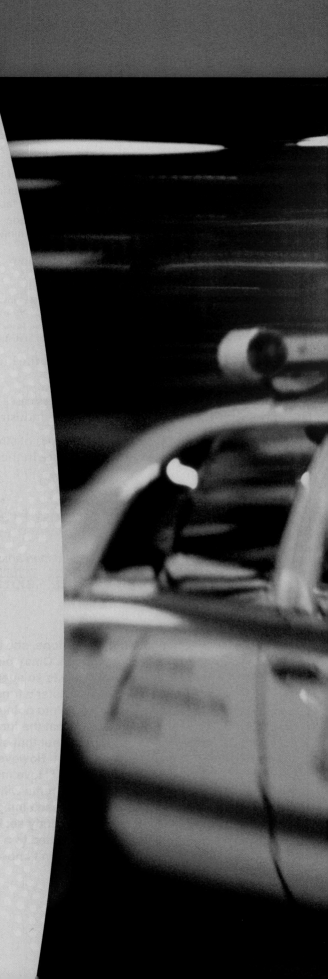

What's Your Health IQ?

BEHAVIOR

Indicate how frequently you engage in each of the following behaviors (1 = never; 2 = occasionally; 3 = most of the time; 4 = all of the time). Total your points, and then turn to p. 642.

1. I calm down before telling someone that what he or she said or did upset me.

2. I respect others even if they are different from me.

3. I don't pick on or tease others.

4. I don't carry weapons.

5. I don't solve arguments with fights.

6. I am assertive and communicate directly and respectfully, not aggressively.

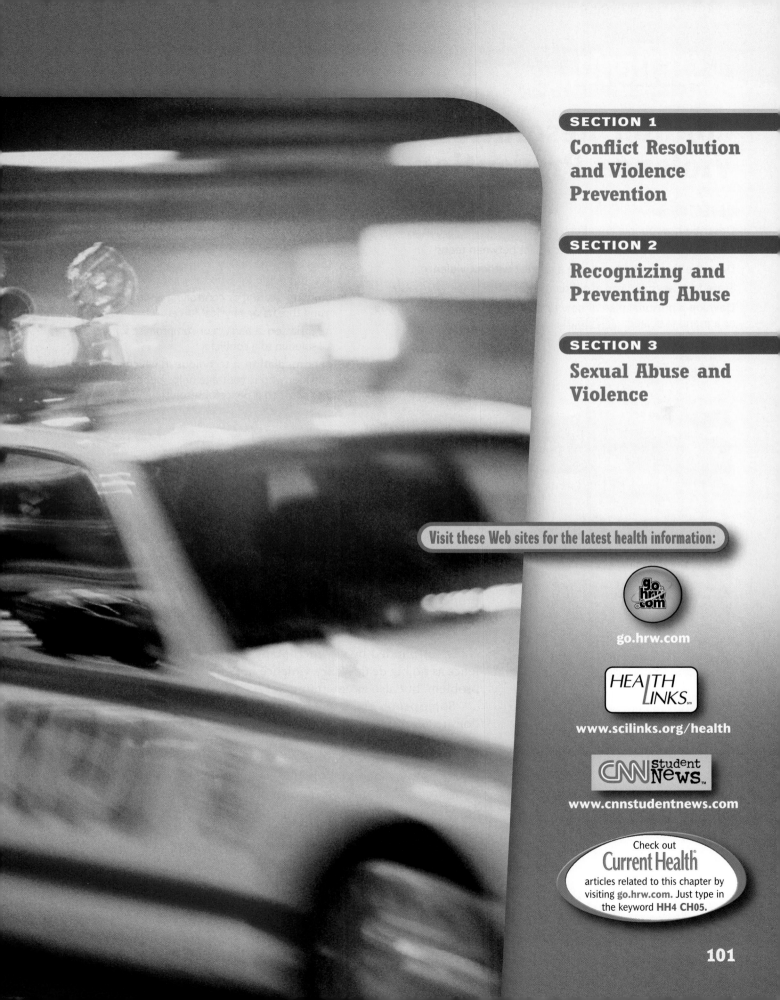

SECTION 1
Conflict Resolution and Violence Prevention

SECTION 2
Recognizing and Preventing Abuse

SECTION 3
Sexual Abuse and Violence

Visit these Web sites for the latest health information:

go.hrw.com

HEALTH LINKSsm

www.scilinks.org/health

CNN student News™

www.cnnstudentnews.com

Check out
Current Health®
articles related to this chapter by
visiting go.hrw.com. Just type in
the keyword **HH4 CH05**.

Conflict Resolution and Violence Prevention

OBJECTIVES

Describe how people are affected by the violence around us.

Identify five factors that lead to conflict between teens.

Describe three ways to resolve a conflict without violence.

State four ways you can avoid dangerous situations. **LIFE SKILL**

Develop a personal plan of how to handle a situation in which you or a friend is bullied. **LIFE SKILL**

KEY TERMS

violence physical force that is used to harm people or damage property

tolerance the ability to overlook differences and accept people for who they are

bullying scaring or controlling another person by using threats or physical force

negotiation a bargain or compromise for a peaceful solution to a conflict

peer mediation a technique in which a trained outsider who is your age helps people in a conflict come to a peaceful resolution

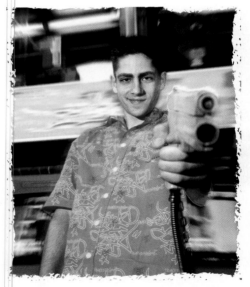

From the games we play to the music we listen to and the movies we see, violence is all around us.

When Milos first moved to his new town, older kids made fun of the way he dressed and how he talked. He was beaten up three times in the first month. He eventually joined a gang for protection. Now, he's pushing others around.

Violence Around Us

Violence is any physical force that is used to harm people or damage property. Unfortunately, violence has started to become a way of life in our society. We see it on TV, in the movies, in the newspaper, in video games, in our schools, and even in our own homes. We are literally surrounded by violence. Many have come to think about violence as no big deal. We see violence not only as a quick solution to a problem, but also as entertainment such as in many action movies.

Some people think that if they don't actually get injured, violence doesn't affect them. This is not true. Seeing and experiencing violence can often make a person insensitive to others who might be in trouble. For example, kids who frequently observe teasing might consider the behavior as normal. When teasing becomes common, it is easier to be *apathetic*, or unconcerned, of others who have been hurt.

Observing and experiencing violence can also make a person more violent towards others. For example, Milos was beaten up when he moved to his town. Now he beats other kids.

Being hardened and becoming violent are responses to experiencing and seeing violence. These responses to violence don't make anyone safer. On the contrary, the responses escalate violence and make society unsafe and helpless to stop the violence.

Factors That Lead to Conflicts Between Teens

A *conflict* is another name for a fight or a disagreement. A conflict can be small, like a disagreement over how to play a game. A conflict can also be large, like the tensions between two countries.

Some people wrongly choose violence to resolve a conflict. Violence does not solve a problem, it makes the problem worse. Violence can lead to injury and even death. Often, violence provokes further violence in the form of revenge. Understanding the factors that can lead to conflict can help prevent conflicts from getting out of control.

Feeling Threatened   The stress from being threatened can often lead to violence. Milos's situation is a good example. He reacted to threats and violence against him with more violence. Violence is never a good solution to a problem. Violence only makes the problem bigger. Bringing a gun or a weapon to school will not protect you. It will put you and others in greater danger.

Unmanaged Anger   Unmanaged anger can also contribute to conflict. Being *fatigued,* or very tired, or living in an over-crowded area can cause a person to be more irritable and act out with anger. However, it is important to deal with anger effectively. If you feel you have problems managing your anger, ask your parents or a trusted adult where you can get help. Remember that only you are responsible for how you express your anger.

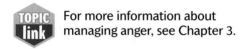 For more information about managing anger, see Chapter 3.

Lack of Respect   Being disrespectful to others can lead to conflict. For example, picking on someone, or destroying one of his or her belongings is one form of disrespect. Having negative opinions about people because of their race, their ethnicity, their gender, their religion, or the way they dress are other ways of being disrespectful.

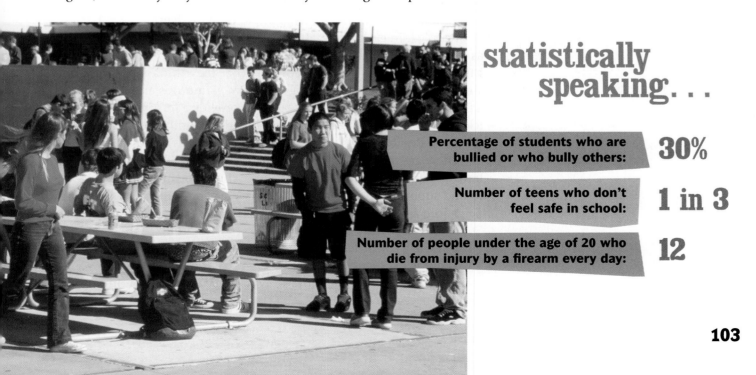

statistically speaking...

Percentage of students who are bullied or who bully others:	**30%**
Number of teens who don't feel safe in school:	**1 in 3**
Number of people under the age of 20 who die from injury by a firearm every day:	**12**

A violent act against someone just because he or she is different in race, religion, culture, or ethnic group, is called a *hate crime*. Many forms of violence could be stopped if people were more tolerant. **Tolerance** is the ability to overlook differences and accept people for who they are.

Bullying Scaring or controlling another person by using threats or physical force is called **bullying.** Bullies can use physical force, such as hitting, kicking, or damaging one's property. Bullies can also use words to hurt or humiliate another person by name-calling, insulting, making racist comments, taunting, or teasing.

Bullies can be manipulative in less obvious ways, such as by spreading nasty rumors. Bullies often form *cliques*. A clique is a close peer group that includes certain people and excludes others.

The following list provides suggestions on how to prevent bullying or being bullied.

▶ Be tolerant of others. Encourage your friends to respect others.
▶ If you see someone being bullied, tell a trusted adult.
▶ Don't be embarrassed to ask for help from friends, teachers, or parents. Bullies won't pick on you if they can't get away with it.
▶ Be assertive, not aggressive. Bullies like to pick on those they think are weak, but responding aggressively to a bully may make the situation worse.
▶ Avoid bullies or any people who are disrespectful or threatening.
▶ Respect yourself. No matter what bullies may say to you, stand by what you believe and be proud of who you are.

Gangs Gangs often cause conflict and violence. A *gang* is a group of peers who claim a territory. Most gangs have a leader and use recognizable symbols or tattoos. Often gangs commit acts of vandalism and carry weapons. They often use drugs, and alcohol, which can play a role in many dangerous situations. Gangs are destructive to the community, the people who live in it, and themselves.

People join gangs for many reasons. Gangs may make people feel as if they fit in or make them feel safe, or powerful. Some people join gangs for excitement, recognition, or what they think is respect. TV shows and movies often make gangs seem glamorous and may make a person want to join a gang. A gang can provide a lonely person with friendship. Teens may join gangs because their family members are in the gang. Regardless of the reason, joining a gang is a bad idea.

There are many other choices besides joining a gang. You do not have to support or take part in violence. The following are other ways to find support and your own place in your community.

▶ join a sports team or school club
▶ volunteer with your neighborhood watch group
▶ coach a sports team for younger kids

There is no excuse for joining a gang. If you feel unsafe in your community, work with community leaders to fight for improvements.

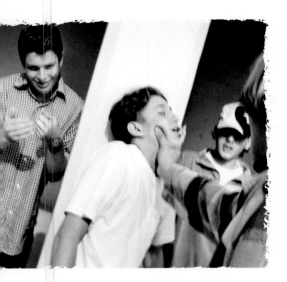

Bullies threaten, hassle, or intimidate smaller or weaker people.

Avoiding Dangerous Situations

To avoid dangerous situations, you should not only stay clear of potentially violent people, but also avoid situations where you might cause conflict or violence. For example, don't join gangs and don't carry weapons. **Figure 1** shows some other ways to avoid conflicts.

Some dangerous situations happen unexpectedly. You may find yourself in a conflict that starts to get out of control and could lead to violence. Follow these steps to avoid dangerous situations.

1. **Recognize the signs.** Part of avoiding dangerous situations is being able to recognize when a situation is getting out of control. People who are beginning to lose control of their anger will show it in the tone and volume of their voice. Nonverbal signs of anger can also appear in body language. For example, clenching one's fists or teeth, getting red in the face, or narrowing one's eyes are signs that anger is getting out of control. Also, look for these signs in yourself.

2. **Calm things down.** If you see signs that a situation might end in conflict, there are things you can do to calm down the situation and avoid a conflict. Always be respectful to the other person. If someone says something that makes you upset, take a deep breath and count to 10 before responding. Use the tips for managing anger and using "I" messages you learned in Building Self-Esteem and Mental Health.

3. **Leave the situation.** If things look like they might get out of control, you can arrange to discuss the matter later when you both cool down. If you no longer feel as if you have control of the situation or of your own anger, you should leave immediately.

4. **Offer alternatives.** Even if someone insists that you fight, you don't have to. Firmly say that you will not fight. You can offer alternatives to a physical battle, such as a basketball contest. You can make an excuse for why you need to leave. Act like the other person is making a big deal over something small. The important thing is to get yourself and others out of danger.

Everyone deserves to feel safe. People should not be so worried about their safety that they are afraid to go to school or take part in their favorite activities. Every teen should feel confident that there are adults and authorities that are committed to protecting him or her. If you feel unsafe and don't know what to do about a situation, these adults and authorities can be your best defense. If someone tells you that he or she is planning a violent act, tell a responsible adult. Even if you believe the person is joking, it is important for your safety and the safety of others that you tell a responsible adult.

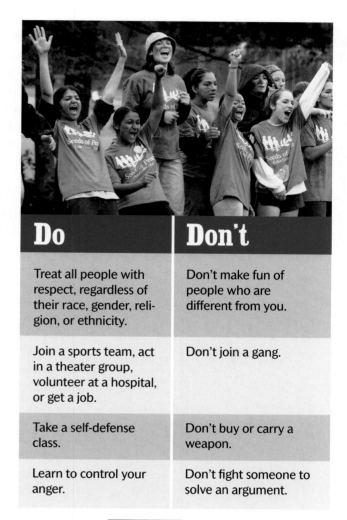

Do	Don't
Treat all people with respect, regardless of their race, gender, religion, or ethnicity.	Don't make fun of people who are different from you.
Join a sports team, act in a theater group, volunteer at a hospital, or get a job.	Don't join a gang.
Take a self-defense class.	Don't buy or carry a weapon.
Learn to control your anger.	Don't fight someone to solve an argument.

Figure 1

These teens from Pakistan, India, the Middle East, and the Balkans respect and support each other as teammates in a soccer game. As indicated in the figure above, showing respect to others who are different from you is one important way to avoid conflict.

Resolving Conflict Without Violence

Let's say you have followed all the steps to avoid dangerous situations yet find yourself in a serious conflict. There are ways to resolve conflicts effectively without using violence, but they require work. It's not easy to work out a problem with someone who has made your blood boil. It's hard to be respectful to someone who hasn't been respectful to you. That's why resolving a conflict nonviolently takes more courage and strength than using violence does.

TOPIC link For more information about communicating effectively, see Chapter 3.

Conflict Resolution Skills   *Conflict resolution* is a nonviolent way to deal with arguments. All people involved in the conflict sit down together and express their points of view. Everyone works together to find a solution acceptable to all parties involved. A common and successful approach is through negotiation. A **negotiation** is a bargain or compromise for a peaceful solution to a conflict.

Being able to successfully negotiate a conflict depends on your communication skills. Here are some tips for communicating effectively to resolve conflicts.

▶ Be respectful, yet be assertive.
▶ Use the steps of the Making GREAT Decisions model.
▶ Don't call each other names or raise your voice.
▶ Allow the other person time to speak.
▶ Don't make assumptions.
▶ Focus on the real issue.
▶ Be open to change and look for shared interests.
▶ Use "I" messages, not "you" messages.
▶ Use listening skills and try to understand what the other person wants.

If negotiating a conflict on your own isn't working, don't give up. You can also try *peer mediation*. **Peer mediation** is a technique in which a trained outsider who is your age helps people in a conflict come to a peaceful resolution.

Peer mediators help people involved in a conflict work out the problem in a nonviolent way.

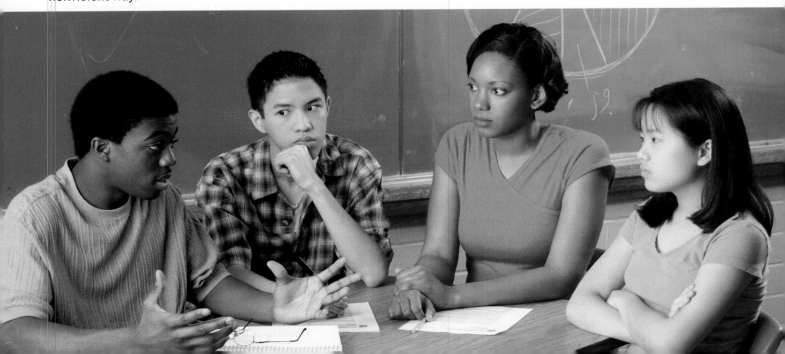

Peer Mediation   Having nonbiased outsiders organize a negotiation for you can be a big help in resolving conflicts. Peer mediators are trained to keep discussions fair. They make sure each person has a chance to speak, and they make sure the discussion focuses on the real issue.

Many schools provide peer mediation services. If students in the school want help solving a conflict, they usually fill out a form describing the problem and submit the form to the mediation program. Sometimes, mediation referrals come from third parties, such as students or teachers who know trouble is brewing between two people.

In peer mediation, each student tells his or her side of the conflict. Students get a chance to vent their feelings and talk to each other if they want to. They can ask questions and clarify facts. The parties brainstorm solutions. Usually, at least two mediators keep track of the solutions that are discussed. However, the mediators don't make suggestions unless they are asked. Their job is to ensure that everyone has a voice to guide the group toward a solution and to make sure things are worked out "fair and square."

Eventually, the arguing students agree to one of the suggestions on their brainstorming list that they created. Both parties sign a contract agreeing to the solution. The peer mediators follow up by checking to see if both sides are following the agreement.

With peer mediation, both parties in a conflict are guaranteed to work out the problem in a safe, nonviolent way. A lot of students like peer mediation because it is run by students. Adults only supervise. Is there a peer mediation program in your school? If not, you may want to talk to a teacher or principal about starting one.

MAKING GREAT DECISIONS

Max and Ryan have been friends since kindergarten. Now they are in high school together. One day, Max and Ryan are talking in the cafeteria. Ryan starts telling Max about some kids who have been bullying him after school. Ryan swears Max to secrecy, unzips his bag, and shows Max a gun. Max asks Ryan why he needs a gun. Ryan says, "Just in case."

Write on a separate piece of paper what you would do if you were in Max's situation. Remember to use the decision-making steps.

G ive thought to the problem.
R eview your choices.
E valuate the consequences of each choice.
A ssess and choose the best choice.
T hink it over afterward.

SECTION 1

REVIEW   *Answer the following questions on a separate piece of paper.*

Using Key Terms

1. **Identify** the term for "the ability to overlook differences and accept people for who they are."
2. **Define** the term *bullying*.
3. **Identify** the term for "a bargain or compromise for a peaceful solution to a conflict."

Understanding Key Ideas

4. **Describe** how violence affects us.
5. **State** five factors that can lead to conflict.

6. **Identify** which of the following is *not* a skill for successfully resolving conflict.
   a. negotiation   c. bullying
   b. peer mediation   d. compromise
7. **Describe** why peer mediation has been successful in high schools.
8. **LIFE SKILL** **Practicing Wellness** List four ways you can avoid dangerous situations.

Critical Thinking

9. **LIFE SKILL** **Coping** Develop a plan on how to handle a situation in which you are being bullied.

SECTION 1   *Conflict Resolution and Violence Prevention*   **107**

Recognizing and Preventing Abuse

OBJECTIVES

Identify abusive behavior.

Describe four types of abuse.

Summarize the effects of abuse.

Identify help that is available for those in abusive relationships.

List actions you can take to protect yourself from abuse.

LIFE SKILL

KEY TERMS

abuse physical or emotional harm to someone

neglect the failure of a caretaker to provide for basic needs, such as food, clothing, or love

domestic violence the use of force to control and maintain power over a spouse in the home

hazing harassing newcomers to a group in an abusive and humiliating way

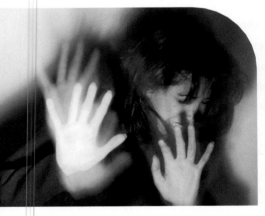

Often, people who are abused are abused by someone they should be able to trust.

Tad was watching TV when he heard screaming from the apartment next door. His neighbors were fighting again, but this time the fight sounded really bad. He could hear furniture being thrown and something breaking. One of the voices sounded very frightened.

What Is Abuse?

Abuse is physical or emotional harm to someone. Abuse can take place anywhere, including at school, on the street, or at home. Unfortunately, the most common forms of abuse come from people one should be able to trust, such as family members, friends, boyfriends, or girlfriends. For this reason, people who are being abused don't feel as if they can leave the abuser or demand to be treated respectfully. However, it is necessary for them to do so. Many forms of abuse are illegal. No one should have to tolerate abuse.

It is difficult to imagine what would make someone inflict harm on a loved one, such as a child, a spouse, a girlfriend, a boyfriend, a peer, or an elderly parent. You may be surprised to find out that the abuser is often someone who was once abused himself or herself. If people grow up in a family in which they were abused, they learn that abusive behavior is the normal response to tension or conflict.

Abusive Behavior Learning to recognize inconsiderate and disrespectful behavior will help you avoid abusive people. For example, an abusive relationship may exist if a person is controlling, obsessive, manipulative, selfish, aggressive, or needy. An abusive person may get jealous easily, have difficulty controlling anger, or demand that the other person not see certain people or wear certain clothes. An abuser will often insult, humiliate, or put down others. Abusers often use *coercion*, which is force or threats. If you know of someone who has been abusive to others, chances are that he or she could be abusive to you, too.

Types of Abuse

There are many types of abuse. The following is a description of the most common types of abuse.

Child Abuse As many as 3 million cases of child abuse are reported every year in the United States. Many more cases never get reported. Children are frequent targets of abuse because they are young and can't or don't know how to respond appropriately. Sometimes one sibling will abuse another. Child abuse is usually categorized in four different ways: physical abuse, emotional abuse, sexual abuse, and neglect. **Neglect** occurs when a caretaker fails to provide basic needs, such as food, clothing, or love.

Domestic Violence The use of force to control and maintain power over a spouse in the home is called **domestic violence.** A former spouse, a fiancé, a boyfriend, or a girlfriend can also commit domestic violence. Women can abuse their male partners, but women are much more likely to be the victims of domestic violence. It is estimated that an act of domestic violence occurs somewhere in the United States every 15 seconds.

Often an abusive relationship goes through a cycle of three stages, as shown in **Figure 2.**
1. **Tension-building phase** A time of emotional abuse such as insults or threats.
2. **Violent episode phase** An act of physical abuse occurs such as choking or hitting.
3. **Honeymoon phase** The time when the couple makes up. This phase is often the reason people stay in abusive relationships.

Figure **2**

Violence in domestic relationships often cycles through three stages. The cycle will often repeat itself continuously, sometimes for years, until the partners get help or the relationship ends.

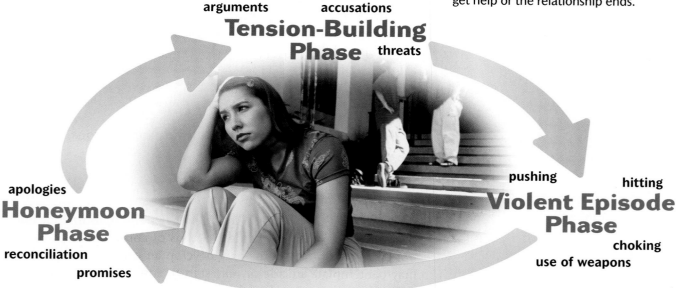

insults
arguments   accusations
Tension-Building Phase   threats

pushing   hitting
Violent Episode Phase
choking
use of weapons

apologies
Honeymoon Phase
reconciliation
promises

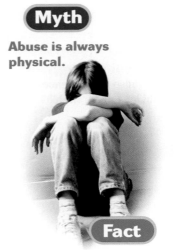

Myth

Abuse is always physical.

Fact

Abuse can be emotional as well as physical.

Elder Abuse   The elderly are often viewed as the wisest people in the community. Unfortunately, elderly people are not always treated with respect by all people. Because elderly people are often frail, they can be easily taken advantage of. For example, people will sometimes steal from them. They may be neglected in nursing homes or in their own homes. Elder abuse can also take the form of physical abuse and emotional abuse.

Hazing   Harassing newcomers to a group in an abusive and humiliating way is called **hazing.** Hazing may happen when people join sports teams, gangs, fraternities, or sororities. The idea behind hazing is that it proves you are truly committed to joining the group. However, hazing is unacceptable. When people are beaten up, sexually taken advantage of, or humiliated, hazing becomes abusive and illegal.

It's important to be able to recognize abusive behavior. Abusive behavior can then be reported to stop the immediate violence and to prevent future violent acts.

Effects of Abuse

After reading about some of the types of abuse, you can imagine that abuse may have an impact on a person's life in more ways than one. If a person is physically harmed, he or she might have obvious physical injuries that need to be tended to. However, the effects of abuse are not merely physical. Abuse affects all parts of a person's health.

Take Rosa, for example. Rosa was hazed during her tryouts for the swim team. She really wanted to make the team, so she went through the process. In addition to the bruises from the paddling, she feels so humiliated and depressed at what the team members made her do. She doesn't think she can ever tell anyone. Now it's all she thinks about—night and day. She feels isolated. How can she turn around and be friends with people who abused her?

The effects of hazing are similar to the effects of other forms of abuse. Some examples of the effects of abuse are as follows:

▶ depression

▶ low self-esteem

▶ poor appetite or overeating

▶ low energy or fatigue

▶ poor concentration and difficulty making decisions

▶ difficulty sleeping

▶ feelings of worthlessness

▶ feelings of guilt, shame, and anxiety

An abused person might lose his or her ability to trust or might develop relationship difficulties. Victims of abuse may turn to alcohol or drugs. Some victims may develop an eating disorder. Others may contemplate suicide or may start to suffer from post-traumatic stress disorder, anxiety disorder, or panic attacks.

Protecting Yourself from Abuse

If anyone abuses you, tell your parents, the police, or other trusted adult. Tell the abuser you will let an authority know about his or her behavior. Many forms of abuse, such as physical and sexual abuse, are illegal. Often, the abuser will stop if you threaten to tell because he or she will be afraid of getting into trouble.

Create a Supportive Network of Friends and Family Make sure there are people you can trust and talk to openly. If abuse does occur, you want people to whom you can turn for help. The more positive relationships you have in your life, the more options you will have in case of abuse.

Avoid Disrespectful People If you know of someone who has been abusive to you or to others, you should stay away from that person. Whenever possible, don't go somewhere if you know that person will be there. Leave where you are if that person arrives. Choose friends who treat you and others with respect. Choose friends who make you feel good about yourself. If you let people know that you respect yourself and expect respect from others, chances are that they will treat you with respect.

Be Assertive Abusers frequently prey on people who appear vulnerable or who have low self-esteem. Assertive people set down boundaries that let others know they will not accept hurtful behavior. Being assertive toward an abuser will make it difficult for him or her to abuse you. However, if you act passively toward an abuser, that person will think he or she can abuse you again and again. If you act aggressively, depending on who the abuser is, that person may become angrier and make the abuse worse. Using assertiveness skills can help you protect yourself from abuse. **Figure 3** has examples of assertive statements.

Figure 3

Assertive statements respectfully tell the other person how you feel.

ACTIVITY *If a boyfriend or girlfriend is wrongfully accusing you of cheating on him or her, how would you respond assertively?*

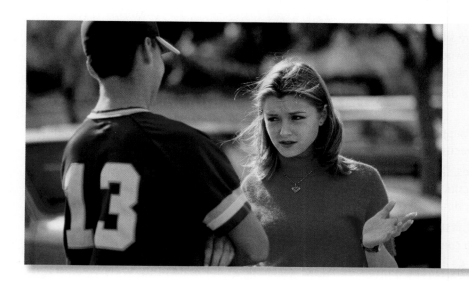

Assertive Statements

"I don't like it when you tell me to whom I can and cannot talk."

"You scare me when you yell like that."

"It hurts when you criticize me and put me down, especially in front of other people."

"I don't want to be around you when you drink or get angry."

HEALTH Handbook For more information about practicing refusal skills, see the Express Lesson on p. 618 of this text.

Show Disapproval If a person does not treat you in an acceptable way, show your disapproval. Showing disapproval lets the abuser know that his or her behavior is not acceptable, that you won't tolerate it, and that you want it to stop.

There are many ways you can show disapproval. One subtle way is to refuse to laugh at an offensive joke. One active way is to yell for help. Earlier you learned about body language, tone of voice, and other means of communication. Use this knowledge to stand up for yourself and to let others know that their behavior is unacceptable. Because you know it is important to behave and speak politely, it can be hard to show disapproval. However, showing disapproval is a necessary part of stopping abuse.

It's important to know that the abuser probably won't stop abusing on his or her own. You may have to tell an abuser more than once that you will not tolerate the hurtful behavior. The refusal skills you learned earlier can be a big help in saying no to abuse. However, it is also important to tell your parents or other trusted adult about the abuse.

LIFE SKILL Activity

Communicating Effectively

Stopping Abuse Before It Starts

Can you think of any situations in which you might need to be assertive or show disapproval? Practicing skills such as showing disapproval and being assertive will help you use these skills confidently.

1. Choose a partner to practice your assertiveness and disapproval skills with.

2. Think of a potentially abusive situation in which you and your partner would like to use assertiveness and disapproval skills.

3. Write down possible things a disrespectful person might say.

4. Write down ways to show disapproval or to be assertive toward the disrespectful person.

5. Now role-play your responses. Decide which partner will be the disrespectful person and which partner will be the victim.

6. After you have gone through all the possible responses, switch roles. If you come up with more responses while role-playing, go ahead and try them. Remember to be assertive, not aggressive.

LIFE SKILL Practicing Wellness Did you find your responses effective as you role-played them? Compare how it felt to take the role of the abusive person to how it felt to take the role of the assertive person.

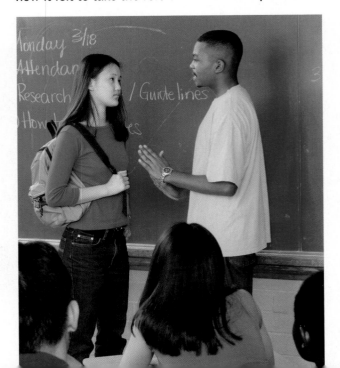

Help for The Abused

Not only is abuse a crime, but *no one* should allow abuse to occur. Something can be done to stop the abuse.

Tell Someone   If you are currently being abused in any way, tell your parents, coach, school administrators, school counselor, or any other trusted adult. The police also have information about shelters and other agencies that help victims of abuse.

Go Somewhere Safe   If you are in immediate danger, leave the situation and go somewhere safe—a friend's or relative's house, the police station, a religious institution, a hospital, a school, or any supervised place where you will be out of harm. Do not think about running away. Running away is not a safe way to escape abuse at home. Runaways almost always find themselves in situations that are worse than the one they left.

Consider Counseling   Abuse leaves mental and emotional scars that last long after the victim is safe. Counselors and other mental health professionals can help victims of abuse deal with low self-esteem, depression, shame, and guilt. Many times, the family of the victim takes part in the therapy, too.

Victims are not the only ones who need help—abusers also need to get help. Abusers need help to realize that their behavior is hurtful, illegal, and unacceptable. There are programs available to help abusers change their behavior.

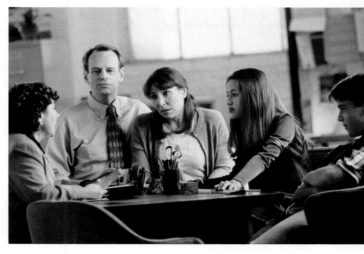

Family counseling can help family members deal with the long-term effects of abuse and can also stop future acts of abuse.

SECTION 2

REVIEW   *Answer the following questions on a separate piece of paper.*

Using Key Terms

1. **Define** the term *neglect*.
2. **Identify** the term for "harassing newcomers to a group in an abusive and humiliating way."

Understanding Key Ideas

3. **List** five examples of inconsiderate and disrespectful behavior abusive people do.
4. **Identify** the form of abuse that occurs between a husband and wife or between a boyfriend and girlfriend.
   - **a.** child abuse
   - **b.** elder abuse
   - **c.** domestic violence
   - **d.** hazing

5. **List** the three phases of the cycle of violence.
6. **Describe** why children and the elderly are especially vulnerable to abuse.
7. **Describe** the effects of abuse.
8. **LIFE SKILL** **Coping** List people you can go to for help if you or someone you know has been abused.
9. **LIFE SKILL** **Practicing Wellness** Describe actions you can take to prevent and avoid abuse.

Critical Thinking

10. Why do you think abused children often have trouble making friends?

Sexual Abuse and Violence

OBJECTIVES

Define sexual abuse.

Describe sexual harassment.

Describe facts about sexual assault and rape.

Name five things a person should do if he or she has been sexually assaulted.

List three ways you can protect yourself from sexual abuse and violence. **LIFE SKILL**

KEY TERMS

sexual abuse any sexual act without consent

incest sexual activity between family members who are not husband and wife

sexual harassment any unwanted remark, behavior, or touch that has sexual content

sexual assault any sexual activity in which force or the threat of force is used

date rape sexual intercourse that is forced on a victim by someone the victim knows

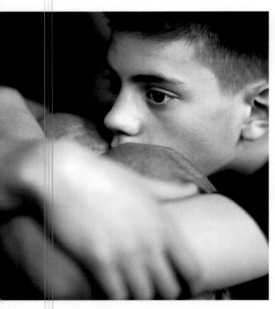

Boys as well as girls are victims of sexual abuse.

Alex was excited when he got his first job at the ice-cream stand. But, now he hates to go to work. His boss sometimes touches him in places he doesn't want to be touched. Tonight, he is really worried. He has to close up the stand alone with the boss.

Sexual Abuse

Sexual abuse is any sexual act without consent. Any act in which a person touches you in a sexual way that makes you feel uncomfortable is an act of sexual abuse. The acts can range from kissing and fondling to forced intercourse. For example, it is considered sexual abuse if the abuser touches the victim in a sexual way or if the victim is forced to touch the abuser in a sexual way. It is also considered sexual abuse if either the victim or abuser is indecently exposed or if the victim is shown pornography.

Children and Sexual Abuse Sexual activity between family members who are not husband and wife is known as **incest.** Incest traumatizes a child not only physically but also emotionally. Because the child is being abused by someone he or she knows and trusts, the child may find it difficult to tell when he or she is being abused.

Another reason children find it hard to admit that they are being sexually abused is that the abuse tends to begin "innocently" with affectionate hugs and kisses. The abuser may manipulate the child into feeling special. The behavior progresses to caresses and sexual teasing and then to sexual activity. Because the behavior started in an innocent fashion, children feel as if they did something to encourage the abuse. They then feel too ashamed to tell someone. However, if no one finds out, the abuse can continue.

Anyone being sexually abused should tell a trusted adult. All forms of sexual abuse are illegal and should be reported to the police.

Sexual Harassment

Every time James sees Tiffany, he has something to say about how she looks. The way he looks up and down her body makes her feel so uncomfortable. She has started wearing baggy clothes. She has even started walking to school the long way just so she doesn't bump into him.

Matt went out with Lydia. The date turned into a bad evening. She kept pressuring him to have sex. He said no many times. Then, she accused him of not liking girls. She became angry and left early. At school today, she avoided him. He saw her whispering to her friends and looking at him from across the room. Matt felt so embarrassed. He couldn't wait for the bell to ring so that he could leave.

The two situations above are examples of sexual harassment. **Sexual harassment** is any unwanted remark, behavior, or touch that has sexual content. Can you identify the harassing behaviors? If the behavior makes your school, home, or work environment intimidating, hostile, or offensive, the behavior is sexual harassment. In the cases of Tiffany and Matt, the harassers were making the school environment uncomfortable.

When people are confronted about sexual harassment, they will often say they were only flirting. How do you feel when someone flirts with you? You might feel flattered, respected, and attractive. But, Tiffany and Matt felt uncomfortable, cornered, and ashamed. Do you see the difference? Whatever intention you may have, if someone tells you that he or she doesn't like your behavior, you are not flirting. If you are unsure how someone feels about your flirting, you can always ask.

Power and Sexual Harassment   Sexual harassment is most dangerous when the harasser holds a position of power, such as a doctor, teacher, boss, or older friend of the family. In such a case, the victim is often afraid to complain about the behavior. He or she doesn't want to risk his or her health, get a bad grade, lose a job, or embarass the family. Victims may even get direct messages, such as "If you have sex with me, I'll give you a raise."

Responding to Sexual Harassment   If you are being sexually harassed, there are things you can do to stop the harassment.

1. **Tell the harasser to stop.** The harasser might not know that he or she is making you feel uncomfortable. If you never say anything, he or she will never know that you disapprove of the behavior.

2. **Report the harassment.** If the harassing continues after you told the person to stop, avoid the person and complain about the harassment to a higher authority. The higher authority might be a parent, guidance counselor, principal, or owner of a business. Sexual harassment is illegal. Most schools and businesses have rules prohibiting sexual harassment. Use those rules and government laws to stop the behavior.

Examples of Sexual Harassment?

▶ Telling unwanted sexual stories or jokes

▶ Making sexual remarks about a person's clothing and the way it fits on the person's body

▶ Staring at a person's body or body parts

▶ Continuously asking a person out or sending gifts, e-mails, or love notes after he or she asked you to stop

▶ Touching, patting, or pinching a person in a sexual way

▶ Standing too close to or brushing up against a person's body

▶ Making sexual gestures

▶ Offering the person something he or she needs in return for sex

Sexual Assault and Rape

Sexual assault is any sexual activity in which force or the threat of force is used. Sexual assault can range from forced kissing to pulling off clothes and grabbing body parts. Forced sexual intercourse, or *rape*, is an extreme form of sexual assault.

Some people think that sexual assault and rape are committed by strangers. The truth is that about 80 percent of victims of sexual assault and rape know their attacker. **Date rape**, also referred to as acquaintance rape, is sexual intercourse that is forced on a victim by someone the victim knows. The rapist uses the trust that he or she has developed with the victim to take advantage of the victim. Rape can also happen between married couples. This is a form of domestic violence. Some people believe that rape occurs because the attacker wants sexual intercourse. However, the real reason that people rape is to gain power and control.

Using alcohol and drugs as well as being around people who use alcohol and drugs can put you in a dangerous situation. About 45 percent of rapists were under the influence of alcohol when they raped somebody. Also, rapists sometimes give alcohol and drugs to victims so that they will be more vulnerable. Rapists have also been known to slip drugs into the victim's drink. These drugs are commonly known as *date-rape drugs*. The drugs cause the victim to lose consciousness. In some cases, date-rape drugs can be fatal.

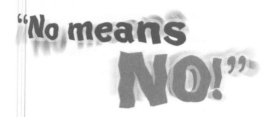

Effects of Sexual Assault and Rape   Like victims of other types of violence, victims of rape and sexual assault suffer both physical and emotional trauma. Survivors may experience injuries such as bruises, cuts, and broken bones. They may also be exposed to pregnancy and sexually transmitted diseases (STDs). Victims may feel guilt and shame about the assault. They may have trouble sleeping or eating. They may even suffer from post-traumatic stress disorder.

Rape and sexual assault are not only morally wrong, they are illegal. Depending on the state, the sentences for a conviction of sexual assault or rape range from fines and community service to years in prison.

Beliefs Vs. Reality

"Only young, beautiful people are raped."	People of all ages are victims of rape.
"Men and boys are never raped."	One out of 10 victims of rape is male.
"People who wear sexy clothes are asking to be raped."	It doesn't matter what a victim wears. No one asks to be raped.
"Rape is an act of sexual frustration."	Rape is an act of power and control.
"Most rapes are committed by someone unknown to the victim."	Most rapes are committed by a person known to the victim.

Protecting Yourself from Sexual Abuse and Violence

There are many things you can do to decrease your risk of sexual abuse and violence. The following are some suggestions.

At Home   You can keep your house safe by making sure all the windows and doors are locked. Don't open the door to strangers. Don't hide a spare key in an obvious place.

Know your neighbors, and make sure your neighbors know you. If everyone knows each other, then people can be on the lookout for strangers in the community.

If you are home alone, make sure you have the phone number where your parents or guardians will be if you need to call them. Do not tell callers that you are home alone. Keep other emergency numbers readily available.

On the Street   The first rule of preventing abuse on the street is don't go out alone, especially at night. Be alert. Walk purposefully, and act as if you know where you are going. If you look lost, you will appear vulnerable. Always make sure you have enough money to make a phone call if you feel threatened. If you do feel threatened, yell and run into a store or other public place.

By People You Know   Most of the sexual violence that occurs comes from someone the victim knows. Preventing sexual abuse and violence from people we know is a little different from preventing it from people we don't know. The people we know don't have to sneak up next to us on the street. Chances are that we let them into our house or are walking with them on the street.

Know signs of abusive people, and don't get involved with those people. Be careful about people you meet on the internet, especially if they discuss or show pornography. Do not agree to meet them in person. Avoid people who are hostile or disrespectful. Rapists are often motivated to make the person feel powerless, degraded, dirty, and ashamed. If someone you know makes you nervous or makes offensive jokes or comments, tell him or her you don't like the behavior and also tell a parent or other trusted adult.

No one, not your friends, your family members, or your boyfriend or girlfriend, has a right to sexually abuse you. Use the communication skills, refusal skills, and decision-making skills you have learned to protect yourself. Use body language and voice tone, volume, and pitch to discourage a sexual offender. Say no clearly and loudly over and over again. Make it clear that you think that the person's behavior is inappropriate.

If you are being attacked, call out for help. Call as much attention to the situation as you can. Break things. Do whatever you can to protect yourself.

Protecting Yourself from Date Rape

▶ **When going on a date, know who the person is, where you are going, and what you will be doing. Make sure friends and family know this information too.**

▶ **Don't be alone with your date. Go on dates in public places.**

▶ **Go on double dates or group dates.**

▶ **Do not accept drugs or alcohol.**

▶ **Do not allow anyone to have an opportunity to put drugs in your beverage.**

▶ **Be wary of meeting anyone on the Internet.**

▶ **Know where a phone is at all times.**

▶ **Set limits, and communicate these limits clearly and firmly ahead of time.**

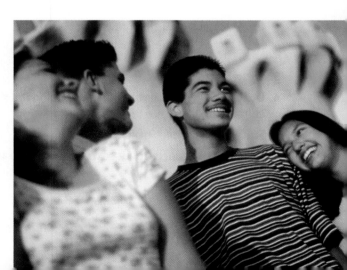

Help After a Sexual Assault

If you have been raped or assaulted, there are several things you should do.

1. Make sure you are away from further harm.

2. Call for help. You can call your family, the police, a neighbor, a friend, or any other trusted adult.

3. Don't change anything about your body or your environment. Don't shower or go to the bathroom. Don't change your clothes or wash or comb your hair. Don't clean up the place where you are. There might be evidence that can be collected by the police or at a hospital. You can cover yourself with a blanket to feel more comfortable.

4. Ask someone to take you to the hospital.

5. Seek therapy or counseling. Remember, abusers want to make the victim feel ashamed and humiliated. Counselors can help reassure victims that they are not to blame for the assault.

Sometimes, people who are sexually assaulted just want to forget the whole incident and put it behind them. There are two problems with forgetting the assault. First, if you are in denial about the incident and don't seek medical care, then you can't get physical or emotional treatment from trained personnel.

The second problem is that if you don't report it, the abuser cannot be stopped. If you report the attack, you may be preventing another person from going through what you did. Many victims do not report crimes because they don't want to go through a trial. However, you can report an assault without prosecuting. This way, the incident is on record, so you can prosecute later. If you do not report the assault immediately and if you destroy any evidence, prosecuting later will be very difficult.

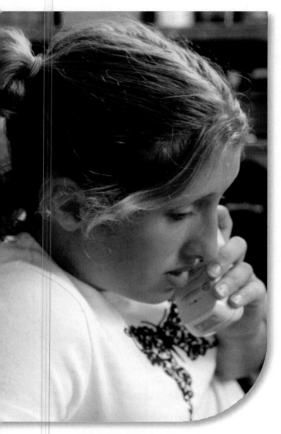

One of the first steps after a sexual assault is calling for help.

SECTION 3

REVIEW
Answer the following questions on a separate piece of paper.

Using Key Terms

1. **Define** the term *sexual harassment*.

2. **Identify** the term for "any sexual activity in which force or the threat of force is used."

Understanding Key Ideas

3. **Describe** sexual abuse.

4. **Describe** why victims of sexual abuse find it difficult to admit they are being abused.

5. **State** five examples of sexual harassment.

6. **Describe** three facts about sexual assault and rape.

7. **Identify** which of the following is *not* a way to protect yourself from date rape.
   a. double dating
   b. going out with people who drink
   c. going on dates in public places
   d. being assertive

8. **List** five things a person should do if he or she has been sexually assaulted.

Critical Thinking

9. **LIFE SKILL** **Practicing Wellness** Describe three ways you can protect yourself from sexual abuse and violence.

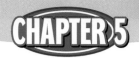

Highlights

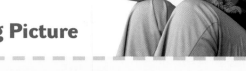

Key Terms

The Big Picture

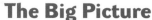

SECTION 1

violence (102)
tolerance (104)
bullying (104)
negotiation (106)
peer mediation (106)

✔ Being exposed to violence can make people fearful, unsympathetic to others, and more likely to use violence themselves.

✔ Factors that lead to violence include feeling threatened, not managing anger, not showing respect for others, bullying, and gangs.

✔ You can avoid dangerous situations by recognizing signs, calming things down, leaving the situation, offering alternatives, avoiding gangs, and avoiding weapons.

✔ Conflict resolution skills, such as negotiation and peer mediation, are effective, nonviolent ways to deal with arguments.

✔ Being assertive and asking for help are two ways you can protect yourself from bullying.

SECTION 2

abuse (108)
neglect (109)
domestic violence (109)
hazing (110)

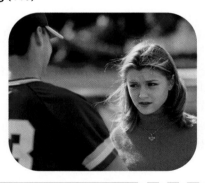

✔ Being able to identify disrespectful and inconsiderate behavior such as selfishness, aggression, and excessive jealousy, will help you avoid abusive people.

✔ Four types of abuse are child abuse, domestic violence, elder abuse, and hazing.

✔ Besides causing physical injury, some effects of abuse are depression, low self-esteem, guilt, shame, anxiety, distrust, and difficulty developing relationships. Many who are abused turn to alcohol or drugs.

✔ Creating a supportive network, avoiding disrespectful people, being assertive, and showing disapproval will help you protect yourself from abuse.

✔ Victims of abuse should tell a trusted adult, go somewhere safe, and get counseling.

SECTION 3

sexual abuse (114)
incest (114)
sexual harassment (115)
sexual assault (116)
date rape (116)

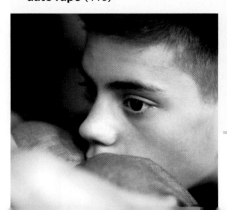

✔ Sexual abuse is any physical sexual act that happens without one's consent. It can cause physical and emotional trauma.

✔ Sexual harassment is unwanted sexual attention, such as telling offensive jokes, staring at someone's body, or touching people in sexual ways.

✔ Most rapes are committed by someone the victim knows.

✔ A few ways you can protect yourself from sexual abuse and violence are keeping your house locked up, not going out alone, and avoiding disrespectful people.

✔ If someone has been sexually assaulted, he or she should find safety, call for help, not clean up, report the incident to the police, and seek counseling.

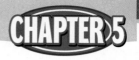

Review

Using Key Terms

abuse (108)
bullying (104)
date rape (116)
domestic violence (109)
hazing (110)
incest (114)
neglect (109)

negotiation (106)
peer mediation (106)
sexual abuse (114)
sexual assault (116)
sexual harassment (115)
tolerance (104)
violence (102)

1. For each definition below, choose the key term that best matches the definition.
   a. a technique in which a trained outsider who is your age helps people in a conflict come to a peaceful resolution
   b. the ability to overlook differences and accept people for who they are
   c. the use of force to control and maintain power over a spouse in the home
   d. sexual activity between family members who are not husband and wife
   e. harassing newcomers to a group in an abusive and humiliating way
   f. sexual intercourse that is forced on a victim by someone the victim knows
   g. any unwanted remarks, behavior, or touch that has sexual content
   h. a bargain or compromise for a peaceful solution to a conflict
   i. any sexual activity that involves the use of force or the threat of force
   j. any sexual act without consent

2. Explain the relationship between the key terms in each of the following pairs.
   a. *bullying* and *violence*
   b. *neglect* and *abuse*

Understanding Key Ideas

Section 1

3. Explain how observing and experiencing violence can cause a person to become apathetic.

4. Which of the following does *not* contribute to conflict?
   a. gangs
   b. feeling threatened
   c. negotiating
   d. bullying

5. Explain how using tolerance can help prevent a conflict.

6. Why might someone join a gang?

7. List the 4 steps for avoiding a dangerous situation in a conflict that is getting out of control.

8. Describe three ways to communicate effectively to resolve conflict. **LIFE SKILL**

9. **CRITICAL THINKING** Create an action plan to help someone who is being bullied.

Section 2

10. Which is *not* a sign of inconsiderate or disrespectful behavior common in abusive people?
    a. manipulation
    b. aggression
    c. obsession
    d. empathy

11. Neglecting an older person is an example of _____ abuse.

12. Why are children frequently targets for abuse?

13. Which of the following is *not* an effect of abuse?
    a. eating disorder
    b. high self-esteem
    c. drug and alcohol abuse
    d. depression

14. Describe how you can show disapproval for inconsiderate and disrespectful behavior. **LIFE SKILL**

15. **CRITICAL THINKING** Create a list of trusted adults you could go to for help if you were being abused.

Section 3

16. Give an example of sexual abuse.

17 Explain effective ways of dealing with sexual harassment.

18. Explain how being around people who drink alcohol and use drugs can put you at risk for sexual assault.

19. Which of the following should you *not* do immediately after you have been sexually assaulted?
    a. call the police
    b. call a trusted adult
    c. get to safety
    d. take a shower

20. What are three ways you can protect yourself from sexual abuse and violence? **LIFE SKILL**

Interpreting Graphics

Study the figure below to answer the questions that follow.

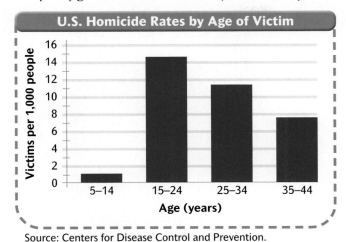

U.S. Homicide Rates by Age of Victim

Source: Centers for Disease Control and Prevention.

21. What is the difference between homicide rates for your age group and homicide rates for 25- to 34-year-olds? **MATH SKILL**

22. CRITICAL THINKING Why do you think 15–24 year-olds have the highest homicide rate?

Activities

23. Health and Your Community Start a neighborhood watch program, or join one that already exists in your community. Work with neighbors to write a plan for contacting authorities if a disturbance occurs.

24. Health and You Describe an example of a conflict that you have recently had. Evaluate your style of resolving the conflict. Now, use the conflict management skills you learned to explain all the possible ways you could improve your style of resolving conflicts.

25. Health and Your Community Meet with a local law enforcement officer to discuss potentially dangerous situations in your community. Write a paper on these potentially dangerous situations and ways you can avoid them.

Action Plan

26. LIFE SKILL Practicing Wellness Develop an action plan to deal with a conflict you might have with a family member or friend.

Standardized Test Prep

Read the passage below, and then answer the questions that follow. **READING SKILL** **WRITING SKILL**

A man moved into the apartment next door to Tasi last week. He makes her nervous. Whenever she passes him in the hall, he looks over her whole body. Yesterday, when Tasi came home from school, the man asked her to come over to his apartment to watch a movie. When she said she didn't want to, he became <u>irate</u>. His voice started getting louder and he moved closer to her. She ran into her apartment. She locked the door and called her father at work.

27. In this passage, the word *irate* means
 A angry.
 B sensitive and caring.
 C silent.
 D playful.

28. What can you infer from reading this passage?
 E The man is happy.
 F Tasi doesn't know how to say no.
 G The man might abuse or assault Tasi.
 H Tasi's father needs a new job.

29. Write a paragraph that describes how Tasi protected herself. Describe what further action Tasi and her father can take in the future to protect Tasi from the man.

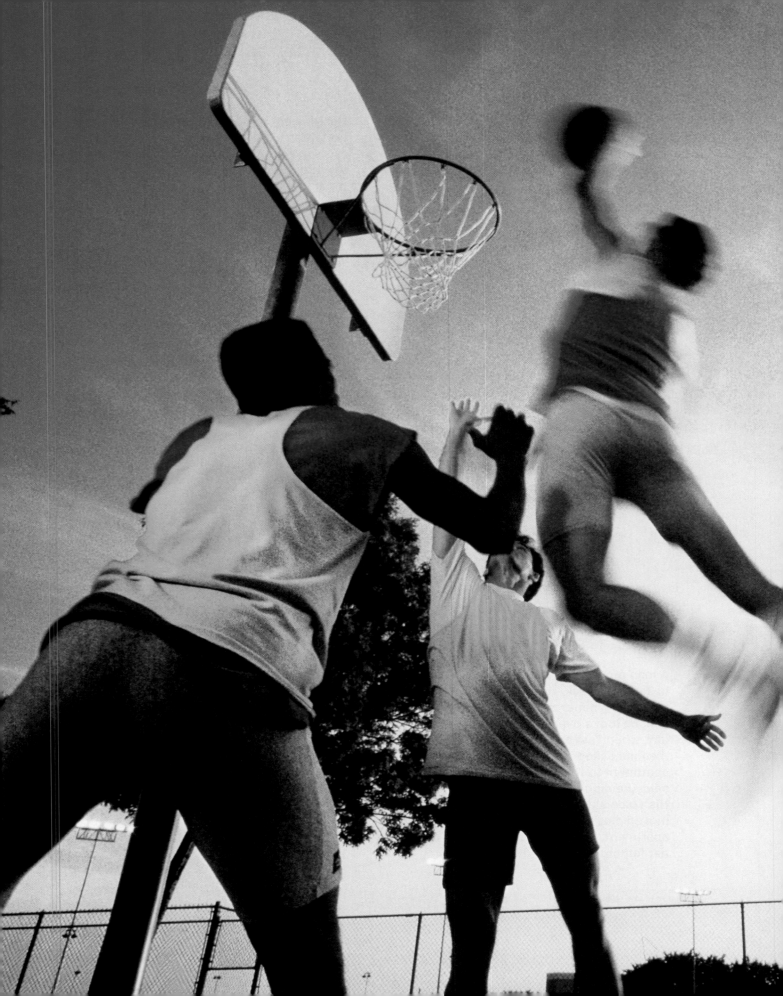

UNIT 2
Health and Your Body

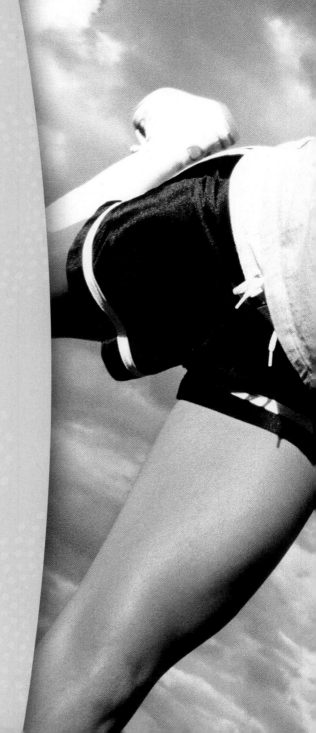

Physical Fitness for Life

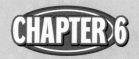

What's Your Health IQ?
KNOWLEDGE

Which of the following statements are true, and which are false? Check your answers on p. 642.

1. To gain the benefits of exercise, you must exercise every day.

2. Exercise can help improve depression.

3. Girls will develop large, manly muscles if they lift weights.

4. Lifting weights develops cardiorespiratory endurance.

5. The longer and harder you train, the better your health will be.

6. Anabolic steroids are illegal drugs.

7. Teens need more sleep than their younger siblings or their parents need.

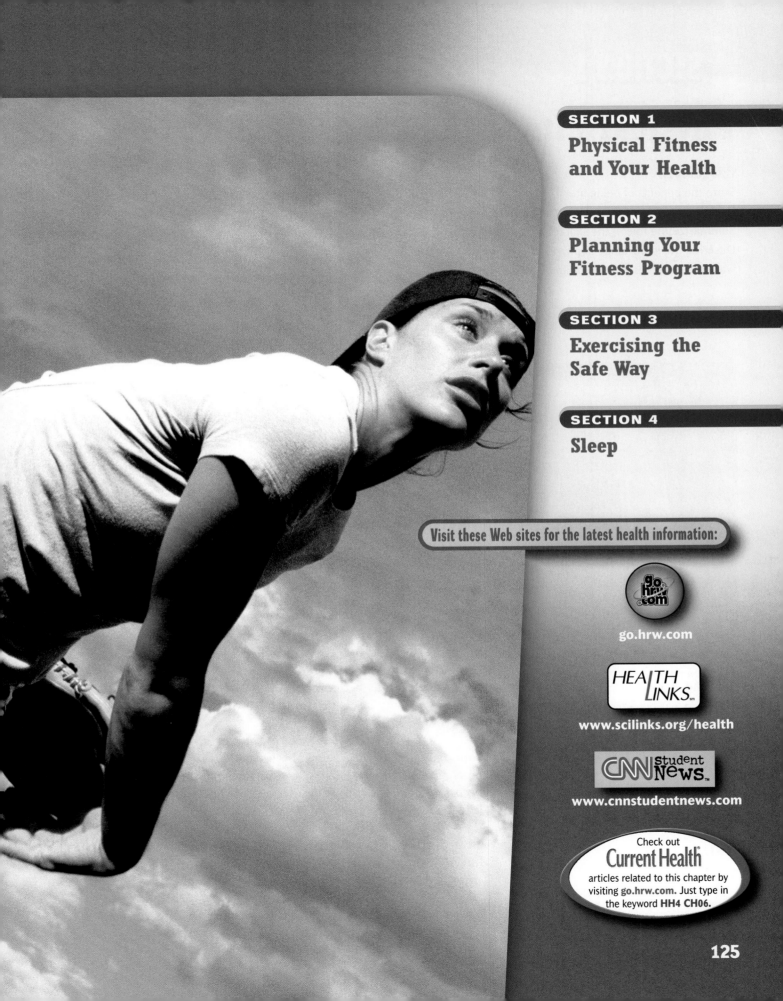

Visit these Web sites for the latest health information:

go.hrw.com

HEALTH LINKSsm

www.scilinks.org/health

CNN student News™

www.cnnstudentnews.com

Check out **Current Health** articles related to this chapter by visiting go.hrw.com. Just type in the keyword **HH4 CH06.**

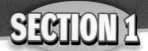

Physical Fitness and Your Health

OBJECTIVES

State the benefits of being fit.

Describe the five health-related components of physical fitness.

Summarize the role of the skill-related fitnesses.

Describe the importance of physical fitness for all ages and abilities.

Name three things you can do to be a good sport. **LIFE SKILL**

KEY TERMS

physical fitness the ability of the body to perform daily physical activities without getting out of breath, sore, or overly tired

chronic disease a disease that develops gradually and continues over a long period of time

health-related fitness fitness qualities that are necessary to maintain and promote a healthy body

resting heart rate (RHR) the number of times the heart beats per minute while at rest

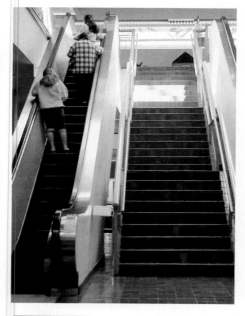

Figure 1

Adding physical activity to your daily life can be easy.

ACTIVITY *How could these people add more physical activity to their daily lives?*

"**M**iracle Life anti-aging pills will keep you feeling young and give you more energy, guaranteed!" You've probably seen or heard ads just like this. The makers of such products claim to have the secret to a long healthy life. Well, the secret is out, and as you'll discover, it's not really much of a secret.

The Benefits of Being Fit

Part of the answer to living a long, healthy life is to be physically fit. **Physical fitness** is the ability of the body to carry out daily physical activities without getting out of breath, sore, or overly tired. Regular physical activity leads to a physically fit body.

A certain amount of physical activity every day has been shown to keep you healthy and lowers your risk of certain diseases. As shown in **Figure 1,** many modern conveniences, such as escalators, cars, computers, and even TV remote controls, have reduced the need for us to be physically active in our daily lives. An overall reduction in the daily activity levels of children, teens, and adults has led to an increasingly unfit population.

Exercise is an excellent way of keeping a high level of activity in your daily life. *Exercise* is any physical activity that improves or maintains physical fitness. Exercise can be a formal set of activities or can be informal play. However, other everyday activities, such as raking leaves and walking to school, can also help keep you fit.

Stay Active, Stay Alive Having a sedentary lifestyle has been linked to an increased risk of developing many illnesses, such as chronic diseases. A **chronic disease** is a disease that develops gradually and continues over a long period of time. A chronic disease can take a long time to treat. Examples of chronic diseases related to lifestyle include cardiovascular (heart) disease, stroke, high blood pressure, type 2 diabetes, and certain forms of cancer. Staying fit through regular exercise has been shown to be a significant factor in preventing the development of some of these chronic diseases.

Physical Benefits Staying fit also has many physical benefits. Most people feel that exercising improves their appearance and makes them feel good about themselves. Exercise also leads to many improvements within your body.

▶ The heart and lungs get stronger, allowing more blood and oxygen to circulate around the body.

▶ Blood cholesterol levels are kept within a healthy range, and blood vessels are kept strong and healthy.

▶ Building muscular strength and endurance and also flexibility of our joints makes our muscles more efficient at controlling our movements and protects against back injuries.

▶ A good ratio of muscle mass to fat mass is maintained.

▶ Metabolic rate is increased. Your metabolic rate is the rate at which your body converts food energy into the energy that keeps you alive.

▶ More Calories are burned because of an increase in muscle mass.

Being fit can increase your enjoyment of life!

Social Benefits
Regular exercise can be a great way to meet people.

Mental Benefits
Exercise can help
▶ reduce anxiety
▶ reduce depression
▶ increase self-confidence
▶ improve self-image

Healthy coronary arteries

Blocked coronary artery

Physical Benefits
Being fit helps prevent the high blood cholesterol levels and coronary plaque buildup that can lead to a heart attack.

Mental Benefits   Many people use regular exercise as a way to feel good mentally. Regular exercise has positive effects on feelings of depression and anxiety. Exercise can help reduce your stress levels and help you sleep better. How? Exercise takes your mind off of your worries and causes the release of certain body chemicals called *endorphins* (en DAWR finz). Endorphins can give you a feeling of wellness and happiness after a good, hard workout. Increased oxygen to the brain during exercise can help you feel more alert. This in turn helps you feel more energized and better able to deal with day-to-day tasks.

Social Benefits   Many people feel increased self-esteem as they exercise to stay fit. Part of this feeling is a result of the positive body changes that occur because of exercise. As a result of the increased self-esteem, such people are more likely to socialize with others.

Engaging in physical activity is also an opportunity to socialize with others who have the same interests. Working together on a team can help you develop your communication skills. It also gives you a chance to interact with many different people of differing abilities.

Five Components of Health-Related Fitness

Physical fitness can be classified into five components. These are commonly called *health-related components of fitness*. **Health-related fitness** describes qualities that are needed to maintain and promote a healthy body. The five components of health-related fitness are muscular strength, muscular endurance, cardiorespiratory endurance, flexibility, and body composition.

Muscular Strength   Muscles move and apply force to objects and to each other by contracting. *Muscular strength* is the amount of force that a muscle can apply in a given contraction. Lifting a weight, climbing the stairs, and pushing a large piece of furniture are acts of muscular strength. During weight (or resistance) training, muscles are challenged to contract more than they are used to doing. The muscle cells themselves become larger in response to this extra work. This growth increases the overall strength of the muscle.

Muscular Endurance   *Muscular endurance* is the ability of the muscles to keep working (contract) over a period of time. Muscular endurance allows you to carry out tasks that require muscles to remain contracted for a period of time. Examples of sports that require good muscular endurance include cross-country skiing and gymnastics. Muscular strength and endurance are closely related; as one improves, the other improves. Both muscular strength and muscular endurance can be developed by regular weight training.

Weight training is considered to be an anaerobic activity. During *anaerobic activity*, muscle cells produce energy without using oxygen. Anaerobic activity is intense and short in duration.

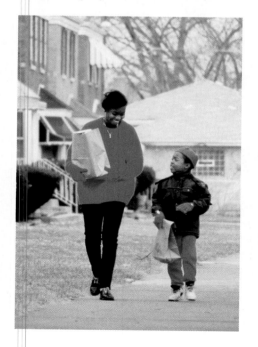

Good muscular strength and endurance are important, even for small, everyday activities.

Cardiorespiratory Endurance

Cardiorespiratory endurance (KAHR dee oh RES puhr uh TAWR ee en DOOR uhns) is the ability of your heart, blood vessels, lungs, and blood to deliver oxygen and nutrients to all of your body's cells while you are being physically active. It is the single most important component of health-related fitness. As your cardiorespiratory endurance increases, your heart beats slower and stronger. An indicator of poor cardiorespiratory endurance is running out of breath while doing strenuous activity.

Resting heart rate and recovery time are indicators of your level of cardiorespiratory endurance. **Resting heart rate (RHR)** is the number of times the heart beats per minute while at rest, such as just before you get up from a good night's sleep. *Recovery time* is the amount of time it takes for the heart to return to RHR after strenuous activity. Good cardiorespiratory endurance reduces recovery time and RHR.

Aerobic activity tends to improve your cardiorespiratory endurance. During *aerobic activity*, muscle cells use oxygen to produce energy for movement. The intensity of aerobic exercise is low enough so that the heart, lungs, blood vessels, and blood are all able to bring enough oxygen to your muscles. This allows your heart and muscles to continue with the activity for a long period of time (at least 20 to 60 minutes). Aerobic activity is continuous, uses large muscle groups, and tends to be rhythmic in nature. Examples include walking, jogging, dancing, swimming, cycling, and jumping rope.

Flexibility

Flexibility is the ability of the joints to move through their full range of motion. Good flexibility keeps joint movements smooth and efficient. Strong and healthy ligaments and tendons allow greater flexibility of a joint. Ligaments are the tissues that hold bones together at a joint. Tendons are the tissues that join muscles to bones. Any activity that involves a joint moving through a full range of motion will help maintain flexibility. As shown in **Figure 2,** stretching exercises, when done correctly, improve flexibility.

Having good flexibility alone is not the most important component of physical fitness. However, keeping a good level of flexibility is important because lack of use can cause joints to become stiffer as you become older.

Together with muscular strength and muscular endurance, flexibility is very important for overall fitness. These three components promote the health of bones and muscles.

Body Composition

Body composition refers to the ratio of lean body tissue (muscle and bone) to body-fat tissue. A healthy body has a high proportion of lean body tissue compared to body-fat tissue. Women have more body fat than men do. Also, body fat increases with age as muscle mass decreases.

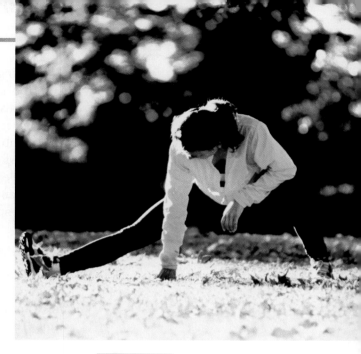

Figure 2

Maintaining good flexibility through regular stretching as a part of warm-ups and cool-downs can reduce the risk of muscle tears, strains, and stress injuries.

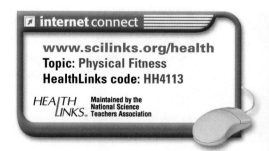

internet connect

www.scilinks.org/health
Topic: Physical Fitness
HealthLinks code: HH4113

HEALTH LINKS. Maintained by the National Science Teachers Association

Having a certain amount of fat is necessary for good health. However, too much body fat increases the risk of getting certain lifestyle-related diseases, such as diabetes and cardiovascular disease. Excess body fat is almost always due to being inactive as well as having poor eating habits. Also, because of the stress of excess weight on the joints, people who have excess body fat are more likely than people who do not have excess body fat to have joint problems and back pain. Regular exercise and good eating habits are the best ways to develop a favorable body composition.

Skills Developed by Fitness

Skill-related fitness describes components of fitness that are important for good athletic performance. The six components of skill-related fitness are coordination, balance, agility, power, speed, and reaction time. The components of skill-related fitness are not as important for developing health as the health-related fitness components are. However, skill-related components are important for good athletic performance. For example, agility, coordination, and power are important in sports such as basketball, karate, football, and soccer. Athletic training concentrates on developing components of skill-related fitness.

Sport and Fitness

A great way to achieve total physical fitness is to get involved in an organized sport. Organized sports allow you to improve your social and communication skills and to interact with people of different abilities. Taking part in sports such as hiking, fishing, or camping will also enable you to explore the natural environment.

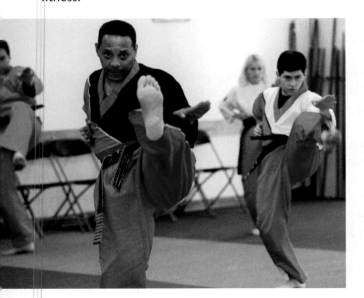

Total fitness can be achieved by taking part in an activity or sport to improve both health-related and skill-related fitness.

What Sport Can You Do?   Sports are not limited to athletes. What sport you enjoy or choose to participate in is up to you. You should consider several things when deciding what sport to take part in.

▶ Do you want to improve your abilities in a sport you have tried in the past or try something completely new?

▶ Do you want to participate in an individual sport or a team sport? Individual sports are suited to people who enjoy one-on-one competition. Team sports allow you to interact with many people at one time. Working as a team helps develop problem-solving and conflict-resolution skills.

▶ What activities are available in your area? Go to your local community center or youth club, and find out what activities are offered. Also, your school may have after-school activity programs that you can join.

▶ What facilities do you need? If facilities such as a pool are needed, make sure they are easy for you to get to.

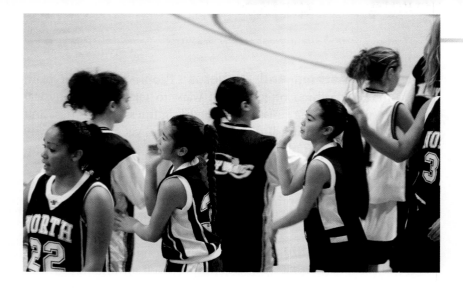

Tips on Being a Good Sport

▶ **Be a gracious winner.** Don't purposely make the other team members feel like losers.

▶ **Be mannerly.** Thank the competing team or individual for a good game when the game is over.

▶ **Be a good loser.** Accept that you will win some and you will lose some.

▶ **Show respect for others' abilities.** Never use foul or abusive language.

▶ **Assume some responsibility.** Do not blame others or their performance if you lose. You are part of a team.

▶ **Be a good fan.** Cheer—don't jeer.

▶ **Above all, remember it is all just for fun!**

Sport and Competition Competition takes different forms—from the informal games between friends to formal competition with official rules and referees or umpires. Whether you compete in informal or formal play, competition will help develop your motivation, leadership, and cooperation skills. These are life skills that will help you in many areas of your daily life. Competition can also be valuable for the enjoyment you can get from just taking part in a sport.

Be a Good Sport To have winners, there must be losers. Losing competitors will naturally be disappointed at the loss. Likewise, winning teams have the right to be excited and proud. However, winning is never an excuse to be inconsiderate or hurtful to the losing team or individual.

Rules and regulations are meant to encourage fair play between competitors. Obeying and respecting game officials' decisions in any sport is necessary for fair play. Few coaches will tolerate disrespect on the field. Being removed from the game will hurt only yourself and your team's chances in competition.

Physical Fitness Is for Everyone

It is never too early for you to develop a healthy lifestyle of lifelong physical activity. However, the benefits of maintaining fitness can be obtained only through a lifetime commitment to regular exercise.

A Lifetime of Physical Fitness Even though a person may begin suffering from cardiovascular disease at the age of 60, he or she likely began to develop the disease at a much earlier age. By beginning good habits in your early years and making a commitment to lifelong activity, you can delay or even prevent some of the chronic diseases associated with growing older. Frequent strength training may help prevent the bone-thinning disease osteoporosis (AHS tee oh puh ROH sis) in later life. Strength training even at an older age will help maintain bone density, muscle tone, muscle strength and endurance, and flexibility. The lifestyle choices you make now will affect your health for the rest of your life.

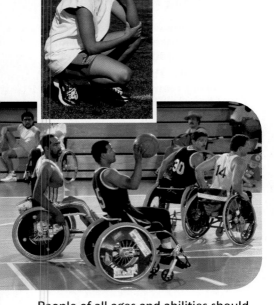

People of all ages and abilities should take part in regular physical activity to reduce their risks of chronic diseases and to help them feel their best.

Fitness and Asthma and Diabetes People who suffer from exercise-induced asthma often do not want to take part in physical activity or sport. Asthma causes a feeling of tightness in the chest and can cause coughing during and after exercise. And yet, physical activity is part of the treatment plan for people who have asthma. Gaining fitness helps decrease the severity of asthma symptoms. Exercise is also a very important part of the treatment plan for people who have diabetes because exercise helps control blood sugar levels. Exercise can also help with weight problems that are often associated with diabetes.

Fitness and Disability Have you ever thought about how you could dribble a basketball while steering yourself around in a wheelchair? How could you sprint 100 meters with an artificial leg? Many individuals have taken on the challenges of physical and mental disabilities and have become great athletes.

The Special Olympics and Paralympics show us that mental and physical disabilities do not stop people from becoming world-class athletes. The *Special Olympics* is an organization that enables and encourages people who are learning disabled to become physically fit. The organization also encourages such people to become more involved in society through sports training and competition. The *Paralympics* are Olympic-style games for athletes with physical disabilities.

No matter what your age or abilities are, being physically active—whether it is done through an exercise program, an organized sport, or just your everyday activity—is of great value to everyone. So, in short, part of the answer to a longer, healthier life is to be active!

SECTION 1

REVIEW *Answer the following questions on a separate piece of paper.*

Using Key Terms

1. **Name** the term that means "the ability of the body to carry out daily activities without getting out of breath, sore, or overly tired."

2. **Identify** which condition is *not* a chronic disease.
   a. diabetes   c. heart disease
   b. cancer   d. cold

3. **Identify** the single most important component of health-related fitness.
   a. muscular strength
   b. body composition
   c. cardiorespiratory endurance
   d. muscular endurance

4. **Define** *resting heart rate*.

Understanding Key Ideas

5. **List** six benefits of being fit.

6. **Name** a health-related component of fitness and a sport that develops that component.

7. **Contrast** the functions of health-related components and skill-related components of fitness.

8. **Name** one common disease for which physical activity can be part of the treatment.

9. **LIFE SKILL** **Communicating Effectively** Identify four ways you can show you are a good sport.

Critical Thinking

10. **LIFE SKILL** **Practicing Wellness** Discuss the statement "Physical activity can actually prevent you from having a heart attack."

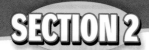

Planning Your Fitness Program

OBJECTIVES

Describe the important factors to think about before starting a fitness program.

Describe the steps involved in designing a fitness program.

Calculate your resting heart rate, target heart rate zone, and maximum heart rate.

Evaluate the use of the FITT formula in fitness training.

Design and implement a personal fitness program and set your fitness goals. **LIFE SKILL**

KEY TERMS

target heart rate zone a heart rate range that should be reached during exercise to gain cardiorespiratory health benefits

FITT a formula made up of four important parts involved in fitness training: **f**requency, **i**ntensity, **t**ime, and **t**ype of exercise

repetitions the number of times an exercise is performed

set a fixed number of repetitions followed by a rest period

Maria's mom has heart disease. Maria has done some research and believes she could develop heart disease, too. Maria also read that regular exercise can help lower her chance of developing heart disease. Now she's determined to become more fit, but she's not sure where to start.

Getting Started with Your Fitness Program

You don't have to be an athlete to be physically fit, and you do not have to be fit to start a fitness program. Before you start any fitness program, however, there are many factors you should consider.

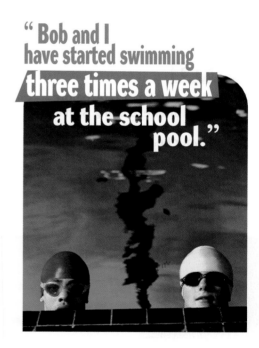

"Bob and I have started swimming three times a week at the school pool."

▶ **Do you have any health concerns, such as diabetes or asthma?** Be sure to consult your doctor about your program if you do have health concerns.

▶ **Are you healthy enough to start a program?** You should schedule a physical examination with your doctor. Your doctor will be able to assess your level of health. He or she will check your heart rate, blood pressure, height, weight, and reflexes and may also check any health concerns you have.

▶ **What types of activities do you enjoy?** Be sure to choose activities that fit into your schedule and that won't bore you easily. Ask a friend to join you.

▶ **How much will your planned activities cost?** Cost is something to think about before choosing an activity. Many fitness activities such as walking or jogging do not require expensive clothing or shoes. However, for activities that require special equipment, you should rent or borrow the equipment from a reliable source. This will allow you to decide if you like the activity before you buy your own equipment. A little research may save you money and time in the long run.

Getting FITT

After you choose an activity you may still have many questions, such as, How many times per week should I do the activity? How hard should the activity be? How long should each workout take? The FITT formula can be used as a helpful guide to answer these questions.

The **FITT** formula is made up of four important parts of fitness training: *frequency*, *intensity*, *time*, and *type*. For exercise to be effective, it must be done enough times per week (*frequency*), hard enough (*intensity*), and for long enough (*time*). Finally, the kind (*type*) of exercise is important. The FITT formula recommendations differ slightly for each health-related component of fitness. **Figure 4** presents many types of activities that develop the health-related components and identifies the frequency with which each activity needs to be done.

Developing Your Cardiorespiratory Endurance
Recommendations for cardiorespiratory fitness are as follows:
- ▶ **Frequency** Exercise must be performed three to five times a week.
- ▶ **Intensity** If you are training at 85 percent of your MHR, 20 minutes per session is enough. If you are training at 50 to 60 percent of your MHR, 60 minutes of training per session is needed to gain health benefits.

Figure 4

The Activity Pyramid can help you develop your fitness program. If you are currently sedentary, begin at the top of the pyramid (everyday activities) and gradually increase your level of activity. If you are already pretty active, you can increase the amount of time you spend doing physical activities.

The Activity Pyramid

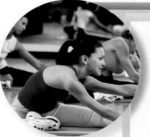
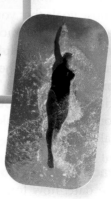
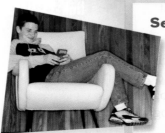

Household and recreational activities
(every day)

walking the dog, gardening, cleaning your room, soccer, sweeping the floor, hiking, dancing, golf, walking or cycling to the store

Muscular strength and endurance, and flexibility
(2 to 5 times a week)

push-ups, curl-ups, ballet, stretching, martial arts, yoga

Cardiorespiratory endurance
(3 to 5 times a week)

swimming, tennis, running, gym aerobics, jumping rope, aerobic dance

Sedentary activities
(seldom)

watching TV, playing computer games, talking on the phone

▶ **Time** Twenty to sixty minutes per session is recommended, depending on the intensity of the exercise. Intensity means how hard your heart is working and how difficult the activity is to do. The higher the intensity of the exercise, the less time you need to do it.

▶ **Type** Any aerobic activity that keeps heart rate within your target heart rate zone is good.

Developing Your Muscles Muscular strength and muscular endurance are closely related. As one improves, so does the other. Training programs are designed to address each of these health related components. FITT recommendations that address muscular development are as follows:

▶ **Frequency** Weight train 2 to 3 times a week.

▶ **Intensity** Select a weight that you can lift at least 8 times but no more than 12 times. The weight being lifted is called the *resistance*. Each lift is called a repetition. **Repetitions** are the number of times an exercise is repeated. A fixed number of repetitions

> There is no difference between the same amount of male muscle and female muscle in terms of strength.

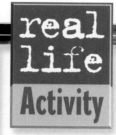

real life Activity

DEVELOP YOUR FITNESS PLAN

LIFE SKILL
Setting Goals

Materials

✔ paper
✔ pencil
✔ ruler

Procedure

1. **Draw** a table that has seven columns. Title the table "Activity Plan for the Week." Label the columns with the days of the week.

2. **Write** your fitness goal below the table. For example, you might write, "I want to run a 5 kilometer race in under 30 minutes."

3. **Create** a week of activities that are based on developing the five components of physical fitness. Remember to include at least 60 minutes of activity daily.

Conclusions

1. **Summarizing Results** What resources in your community can you use to carry out your fitness plan?

2. **Applying Information** Describe how your fitness plan will help you reach your goal.

3. **CRITICAL THINKING** Develop ways to address possible barriers to your training program, such as bad weather, expensive equipment, or lack of time.

4. **CRITICAL THINKING** Identify ways you can assess your progress.

5. **CRITICAL THINKING** How can you reward yourself for following your plan?

Activity Plan for the

Mon.	Tue.	Wed.

Tips to Keep You Motivated

▶ **Look at it as down time. Training can be the perfect "time out" from a busy day.**

▶ **Train with a friend. A training partner will keep you company and may introduce some healthy competition.**

▶ **Set realistic goals. Make a contract for yourself, and reward yourself often for sticking with your program.**

▶ **Understand that you'll have bad days. When you don't reach a day's workout goals do not be discouraged—just start up again the next day.**

▶ **Keep the appointment. Consider your workout an important appointment that you cannot miss, and you'll be more likely to keep to it.**

followed by a rest period is called a **set.** Rest periods between sets are between 1 and 3 minutes long. Do one to three sets of 8 to 12 repetitions for all the major muscle groups.

▶ **Time** A total workout can be about 30 minutes long but should not be longer than 60 minutes.

▶ **Type** Anaerobic activities such as weight lifting and sit-ups tend to develop muscular strength and endurance. To build muscular endurance, you lift lighter weights (less resistance) with more (8 to 15) repetitions. To build strength, you should lift heavier weights (more resistance) with fewer (3 to 8) repetitions.

Increasing Your Flexibility   The following are FITT recommendations for flexibility:

▶ **Frequency** Perform stretching 3 to 5 days a week. For the best results, stretch daily.

▶ **Intensity** Stretch muscles, and hold at a comfortable stretch for about 15 to 30 seconds. Relax into the stretch, and as you breath out, you will stretch a little further. Never bounce as you stretch. Repeat each stretch three to five times.

▶ **Time** Stretch for 15 to 30 minutes.

▶ **Type** Stretching can be done on its own or as part of a warm-up and cool-down. Yoga is also a popular form of flexibility exercise.

When Will I See Changes?   The length of time it takes to see a difference varies from person to person. On average, it takes about 6 weeks to really notice the difference in the health-related components. So, don't get discouraged!

SECTION 2

REVIEW   *Answer the following questions on a separate piece of paper.*

Using Key Terms

1. **Define** the term *target heart rate zone.*

2. **List** the four parts of fitness training that FITT stands for.

3. **Name** the term that refers to the number of times an exercise is performed.

4. **Identify** the term that means "a fixed number of repetitions followed by a rest period."
   a. frequency   c. repetition
   b. intensity   d. set

Understanding Key Ideas

5. **List** the important things to consider before beginning a fitness program.

6. **Summarize** the steps to designing a fitness program.

7. **List** the steps of how to calculate your target heart rate zone.

8. **Identify** what each letter of the acronym FITT means in relation to a fitness plan.

Critical Thinking

9. **LIFE SKILL** **Practicing Wellness** Is it a good idea to do both aerobic exercises and anaerobic exercises as parts of a fitness program? Explain.

10. Why is it important to monitor your heart rate before, during, and after exercising or training.

Exercising the Safe Way

OBJECTIVES

Describe six ways to avoid sport injuries.

Identify four signs of overtraining.

Describe the RICE method of treating minor sports injuries.

State the dangers posed by the use of performance enhancing drugs.

Summarize the importance of wearing safety equipment to prevent sports injuries. **LIFE SKILL**

KEY TERMS

dehydration a state in which the body has lost more water than has been taken in

overtraining a condition that occurs as a result of exceeding the recommendations of the FITT formula

dietary supplement any product that is taken by mouth that can contain a dietary ingredient and is also labeled as a dietary supplement

anabolic steroid a synthetic version of the male hormone testosterone used for promoting muscle development

"An ounce of prevention is worth a pound of cure." These words are cold comfort to someone who has pulled a muscle or strained a tendon. However, most sports injuries are easy to prevent.

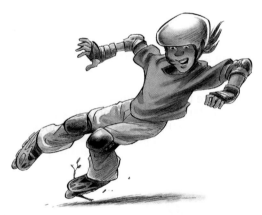

Avoiding Sports Injuries

The most common sports injuries are injuries to muscles, tendons, ligaments, and bones. These injuries are classified as either acute—having a sudden onset and short duration—or chronic—having a gradual onset and long-term effects.

Most acute injuries are minor bumps and scrapes that heal quickly and don't require much treatment. However, some acute injuries are more serious. Prompt medical attention is always required for a serious injury such as a fracture or concussion. Chronic injuries can take months or even years to treat.

Beliefs Vs. Reality

"No pain, no gain."	Exercise can sometimes be uncomfortable but should never be painful. Pain means injury.
"Doing two or three 30-minute cardiovascular workouts a day will help me lose those extra pounds."	Not allowing your body to rest between training sessions will cause injury. Also, it is wise to review your eating habits as part of any fitness program.
"Working out in heavy sweats will help burn fat quicker."	Wearing excess clothing during a workout increases water loss and the chance of heat exhaustion or even heatstroke.

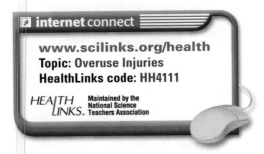
This damage results in chronic injury. Continued stress on the tissue can lead to weakness, loss of flexibility, and chronic pain.

Overuse injuries are becoming more common in adolescents, particularly in adolescents who are gymnasts, runners, or swimmers. Children and adolescents are very prone to overuse injuries because their bones are still growing. Damage to growing bones and other tissues can cause lifelong weakness and loss of flexibility. Treatment of overuse injuries should include resting the injured site, applying ice or heat as required, and undergoing physical therapy and rehabilitation to rebuild strength and flexibility at the site of injury.

Choose the Correct Equipment and Clothing

▶ **Wear comfortable clothing.** Your clothing should allow free movement of your body. Choose fabrics that draw moisture away from the skin.

▶ **Dress suitably for the weather and exercise intensity.** Many thin layers together insulate better than one or two thick layers. In cold weather, wear thin layers that can be removed if you get too warm. Wearing a brimmed hat, sunscreen, and sunglasses are musts when exercising outdoors, even in winter!

▶ **Always wear safety equipment, and wear it correctly.** Get training or advice from a reliable person on the correct use and fit of safety equipment.

▶ **Choose shoes that are made for your activity.** Good shoes play a very important role in preventing injury. However, you do not need an expensive pair of shoes unless you are training a lot or have a diagnosed foot problem. Ask for advice from a person who works in a specialty shoe store.

▶ **Make sure you can be seen.** Wear bright, reflective clothing if training at night.

▶ **Obey laws, regulations, and warning signs.** Ignoring these could lead to injury or even death.

Treating Minor Sports Injuries

Most injuries, regardless of type, have one thing in common: swelling. Swelling causes pressure in the injured area, and this increase in pressure causes pain. You must quickly control swelling because swelling slows down the healing process.

Apply the RICE principle to control swelling: rest, ice, compression, and elevation. As shown in **Table 2,** the RICE principle can be applied to both acute and chronic injuries.

▶ **Rest** It is important to protect the injured muscle, ligament, tendon, or other tissue from further injury.

▶ **Ice** Apply ice bags or cold packs to the injured site, and leave the ice on the injured site for no longer than 15 to 20 minutes. Leaving ice on any longer or placing ice directly on the skin can damage the skin.

Rest
Ice
Compression
Elevation

The RICE technique is used for the early treatment of sports-related injuries. RICE plays a critical role in limiting swelling.

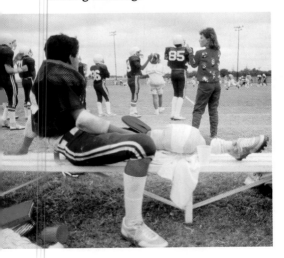

▶ **Compression** Compression reduces swelling. Wrap a cloth bandage around the affected area. If you feel a throbbing or the bandage is too tight, remove the bandage and reapply it.

▶ **Elevation** Raising the injured site above heart level when possible can help reduce swelling.

Medical advice must be sought immediately if there is unconsciousness or persistent pain or bleeding. It would be a wise decision to get certified in first aid so that you can confidently and correctly treat an injury until you get to a doctor or hospital.

Recovery from Injury The RICE principle is applied as first aid when an injury occurs, but it is also useful during recovery. Muscles in an injured limb lose strength and flexibility when they are not used. Rehabilitation is the process of regaining strength and coordination during recovery from an injury. Returning to activity before an injury is fully healed and rehabilitated puts you at risk of reinjury. Therefore you should always let an injury completely heal before attempting any activity that may stress the injured site. However, to keep doing activities that do not stress the injury is also important.

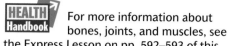 For more information about bones, joints, and muscles, see the Express Lesson on pp. 592–593 of this text.

Table 2 Common Injuries and Treatments

Injury	Cause	Treatment
Sunburn (acute)	overexposure of the skin to ultraviolet (UV) rays in sunlight	drinking plenty of fluids; applying light moisturizer; prevention-wearing sunscreen and protective clothing
Tendon and muscle strain (acute)	overstretching or over contraction of muscles causes muscle fibers or tendons to tear	rest and immobilization (a mildly pulled muscle can recover in as little as a week; tendons can take longer)
Ligament sprain (acute)	forcing a joint to move beyond its normal limits can cause ligament fibers to tear	RICE and strengthening of the muscles and tendons around the joint through rehabilitation
Fracture (acute)	extreme stress and strain causes cracks in bone	immediate medical attention; rest and immobilization for 6 to 8 weeks
Heat exhaustion (acute)	training in hot or humid weather; extreme dehydration	immediate medical attention; moving to a shady spot, drinking plenty of cool water, and applying cool water to body
Concussion (acute)	a blow to the head, face, or jaw that causes the brain to be shaken in the skull	rest under observation; immediate medical attention if there is unconsciousness, vomiting, a seizure, or a change in the size of the pupils
Tendinitis (chronic)	inflammation of a tendon due to trauma or overuse	RICE (healing can take from 6 to 8 weeks); apply heat after 36 to 48 hours if swelling is gone
Stress fracture (chronic)	repeated stress or overuse causes tiny fractures in the bone	RICE and sometimes immobilization; female athletes with a stress fracture may need a bone scan
Shin splint (chronic)	straining of muscles that are attached to the shin bone	RICE; applying ice several times a day; strengthening of the lower leg muscles

Supplements, Drugs, and Athletic Performance

Some athletes feel that taking dietary supplements or drugs gives them a competitive edge. A **dietary supplement** is any product that is taken by mouth that can contain a dietary ingredient, and is also labeled as a dietary supplement. Makers of these supplements can claim that their dietary supplement helps improve athletic performance. For example, some protein supplements are advertised as helping to increase muscle mass. **Table 3** summarizes some common ingredients of dietary supplements and drugs used by some athletes.

Dietary Supplements   Supplements are not regulated by the Food and Drug Administration (FDA). Makers of these products can make claims for their product without any scientific proof. The strength of a supplement can vary widely. Claims that dietary supplements improve performance are often based on improvements that are the result of training, not a result of taking supplements. Some supplements that contain non-nutrient ingredients, such as caffeine, ephedrine, andro, or GBL, may have dangerous side effects or are banned by certain athletic associations. Athletes and non athletes who have a wholesome well-balanced diet do not need such supplements.

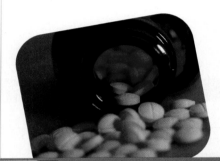

Table 3 Common Supplement Ingredients and Drugs

Name	How does it affect the body?	Dangers
Caffeine	a central nervous system stimulant that makes you feel awake and alert	raises blood pressure and heart rate if used in excess; affects sleep, mood, and behavior; can lead to dehydration by increasing urination
Amphetamines	mask fatigue, increase sense of well-being and mental alertness	raise blood pressure, increase aggressiveness, increase risk of injury, and circulatory collapse (shock)
Ephedrine (ephedra, ma huang)	stimulates the brain and nervous system, increases alertness, and may mask signs of fatigue	may lead to abnormal heartbeat, dizziness, psychiatric episodes, and seizures
Adrenal androgens (includes DHEA and Andro)	claimed to increase muscle strength and improve athletic performance when taken as a supplement	can cause behavioral, sexual, and reproductive problems; causes liver damage, muscle disorders, and increased risk of heart disease; can stunt growth in teens
Gamma-butyrolactone (GBL)	claimed to induce sleep, release growth hormone, increase athletic performance, and relieve stress	can cause vomiting, an increase in aggression, tremors, slow heartbeat, seizures, breathing difficulties, and coma
Anabolic steroids	increase muscle size and strength	increase aggressive behavior, cholesterol levels, and risk of kidney tumors; can cause severe acne, testicular shrinkage, liver cysts, and fatal damage to heart muscle; can stunt growth in teens

Anabolic Steroids Anabolic steroids are synthetic compounds that resemble the male hormone *testosterone*. Doctors use small amounts of anabolic steroids to treat some conditions, such as muscle disease, kidney disease, and breast cancer. Men normally produce about 2.5 to 11 mg of testosterone a day. A steroid abuser may take as much as 100 mg a day.

Despite the harmful effects of anabolic steroids and the fact that abusing them is illegal, many men, women, and teens use them. It is estimated that more than a million male and female athletes are taking or have taken anabolic steroids. Reported effects for females include excessive growth of facial and body hair, baldness, increased risk of cancer, and menstrual problems.

These effects are in addition to the side effects that affect both males and females that are listed in **Table 3**. Nevertheless, the incidence of steroid use among high school athletes is estimated to be 6 to 11 percent. Many athletes who abuse anabolic steroids start using the drugs as early as age 15.

Playing It Safe!

Exercising is a great way to stay physically fit. If you follow the basic rules to avoid sport injuries and avoid supplements and drugs, you will find out how much fun it can be to exercise and be fit.

In addition, remember to exercise or train in open areas that have good lighting, bring a friend, and always let someone know where you'll be and what time you'll return.

MAKING GREAT DECISIONS

A close friend of yours has always been into bodybuilding and weight lifting. Over the last few months, he has not been doing well in his competitions. He has a few friends who have suggested that taking a steroid will give him a competitive edge and will put him back on top.

Write on a separate piece of paper the advice that you would give your friend. Remember to use the decision-making steps.

Give thought to the problem.
Review your choices.
Evaluate the consequences of each choice.
Assess and choose the best choice.
Think it over afterward.

SECTION 3

REVIEW *Answer the following questions on a separate piece of paper.*

Using Key Terms

1. **Identify** the term for "a state in which the body has lost more water than has been taken in."
   a. chronic injury
   b. dehydration
   c. overtraining
   d. testosterone

2. **Define** *overtraining*.

3. **Define** what an anabolic steroid is.

Understanding Key Ideas

4. **Identify** three ways to prevent sports injuries.

5. **Describe** how overtraining can lead to chronic injury.

6. **State** why it is important to follow the RICE steps right after an injury.

7. **Evaluate** the statement "All athletes need to take some kind of supplement."

Critical Thinking

8. **LIFE SKILL** **Practicing Wellness** How could wearing the wrong type or size of safety equipment lead to an injury?

9. What advice would you give a friend who started exercising hard every day and whose body now hurts too much to move?

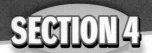

Sleep

OBJECTIVES

Describe why sleep is an important part of your health.

List the effects of sleep deprivation.

Compare how the amount of sleep needed by teens differs from the amount needed by adults or children.

Identify the two different types of sleep.

List three ways that you can improve your sleeping habits. **LIFE SKILL**

KEY TERMS

sleep deprivation a lack of sleep

circadian rhythm the body's internal system for regulating sleeping and waking patterns

insomnia an inability to sleep, even if one is physically exhausted

sleep apnea a sleeping disorder characterized by interruptions of normal breathing patterns during sleep

" **I should have stopped playing video games earlier** last night. "

Can you remember a time when you were so tired that you couldn't concentrate in class? When you are tired, your concentration declines, it's hard to finish your tasks, and you are less able to handle stressful situations.

Sleep: Too Little, Too Often

A recent poll conducted by the National Sleep Foundation, "Sleep in America," found that over 60 percent of adults in the United States experience sleep problems. Sleep is not just a "time out"; it is essential for your health and safety. You need sleep for good health, and you need to get enough of it.

What is sleep, and why do we need it? The answer is not completely clear, but we do know that sleep is needed by the brain. Even mild sleepiness has been shown to hurt all types of performance—in school, sports, and even when playing video games!

Sleep deprivation is a lack of sleep. People who are sleep deprived over a long period of time suffer many problems. For example, they may have the following problems:

▶ **Stress-related problems** Even occasional periods of sleep deprivation can make everyday life seem more stressful and can cause you to be less productive.

▶ **Increased risk for getting sick** Long-term sleep deprivation decreases the body's ability to fight infections.

▶ **Increased risk for dangerous accidents** Sleepiness can cause a lack of concentration and a slow reaction time which can lead to dangerous and even fatal accidents. For example, drowsy driving is a major problem for drivers aged 25 or under.

Getting enough good quality sleep is as important as being physically fit and having good nutrition. The amount of sleep a person needs varies. Most adults need an average of 8 hours of sleep per night. But some adults need as little as 6 hours; others need 10 hours.

Teens and Sleep

Teens need more sleep than their parents and younger siblings do. Teens need about 9 hours and 15 minutes of sleep a night.

Why do teens need more sleep? When puberty takes place, the timing of a teen's circadian rhythm is delayed. The **circadian rhythm** (also known as a circadian clock or body clock) is the body's internal system for regulating sleeping and waking patterns. In general, our circadian rhythm is timed so that we sleep at night and wake during the day. When the rhythm is delayed at puberty, the body naturally wants to go to sleep later at night and wake up later in the morning. So, teens usually have more difficulty falling asleep until late at night and have a little more difficulty waking up early in the morning. Many teenagers are not alert until after the typical high school day has already begun.

The good news is that you can adjust your circadian clocks for the school year. This process may take several weeks but it is worth the time. Adjusting your circadian rhythm to fit your schedule can reduce morning crankiness, make you feel happier, and help you face the day ahead.

Myth

I need only 6 hours of sleep a night.

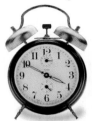

Fact

Teens need between 8.5 and 9.25 hours of sleep every night.

LIFE SKILL Activity

Practicing Wellness

Getting Enough Sleep

Does the following passage sound familiar?

Greg rolled out of bed after hitting the snooze button for the 10th time. As he shuffled out of the room, he turned off the TV—he had left it on all night. His shower woke him up long enough to grab a muffin and get to school. Greg's first class period was a blur. All he could think of was sleeping. After class, he couldn't remember a thing the teacher said. He grabbed a soda from the vending machine to help himself wake up. He had a busy day, but when bedtime arrived, he just couldn't sleep!

You can develop better sleeping habits. Begin by keeping a week-long sleep log that records the following information:

1 The times you go to sleep and wake up

2 The things that affect your sleeping patterns

3 The reasons you cannot fall asleep or do not sleep well

4 The ways in which lack of sleep affects your activities or behaviors during the day

LIFE SKILL Assessing Your Health

1. What patterns did you find from your sleep log?

2. What types of things affect your sleep patterns?

3. Write down three things you can do to improve your sleeping habits.

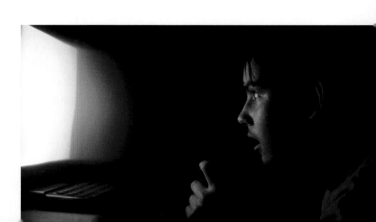

Six Tips for Getting a Good Night's Sleep

1 Develop a routine. Go to bed and get up at the same time, even on weekends!

2 Exercise every day. The best time is in the late afternoon or early evening, but not too close to bedtime.

3 Limit caffeine. After about lunch time, stay away from coffee, colas, or foods with caffeine.

4 Relax. Avoid heavy reading, studying, and computer games within 1 hour of bedtime.

5 Say no to all-nighters. Staying up all night, even to study for an exam, will disturb your sleep pattern and your ability to function the next day.

6 Your bed is for sleep. Do not eat, watch TV, or study in bed.

The Stages of Sleep

While you sleep, your brain and body go through cycles of deep and light sleep. These two types of sleep are called NREM and REM. NREM stands for "nonrapid eye movement," and REM stands for "rapid eye movement."

In the beginning of a sleep cycle, we go into NREM sleep. The body recovers from the stress of the day's activities during this part of the sleep cycle. Brain activity is at its lowest during NREM sleep. The REM portion of the sleep cycle is called *dream sleep*. It first happens about 1.5 hours into sleep. REM sleep got its name from the rapid movement of the eyes during this phase of sleep. During a normal sleep cycle, periods of NREM sleep alternate with periods of REM sleep. Both types of sleep are essential in helping us lead healthy, active lives.

Insomnia and Other Sleep Disorders Sleep deprivation can result from insomnia. **Insomnia** is an inability to sleep, even if one is physically exhausted. Caffeine, alcohol, smoking, stress, and lack of exercise are all common causes of insomnia. Insomnia seems to become more of a problem as we age. Insomnia can often be treated by a simple change in daily habits, such as limiting caffeine late in the day.

Sleep apnea is a serious sleeping disorder in which there are interruptions in normal breathing patterns during sleep. These pauses in breathing can put great stress on the heart. People with sleep apnea can be constantly tired because of nights of disturbed sleep. Sleep apnea is most common in older people and people who are obese. See your doctor if you have sleeping problems for 3 weeks or longer or if you fall asleep during the day.

SECTION 4

REVIEW
Answer the following questions on a separate piece of paper.

Using Key Terms

1. **Name** the term that means "lack of sleep."

2. **Define** *circadian rhythm.*

3. **Identify** the term that means "the inability to fall asleep even if one is physically exhausted."
   a. sleep deprivation   c. circadian rhythm
   b. insomnia   d. sleep apnea

4. **Name** the condition in which a person has an interrupted breathing pattern during sleep.

Understanding Key Ideas

5. **List** the effects of sleep deprivation on your health.

6. **Describe** how sleep deprivation can affect daily life.

7. **Describe** what happens during NREM and REM sleep.

8. **LIFE SKILL** **Assessing Your Health** Which common causes of insomnia can you control? What changes would make the most improvement to your sleep?

Critical Thinking

9. Do you think insomnia can affect teens? Explain.

10. Give reasons why teens need more sleep than adults do.

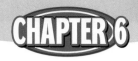

CHAPTER 6

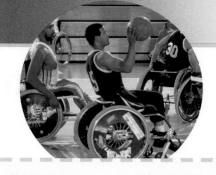

Highlights

Key Terms

The Big Picture

SECTION 1

physical fitness (126)
chronic disease (126)
health-related fitness (128)
resting heart rate (RHR) (129)

✔ Staying physically fit reduces the risk for certain chronic diseases.

✔ There are five components to health-related fitness; muscular endurance, muscular strength, cardiorespiratory endurance, flexibility, and body composition.

✔ Developing skill-related fitness is important for good athletic performance.

✔ People of all ages can benefit from regular physical activity.

SECTION 2

target heart rate zone (134)
FITT (136)
repetitions (137)
set (138)

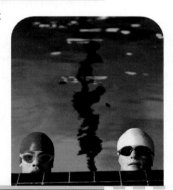

✔ A fitness program must be suited to your abilities, your level of fitness, and your access to facilities and equipment.

✔ Calculating your resting heart rate (RHR) and your target heart rate zone are some of the first steps to designing a fitness program.

✔ Monitoring your heart rate during cardiorespiratory exercise is one of the best ways to monitor the intensity of the activity.

✔ Following the FITT formula can help you develop a safe and effective fitness program.

✔ Setting realistic fitness goals is the foundation of any fitness program.

SECTION 3

dehydration (141)
overtraining (141)
dietary supplement (144)
anabolic steroid (145)

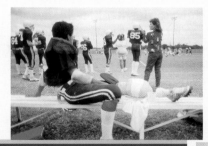

✔ Most sports injuries can be avoided by proper conditioning, warming up and cooling down, stretching, avoiding dehydration, wearing safety equipment, and wearing the correct clothing and shoes.

✔ The damaging effects of overtraining and overuse can be long term.

✔ Most acute injuries should be treated immediately before swelling sets in. Rest, ice, compression, and elevation (RICE) is the most effective treatment.

✔ The usefulness of dietary supplements in improving athletic performance is not scientifically proven. The use of anabolic steroids for enhancing athletic performance is illegal.

SECTION 4

sleep deprivation (146)
circadian rhythm (147)
insomnia (148)
sleep apnea (148)

✔ Sleep deprivation can increase stress, reduce productivity, lead to illness, and cause accidents.

✔ Teens need more sleep that children and adults.

✔ People with normal sleep patterns have a predictable alternating pattern of REM (dream sleep) and NREM (nondreaming) sleep.

✔ Sleeping habits can be improved by making simple dietary changes and by having a quiet, restful place to sleep.

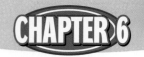

Review

Using Key Terms

anabolic steroid (145)
chronic disease (126)
circadian rhythm (147)
dehydration (141)
dietary supplement (144)
FITT (136)
health-related fitness (128)
insomnia (148)
overtraining (141)
physical fitness (126)

repetitions (137)
resting heart rate (RHR) (129)
set (138)
sleep apnea (148)
sleep deprivation (146)
target heart rate zone (134)

1. For each definition below, choose the key term that best matches the definition.
   a. a fixed number of repetitions followed by a rest period
   b. synthetic form of the male hormone testosterone
   c. a disease that develops over a long period of time and, if treatable, takes a long time to treat
   d. the body's internal "clock"
   e. a formula used to assess how long, how often, and how hard you should exercise
   f. the number of times an exercise is performed

2. Explain the relationship between the key terms in each of the following pairs.
   a. *physical fitness* and *chronic disease*
   b. *overtraining* and *RICE*
   c. *sleep apnea* and *sleep deprivation*
   d. *RHR* and *target heart rate zone*

Understanding Key Ideas

Section 1

3. Describe five benefits of being physically fit.

4. List the five health-related components of fitness and an activity that develops each component.

5. What is the importance of skill-related fitness?

6. Explain how being a good sport can help you develop healthy life skills. **LIFE SKILL**

7. **CRITICAL THINKING** A friend says, "I don't have to bother to exercise. There'll be a cure for all of those diseases by the time I'm old!" Reply to these comments.

Section 2

8. What are the important factors to consider before starting a fitness program?

9. Describe each step in designing a fitness program.

10. Calculate the target heart rate zone of a 15-year-old.

11. Explain how the FITT formula can act as a guide when you are developing a fitness program.

12. In which of the following is the term *repetitions* used?
    a. running   c. weight lifting
    b. cycling   d. swimming

13. **CRITICAL THINKING** Explain the role of health fitness standards in designing a fitness program.

Section 3

14. What can you do to help prevent a sports injury?

15. List three signs of overtraining.

16. Describe the first steps in treating a minor sports injury.

17. Identify the effects of abusing anabolic steroids.

18. How can the FITT formula help you in avoiding a sports injury.

19. **CRITICAL THINKING** Your little sister who has just learned how to ride her bicycle says she no longer wants to wear her bicycle helmet because she "looks like a baby" while wearing it. What can you say to your sister to highlight the importance of wearing her bicycle helmet? **LIFE SKILL**

Section 4

20. Why is sleep so important?

21. Describe four consequences of not getting enough sleep.

22. How many hours of sleep a night do teens need?

23. In what phase of sleep does dreaming occur?

24. Identify four things you can do to get a good night's sleep. **LIFE SKILL**

Interpreting Graphics

Study the figure below to answer the questions that follow.

Six Leading Causes of Death

Cause of death	Percentage of total deaths	Lifestyle factors*
Heart disease	30	I, D, S
Cancer	23	I, D, S, A
Stroke	7	I, D, S
Respiratory disease	5	S
Accidents	4	
Diabetes	3	I, D

* I = inactivity, D = diet, S = smoking, A = alcohol

Source: Centers for Disease Control and Prevention.

25. Equal numbers of people die from heart disease as die from cancer, accidents, and diabetes combined. How can you determine this information from the graph? **MATH SKILL**

26. CRITICAL THINKING Based on the information in this chart, what is one of the most important lifestyle changes you can make to prevent heart disease?

Activities

27. Health and You Identify your target heart rate zone. Identify the purpose of knowing your target heart rate zone.

28. Health and You Keep an activity log for 1 day. Write down everything you do in a day and the length of time you do each activity. Identify wasted time, and see if you can fit in exercise time and more sleep time.

29. Health and Your Community Prepare a brochure that identifies locations in your community in which people of all ages can exercise regularly and safely. Include facility information, available classes, and fees.

Action Plan

30. LIFE SKILL Setting Goals Write a list of reasons you want to get more fit. Identify your short- and long-term goals. Write out an exercise contract that shows when, where, and what your program will be. Write down the day you will start.

Standardized Test Prep

Read the passage below, and then answer the questions that follow. **READING SKILL WRITING SKILL**

Jorge was always tired. He felt that he was always studying for an exam or writing reports for school. He was also depressed because his dad had some kind of heart disease and was in and out of the hospital. Jorge was often so tired after school that all he wanted to do was to flop down in front of the TV. Although he was exhausted, he found it difficult to fall asleep before midnight. However, he would often fall asleep much later in front of the flickering TV. He was on the school track team but had not been making training recently. The quality of his school work was also <u>deteriorating</u> and he was really fed up.

31. In this passage, the word *deteriorating* means
  A staying the same.
  B getting better.
  C getting worse.
  D often on time.

32. What can you infer from reading this passage?
  E Jorge is depressed.
  F Jorge is sleep deprived.
  G Jorge is probably going to lose his place on the track team.
  H all of the above

33. Write a paragraph describing how Jorge could change his life for the better. Suggest healthful changes Jorge can make in his lifestyle to feel better both physically and emotionally.

34. If Jorge sleeps an average of four and a half hours a night, how much sleep is he missing out on to get the recommended amount of sleep for teens? **MATH SKILL**

CHAPTER 7

Nutrition for Life

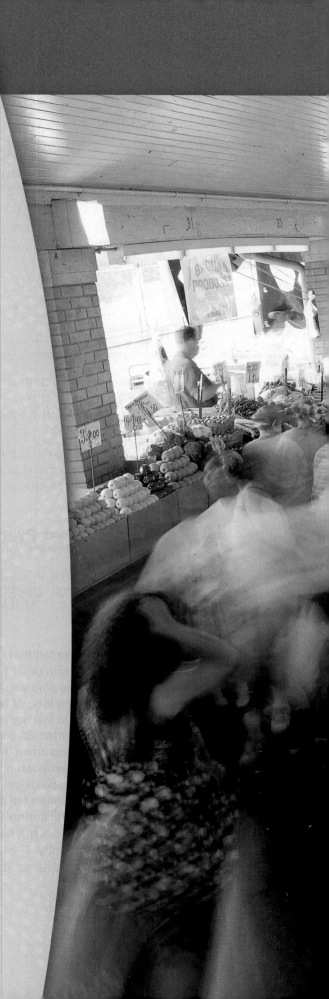

What's Your Health IQ?
KNOWLEDGE

Which of the statements below are true, and which are false? Check your answers on p. 642.

1. Eating too much protein, carbohydrate, or fat will make you gain weight.

2. Peanut butter and potato chips are high in cholesterol.

3. Fiber isn't important because it cannot be absorbed.

4. You don't need to worry about getting enough vitamins and minerals because they are needed in such small amounts.

5. Water is a nutrient.

6. The Recommended Dietary Allowances are guidelines for the amounts of nutrients we need.

7. Snacking is bad for you.

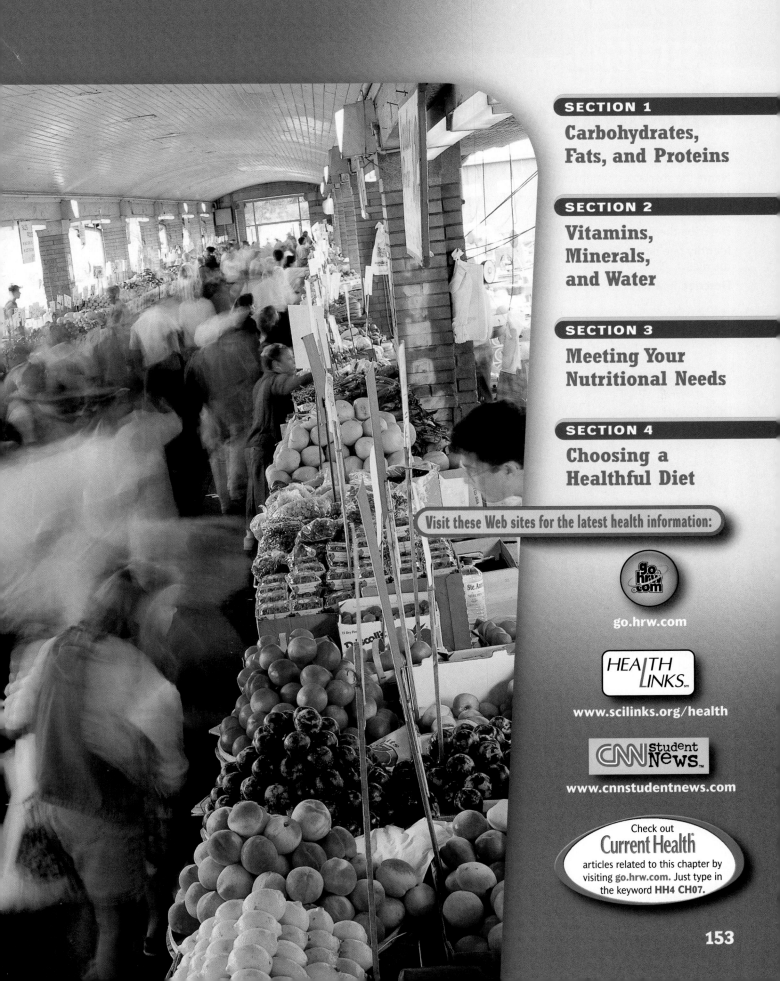

Visit these Web sites for the latest health information:

go.hrw.com

go.hrw.com

HEALTH LINKS.

www.scilinks.org/health

CNN student News.

www.cnnstudentnews.com

Check out **Current Health** articles related to this chapter by visiting **go.hrw.com**. Just type in the keyword **HH4 CH07.**

Carbohydrates, Fats, and Proteins

OBJECTIVES

Name the six classes of nutrients.

Identify the functions and food sources of carbohydrates, proteins, and fats.

Describe the need for enough fiber in your diet.

Identify one health disorder linked to high levels of saturated fats in the diet.

Describe how diet can influence health. **LIFE SKILL**

KEY TERMS

nutrition the science or study of food and the ways in which the body uses food

nutrient a substance in food that provides energy or helps form body tissues and that is necessary for life and growth

carbohydrate a class of energy-giving nutrients that includes sugars, starches, and fiber

fat a class of energy-giving nutrients; also the main form of energy storage in the body

protein a class of nutrients that are made up of amino acids, which are needed to build and repair body structures and to regulate processes in the body

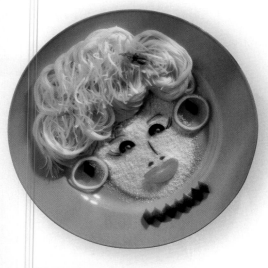

The saying "You are what you eat" reflects the idea that the food you eat affects how healthy you are.

Would you rather eat spinach, a cheeseburger, or a hot fudge sundae? Each choice contains different amounts and combinations of the nutrients you need to stay healthy. But no one food provides them all.

What Is Nutrition?

How do you know if you are eating a balanced, healthy diet? **Nutrition** is the science or study of food and the ways in which the body uses food. It is also the study of how and why we make food choices. Nutrition is also the study of the nutrients foods contain. **Nutrients** are substances in food that provide energy or help form body tissues and are necessary for life and growth.

Six Classes of Nutrients There are six classes of nutrients in food—carbohydrates, fats, proteins, vitamins, minerals, and water. **Carbohydrates** are a class of energy-giving nutrients that include sugars, starches, and fiber. **Fats** are a class of energy-giving nutrients that are also the main form of energy storage in the body. **Proteins** (PROH teens) are a class of nutrients made up of amino acids, which are needed to build and repair body structures and to regulate processes in the body.

A Balanced Diet Keeps You Healthy To stay alive, healthy, and growing, a person must eat and drink the right amounts of nutrients. Eating too little food causes weight loss, poor growth, and if severe enough, death. But eating too much food can also cause illness. When too much fat, carbohydrate, or protein is taken into the body, the extra energy is stored as body fat. Excess body fat increases the risks of developing heart disease, high blood pressure, and many other chronic diseases and disorders linked to poor nutrition. Thus, if you eat a healthy diet, you are more likely to be healthy and stay healthy.

What you eat today not only affects how you look and feel right now but also can affect your health in the long term. The diet you eat during your teens can affect your risk of developing obesity, heart disease, diabetes, osteoporosis, and cancer when you are in your 30s, 40s, or 50s. These diseases, which are common causes of death in the United States, are affected by diet.

Food Has Fuel for Your Body   Food provides the fuel that runs your body. The sum of the chemical processes that take place in your body to keep you alive and active is called *metabolism*. Metabolism requires energy and nutrients. The nutrients in food that provide energy are carbohydrates, fats, and proteins. In this section, we will look at carbohydrates, proteins, and fats. Vitamins, minerals, and water are also nutrients needed for metabolism, but they do not provide energy. These nutrients are discussed in the next section.

The energy in food is measured in Calories. **Figure 1** shows the amount of energy, in Calories, that certain foods offer. Carbohydrate and protein each provide 4 Calories per gram. Each gram of fat provides 9 Calories. So, 100 grams of bread, which is mostly carbohydrate, provides about 250 Calories. But 100 grams of chocolate cake, which contains a large amount of fat, provides about 600 Calories.

Figure 1

The number of Calories in a food depends on the amount of carbohydrate, fat, and protein it contains.

1/2 cup of ice cream: 178 Calories

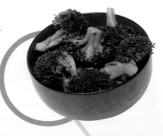

1 cup of broccoli: 27 Calories

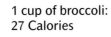

Flour tortilla with beans and rice: 218 Calories

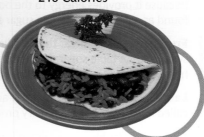

How Much Energy?

1 cup of low-fat fruit yogurt: 231 Calories
3 slices of Cheddar cheese: 154 Calories

1 apple: 81 Calories

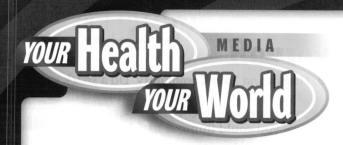

Healthy Meal— or Good Deal?

Restaurant and fast-food serving sizes are increasing dramatically. We are told that we can eat more food for less money. But is all of this food making us less healthy?

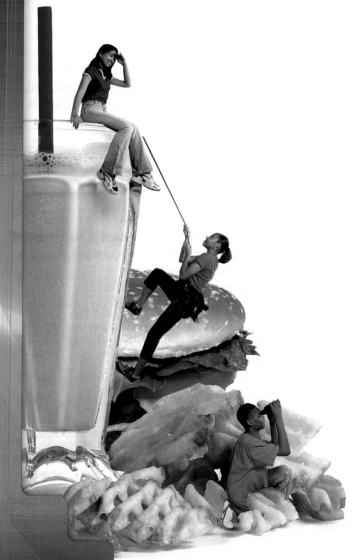

The last time you went into a restaurant and ordered a hamburger or a fish sandwich, did someone ask you if you wanted a bigger size for just a few pennies more? Did you order the "Super Portion" or the "Gigantic Burger?" Did the waitperson bring you a plate that had enough food to feed a football team? Many of us would answer yes to these questions.

Big—and Bigger

Study after study has shown that the average size of a serving in a restaurant, fast-food establishment, or convenience store has skyrocketed over the past 10 years. The message is *More is better.* In the past, the average soda serving was about 8 ounces. Today, a 20-ounce soda is not unusual. It's almost impossible to find an 8-ounce soda. One convenience store now sells a soda portion that is 64 ounces—a half gallon—and that contains more than 600 Calories. Most fast-food restaurants offer super or extra-large portions that were unheard of even 5 years ago.

Think Before You Buy

The excessiveness of our food culture is also reflected in advertising. The food industry spends more than $7 billion a year on food advertisements. The majority of this money goes to promote processed foods. For example, hardly anyone advertises potatoes, yet millions of dollars are spent to advertise potato chips. For food companies, processed foods bring in much more profit than nonprocessed foods do.

When you see food advertisements, pay attention to what they are trying to tell you. Most people know a chicken sandwich tastes good, so the ads often sell you something else. "Triple-burger for just 99 cents; extra-large fries for only 29 cents more." How many ads are actually telling you that what you're buying is not a good meal but a good deal?

Portion Sizes Affect People

Doctors, nutritionists, and health experts argue that people are at greater of obesity and other disorders when they are constantly bombarded with messages to eat more food. In fact, many people are eating more because they don't know when to stop. For example, people who are served large food portions often eat all that they are served. This tendency may reflect our cultural training to "clean one's plate." Many doctors and nutritionists suggest that the food portions served greatly exceed the amounts that a person needs for good health.

Eating Smart in a Huge Food Culture

Healthful living is about making smart choices. Having some good strategies for eating helps you stay healthy in a world of giant-sized portions. Nutritionists have some good advice that you may consider as you make your choices about how much food to eat.

▶ **Serve yourself.** If possible, be the one to put your food on your plate. You can ask your parents to place all of the food on the table "family style." This way, each member of the family can put food on his or her own plate. This approach greatly reduces overeating.

▶ **Be aware of portion sizes.** Recognize that the modern world is telling you to eat, eat, eat. Ads often direct you to spend less to eat more. What you have to do is see through all of this advertising and make smart eating choices. Take control of your health by making your own decisions on how much you eat. If you have doubts about how much you eat, talk about your eating with someone you trust.

▶ **Be aware of messages to eat more.** Messages to eat more food are all around you. To make yourself more aware, keep a list of all of the ads and cultural messages that you see in a week. Awareness of how our culture affects us is a great tool that you can use to stay healthy.

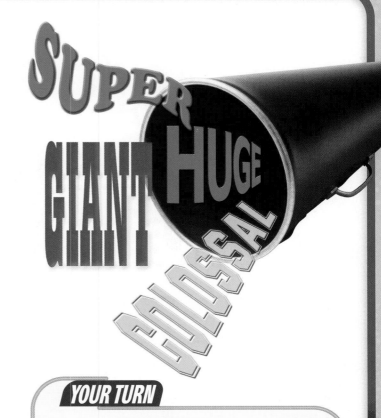

YOUR TURN

1. **Summarizing Information** In what three ways may modern food ads take your attention away from healthful eating choices?

2. **Inferring Relationships** Name three things in our culture other than food ads that encourage overeating.

3. **CRITICAL THINKING** Find one food ad that stresses large portions. Discuss how the ad goes about influencing the amount that people eat.

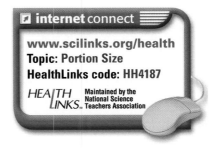

internet connect

www.scilinks.org/health
Topic: Portion Size
HealthLinks code: HH4187

HEALTH LINKS™ Maintained by the National Science Teachers Association

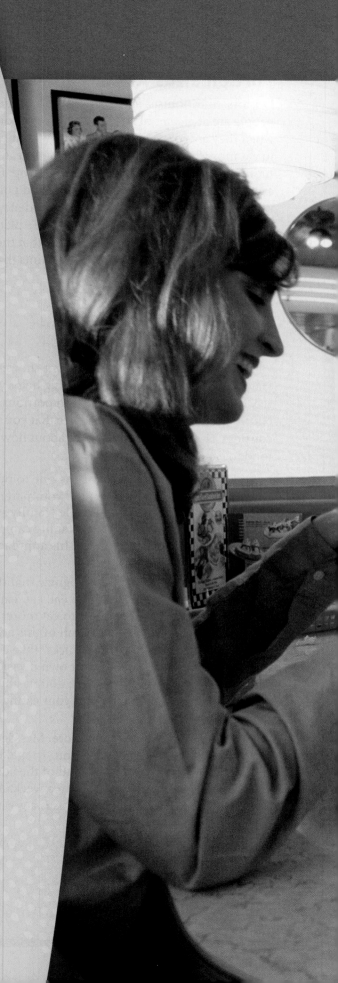

CHAPTER 8

Weight Management and Eating Behaviors

What's Your Health IQ?
KNOWLEDGE

Which of the statements below are true, and which are false? Check your answers on p. 642.

1. Your friends, family, and environment can influence what foods you eat.

2. Eating breakfast can help your performance in school.

3. It is possible for a person with a high body weight to have a healthy level of body fat.

4. Weight loss is the focus of any weight management plan.

5. Eating disorders are serious problems that require medical help.

6. Diarrhea can be life threatening.

7. Most food-borne illnesses are caused by food eaten at restaurants.

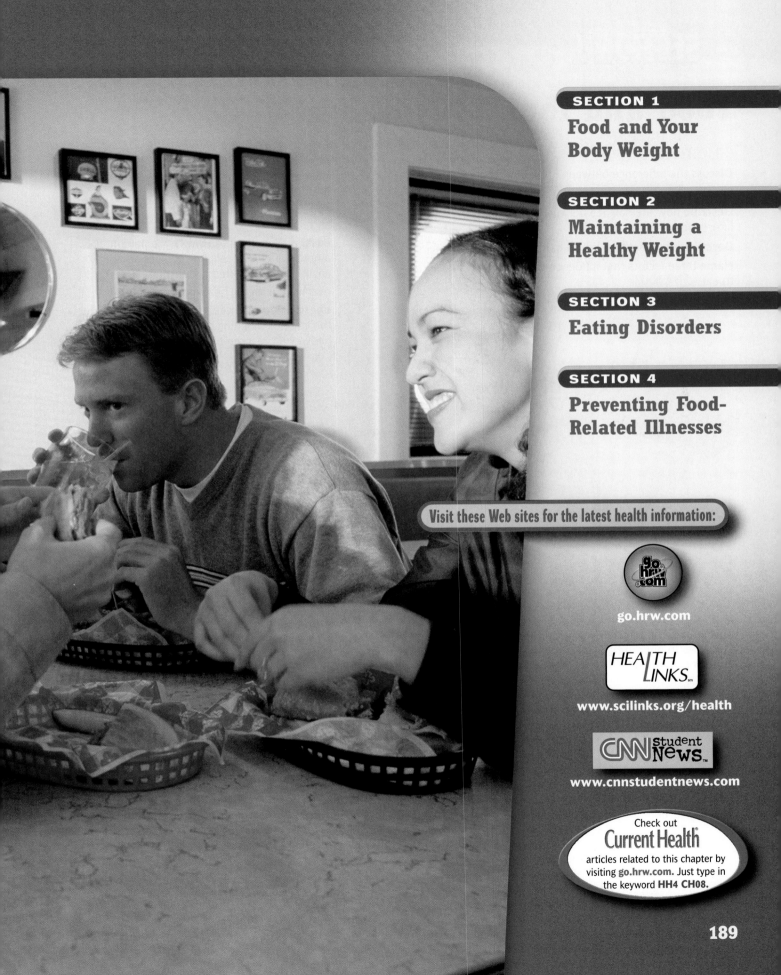

Visit these Web sites for the latest health information:

go.hrw.com

HEALTH LINKS

www.scilinks.org/health

CNN student News

www.cnnstudentnews.com

Check out **Current Health** articles related to this chapter by visiting **go.hrw.com**. Just type in the keyword **HH4 CH08.**

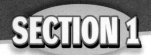

Food and Your Body Weight

OBJECTIVES

Discuss the difference between hunger and appetite.

Summarize why eating a healthy breakfast is important.

Describe how the balance between food intake and exercise affects body weight.

Describe how obesity is linked to poor health.

Name three factors that influence the foods you choose to eat. **LIFE SKILL**

KEY TERMS

hunger the body's physical response to the need for food

appetite the desire, rather than the need, to eat certain foods

basal metabolic rate (BMR) the minimum amount of energy required to keep the body alive when in a rested and fasting state

overweight being heavy for one's height

obesity having excess body fat for one's weight; the state of weighing more than 20 percent above your recommended body weight

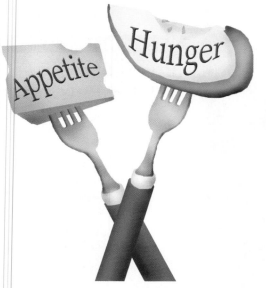

Both hunger and appetite play important roles in our eating habits. An imbalance between the two can lead to health problems.

Have you ever found yourself feeling full after a meal and then digging into a piece of pie for dessert? You've probably never thought of how you seem to make room for more food, even when you feel full. Many things influence why and when you eat.

Why Do You Eat?

Why do people eat even when they aren't hungry? **Hunger** is the body's physical response to the need for food. It is triggered by signals in your body that tell you to eat. The food you eat provides you with energy and nutrients that you need to remain healthy.

Are You Really Hungry? But most people don't eat just to stay healthy. Most people also eat because of their appetite. **Appetite** is a desire, rather than a need, to eat certain types of foods. For example, the decision to eat an ice-cream cone with your friends, even though you just ate a meal, was triggered by appetite rather than hunger. Appetite may be triggered by many factors, including the sight or smell of food, the time of day, or the time of year. What your friends are eating—and even what mood you are in—can trigger your appetite.

You skipped breakfast because you got up late. You're in class, and your stomach is growling. It is almost lunchtime, and you are feeling a little lightheaded and are unable to concentrate. These feelings are your body's way of telling you that you are hungry and your body needs fuel. They are caused by a number of different signals in your body.

Some of these signals come from your digestive tract, and some come from other parts of your body. For example, your empty

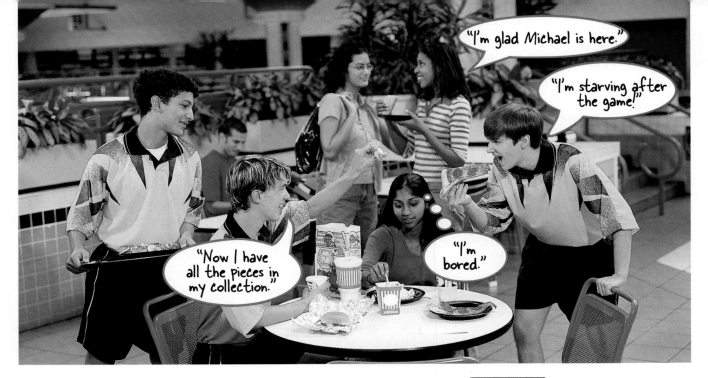

Figure 1

There are many reasons for choosing the foods we eat. Some of these reasons can lead you to choose healthy or unhealthy foods.

ACTIVITY *List the reasons why these teens are eating. Did they make healthy choices?*

stomach tells you to eat by sending messages to your brain. The levels of nutrients and other substances in your bloodstream also signal the brain that you need to eat. When you have eaten enough, other signals from the brain and digestive system make you feel full and satisfied. This full feeling is called *satiety* (suh TIE uh tee). Food in your stomach causes the stomach to stretch. This stretching is sensed by nerves, which send a "stop eating" message to the brain. The sensations of hunger and satiety help you eat the right amount to feed your body and to stay at a healthy weight.

What Foods Do You Choose? The amount and type of food you choose to eat are affected by many factors as shown in **Figure 1.** These factors include

- the smell and taste of the food
- mood
- family traditions and ethnic background
- social occasions
- religious traditions
- health concerns
- advertising
- cost and availability

For example, you may eat sandwiches for lunch because they are easy to carry to school. Americans often eat turkey on Thanksgiving day because of tradition. Where you grew up also plays a role in what you generally eat. If you grew up in the southwestern United States, you may eat Mexican food regularly, even if it isn't part of your ethnic background. And someone who is growing up on the East Coast may eat more seafood than someone in the Midwest does. Some of us eat when we are bored or upset. We also avoid foods because we think they are unhealthy.

How Excess Food Energy Is Stored

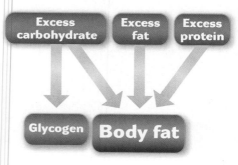

Figure 2

Excess dietary fats and proteins are stored in the body as fat. When glycogen stores are full, excess dietary carbohydrates are then stored as fat.

TOPIC link For more information about exercising and keeping fit, see Chapter 6.

Food Provides Energy

Carbohydrates, fats, and proteins are the energy-giving nutrients. This energy is measured in units called *Calories*. The amount of energy in a certain food depends on how much carbohydrate, fat, and protein the food contains. Carbohydrates and proteins each provide 4 Calories per gram. Fats provide 9 Calories per gram. Foods high in fat are high in Calories because fat provides the most Calories per gram.

After you have eaten a meal, your digestive system breaks down the food. Some of the energy released from food is used almost immediately to fuel the thousands of reactions in your body that keep you alive. Extra food energy that is not needed immediately is stored by the body in two forms—glycogen and fat. **Figure 2** shows how excess food energy is stored by the body. Most of the energy stored in the body is stored as fat. Fat can provide most of the body's energy, but small amounts of glucose are also needed. Glycogen can be broken down quickly to glucose. When the limited glycogen stores are used up, body proteins are needed to form glucose.

The Right Breakfast Keeps You Going When you wake up in the morning, you usually haven't eaten for 10 to 12 hours. If you go to school without breakfast, you must depend on stored energy to fuel your body and brain. By lunchtime, you may not have eaten for more than 16 hours! The food you eat at breakfast gives you a quick source of energy for your body and glucose for your brain.

How long your breakfast or any other meal keeps you going depends on how much you have eaten and what foods you eat. Meals with fat and protein keep you feeling full longer than meals made of mostly carbohydrates. So a slice of dry toast and orange juice for breakfast will likely cause you to feel hungry long before lunchtime. However, a meal with a mixture of carbohydrate, protein, and some fat, such as yogurt, cereal, and fruit, will keep you feeling full and energized longer.

How Much Energy Do You Need? How much food energy, or Calories, you need depends on how much energy your body is using. Everyone knows you need energy for running, swimming, and playing basketball. But did you know that your body needs energy even when you aren't moving?

Most of the food energy the body needs is used for basic functions, such as breathing, circulating blood, and growing. The amount of energy needed for these basic functions is called the basal metabolic rate. **Basal metabolic rate (BMR)** is the minimum amount of energy needed to keep you alive when you are in a rested, fasting state, such as just after you wake up in the morning. The amount of energy that is used for BMR is different for each person.

Also, the Calorie requirements of boys and girls differ. On average, boys require more Calories per day than girls do. For example, active 15-year-old boys need about 3,000 Calories per day, and active 15-year-old girls need about 2,300 Calories per day.

The more active you are, the more energy your body uses. **Figure 3** provides several examples of the amount of energy burned during different activities. For example, it takes more energy for a person to run for 15 minutes than to walk for the same amount of time. But if you walk for an hour, you may use more energy than you would during a 15-minute run. The amount of energy needed for an activity also increases as body weight increases. For example, it takes more energy for a 130-pound person to walk a mile than for a 110-pound person to walk the same distance.

Balancing Energy Intake with Energy Used

When the amount of food energy you take in is equal to the amount of energy you use, you are in *energy balance*. Eating more or less food than you need will cause you to be out of energy balance. Eating extra food energy increases the body's fat stores and causes weight gain. Eating less food than you need decreases the body's fat stores and causes weight loss.

Some body fat is essential for health. It is needed for normal body structures and functions, as an energy store, for insulation, and for protection of the body's internal organs. A healthy amount of body fat for young women is 20 to 30 percent of body weight. For young men, the amount is 12 to 20 percent of body weight. We build up storage fat when we put on weight. Most people who are overweight have excess stored fat.

Overweight is the term used to describe a person who is heavy for his or her height. Generally, people who are overweight have excess body fat.

Research has shown that students who eat breakfast perform better in school than those who skip breakfast.

Figure 3

Different activities have different energy demands. The more intense the activity level, the greater the number of Calories that are burned per hour.

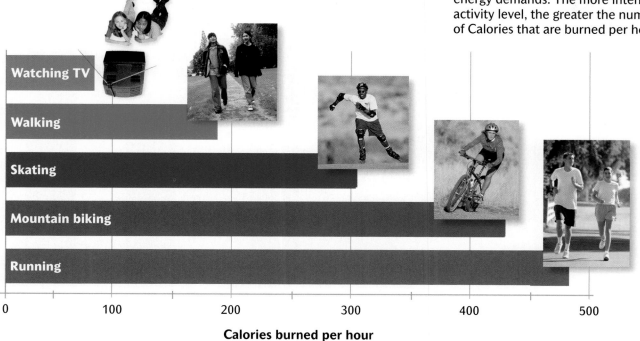

Calories burned per hour

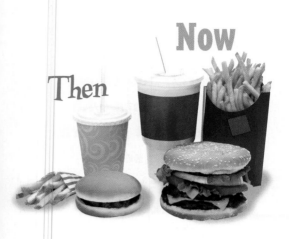

Figure 4

Over the years, the size and the number of Calories in a fast-food meal have increased dramatically.

ACTIVITY *Use the Calorie table on pp. 622–627 to compare the Calories in a plain, single-patty hamburger, a small order of fries, and a small soda with the Calories in an extra large meal.* **MATH SKILL**

Figure 5

Lack of physical activity and poor dietary habits have lead to an increase in the percentage of people who are overweight or obese.

Being Overweight Can Cause Health Problems Having excess body fat increases the risk of suffering from many long-term diseases. Some of these health problems include

▶ heart disease and high blood pressure
▶ certain forms of cancer, including prostate, colon, and breast cancer
▶ type 2 diabetes
▶ sleeping problems such as sleep apnea

Overweight and Obesity: A Growing Problem

Obesity (oh BEE suh tee) is a condition in which there is an excess of body fat for one's weight. A person is considered obese if he or she weighs more than 20 percent above his or her recommended weight range. Being obese or being overweight is most common in developed countries, such as the United States.

More people are overweight or obese than ever before. As **Figure 5** shows, more than 60 percent of all adult Americans are currently overweight, and almost 30 percent of those who are overweight are obese. Adults are not the only ones getting heavier. About 14 percent of children and teenagers in the United States are overweight. This trend is worrisome because being overweight, especially when young, increases the risk of suffering from chronic diseases such as diabetes and heart disease. Overall, physical inactivity and poor diet pose the greatest risk to health. However, an overweight person who is active regularly is at lower risk than a person of correct weight who is not active.

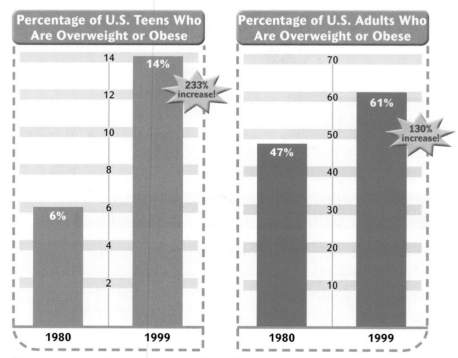

Percentage of U.S. Teens Who Are Overweight or Obese

1980: 6%
1999: 14%
233% increase!

Percentage of U.S. Adults Who Are Overweight or Obese

1980: 47%
1999: 61%
130% increase!

Source: Centers for Disease Control and Prevention and National Center for Health Statistics.

Why Are So Many People Overweight? There are two main reasons why increasing numbers of Americans are overweight. The first reason is our lack of physical activity. Many modern conveniences have helped decrease our daily levels of activity. We drive more often than we walk, and we play video games and watch TV more often than we ride our bikes.

The second reason people are gaining so much body fat is our changing diet. Many Americans eat more food than they need to, and choose foods high in fat and sugar. Supermarkets, fast-food restaurants, and all-night shopping marts provide easy access to food. High-Calorie snack foods, drinks, baked goods, and candy tempt us at the checkout counter of the supermarket. In these busy days, grabbing a snack from the vending machine or buying lunch at a fast-food restaurant is far more convenient for many people than preparing a healthy meal is.

What Can You Do? With a little preplanning and goal setting, maintaining a healthy weight is something everyone can do. It is important to avoid becoming overweight in the first place. Exercise and a healthy diet can help you stay in a healthy weight range.

Every year, about 44 percent of American women and 29 percent of American men try to lose weight. Many never lose any weight, and most who do lose weight eventually regain it. When trying to lose weight, people often have unrealistic goals (such as losing 7 pounds per week) and try very strict diets. Failure to achieve these unrealistic goals often causes a cycle of dieting and disappointment throughout life. A weight management plan that is suited just to you will have the most success.

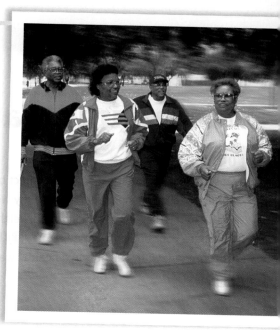

Regardless of age or level of fitness, everyone can benefit from regular exercise.

SECTION 1

REVIEW *Answer the following questions on a separate piece of paper.*

Using Key Terms

1. **Identify** the term that means "the body's physical response to the need for food."
   a. appetite
   b. obesity
   c. basal metabolic rate
   d. hunger

2. **Name** the term used to describe the minimum amount of energy that is needed to keep you alive when your body is in a rested and fasting state.

3. **Compare** the terms *overweight* and *obesity*.

Understanding Key Ideas

4. **Summarize** why appetite is more likely to lead to overeating than hunger is.

5. **State** the advantages of eating breakfast.

6. **Describe** how your energy balance and body weight would be affected if you walked home from school every day instead of taking the bus.

7. **Describe** what happens when energy intake exceeds the body's energy needs.

8. **Describe** how excess body fat affects health.

9. **Name** two reasons for the increase in the number of overweight or obese people.

Critical Thinking

10. **LIFE SKILL** **Being a Wise Consumer** You are cooking dinner for your family. You go to the grocery store to buy the ingredients. List four factors that may influence your food choices.

Children, Teens, and BMI Adult BMI guidelines are not suitable for people younger than 20 years old. The definitions of *overweight* and *underweight* for children and adolescents are less clear because young people grow and develop at such different rates. A chart that compares BMI to age has been developed specifically for children and teens to account for changing body shapes and sizes. One chart is used for boys, and another chart is used for girls.

A Healthy Weight Management Plan

Once you have determined whether you are within a healthy weight range, you can develop your weight management plan. **Weight management** is a program of sensible eating and exercise habits that will help keep weight at a healthy level. For most overweight children and teens, the focus of weight management programs should be to slow or stop weight gain, not to cause weight loss. This approach allows the child or teen to continue to grow in height so they "grow into" their weight. Weight loss in children and teens is recommended only for those whose excess weight has caused health problems such as high blood pressure or difficulty breathing. Regular exercise in a weight management plan is just as important as a healthful diet.

Analyzing DATA

Understanding Body Mass Index

1 Malik is 15. He is 5 feet 8 inches tall and weighs 158 pounds. He wants to find out if he is at a healthy weight. To do this, he needs to find his BMI by using the following equation:

$$BMI = weight \text{ (lb)} \div height \text{ (in.)} \div height \text{ (in.)} \times 703$$

Malik's BMI calculations would be

$$158 \div 68 \div 68 \times 703 = 24.0$$

Malik has a BMI of 24.

2 Malik now needs to find the healthy BMI range for 15-year-old boys.

3 His BMI of 24 is higher than the healthy range for his age. If he has a lot of muscle mass, the BMI chart may not be right for him. If he does not have a lot of muscle mass, he should then change factors such as his activity level and his snacking habits. Doing so will help him grow in height without growing in weight.

Healthy BMI Range		
Age	Boys	Girls
12	14.9–21	14.8–21.6
13	15.4–21.8	15.3–22.5
14	15.9–22.6	15.8–23.3
15	16.5–23.4	16.2–24
16	17.1–24.2	16.7–24.6
17	17.6–25	17.3–25.2
18	17.8–25.6	17.5–25.7

Source: National Center for Health Statistics and National Center for Chronic Disease Prevention and Health Promotion.

Your Turn

1. Calculate your BMI. **MATH SKILL**

2. Is your BMI in the healthy range?

3. Why is the healthy BMI range different for each age group?

4. **CRITICAL THINKING** Let's say your BMI is slightly above the healthy range for your age. Predict what will happen to your BMI over the next year if your weight remains the same, but you grow an inch taller.

Eat Smart, Exercise More The simplest and healthiest way to decrease the number of Calories you eat is to reduce portion sizes and to keep high-Calorie choices as a treat. This decision can be difficult to make if your friends are going out for ice cream. Sometimes the best way to avoid excess Calories is to skip the outing. But another way is to learn some lower-Calorie options. For example, instead of a double scoop ice cream, choose an ice pop, low-fat frozen yogurt, or sherbet. These options have fewer Calories than ice cream does.

Exercise increases your energy needs and makes managing your weight easier. Even small changes in activity levels, as shown in **Figure 6,** can result in weight loss. Exercise will also increase your muscle strength, improve fitness, and relieve boredom and stress. The recommended exercise goal for teens is at least 60 minutes of moderate activity daily.

Changing either eating habits or exercise involves changing your behavior. Keeping a log of your food intake and exercise may help you to make such changes. You can then review the log to see when you are likely to eat more than you intend or to see what prevents you from getting the exercise you planned.

Lose Fat, Not Muscle! For those who need to lose weight, the goal for weight loss is to lose fat without losing muscle. A weight-loss rate of a half pound to one pound per week is recommended to prevent the loss of muscle. Faster weight loss is usually due to the loss of water and muscle, not fat. To lose a pound a week, an average person would need to eat 500 fewer Calories each day or burn 500 more Calories each day. Weight loss while dieting often stops and starts. Weight can drop one week and stay the same the next. This process can be frustrating to the dieter and can sometimes lead to dangerous weight-loss practices.

> **"Your choice of diet can influence your long-term health prospects more than any other action you can take."**
>
> —Former Surgeon General
> C. Everett Koop

Figure 6

Even small changes in your daily activity levels can lead to weight loss.
ACTIVITY *Record and analyze your food intake and level of activity for a week. Do you need to make changes to improve your activity levels and eating habits?*

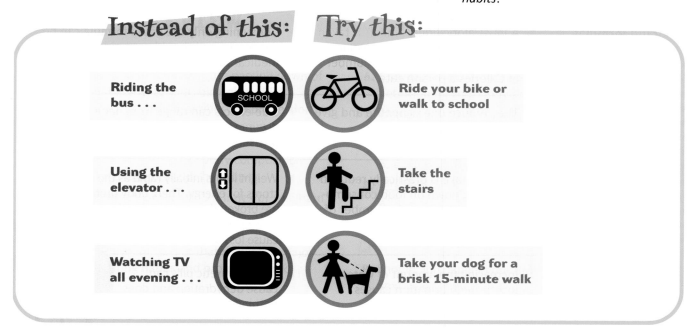

Instead of this: Try this:

Riding the bus . . . — Ride your bike or walk to school

Using the elevator . . . — Take the stairs

Watching TV all evening . . . — Take your dog for a brisk 15-minute walk

Eating Disorders

OBJECTIVES

Discuss the relationship between body image and eating disorders.

Describe the type of individual who is most at risk for an eating disorder.

List the symptoms and health dangers of the most common eating disorders.

Identify ways to help a friend who you think is developing an eating disorder. **LIFE SKILL**

Identify health organizations in your community that help people with eating disorders. **LIFE SKILL**

KEY TERMS

body image how you see and feel about your appearance and how comfortable you are with your body

anorexia nervosa an eating disorder that involves self-starvation, a distorted body image, and low body weight

bulimia nervosa an eating disorder in which the individual repeatedly eats large amounts of food and then uses behaviors such as vomiting or using laxatives to rid the body of the food

binge eating/bingeing eating a large amount of food in one sitting; usually accompanied by a feeling of being out of control

purging engaging in behaviors such as vomiting or misusing laxatives to rid the body of food

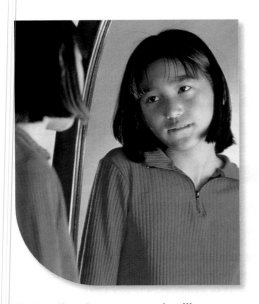

Eating disorders are complex illnesses that can involve having a distorted body image.

TOPIC link For more information about self-concept, see Chapter 2.

Jenny had carried her dieting too far. She barely ate a thing and exercised all the time. When she was rushed to the hospital after fainting, she weighed only 85 pounds. Jenny didn't listen when her friends said that she was too thin. She hated how "fat" she looked.

What Are Eating Disorders?

Normally we eat when we are hungry and stop eating when we are full. However, eating patterns that are inflexible and highly structured are not normal. Abnormal eating patterns may include never eating enough, dieting excessively, eating only certain types of foods, eating too much, and not responding to natural feelings of fullness or hunger. These patterns may be warning signs of an eating disorder.

Eating disorders are conditions that involve an unhealthy degree of concern about body weight and shape and that may lead to efforts to control weight by unhealthy means. Examples of eating disorders include starving oneself, overeating, and forcefully ridding the body of food by vomiting or using laxatives. Eating disorders greatly affect all aspects of the sufferer's life and the lives of his or her loved ones.

Body Image and Eating Disorders Your **body image** is how you see and feel about your appearance and how comfortable you are with your body. Your body image can change with your mood, your environment, and your experiences. Your body image can also affect your eating habits and health. People who believe they are too fat may limit the food they eat even if they are not overweight. People with eating disorders often do not see themselves as they really are. In other words, they have a distorted body image.

Culture and society often define what we think of as a perfect body. In the 1950s, many women wanted to look like Marilyn Monroe—curvy and full figured. In the United States today, clothing styles and fashion models on television and in magazines suggest that thin is in and a perfectly toned, muscular body is best. The models we see in magazines and on television act as a standard for attractiveness and acceptability. But in fact, the women and men on magazine covers represent less than 1 percent of the population!

A Healthy Body Image   Having a healthy body image means you accept your body's appearance and abilities. It also means that you listen to what your body tells you. Developing a healthier body image requires paying attention to, appreciating, and caring for your body. You should have realistic expectations about your size that are based on your heredity and should realize that weight and body shape can change frequently and rapidly in teens.

The men and women on magazine covers represent less than 1 percent of the population.

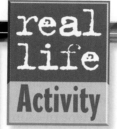

real life Activity

SOCIETY AND BODY IMAGE

LIFE SKILL
Evaluating Media Messages

Materials

✔ colored paper
✔ teen, fashion, and fitness magazines
✔ scissors
✔ paste

Procedure

1. **Cut** out images of teenage girls and boys from the magazines.
2. **Paste** the images onto the colored paper to create a collage.

Conclusions

1. **Summarizing Results** Describe the body sizes and shapes in the images that you have collected.

2. **Comparing Information** How are these images like those of your friends and classmates? How are they different?

3. **Analyzing Results** Are these images used to sell a product? If so, what product is each image selling?

4. **CRITICAL THINKING** How can behaviors such as drug use and dieting develop from having an unrealistic body image?

5. **CRITICAL THINKING** From what other sources do you get messages about body image?

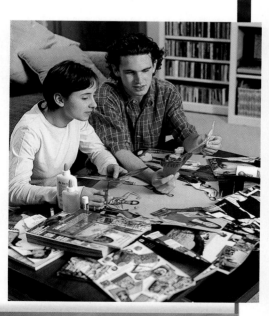

A Closer Look at Eating Disorders

Thousands of people die each year from complications related to eating disorders. Eating disorders often develop during adolescence, when children's bodies and responsibilities change from those of children to those of adults.

Many factors contribute to the development of eating disorders. Genetics, culture, personality, emotions, and family are all believed to play a role. Eating disorders are on the rise among athletes in sports that require athletes to be thin, such as gymnastics and figure skating. Eating disorders are also found in athletes who must fit into a particular weight class, such as wrestlers. Eating disorders are most common in young women, overachievers, perfectionists, and adolescents who have a difficult family life. Eating disorders are also most common in people from cultures in which being thin is equated with being attractive, successful, and intelligent and also in people whose jobs depend on their body shape and weight, such as dancers, gymnasts, and models.

Common Eating Disorders Three of the most common eating disorders, anorexia nervosa, bulimia nervosa, and binge eating disorder are summarized in **Table 2.**

Anorexia nervosa is an eating disorder that involves self-starvation, a distorted body image, and low body weight. **Bulimia nervosa** is an eating disorder in which an individual repeatedly eats large amounts of food and then uses behaviors such as vomiting or using laxatives to rid the body of the food. **Bingeing** or **binge eating** is eating of a large amount of food in one sitting. Depending on the type of eating disorder, bingeing may be followed by purging. **Purging** is behavior that involves vomiting or misusing laxatives to rid the body of food.

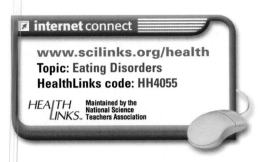
Dangers of Eating Disorders

- ▶ Hair loss
- ▶ Dental problems
- ▶ Broken blood vessels in the face and eyes
- ▶ Dry, scaly skin
- ▶ Severe dehydration
- ▶ Rectal bleeding from laxative abuse
- ▶ Heart irregularities
- ▶ Organ failure
- ▶ Death

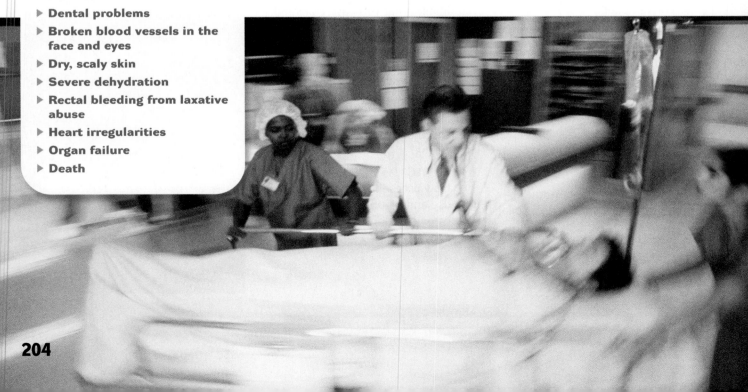

Table 2   Common Eating Disorders

What is it?	Signs and symptoms	Treatment
Anorexia nervosa is an obsession with being thin that leads to extreme weight loss. Some people with anorexia binge and then purge as a means of weight control. Sufferers often have very low self-esteem and feel controlled by others. The average teen consumes about 2,500 Calories per day. But someone with anorexia may consume only a few hundred Calories.	▶ intense fear of weight gain ▶ overexercising ▶ preferring to eat alone ▶ preoccupation with Calories ▶ extreme weight loss ▶ loss of menstrual periods for at least 3 months ▶ hair loss on head ▶ depression and anxiety ▶ weakness and exhaustion Extreme weight loss	▶ medical, psychological, and nutritional therapy to help the person regain health and develop healthy eating behaviors ▶ family counseling 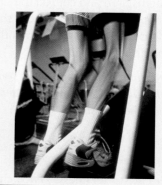
Bulimia nervosa is a disorder that involves frequent episodes of binge eating that are almost always followed by behaviors such as vomiting, using laxatives, fasting or overexercising. A person with bulimia may consume as many as 20,000 Calories in binges that last as long as 8 hours.	▶ preoccupation with body weight ▶ bingeing with or without purging ▶ bloodshot eyes and sore throat ▶ dental problems ▶ irregular menstrual periods ▶ depression and mood swings ▶ feeling out of control ▶ at least two bulimic episodes per week for at least 3 months	▶ therapy to separate eating from emotions and to promote eating in response to hunger and satiety ▶ nutritional counseling to review nutrient needs and ways to meet them
Binge eating disorder is a disorder that involves frequent binge eating but no purging. It is frequently undiagnosed. About one-quarter to one-third of people who go to weight-loss clinics may have binge eating disorder.	▶ above-normal body weight ▶ bingeing episodes accompanied by feelings of guilt, shame, and loss of control	▶ psychological and nutritional counseling
Disordered eating patterns are disordered eating behaviors that are not severe enough to be classified as a specific eating disorder. They are often referred to as "disordered eating behaviors." Many teens are believed to have disordered eating behaviors that could lead to serious health problems.	▶ weight loss (less than anorexia) ▶ bingeing and purging less frequently than in bulimia ▶ purging after eating small amounts of food ▶ deliberate dehydration for weight loss ▶ hiding food ▶ overexercising ▶ constant dissatisfaction with physical appearance	▶ psychological and nutritional counseling

MAKING GREAT DECISIONS

You're worried about your best friend, Samantha. When she goes out to eat with you and your other friends, she talks about food a lot, but all she ever orders is a diet soda. She has lost weight and seems tired and cold all the time. You tell her that she looks too thin, but she complains that she is fat. You suspect Samantha may have an eating disorder.

Write on a separate sheet of paper the steps that you would take to help your friend. Remember to use the decision-making steps.

Give thought to the problem.

Review your choices.

Evaluate the consequences of each choice.

Assess and choose the best choice.

Think it over afterward.

Could You Be at Risk? People at risk of developing an eating disorder may find they have traits such as preferring to eat alone, being overly critical about their body size and shape, thinking about food often, weighing themselves every day, and/or eating a lot of "diet" foods. If your concerns about food or your appearance have led to trouble in school, at home, or with your friends, you should discuss your situation with a parent, a school nurse, a counselor, a doctor, or another trusted adult.

Getting Help Professional help from physicians, psychologists, and nutritionists is essential to manage and recover from an eating disorder. Unfortunately, people with eating disorders often deny that they have a problem and believe that their behavior is normal and a chosen lifestyle. As a result, they may not seek help early on when treatment can help prevent severe physical problems.

If you believe a friend has an eating disorder, it is important to encourage your friend to seek help. In private, let your friend know of your concern for his or her health. Listen to your friend. If you are unsuccessful, tell a trusted adult, or contact an agency that provides eating disorder counseling in your area. Remember, even if you are sworn to secrecy by your friend, it is important that a responsible adult knows about your fears. When a life is in danger, there is no confidentiality to keep.

SECTION 3

REVIEW
Answer the following questions on a separate piece of paper.

Using Key Terms

1. **Define** the term *body image*.

2. **Identify** the eating disorder that involves extreme weight loss.
   a. anorexia nervosa
   b. bulimia nervosa
   c. purging
   d. binge eating disorder

3. **List** the symptoms of bulimia nervosa.

4. **Name** the term that means "a rapid consumption of a large amount of food."

Understanding Key Ideas

5. **Describe** how a negative body image can affect eating behavior.

6. **Describe** how you could tell if a friend or family member was at risk of an eating disorder.

7. **Compare** the symptoms of anorexia with those of bulimia, and describe how the disorders affect health.

8. **LIFE SKILL** **Communicating Effectively** Describe how you could help a friend you think is developing an eating disorder.

9. **LIFE SKILL** **Using Community Resources** Identify resources in your local community that help people with eating disorders or their families.

Critical Thinking

10. Should someone who binges and purges about once a month be worried about the consequences of bulimia? Explain.

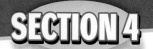

SECTION 4

Preventing Food-Related Illnesses

OBJECTIVES

Describe three of the most common digestive disorders.

Describe how diarrhea can be life threatening.

Discuss how food allergies can affect health.

Identify a common cause of food intolerances.

List things you can do to reduce your chances of getting a food-borne illness. **LIFE SKILL**

KEY TERMS

food allergy an abnormal response to a food that is triggered by the immune system

lactose intolerance the inability to completely digest the milk sugar lactose

food-borne illness an illness caused by eating or drinking a food that contains a toxin or disease-causing microorganism

cross-contamination the transfer of contaminants from one food to another

W hile in the library, Aaron started to feel bad. His stomach hurt, and he felt a little sick. It couldn't have been the burger he'd had for lunch—it was so good! He had barely packed up his bag before he had to run for the bathroom.

Food and Digestive Problems

To provide the body with nutrients, food must be digested and then the nutrients must be absorbed. Problems in any part of the digestive system can affect your health. Most digestive problems like Aaron's are not serious. But if you have severe or persistent symptoms, you should see a doctor.

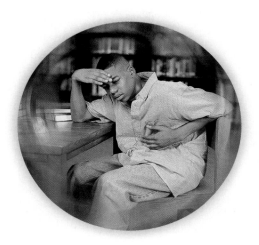

Digestive problems can sometimes develop quickly.

Heartburn   Have you ever had a burning feeling in your chest after a large meal? This burning feeling is called *heartburn* and is caused by stomach acid leaking into the esophagus. The esophagus is the tube that connects your throat with your stomach. The main cause of heartburn is overeating foods that are high in fat. Stress and anxiety can also cause heartburn by increasing the amount of acid made by the stomach. Heartburn is usually a minor problem that can be prevented by eating small, low-fat meals frequently and by not lying down soon after eating.

Ulcers   Pain after eating can also be a symptom of a more serious ailment, such as an ulcer. Ulcers are open sores in the lining of the stomach or intestine. Recent studies have shown that most ulcers are caused by a bacterial infection of the stomach lining. Fortunately, the infection is treatable with antibiotics. Stress and an unhealthy diet can make ulcers worse.

Embarrassing Digestive Problems Some intestinal problems are as embarrassing as they are uncomfortable. Gas, diarrhea, and constipation can be difficult to discuss. However, they can often be avoided by changes in the diet.

Gas is produced when bacteria living in the large intestine break down undigested food. Normally, you don't notice the daily activities of these bacteria. Some foods, such as beans, contain a large amount of indigestible material. Although you cannot digest this material, it acts as a huge meal for the millions of bacteria that live in your large intestine. The bacteria produce a lot of gas while feasting on the beans. The end result for you is gas, or flatus. The buildup of this gas can make you feel bloated and can give you *flatulence.*

Diarrhea refers to frequent watery stools. Diarrhea can be caused by infections, medications, or reactions to foods. Occasional diarrhea is common and mostly harmless. But because diarrhea increases water loss from the body, prolonged diarrhea can lead to dehydration. Dehydration occurs when the amount of water in the body decreases enough to cause a drop in blood volume. Dehydration can make it difficult for the blood to carry nutrients and oxygen around the body and can become life threatening. Every year dehydration from diarrhea kills millions of children in the developing world. If you experience diarrhea, drink a lot of fluid, such as water or sports drinks, to replace lost water.

Constipation is difficulty in having bowel movements or is having dry, hard stools. Constipation can be caused by weak intestinal muscles or by a diet that is low in fiber or fluid. It can be prevented by getting plenty of exercise, drinking a lot of water (at least eight glasses a day), and eating a diet high in whole grains, fruits, and vegetables.

Food Allergies

A **food allergy** is an abnormal response to a food that is triggered by the body's immune system. The immune system reacts to the food as if it were a harmful microorganism. The allergic reaction can cause symptoms throughout the body. Sometimes reactions are mild, but they can be life threatening. An upset stomach, hives, a runny nose, body aches, difficulty breathing, and a drop in blood pressure can all be food allergy symptoms. In some cases, these symptoms appear immediately. In others, they take up to 24 hours to appear.

Is It a Food Allergy? True food allergies are relatively rare. To find out if symptoms are due to a specific food, you must cut from your diet for 2 to 4 weeks all foods suspected of causing an allergic reaction. Then, a "food challenge" can be done by eating a small amount of one suspected food. You should do a food challenge in a doctor's office in case you have a serious reaction. If a reaction occurs, a diagnosis of a food allergy can be made. If no reaction occurs, a larger amount of the food can be eaten. If you still have no reaction, then an allergy to that food may be ruled out.

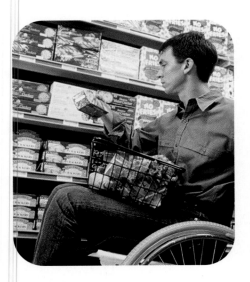

Common Causes of Food Allergies

▶ **Peanuts**
▶ **Eggs**
▶ **Wheat**
▶ **Strawberries**
▶ **Soy foods**
▶ **Seafood**
▶ **Milk**

A food challenge should not be done with a suspected allergy to peanuts because reactions to peanuts can be deadly. Individuals who are allergic to peanuts can be so sensitive that exposure to tiny amounts, such as contamination from peanut-containing foods nearby, can cause serious reactions. Once this allergy is suspected, peanuts must be avoided.

Managing Food Allergies   The best way to prevent an allergic reaction to food is to avoid eating the food to which you are allergic. Don't be afraid to ask about ingredients in food served in restaurants or at a friend's house. Food labels can help you find out if a food contains the ingredient. Individuals who have serious food allergies need to carry *epinephrine* with them. Injecting themselves with this hormone after exposure to the food can prevent a fatal reaction.

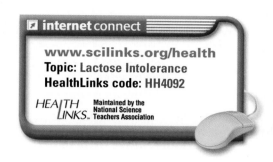

Food Intolerances

Although the symptoms of a food intolerance can be similar to those of a food allergy, food intolerances do not cause a specific reaction of the immune system. Food intolerances can be caused by eating foods or ingredients in a meal that irritate the intestine (such as onions).

An example of a food intolerance is lactose intolerance. **Lactose intolerance** is a reduced ability to digest the milk sugar lactose. It is not an allergy to milk. Lactose is found in dairy products, such as milk and cheese. Lactose intolerance causes gas, cramps, and diarrhea. These symptoms occur because undigested lactose passes into the large intestine, where it is digested by bacteria that produce acids and gas from the lactose. Lactose intolerance is rare in children but affects about a quarter of the American adult population. The incidence of lactose intolerance varies worldwide. Lactose intolerance affects less than 5 percent of people in northwestern Europe but nearly 100 percent of people in some parts of Asia and Africa.

Food-Borne Illness

A **food-borne illness** is an illness caused by eating or drinking a food that contains a toxin or disease-causing microorganism. Each year, about 76 million people in the United States suffer from food-borne illness. Food-borne illness can be caused by any kind of contamination in food. However, most food-borne illnesses in the United States are caused by eating food contaminated with pathogens, such as bacteria, viruses, fungi, or parasites. Many cases of food-borne illness are so mild that they are not reported to a doctor. So, in most cases the cause of the food-borne illness is never discovered. Most cases of food-borne illness are due to foods that are prepared or eaten at home.

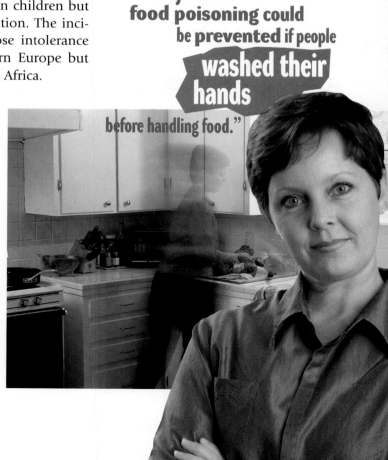

"**Many** cases of food poisoning could be prevented if people **washed their hands** before handling food."

Selecting and Storing Foods Safely

▶ Avoid dented, rusting, or bulging cans.

▶ Meat and fish should be very fresh and free of odor.

▶ Refrigerate leftovers promptly.

▶ Store eggs in the refrigerator.

▶ Never defrost foods at room temperature. Leave them in the refrigerator to defrost overnight.

▶ If you suspect a food is unsafe, play it safe. When in doubt, throw it out.

Is It the Flu?   Symptoms of food-borne illness (nausea, vomiting, and diarrhea) are often thought to be a stomach flu. These symptoms may appear as soon as 30 minutes after eating a contaminated food, or they may take several days or weeks to appear. When treated with rest and a lot of fluids the symptoms usually last only a day or two. However, sometimes food-borne illnesses can be life threatening, especially for young children, pregnant women, the elderly, and the ill. When symptoms are severe, the patient should see a doctor as soon as possible.

Preventing Food-Borne Illness   The majority of food-borne illnesses can be avoided by selecting, storing, cooking, and handling food properly. Proper handling and storage of food is vital to avoid cross-contamination. **Cross-contamination** is the transfer of contaminants from one food to another. Cross-contamination can occur at home, for example, if the same cutting board is used to cut up raw chicken and to prepare vegetables for a salad or if raw and cooked foods are stored together. Cross-contamination can also happen in food-processing plants and restaurants. Contamination of foods in these locations could potentially affect hundreds of people. Therefore, there are many strict federal hygiene regulations that apply to food-processing plants and restaurants and that aim to minimize health risks to the public.

To reduce the risk of food-borne illness in the kitchen
▶ replace and wash dishcloths and hand towels frequently
▶ keep your refrigerator at 41°F
▶ wash your hands, cooking utensils, and surfaces with warm soapy water between each food preparation step
▶ cook food to the recommended temperatures to kill microorganisms

SECTION 4

REVIEW   *Answer the following questions on a separate piece of paper.*

Using Key Terms

1. **Identify** the term used to describe an abnormal response to a food that is triggered by the immune system.
   a. food allergy   c. constipation
   b. lactose intolerance   d. food intolerance

2. **Write** the term that means "an inability to digest lactose."

3. **Name** the term for "an illness caused by eating a food that contains a contaminant such as a microorganism."

4. **Define** *cross-contamination*.

Understanding Key Ideas

5. **Describe** how excess gas can form in the intestines.

6. **Describe** how diarrhea can cause dehydration.

7. **Compare** the symptoms of a food allergy to the symptoms of a food intolerance.

8. **LIFE SKILL** **Practicing Wellness** Identify steps to reduce your chances of getting a food borne illness.

Critical Thinking

9. Can the bacteria on raw chicken that you buy from the store end up in your fresh fruit salad? Explain your answer.

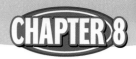

Highlights

Key Terms

SECTION 1

hunger (190)
appetite (190)
basal metabolic rate (BMR) (192)
overweight (193)
obesity (194)

SECTION 2

heredity (196)
body composition (197)
body mass index (BMI) (197)
weight management (198)
fad diet (200)

SECTION 3

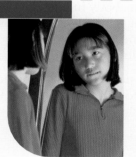

body image (202)
anorexia nervosa (204)
bulimia nervosa (204)
binge eating (bingeing) (204)
purging (204)

SECTION 4

food allergy (208)
lactose intolerance (209)
food-borne illness (209)
cross-contamination (210)

The Big Picture

✔ What you eat and how much you eat are affected by both hunger and appetite.

✔ Personal choices as well as friends, tradition, ethnic background, availability of food, and emotions affect food choices.

✔ Your body weight is affected by your food intake and by your activity levels.

✔ Eating breakfast every day is important for good health.

✔ Being overweight or obese increases the risk of heart disease, diabetes, cancer, and other chronic diseases.

✔ The genes you inherit from your parents and your lifestyle choices determine your body size and shape.

✔ Body mass index is an index of weight in relation to height that is used to assess healthy body weight.

✔ Keeping body weight in the healthy range requires a plan that encourages healthy food choices and good exercise habits.

✔ Fad diets may cause initial weight loss but can be dangerous and do not promote behaviors for long-term weight management.

✔ Individuals with eating disorders often have a distorted body image.

✔ Eating disorders are more common in teenage girls, especially overachievers who have a poor self-image, and in athletes who must restrict their weight.

✔ Anorexia nervosa is an overwhelming fear of gaining weight and can result in self-starvation. Bulimia nervosa involves frequent bingeing and purging, which can cause many health problems.

✔ Eating disorders should be identified and treated early to avoid long-term health problems.

✔ Common digestive disorders include heartburn, ulcers, constipation, diarrhea, and flatulence.

✔ Diarrhea causes water loss and can result in dehydration, which is very dangerous, especially to children and the elderly.

✔ A food allergy involves a reaction by the body's immune system to particular foods. A food intolerance may cause symptoms similar to those of an allergic reaction, but it is not a specific immune reaction.

✔ Proper handling and storage of food can prevent a food-borne illness.

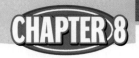

Review

Using Key Terms

anorexia nervosa (204)

appetite (190)

basal metabolic rate (BMR) (192)

binge eating/bingeing (204)

body composition (197)

body image (202)

body mass index (197)

bulimia nervosa (204)

cross-contamination (210)

fad diet (200)

food allergy (208)

food-borne illness (209)

heredity (196)

hunger (190)

lactose intolerance (209)

obesity (194)

overweight (193)

purging (204)

weight management (198)

1. For each definition below, choose the key term that best matches the definition.
   a. eating a large amount of food at one time
   b. forcefully ridding the body of Calories
   c. heavy for one's height
   d. how you see and feel about your appearance
   e. sensible eating and exercise habits that keep weight at a healthy level
   f. a diet that promises quick weight loss

2. Explain the relationship between the key terms in each of the following pairs.
   a. *anorexia nervosa* and *bulimia nervosa*
   b. *hunger* and *appetite*
   c. *obesity* and *body mass index*
   d. *food allergy* and *lactose intolerance*
   e. *cross-contamination* and *food-borne illness*
   f. *body composition* and *heredity*

Understanding Key Ideas

Section 1

3. Is eating a piece of chocolate cake for dessert after a big dinner more likely to be motivated by hunger or by appetite? Explain your answer.

4. Why does eating breakfast each morning help you perform better in school?

5. Explain what happens to the extra energy if you eat more food than your body needs.

6. For what health conditions are people with excess body fat at increased risk?

7. What is the best plan for avoiding obesity?

Section 2

8. Explain why a person whose parents are obese may not necessarily become obese.

9. What is the BMI of an individual who is 5 feet 1 inch tall and weighs 127 pounds?

10. Explain why following a weight management plan that has a menu for only one week of meals is unlikely to promote long-term weight loss.

11. **CRITICAL THINKING** A magazine features the "tomato and lemon juice" diet. The diet promises a weight loss of 5 pounds a week. Why is this diet not a good way to manage weight?

Section 3

12. Explain why someone who has a poor body image is more likely to develop an eating disorder.

13. What types of individuals are most at risk for eating disorders?

14. Which of the following is *not* a symptom of an eating disorder?
    a. healthy body image
    b. fear of gaining weight
    c. extreme weight loss
    d. bingeing and purging

15. Identify people or health organizations you could look to for help with a friend who has an eating disorder. **LIFE SKILL**

Section 4

16. Identify actions you can take to help prevent heartburn and constipation. **LIFE SKILL**

17. Identify the main reason why diarrhea can be life threatening.

18. Identify ways you can avoid having a food intolerance. **LIFE SKILL**

19. Describe how washing your hands can protect you from food-borne illness.

20. **CRITICAL THINKING** You are at camp with a friend who is allergic to peanuts. How can you help determine which foods are safe for him to eat?

Interpreting Graphics

Study the figure below to answer the questions that follow.

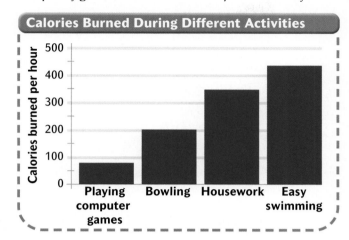

Calories Burned During Different Activities

21. Which of these activities requires the least bodily movement?

22. Estimate how many Calories in total are burned during 30 minutes of housework and 30 minutes of swimming. **MATH SKILL**

23. **CRITICAL THINKING** Which of these activities would be most effective as part of your weight management plan?

Activities

24. **Health and You** Find an advertisement for a diet plan in a magazine or in another source. Does the diet contain all of the components of a healthy weight management plan? Would it be safe to follow this plan for an extended period of time?

25. **Health and Your Community** Prepare a poster display that explores how body images have changed over the past 30 years.

26. **Health and Your Family** Write a short report that describes ways to avoid a food-borne illness in a home kitchen.

27. **Health and You** Think about how the availability of food can affect what you eat and when you eat. Write a healthy meal plan from what is on your school's lunch menu today. **WRITING SKILL**

Action Plan

28. **LIFE SKILL** **Assessing Your Health** List five things that you can do to improve your body image and to keep your weight in the healthy range.

Standardized Test Prep

Read the passage below, and then answer the questions that follow. **READING SKILL** **WRITING SKILL** **MATH SKILL**

> Ann is studying for a history test. She had to cancel tennis after school because she needed the time to study. But now she is bored. To help apply herself to her studies she makes a bowl of buttery popcorn. When that is gone, she gets a bag of chips from the kitchen. When she discovers she has finished off the bag of chips too, she is angry with herself. She has been putting on weight lately. Skipping tennis and eating all this junk food is going to add to her weight gain. She decides that she needs a plan to help her focus on studying without gaining weight.

29. In the passage, the word *apply* means
   - A to put into action or use.
   - B to concentrate one's efforts.
   - C to ask for something.
   - D to select something.

30. What can you infer from reading this passage?
   - E Ann has an eating disorder.
   - F Ann is obese.
   - G Ann eats junk food when she is bored.
   - H Ann is not a good cook.

31. By skipping tennis, Ann uses 150 fewer Calories than usual that day. By eating popcorn and a bag of chips, she eats about 500 extra Calories. What has that done to her energy balance that day?

32. Write a paragraph describing some of the things Ann can do to help her study without gaining weight.

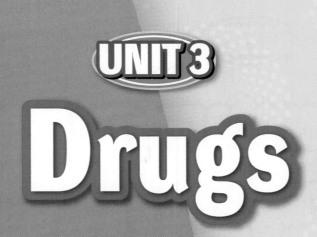

UNIT 3
Drugs

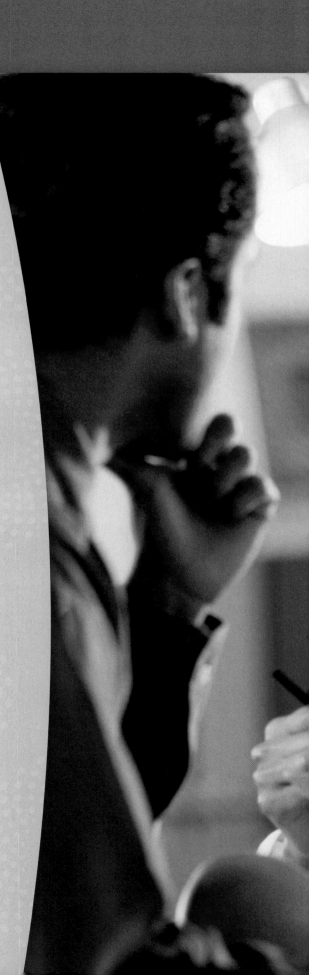

CHAPTER 9

Understanding Drugs and Medicines

What's Your Health IQ?
KNOWLEDGE

Which of the statements below are true, and which are false? Check your answers on p. 642.

1. Side effects of over-the-counter medicines are rare.

2. Cold medicines can cause drowsiness when they are taken with antihistamines.

3. Not following doctor's orders while taking a prescription medicine can be dangerous.

4. Generic drugs work equally as well as brand-name drugs.

5. Nutritional supplements are not approved by the Food and Drug Administration, as are medicines.

6. Drugs that come from natural products are safer than drugs made from chemicals.

7. People cannot become addicted to prescription drugs.

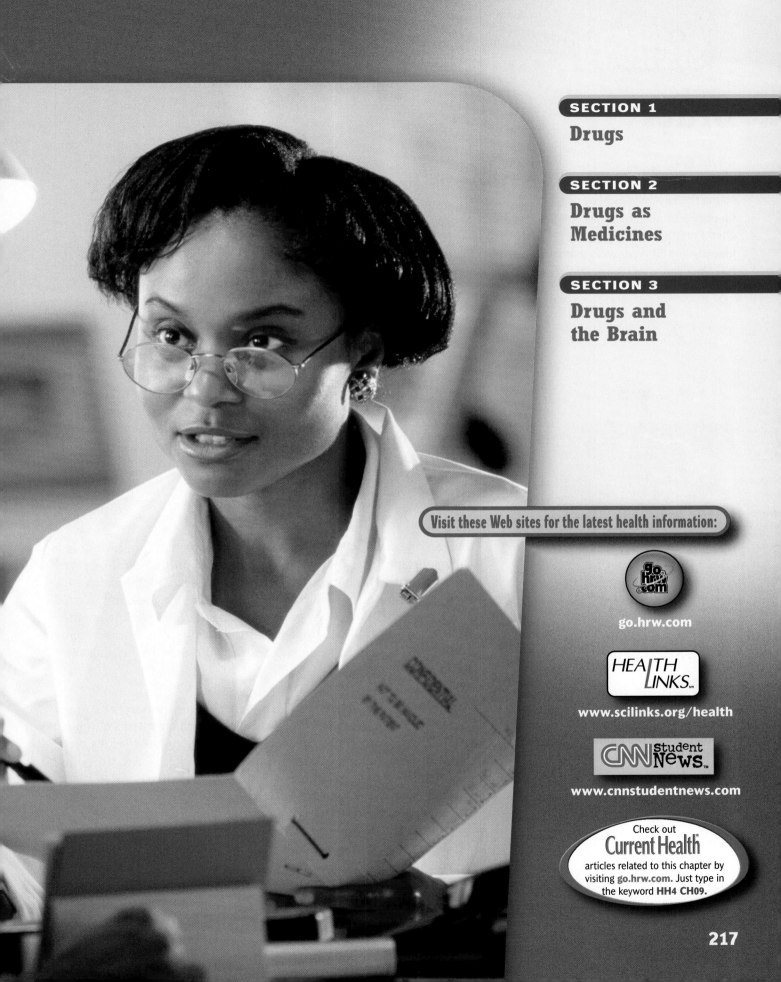

Visit these Web sites for the latest health information:

go.hrw.com

HEALTH LINKS.sm
www.scilinks.org/health

CNN student News™
www.cnnstudentnews.com

Check out
Current Health
articles related to this chapter by
visiting go.hrw.com. Just type in
the keyword **HH4 CH09.**

217

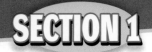

Drugs

OBJECTIVES

List three qualities that make a drug useful as a medicine.

Name the two sources of all drugs.

Identify four different types of medicines and their effects on the body.

Identify five different ways that drugs can enter the body.

Describe why some drugs are considered drugs of abuse.

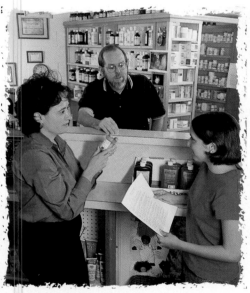

Taking medicine is serious business. Always make sure you are well informed about the medicines you are taking or need to take.

What do aspirin, caffeine, cortisone, and cocaine all have in common? They are all drugs. You encounter some drugs every day. Some drugs help sick people feel better. Some of these drugs you can get only from a doctor. Still, other drugs are taken for their effect on the brain.

What Are Drugs?

How can one class of substances be so many different things? A **drug** is any substance that causes a change in a person's physical or psychological state. Thousands of different drugs exist and they can have many different kinds of effects. Some drugs have one specific effect, while other drugs have many effects. Some drugs kill invading organisms. Other drugs, like the ones used for treating cancer, may even make someone who has cancer feel sick while they are helping the person to get better.

Some Drugs Are Medicines Any drug that is used to cure, prevent, or treat illness or discomfort is called a **medicine.** For example, the antibiotic penicillin is considered a medicine because it kills certain types of bacteria that can infect us and make us sick. To be a good medicine, a drug must have the following qualities:

▶ **Effectiveness** When a medicine is good at carrying out its task, doctors say it is *effective.* For example, penicillin is effective at killing certain types of bacteria.

▶ **Safety** Good medicines also have to be safe. For example, penicillin wouldn't be very useful if it damaged the heart while it was killing bacteria. But penicillin does not damage the heart. So for most people, penicillin is safe to use.

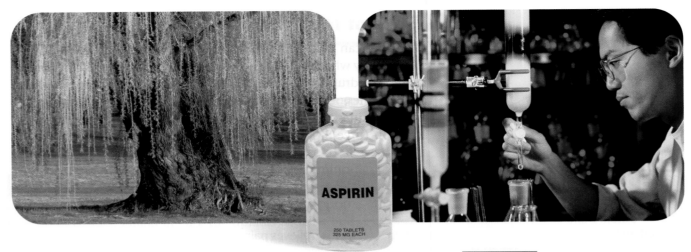

Figure 1

Some medicines, such as aspirin, were originally developed from substances produced by plants. Today many medicines, including aspirin, are created by scientists in laboratories and are made by drug companies.

▶ **Minor side effects** No medicine is perfectly safe for everyone. Any effect that is caused by a drug and that is different from the drug's intended effect is called a **side effect.** Common side effects of medicines include headache, sleepiness, or diarrhea. Most drugs have very minor side effects. If a medicine has too many side effects or if the side effects are too severe, the medicine may not be safe to use, at least not by everyone. For example, some people can have an allergic reaction to penicillin. The reactions to penicillin can range from a rash to a fever and, very rarely, to death.

Some Drugs Are "Drugs of Abuse"

Drugs that are not medicines, such as cocaine, nicotine, alcohol, and marijuana, change the way the brain works in ways that are not healthy. A person takes drugs like these to change how he or she feels or how he or she senses the world. The person may want to feel happier, or less sad or less anxious. Drugs that people take for mind-altering effects that have no medical purpose are called *drugs of abuse.*

Drugs that dramatically change your mood can be very dangerous. Over time, any drug that affects the brain can change your behavior so that you can't control your behavior. This loss of control can lead to serious long-term health problems.

Where Do Drugs Come From?

Despite their differences, all drugs have one thing in common—they are all chemicals. In the past, all drugs came from natural sources such as plants, animals, and fungi. For example, opium, which has been used for thousands of years to treat pain and diarrhea, comes from the unripe seed capsules of the opium poppy. **Figure 1** shows a willow tree, the bark of which is the source of salicin, the chemical from which aspirin was developed.

Many drugs are now created by scientists working in laboratories. Scientists can work on the structure of chemicals to change existing drugs or develop new drugs. Every year, drug companies test thousands of new chemicals to see if the chemicals might be effective as drugs.

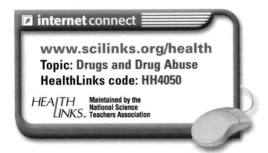

☐ internet connect

www.scilinks.org/health
Topic: Drugs and Drug Abuse
HealthLinks code: HH4050

HEALTH
LINKS. Maintained by the National Science Teachers Association

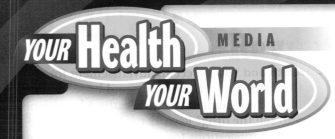
Prescription Drugs and the Media

There was a time when drug companies did not advertise prescription drugs on TV or in magazines. Now, we see such ads often. But are these advertisements good for your health?

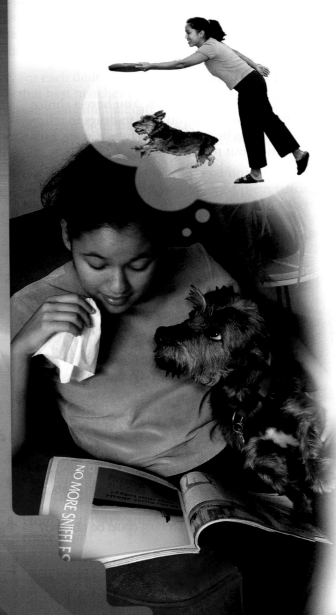

In 1555, the Royal College of Physicians in London declared that no doctor could tell a patient anything about a medicine, including its name. Doctors in those days were concerned that patients would hurt themselves by using medicines unwisely. This cautious attitude persisted in the medical community for more than 450 years, but things have changed in modern times.

Direct-to-Consumer Advertising

Prescription drugs are now so widely advertised in magazines, on the Internet, on the radio, and especially on TV that they affect every person living in this country. This kind of advertising is called *direct-to-consumer (DTC) advertising.* In 2001, the pharmaceutical industry spent $2.5 billion on DTC advertising in the United States. Pharmaceutical companies spent $1.5 billion on TV advertising alone.

Drug Advertising Affects People's Actions

In 1999, one national newsmagazine contained more than 18 pages of advertisements for prescription drugs. Does all of this advertising affect people's choices about medicine? The answer appears to be yes. Thirty percent of all people who see these ads and then go to a doctor ask for an advertised product. More astoundingly, almost half of the doctors give the patient a prescription for the specific drug requested. Only one in four doctors recommends another drug. In short, people are motivated by the ads, and their doctors are likely to give them requested drugs.

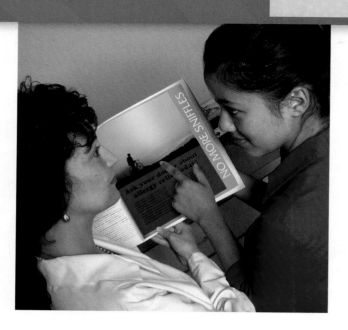

Advertising Prescription Drugs Has Benefits

Many people in the drug and medical field suggest that these ads provide great benefits to you, the consumer. They argue that a consumer has a right to learn about the drugs that are available to treat a symptom. Advertising, they say, is a form of education. If you have asthma, for example, shouldn't you have a right to know which asthma drugs you can use? Why should only a doctor have access to such information?

Another argument in favor of DTC advertising is that it makes money for the pharmaceutical industry. This money, supporters of DTC argue, helps pay for the costly development of current drugs and for the development of new drugs.

Drug Advertising Has Drawbacks

Along with the growth in drug advertising has come a steady growth of criticism. Consumer groups and physicians have complained that advertising sometimes causes people to make bad choices. One argument is that drug ads blur the distinction between providing information and promoting good healthcare. When doctors tell patients that the specific drug they asked for may not be good for them, the patients often react with anger and frustration. They may demand a specific drug even when another is as good, better, or even cheaper. Many doctors say that they feel pressured by patients who had read ads.

Being Aware of the Media's Influence

The media—TV, radio, Internet, newspapers, and magazines—affects everybody's life. The sudden growth in DTC advertising of prescription drugs means that all of us must become wise consumers. Advertising should not be accepted without question.

Your best course of action is to use your physician as a partner in your healthcare. Ask your doctor questions, and listen responsibly to the answers and suggestions. Likewise, all of us must bring skepticism to what we see and hear, especially when someone is trying to sell us something. Drug advertisements may indeed help us make better choices, but if used unwisely, they may compromise our health.

YOUR TURN

1. **Summarizing Information** Give one argument for and one argument against advertising prescription drugs.

2. **Analyzing Methods** Check some current magazines in terms of numbers and types of drug advertisements. How does each ad attempt to sell the drug? Discuss your findings.

3. **CRITICAL THINKING** How can you determine if a drug advertisement is telling you all of the facts about treating a specific illness or using a specific drug?

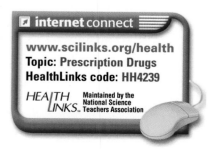

internet connect

www.scilinks.org/health
Topic: Prescription Drugs
HealthLinks code: HH4239

HEALTH LINKS. Maintained by the National Science Teachers Association

CHAPTER 10
Alcohol

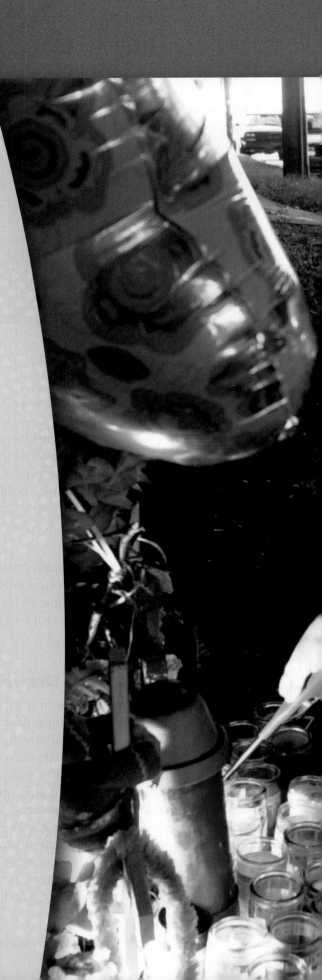

What's Your Health IQ?
KNOWLEDGE

Which of the statements below are true, and which are false? Check your answers on p. 642.

1. A shot of vodka has the same amount of alcohol that a can of beer has.

2. Most of the problems caused by alcohol are due to loss of judgment.

3. One drink can affect a person's ability to drive.

4. Alcohol overdose can be fatal.

5. Children of alcoholics have an increased risk of becoming alcoholics.

6. Alcoholism affects only the alcoholic.

7. Drunk driving is the No. 1 cause of death among teens in the United States.

Visit these Web sites for the latest health information:

go.hrw.com

www.scilinks.org/health

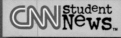

www.cnnstudentnews.com

Check out
Current Health
articles related to this chapter by
visiting **go.hrw.com.** Just type in
the keyword **HH4 CH10.**

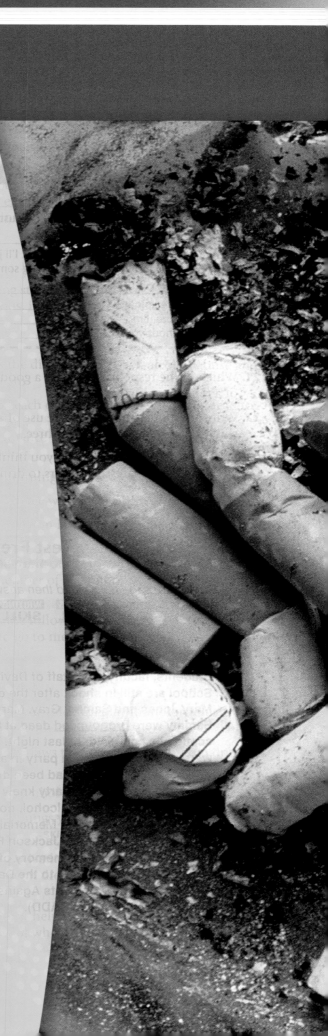

Tobacco

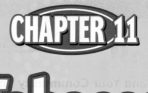

What's Your Health IQ?
KNOWLEDGE

Which of the following statements are true, and which are false? Check your answers on p. 642.

1. At high doses, nicotine is a nerve poison.

2. Chewing tobacco is safer than smoking tobacco because no smoke gets into the lungs.

3. Herbal cigarettes are safer than tobacco cigarettes because they don't contain tobacco.

4. You can smoke for many years before you start to harm your lungs.

5. The smoke that escapes from a burning cigarette is dangerous to others.

6. The placenta protects a fetus from smoke in women that smoke during pregnancy.

7. Nonsmokers get fewer colds than smokers.

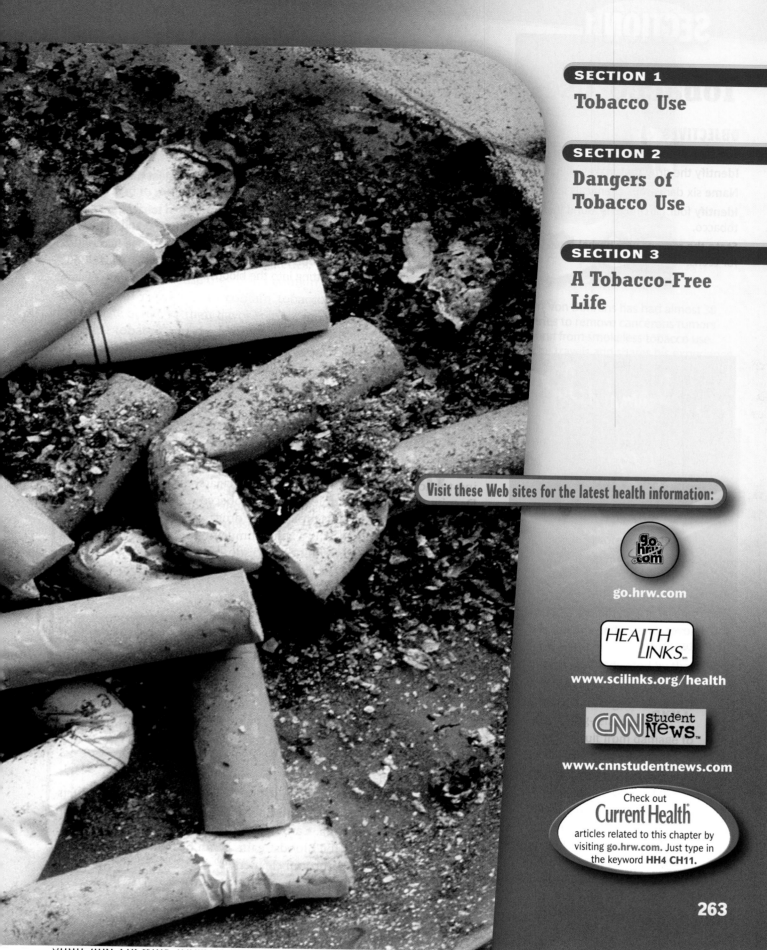

Visit these Web sites for the latest health information:

go.hrw.com

HEALTH LINKS℠
www.scilinks.org/health

CNN student news℠
www.cnnstudentnews.com

Check out
Current Health
articles related to this chapter by
visiting go.hrw.com. Just type in
the keyword **HH4 CH11**.

263

snuff and chewing tobacco also cause you to spit often. None of these effects are very attractive.

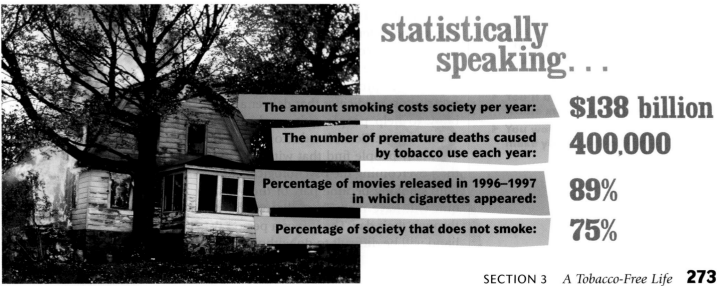

statistically speaking. . .

The amount smoking costs society per year:	**$138 billion**
The number of premature deaths caused by tobacco use each year:	**400,000**
Percentage of movies released in 1996–1997 in which cigarettes appeared:	**89%**
Percentage of society that does not smoke:	**75%**

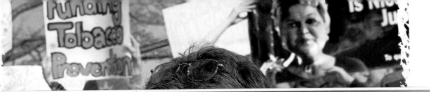

SECTION 3

A Tobacco-Free Life

OBJECTIVES

Discuss the factors that contribute to tobacco use.

Summarize three ways that tobacco use affects families and society.

List four things a person can do to make quitting smoking easier.

Name five benefits of being tobacco free.

List five ways to refuse tobacco products if they're offered to you. **LIFE SKILL**

> **KEY TERMS**
>
> **nicotine substitutes** medicines that deliver small amounts of nicotine to the body to help a person quit using tobacco

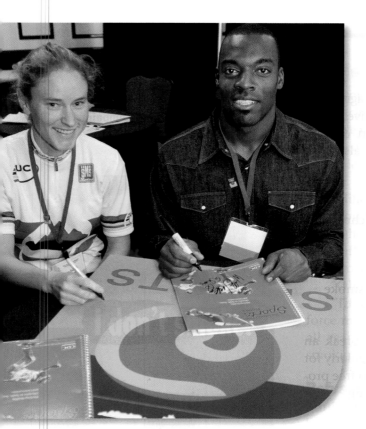

World Cup Mountain Bike Champion Alison Dunlap and New Orleans Saints wide receiver Willie Jackson sign copies of a book that promotes a healthy lifestyle as an alternative to tobacco use for young people.

Life Without Tobacco What does it mean if you've used tobacco? Is it too late to protect your health? Studies show that the sooner you quit using tobacco, the sooner your body can get back to normal.

Within half an hour after quitting smoking, your blood pressure and heart rate will fall back to normal. Eight hours later, you will have rid the carbon monoxide from your bloodstream, and you will have normal blood-oxygen levels. Within a few days, your sense of smell and taste will improve, and breathing will be easier.

During the following months, your lung health will improve, and you won't be short of breath anymore. You'll be reducing your risk of lung cancer by about 10 times, the threat of emphysema will almost disappear, and your risk of heart disease will decrease as well. Even in such a short time, living without tobacco makes a big difference.

Live Healthy and Tobacco Free Life is better without tobacco. The 80 percent of teens who *don't* smoke agree. Tobacco is a dangerous and addictive drug. All forms of tobacco have been proven to cause major health problems that can be deadly. As a result of lawsuits, tobacco companies have paid billions of dollars to the states for exactly that reason.

People may have many reasons for trying tobacco. Friends, family, media influence, rebellion, boredom, and curiosity are all reasons people may smoke or dip for the first time. Most tobacco users generally have only one reason for continuing to use tobacco—addiction. And the best reason for staying tobacco free is life. Your life, your friends' lives, and the lives of all your loved ones will be better without tobacco.

SECTION 3

REVIEW *Answer the following questions on a separate piece of paper.*

Using Key Terms

1. **Define** *nicotine substitute*.

Understanding Key Ideas

2. **List** three reasons people may begin using tobacco.

3. **State** two ways that tobacco use affects families and society.

4. **Identify** which of the following is *not* a cost of tobacco use to society.
   a. tobacco products
   b. funeral costs
   c. fetal alcohol syndrome
   d. medical costs

5. **Describe** a strategy a person could use to make quitting smoking easier.

6. **Identify** five benefits of living tobacco free.

Critical Thinking

7. **LIFE SKILL** **Using Refusal Skills** List five reasons you can give for refusing to use tobacco. Which of these reasons is most important to you?

8. **LIFE SKILL** **Communicating Effectively** Imagine that you have a family member who smokes heavily. What do you think would be the best way to try to convince them to quit smoking?

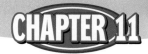
Highlights

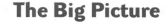

Key Terms

The Big Picture

SECTION 1

nicotine (264)
carcinogen (264)
tar (264)
carbon monoxide (264)

✔ There are many kinds of tobacco products, such as cigarettes, dip, snuff, chew, bidis, kreteks, and pipe tobacco.

✔ All forms of tobacco are dangerous because they contain many harmful chemicals and carcinogens, including nicotine, tar, carbon monoxide, cyanide, and formaldehyde.

✔ Nicotine can enter the body through the lungs, the gums, and the skin.

✔ Herbal cigarettes are thought to be more healthy but are actually just as dangerous as conventional cigarettes.

✔ People who use tobacco products find it very hard to quit because nicotine is a highly addictive drug.

SECTION 2

emphysema (268)
sidestream smoke (270)
mainstream smoke (270)
environmental tobacco smoke (secondhand smoke) (270)

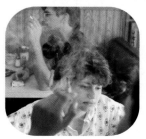

✔ The short-term effects of tobacco use include increases in heart rate, blood pressure, and breathing rate, as well as a reduction in the amount of oxygen that reaches the brain.

✔ Long-term tobacco use leads to oral and lung cancer, bronchitis, emphysema, heart disease, artery disease, and other health problems.

✔ People who breathe environmental tobacco smoke are exposed to the same dangerous chemicals as smokers.

✔ Smoking while pregnant can lead to several kinds of problems for the infant, including miscarriage, developmental difficulties, and SIDS.

✔ There are many reasons not to smoke, including protecting your family, friends, and loved ones from the harmful effects of environmental tobacco smoke.

SECTION 3

nicotine substitutes (274)

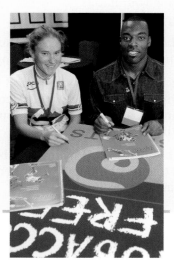

✔ People begin smoking for many reasons. Some want to fit in with friends who smoke, some find it normal after growing up around family members who smoke, and others want to look cool.

✔ Using tobacco is expensive. It costs families and society billions of dollars each year in healthcare and lost productivity.

✔ Quitting smoking can be difficult, but setting a quitting date, marking your progress, getting involved in other activities, and rewarding yourself can help make quitting easier.

✔ Refusing tobacco may be difficult, but practicing effective refusal skills makes it easier to resist pressure.

✔ There are many benefits to being tobacco free, including looking younger, feeling healthier, and living longer than you would if you used tobacco.

✔ Whether a person has used tobacco or not, choosing to live without tobacco dramatically improves a person's quality of life.

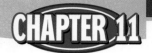

Review

Using Key Terms

carbon monoxide (264)
carcinogen (264)
emphysema (268)
environmental tobacco smoke (secondhand smoke) (270)
mainstream smoke (270)
nicotine (264)
nicotine substitutes (274)
sidestream smoke (270)
tar (264)

1. For each definition below, choose the key term that best matches the definition.
  a. the smoke inhaled and exhaled by the smoker
  b. a gas that blocks oxygen from entering the bloodstream
  c. a lung disease in which the alveoli lose their elasticity or become blocked
  d. any chemical or agent that causes cancer
  e. a sticky substance in tobacco smoke that coats the inside of the airway and contains many carcinogens
  f. the addictive drug found in tobacco

2. Explain the relationship between the key terms in each of the following pairs.
  a. *nicotine* and *carbon monoxide*
  b. *tar* and *emphysema*
  c. *environmental tobacco smoke* and *carcinogen*
  d. *mainstream smoke* and *sidestream smoke*

Understanding Key Ideas
Section 1

3. Name four types of tobacco products.

4. State the reason it is difficult for people to quit using tobacco products.

5. Identify the carcinogens found in tobacco.
  a. benzene   **c.** vinyl chloride
  b. formaldehyde   **d.** all of the above

6. Compare the amount of nicotine in snuff with the amount in cigarette smoke.

7. Are herbal cigarettes safer than regular cigarettes?

8. CRITICAL THINKING Would you consider nicotine a dangerous drug? Explain.

Section 2

9. List three short-term effects of tobacco use.

10. Which of the following is a long-term effect of tobacco use?
  a. heart and artery disease
  b. cancer
  c. receding gums and mouth sores
  d. all of the above

11. Why is smoking dangerous to nonsmokers?

12. Women who smoke while pregnant are more likely to
  a. suffer miscarriage.   **c.** cause SIDS.
  b. have bronchitis.   **d.** All of the above

13. List four reasons not to smoke that you could give to a friend. **LIFE SKILL**

14. CRITICAL THINKING One of the negative aspects of smoking is that the clothes of smokers usually smell like tobacco smoke. Explain why smokers generally cannot smell tobacco smoke on their clothes.

Section 3

15. What factors do you think contribute to people using tobacco in your school? **LIFE SKILL**

16. Describe the financial and health costs of smoking on both the family and the community.

17. Which technique does *not* help a person quit smoking?
  a. setting a goal
  b. punishing yourself for failing
  c. changing your habits
  d. getting support

18. List five benefits both smokers and smokeless tobacco users can expect after quitting.

19. Describe an effective refusal method you could use if someone were to tell you, "Here, try these new cigarettes, almost everyone in our school smokes these." **LIFE SKILL**

20. CRITICAL THINKING Why might it be harder for a person to quit smoking if his or her friends and parents smoke?

Interpreting Graphics

Study the figure below to answer the questions that follow.

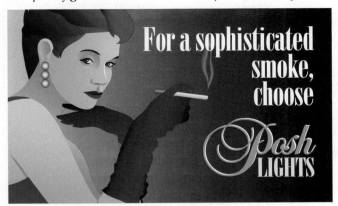

For a sophisticated smoke, choose *Posh* LIGHTS

21. What do you think the word *sophisticated,* as used in the ad above, means? **READING SKILL**

22. What message is this ad trying to convey about tobacco use?

23. CRITICAL THINKING Do you think this ad might encourage a young person to smoke? Explain.

Activities

24. Health and You Imagine you are riding in a car with someone who smokes. **WRITING SKILL** Write a paragraph explaining how you might politely and effectively ask the person not to smoke in the car.

25. Health and Your Community Environmental tobacco smoke is just as dangerous as mainstream smoke. Write a one-page **WRITING SKILL** report advocating for smoke-free environments for nonsmokers.

26. Health and You Write a reply to the following statement: "Just try this cigarette once; one try won't harm you. It's not like you'll become an addict."

Action Plan

27. Take Charge of Your Health Use of clove cigarettes, bidis, and kreteks has become more popular among teens. Research these products, and write a one-page report explaining why teens use these tobacco products.

Standardized Test Prep

Read the passage below, and then answer the questions that follow. **READING SKILL** **WRITING SKILL**

> Cameron and Tony walked up to the counter at the convenient store. "What are you getting?" asked Tony. "Nothing. I'm out of cash," replied Cameron. "Didn't you have a bunch of money last week?" asked Tony. "Yeah, but I spent it on cigarettes." "Man, that just doesn't seem worth it. If you have a <u>finite</u> income, you should save it for the stereo system you want." "I know. Cigarettes keep getting more and more expensive, but I've been smoking for years. I can't stop," said Cameron. "It's not like quitting is impossible," replied Tony.

28. In this paragraph, the word *finite* means
  A limited.
  B endless.
  C spendable.
  D free.

29. What can you infer from reading this paragraph?
  E Tobacco products are cheap.
  F Tony makes more money than Cameron does.
  G Tony thinks tobacco is worth the expense.
  H Cameron is probably addicted to nicotine.

30. Write a paragraph discussing things that Cameron could do to make quitting easier. What could Tony do to help his friend quit smoking?

31. CRITICAL THINKING One reason that tobacco products are so expensive is that the U.S. government charges taxes that consumers must pay when they buy tobacco. Why do you think the government keeps raising these taxes?

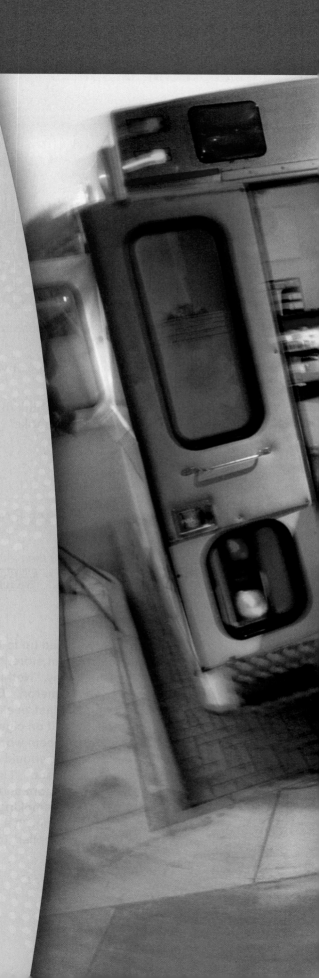

CHAPTER 12

Illegal Drugs

What's Your Health IQ?
KNOWLEDGE

Which of the statements below are true, and which are false? Check your answers on p. 642.

1. If illegal drugs were really dangerous, people wouldn't use them.

2. People can't get addicted to marijuana.

3. Stimulants can help you study more effectively.

4. Anabolic steroids are male hormones, so they should make guys appear more masculine.

5. Barbiturates are safe because they're used as medicine.

6. Most prison inmates committed their crime while high on drugs.

7. Because I'm young, any damage drugs do to my brain will heal by the time I'm an adult.

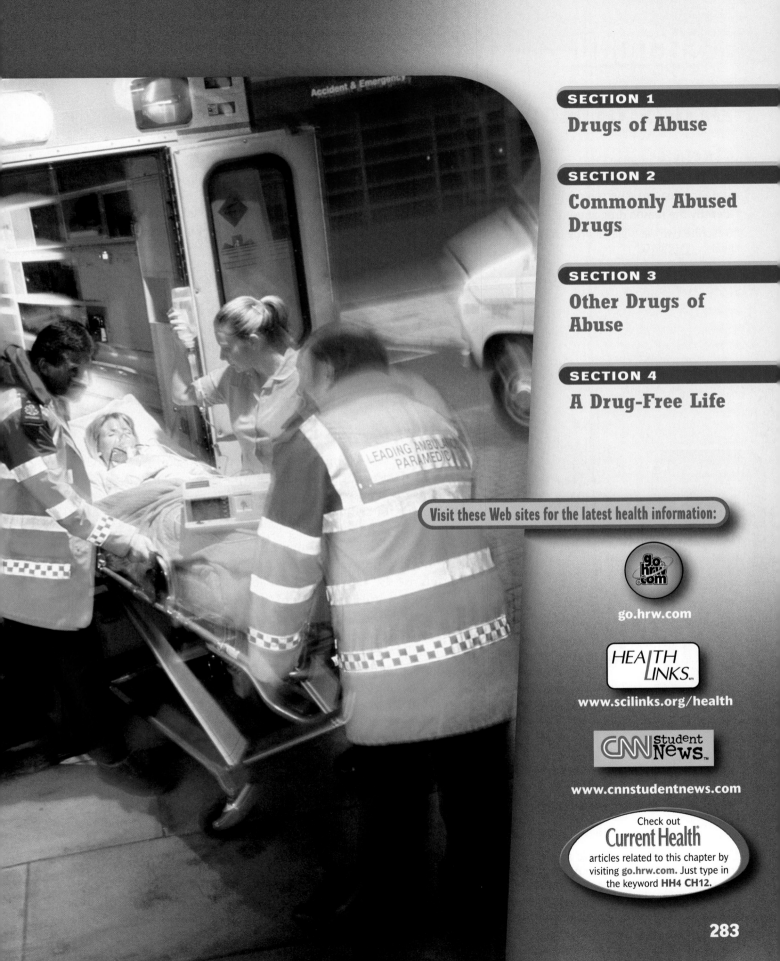

Visit these Web sites for the latest health information:

go.hrw.com

HEALTH LINKS.

www.scilinks.org/health

CNN student News.

www.cnnstudentnews.com

Check out **Current Health** articles related to this chapter by visiting **go.hrw.com**. Just type in the keyword **HH4 CH12.**

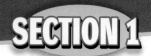
Drugs of Abuse

OBJECTIVES

List six ways illegal drug use can be dangerous.

State five reasons a person might try illegal drugs.

Identify the reason drug abuse is especially dangerous to teens.

Describe two ways illegal drug use conflicts with your values and goals. **LIFE SKILL**

KEY TERMS

drug abuse the intentional improper or unsafe use of a drug

overdose the taking of too much of a drug, which causes sickness, loss of consciousness, permanent damage, or even death

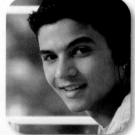

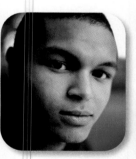

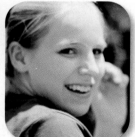

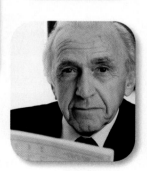

Drug abusers can be any age and be from any background. Each has a different reason for using drugs.

Tonya was the best point guard on the team until she tried cocaine. She liked how it made her feel, so she tried it again. Soon she was spending up to $100 a day on crack. When the team went to the state championship, Tonya couldn't go. She had been arrested for stealing. She had stolen to support her drug habit.

Illegal Drug Use Is Dangerous

Drug abuse is the intentional improper or unsafe use of a drug. Drugs that are used for recreational purposes are called *drugs of abuse*. Many drugs of abuse are *illegal drugs*. This means that possessing, using, buying, or selling these drugs is against the law for people of any age.

It may sometimes seem that our society is full of messages that tell us illegal drug use is normal and not dangerous. For example, characters in the movies and on television can make it seem as though illegal drug use is "cool." Many popular rock bands sing about illegal drugs. You can buy clothes and posters showing illegal drugs. But using illegal drugs is very dangerous for several reasons:

▶ Illegal drugs can have dangerous and permanent effects on the brain and the body.

▶ You can become addicted to almost all illegal drugs.

▶ Illegal drugs are a major factor in many suicides, motor vehicle accidents, and crimes.

▶ With illegal drug use that involves sharing needles, there is also the risk of catching infectious diseases such as hepatitis B and human immunodeficiency virus (HIV).

▶ Illegal drug use can result in overdose. **Overdose** is the taking of too much of a drug, which causes sickness, loss of consciousness, permanent health damage, or even death.

▶ While using illegal drugs, a person loses the ability to make responsible decisions. Having poor judgement while on drugs can result in risky sexual behavior, sexually transmitted diseases, car accidents, and other unsafe situations.

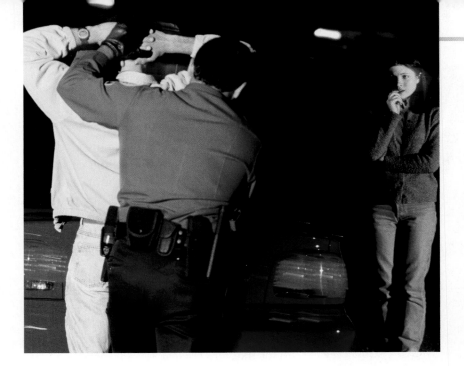

Being caught in possession of illegal drugs is a crime that has serious penalties.

Why Do People Begin Using Drugs?

If illegal drug use is so dangerous, why does anyone even try illegal drugs? People try illegal drugs for many reasons, including the following:

▶ desire to experiment
▶ desire to escape from depression or boredom
▶ enjoyment of risk-taking behaviors
▶ belief that drugs solve personal, social, or medical problems
▶ peer pressure
▶ glamorization of drug use by the media

Often, people begin taking a drug because they like the way it makes them feel. Soon, however, they may find that they must keep taking the drug just to feel normal. Repeated use of drugs that change how the brain works can lead to addiction. Addiction to an illegal drug can be very difficult to overcome.

Regardless of a person's reason for trying an illegal drug, one thing remains the same—the physical, mental, social, and legal consequences for illegal drug use make it not worth the risk.

Teens and Illegal Drug Use   Teens face many challenges during adolescence. These challenges include expectations on the part of parents and teachers and the desire for more freedom and responsibility. These challenges can make adolescence a very stressful time of life and can put teens at a greater risk for abusing illegal drugs.

Other challenges that teens face are intense peer pressure and a strong desire to fit in. There are many other reasons that teens might be tempted to try illegal drugs. The most common reasons that teens give for trying illegal drugs are listed below.

▶ Sometimes, just being around a group of people using drugs creates pressure to join in. This is a common type of peer pressure that doesn't involve direct pressure. Teens may give in and try a drug when they feel everyone else is trying drugs.

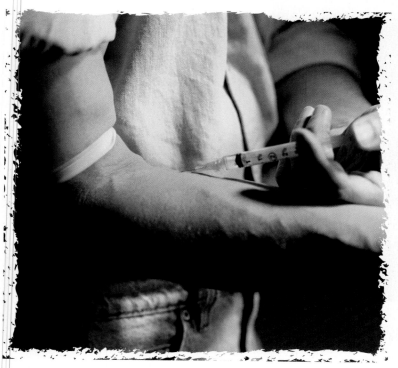

Some people start using drugs to get away from their problems and then can't get away from their drug problem.

▶ When faced with direct pressure to use drugs, teens who lack refusal skills or who feel intimidated may give in to pressure and use drugs.

▶ Many teens think that using illegal drugs is a way to escape from feelings of stress, anger, depression, or frustration. However, after a teen takes drugs, the problem that caused the negative feeling is still there, but now the teen may also have to deal with the consequences of drug use.

▶ Many teens try drugs out of curiosity. This seems natural when the media gives so much attention to drug abuse. Teens may see or hear of another person's experiences with drug use and wonder what it's like.

▶ Other teens may try drugs because they are risk takers or thrill seekers searching for a way to satisfy their desire for new experiences.

Unfortunately, teens have a higher risk of addiction to drugs than adults do. The risk of addiction is higher because young brains are still developing. Drug use or abuse can have irreversible effects on the function of the brain. Altering brain development with drug use can result in a lifetime of struggle to overcome addiction and to remain drug free.

SECTION 1

REVIEW *Answer the following questions on a separate piece of paper.*

Using Key Terms

1. **Define** the term *drug abuse*.

2. **Identify** the term for "the taking of too much of a drug, which causes sickness, loss of consciousness, permanent damage, or even death."

Understanding Key Ideas

3. **Identify** which of the following is a type of media that seems to advocate drug use.
   a. music
   b. movies
   c. television
   d. all of the above

4. **Identify** the reasons illegal drugs are dangerous.

5. **Name** five factors that influence a person's choice to use illegal drugs.

6. **State** the reasons why teens might try illegal drugs.

7. **Defend** the statement that teens should never use illegal drugs.

8. **Predict** the outcome of using an illegal drug to escape from personal problems.

9. **LIFE SKILL** **Setting Goals** Describe two ways illegal drug use would affect your personal values and goals.

Critical Thinking

10. **LIFE SKILL** **Practicing Wellness** Why is it important to have healthy alternatives to drug use?

Commonly Abused Drugs

OBJECTIVES

List three things all types of illegal drugs have in common.

Summarize the effects of four commonly abused illegal drugs on the body.

Describe the effects of marijuana on a person's behavior.

Identify the reason abusing inhalants can be deadly after only one use.

Compare the dangerous effects of five types of club drugs.

Summarize the dangerous effects of anabolic steroids.

KEY TERMS

marijuana the dried flowers and leaves of the plant *Cannabis sativa* that are smoked or mixed in food and eaten for intoxicating effects

inhalant a drug that is inhaled as a vapor

club (designer) drug a drug made to closely resemble a common illegal drug in chemical structure and effect

anabolic steroid a synthetic version of the male hormone testosterone that is used to promote muscle development

"Hey, you want a hit of this joint?" offered Randall. "No way. Do you know what that stuff can do to you?" Jen replied. Randall looked surprised. "Pot isn't dangerous, is it?" "It's dangerous" said Jen, "and it's addictive. Why would I want that?"

Types of Illegal Drugs

There are many types of illegal drugs. As shown in **Table 1,** each type of illegal drug has different effects on the body and the brain. Despite the differences in their effects, all illegal drugs have three things in common.

1. They affect the function of the brain.
2. They are dangerous to your health.
3. They can result in drug dependence and addiction.

Four commonly abused illegal drugs—marijuana, inhalants, club drugs, and anabolic steroids—will be described in this section.

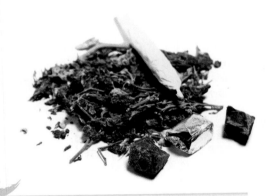

Beliefs Vs. Reality

"Marijuana is a safe drug."	Driving high on marijuana can be just as dangerous as driving drunk.
"It's okay to try a drug just once."	Some drugs, such as crack cocaine or inhalants, can be fatal the first time they are used.
"I can stop any time I want."	The more often you use drugs, the more difficult it can be to stop.
"If I want to use drugs, I only affect myself."	Drug use affects you, your family, your friends, and society.

Table 1   Common Illegal Drugs and Their Effects

Drug and common or street names	How it is taken	Possible intoxication effects	Possible health consequences*
Marijuana *pot, weed, dope, blunt, grass, reefer, Mary Jane* **Hashish** *boom, chronic, hash, hemp*	smoked or mixed in food and eaten	▸ relaxation ▸ feelings of well being ▸ distortion of time and distance ▸ loss of short-term memory ▸ loss of balance and coordination ▸ increased appetite	▸ frequent respiratory infection ▸ impaired learning and memory ▸ panic attack
Inhalants *glue, paint thinner, propane, nitrous oxide, NO, poppers, snappers, whippets*	inhaled	▸ stimulation ▸ loss of inhibitions ▸ dizziness ▸ loss of coordination ▸ nausea and vomiting ▸ headache	▸ heart attack ▸ liver damage ▸ kidney damage ▸ brain damage ▸ coma ▸ death
Club (designer) drugs			
Ecstasy *MDMA, Ecstasy, X, XTC, Adam*	swallowed or snorted	▸ increased awareness of senses ▸ mild hallucinations ▸ increased energy ▸ loss of judgment	▸ impaired learning and memory ▸ hyperthermia (overheating) ▸ rapid or irregular heartbeat ▸ high blood pressure ▸ heart attack ▸ death
GHB *G, liquid X, grievous bodily harm*	swallowed or snorted	▸ relaxation ▸ nausea ▸ loss of inhibitions ▸ euphoria	▸ dangerously slowed breathing ▸ seizures ▸ coma
Ketamine and PCP *Special K, K, Vitamin K, angel dust (PCP)*	injected, snorted, or smoked	▸ confusion ▸ distortions of reality ▸ numbness	▸ loss of memory ▸ loss of muscle control ▸ dangerously slowed breathing
Anabolic steroids *roids, juice*	swallowed or injected	▸ no intoxication effects	▸ increased aggression ▸ shrinking of testes ▸ infertility ▸ growth of breasts in men ▸ growth of facial hair in women ▸ deepening of voice in women ▸ liver rupture/liver cancer ▸ heart damage/heart attack

*All of the drugs listed in this table can result in physical dependence, and some can result in addiction.

Marijuana

Marijuana (MAR uh WAH nuh), also called *pot, weed, reefer,* or *dope,* is the dried flowers and leaves from the plant *Cannabis sativa.* The active chemical in marijuana is *tetrahydrocannabinol* (THC). THC can be detected in the urine for up to several weeks after use. Different marijuana plants may contain very different levels of THC. Marijuana is usually smoked, but it can also be mixed with food and eaten.

Effects of Marijuana   The effects of smoked marijuana are felt within minutes and may last for 2 or 3 hours. The effects of swallowed marijuana are felt within 30 to 60 minutes. Although the short-term effects of marijuana differ depending on the person and the strength of the drug, they can include the following:

- ▶ slowed thinking ability
- ▶ difficulty paying attention
- ▶ distorted sense of time and distance
- ▶ giddiness
- ▶ loss of short-term memory
- ▶ loss of balance and coordination
- ▶ increased appetite
- ▶ anxiety
- ▶ panic attack

Smoking marijuana over a long period of time can cause some of the same health effects as smoking cigarettes. Marijuana smoke has been found to contain many of the same carcinogens as cigarette smoke. Long-term marijuana use may lead to chronic bronchitis, damaged lung tissue, and increased risk of lung cancer.

Marijuana use has a negative effect on learning and social behavior. THC changes the way sensory information gets into the brain. Long-term marijuana use can cause difficulty in remembering, processing, and using information. Marijuana users can have difficulty maintaining attention and shifting attention to meet changing demands in the environment.

Stopping marijuana growers is a major part of the war on drugs. Law enforcement officials frequently destroy large fields of marijuana.

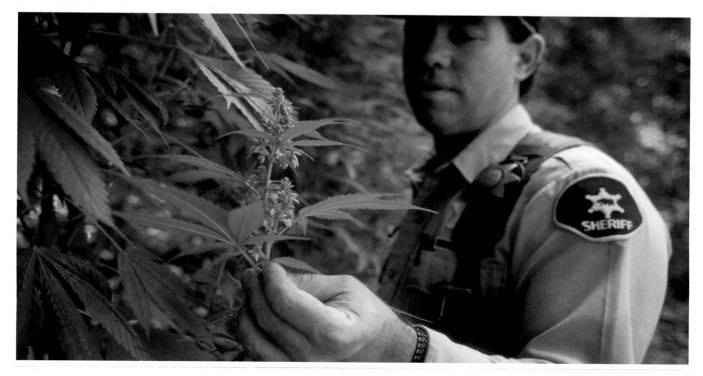

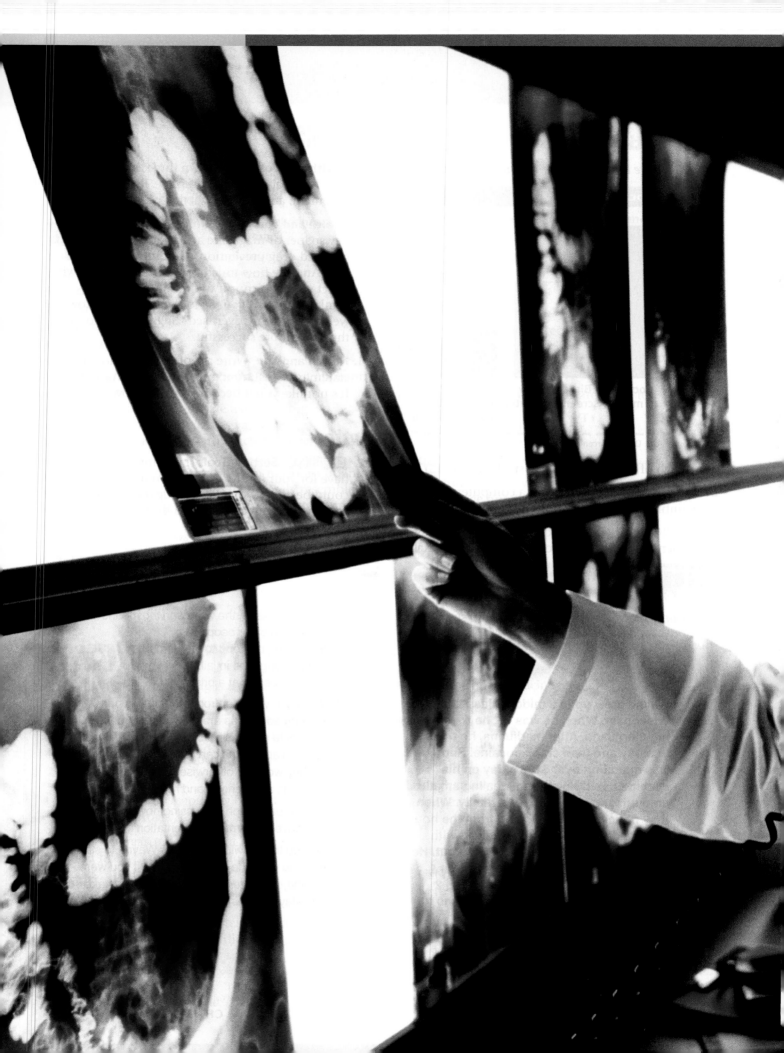

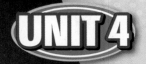

UNIT 4

Diseases and Disorders

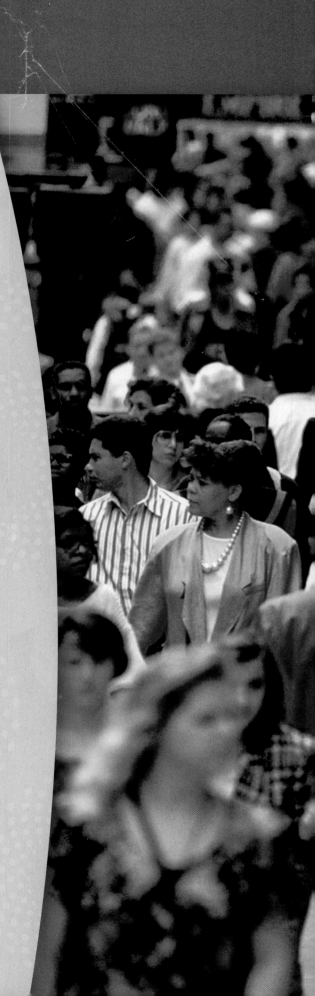

CHAPTER 13

Preventing Infectious Diseases

What's Your Health IQ?
BEHAVIOR

Indicate how frequently you engage in each of the following behaviors (1=never; 2=occasionally; 3=most of the time; 4=all of the time). Total your points, and then turn to p. 642.

1. I cover my mouth while sneezing or coughing.

2. I eat at least five servings of fruits and vegetables each day.

3. I exercise at least five times a week.

4. I have regular check-ups with my dentist and doctor.

5. I wash my hands before eating a meal.

6. When my doctor prescribes antibiotics, I follow and complete the prescription.

7. I drink 8 to 10 glasses of water each day.

8. I get extra sleep when I am sick.

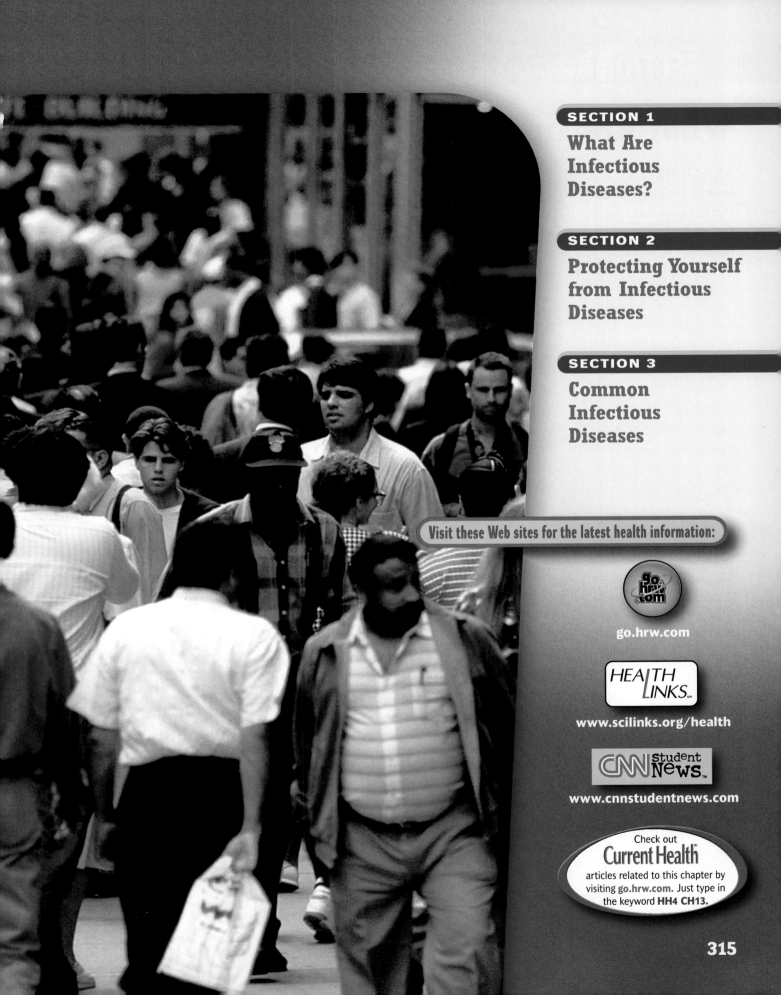

Visit these Web sites for the latest health information:

go.
hrw.
com

go.hrw.com

HEALTH
LINKS.sm

www.scilinks.org/health

CNN student
News.TM

www.cnnstudentnews.com

Check out
Current Health
articles related to this chapter by
visiting **go.hrw.com.** Just type in
the keyword **HH4 CH13.**

What Are Infectious Diseases?

OBJECTIVES

Identify five different agents that can cause infectious diseases.

List four ways that infectious diseases spread.

Describe two different treatments for infectious diseases.

Name two ways you can help prevent the development of antibiotic resistant bacteria. **LIFE SKILL**

While walking to his friend's house, Paul stepped on a rock and cut his foot. Because the cut was small, Paul just kept on walking. Paul didn't know, however, that a hidden army of organisms was starting an attack on his cut.

What Causes Infectious Diseases?

An **infectious disease** (in FEK shuhs di ZEEZ) is any disease that is caused by an agent that has invaded the body. Infectious diseases may be passed to a person from another person, from food or water, from animals, or from something in the environment. Colds, the flu, head lice, and tuberculosis (TB) are examples of infectious diseases.

Figure 1

Infectious diseases are caused by many different pathogens, such as viruses, bacteria, fungi, protozoa, and animal parasites.

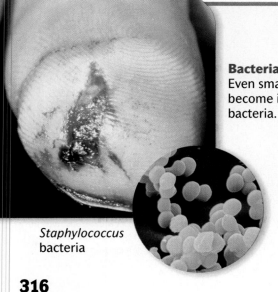

Bacteria
Even small cuts can become infected by bacteria.

Staphylococcus bacteria

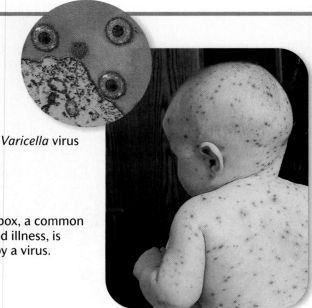

Varicella virus

Virus
Chickenpox, a common childhood illness, is caused by a virus.

All infectious diseases are caused by pathogens. A **pathogen** is any agent that causes disease. **Figure 1** shows some of the different kinds of pathogens that cause infectious diseases.

Bacteria Individually, bacteria are too small to be seen without a microscope. **Bacteria** are tiny, single-celled organisms, some of which can cause disease. Bacteria live almost everywhere on Earth. Some bacteria are even found in the frozen Arctic and in the boiling waters of hot springs.

You have more than 300 kinds of bacteria living in your mouth right now! There's no need to reach for the mouthwash, though, because most bacteria are harmless. Many are actually helpful. For example, bacteria living in your intestines make vitamins that you need to live. However, some kinds of bacteria make you sick when they grow on or inside your body. Some bacteria give off poisons, while other bacteria enter and damage cells. Tuberculosis, tetanus, and sinus infections are examples of diseases caused by bacteria.

Viruses Viruses are even smaller than bacteria. **Viruses** are tiny disease-causing particles made up of genetic material and a protein coat. The genetic material in the virus contains the instructions for making more viruses. Viruses survive and replicate only inside living cells. They reproduce by taking control of body cells and forcing them to make many new viruses. After escaping from the cell, these new viruses seek out other cells to attack. Diseases caused by viruses include chicken pox, colds, the flu, measles, and AIDS.

Fungi Organisms that absorbs and uses the nutrients of living or dead organisms are called **fungi** (singular fungus). The mushrooms in your salad are fungi. They don't cause disease, but other fungi do. Maybe you've had athlete's foot, which is caused by a fungus that lives and feeds on your feet and makes them burn and itch. A fungus, not a worm, is also responsible for the scaly, circular rash known as ringworm.

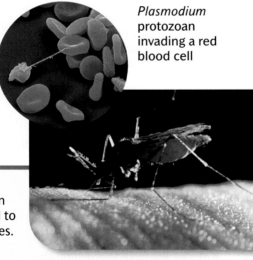

Plasmodium protozoan invading a red blood cell

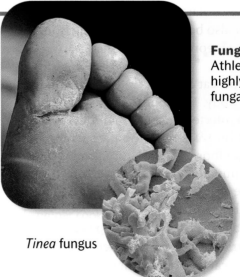

Fungus
Athlete's foot is a highly contagious fungal disease.

Tinea fungus

Protozoan
Malaria is a protozoan disease that is spread to humans by mosquitoes.

Parasite
Lice are parasites that attach to the hair on a person's head and cause itching.

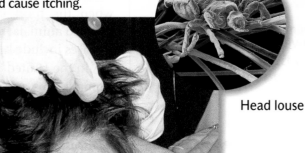

Head louse

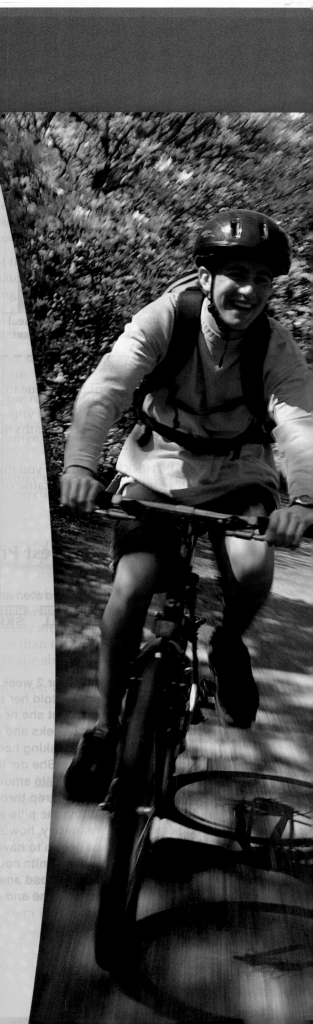

CHAPTER 14
Lifestyle Diseases

What's Your Health IQ?
BEHAVIOR

Indicate how frequently you engage in each of the following behaviors (1 = never; 2 = occasionally; 3 = most of the time; 4 = all of the time). Total your points, and then turn to p. 642.

1. I eat foods that are low in saturated fats and high in fiber.

2. I eat and drink foods that are low in added salt and sugar.

3. I exercise at least 60 minutes every day.

4. I avoid tobacco products and being in smoky environments.

5. I have yearly medical exams.

6. When outside, I wear sunscreen.

7. I eat at least 2 servings of fruit a day.

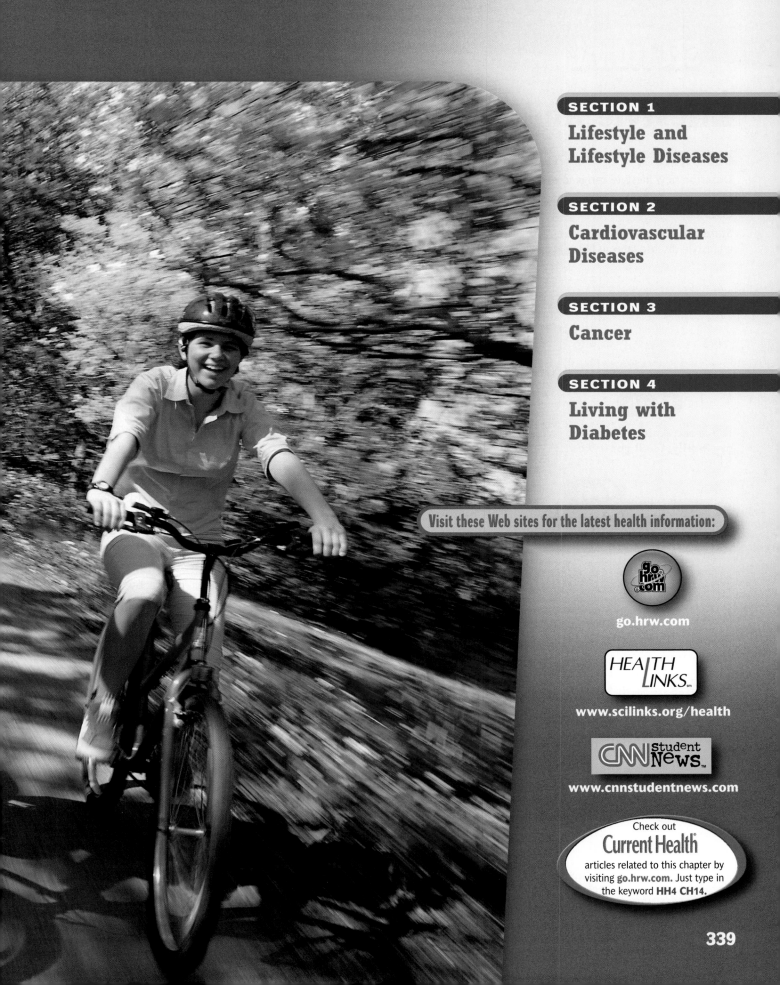

Visit these Web sites for the latest health information:

go.hrw.com

HEALTH LINKS℠

www.scilinks.org/health

CNN student News™

www.cnnstudentnews.com

Check out **Current Health** articles related to this chapter by visiting **go.hrw.com**. Just type in the keyword **HH4 CH14**.

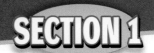

Lifestyle and Lifestyle Diseases

OBJECTIVES

Describe how lifestyle can lead to diseases.

List four controllable and four uncontrollable risk factors for lifestyle diseases.

State two actions you can take now to lower your risk for developing a lifestyle disease later in life. **LIFE SKILL**

KEY TERMS

lifestyle disease a disease that is caused partly by unhealthy behaviors and partly by other factors

Because diabetes runs in my family, I will get it, too.

Many factors, some of which you can control, contribute to diabetes.

E ven though Devon is only 16 years old, he is worried about his health. Both his father and one of his grandfathers have diabetes. Devon worries that he will also develop diabetes, but he doesn't know what to do. He decides to talk to his doctor about ways to reduce his risk.

What Are Lifestyle Diseases?

A hundred years ago, the main causes of death in the United States were infectious diseases, such as tuberculosis (TB) and the flu. Today, however, we are better protected from infections because of good hygiene practices, better living conditions, and medical advances. So, although infectious diseases are still a serious health problem, the top causes of death in the United States today are lifestyle diseases. **Lifestyle diseases** are diseases that are caused partly by unhealthy behaviors and partly by other factors.

What Causes Lifestyle Diseases? Lifestyle diseases are so called because a person's lifestyle (habits, behaviors, and practices) largely determine whether the person develops a lifestyle disease. Lifestyle diseases include cardiovascular disease, many forms of cancer, and two types of diabetes.

Personal habits, behaviors, and practices, however, are not the only factors that determine whether a person develops a lifestyle disease. Other factors that we cannot control, such as age, gender, and genes, also contribute to a person's chances of developing a lifestyle disease.

It is important to know the factors that contribute to lifestyle diseases, because behaviors that lead to lifestyle diseases later in life can start when you are very young. In Devon's case, diabetes runs in his family. The chance that Devon will develop diabetes is greater than it would be if there was not a history of diabetes in his family. However, by practicing a healthy lifestyle now, Devon can reduce his risk of developing diabetes.

340 CHAPTER 14 *Lifestyle Diseases*

Risk Factors for Lifestyle Diseases

When determining if a person might develop a disease, a doctor looks at the person's risk factors. A *risk factor* is anything that increases the likelihood of injury, disease, or other health problems.

Controllable Risk Factors   Taking charge of the risk factors that you can control may greatly decrease your chances of developing a lifestyle disease. Controllable risk factors include habits, behaviors, and practices that you can change, as shown in **Figure 1.** For example, controllable risk factors include

▶ your diet and body weight
▶ your daily levels of physical activity
▶ your level of sun exposure
▶ smoking and alcohol abuse

Thus, exercising regularly, eating a healthy diet, and not smoking will help you reduce your risk of lifestyle diseases later in life. Because there are many risk factors that you have little or no control over, it is important to start healthy habits that you can control early.

Uncontrollable Risk Factors   Some risk factors that contribute to your chances of developing a lifestyle disease are out of your control. However, it is important to understand what these factors are and how they affect your health. Uncontrollable risk factors include

▶ **Age** As you age, your body begins to change. As a result of aging, the body has a harder time protecting itself. Therefore, the chances of developing a lifestyle disease increase as you age.

Figure 1

Some of the risk factors for lifestyle diseases are beyond your control. But you can control many risk factors, such as smoking, physical activity, sun exposure, and diet.

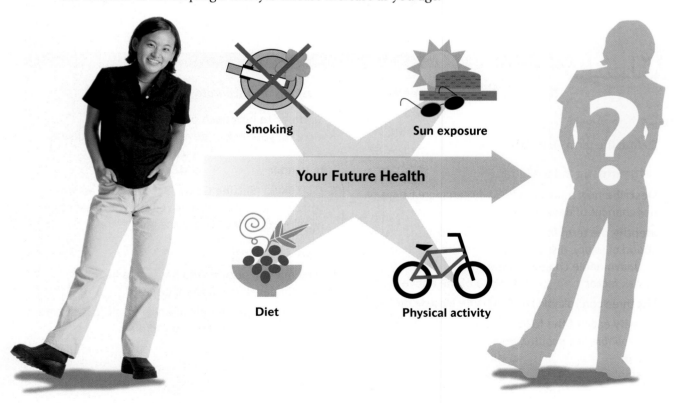

Smoking

Sun exposure

Your Future Health

Diet

Physical activity

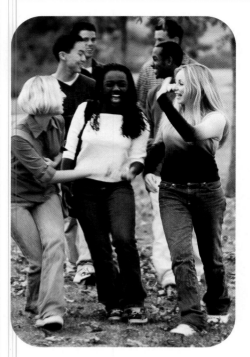

Although we all have uncontrollable risk factors such as age, gender, ethnicity, and heredity, there are still many behaviors you can practice to help lower your risk of developing a lifestyle disease.

▶ **Gender** Certain diseases are more common among members of one gender. For example, men have a greater risk of heart disease than women do, especially earlier in life. Women have a greater risk of breast cancer than men do.

▶ **Ethnicity** Your ethnicity can also influence your chances of developing a lifestyle disease. For example, African Americans are more likely to develop high blood pressure than individuals of European descent are. Mexican Americans have a higher risk of developing diabetes than individuals of European descent do. Asian Americans historically have had a lower incidence of heart disease than people of European decent have had. However, Asian Americans have recently begun to develop heart disease in greater numbers. It is believed that a change to eating a high-fat, low-fiber diet is the main reason for the increase.

▶ **Heredity** In the same way that genes determine your natural hair color, genes can also determine your chances of developing certain lifestyle diseases. For example, in some families heredity may increase the chances that a family member will develop cancer.

However, it is important to remember that just because you have an uncontrollable risk factor for a lifestyle disease, you will not necessarily develop that disease. For example, if you have a hereditary tendency to develop heart disease, you can make healthy food choices and exercise regularly and you may never develop heart disease. You may, however, need to work harder to prevent heart problems than other people do.

SECTION 1

REVIEW   *Answer the following questions on a separate piece of paper.*

Using Key Terms

1. **Define** the term *lifestyle disease*.

Understanding Key Ideas

2. **Describe** how a person's lifestyle can increase his or her chances of developing a lifestyle disease.

3. **Identify** the term for "anything that increases the likelihood of injury, disease or other health problems."
   a. unavoidable chance   c. hereditary tendency
   b. risk factor   d. none of the above

4. **List** three controllable risk factors for lifestyle diseases.

5. **Classify** each of the following risk factors as *controllable* or *uncontrollable*.
   a. age   c. diet
   b. smoking   d. genes

6. **Summarize** how each of the following can increase your risk of developing a lifestyle disease.
   a. age   c. ethnicity
   b. gender   d. heredity

7. **LIFE SKILL** **Setting Goals** Describe two actions you can take today to help reduce your chances of developing a lifestyle disease.

Critical Thinking

8. Why might a person who has lead a healthy lifestyle develop a lifestyle disease?

9. Do people have an obligation to take the best care of themselves that they can? Explain.

Cardiovascular Diseases

OBJECTIVES

Summarize how one's lifestyle can contribute to cardiovascular diseases.

Describe four types of cardiovascular diseases.

Identify two ways to detect and two ways to treat cardiovascular diseases.

List four things you can do to lower your risk for cardiovascular diseases. **LIFE SKILL**

KEY TERMS

cardiovascular disease (CVD) a disease or disorder that results from progressive damage to the heart and blood vessels

stroke a sudden attack of weakness or paralysis that occurs when blood flow to an area of the brain is interrupted

blood pressure the force that blood exerts against the inside walls of a blood vessel

heart attack the damage and loss of function of an area of the heart muscle

atherosclerosis a disease characterized by the buildup of fatty materials on the inside walls of the arteries

X avier just got back from a physical exam. The doctor told Xavier that he had high blood pressure. Xavier knew that high blood pressure was common in his family. He felt that he had already taken some steps to lower his risk.

What Are Cardiovascular Diseases?

Together, the heart and blood vessels make up the cardiovascular system. The diseases and disorders that result from progressive damage to the heart and blood vessels are called **cardiovascular diseases (CVDs).** You may not have heard that term before, but you've probably heard of some kinds of cardiovascular disease: heart attack, stroke, atherosclerosis, and high blood pressure.

Cardiovascular disease is the leading cause of death in the United States. Nearly all of the people who die from CVD are over the age of 40. So why should you worry about CVD now? The damage that leads to CVD builds up over many years and may begin as early as childhood. So, the sooner you start taking care of your heart and blood vessels, the more likely you are to avoid developing a CVD.

Lifestyle and Cardiovascular Disease Why do some people die from cardiovascular disease while others never have any problems? Genetic differences between people are one reason. But whether you develop a cardiovascular disease and how serious it becomes also depend on how you live. For example, smoking, being overweight, having high blood pressure, having high blood cholesterol, or having diabetes greatly increase your risk of developing a cardiovascular disease.

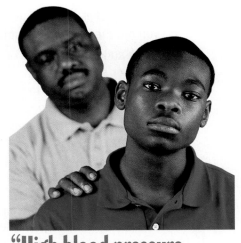

"High blood pressure runs in my family. So, my dad and I are cutting down on the amount of salt we eat."

Types of Cardiovascular Diseases

About 60 million Americans have some form of cardiovascular disease. Heart attacks, strokes, and other kinds of cardiovascular disease kill about 1 million Americans every year. This number is twice the number of people who die from cancer.

Stroke

Each year about 160,000 people die from strokes. **Strokes** are sudden attacks of weakness or paralysis that occur when blood flow to an area of the brain is interrupted. In some cases, a blood clot (shown in yellow) lodges in one of the arteries in the brain. The clot cuts off circulation to nearby brain cells. If the clot isn't removed, the cells begin to die. Strokes can also occur when a hole forms in one of the vessels inside the skull, and blood leaks into the brain. Internal bleeding can severly damage the brain.

Get medical help immediately if you or anyone around you has the following symptoms:

▶ sudden numbness or weakness of the face, an arm, or a leg
▶ trouble seeing in one or both eyes
▶ sudden dizziness or loss of coordination
▶ sudden, severe headache with no known cause

High Blood Pressure

Doctors call *high blood pressure,* or *hypertension,* the silent killer, because many people don't know that their blood pressure is high until they have a heart attack or stroke. **Blood pressure** is the force that blood exerts against the inside walls of a blood vessel. When blood pressure is too high, it puts extra strain on the walls of the vessels and on the heart.

High blood pressure can injure the walls of the blood vessels, which can lead to other cardiovascular diseases. It also makes the heart work harder, which can cause the heart to weaken or fail. High blood pressure can eventually damage the kidneys and eyes, too.

Heart Attack

The narrow *coronary arteries* that cover the heart deliver the nutrients and oxygen that the cells of the hard-working heart require. If a blood clot gets stuck in one of the coronary arteries, it can sharply reduce or shut off blood flow to the heart. As the heart cells die from lack of oxygen, the victim often has a crushing pain in the chest. The result of the reduced blood flow is a heart attack. A **heart attack** is the damage and loss of function of an area of the heart muscle. About one-third of heart attacks injure the heart so badly that they are fatal. Heart attacks can happen at any time, and sometimes they happen without any previous symptoms. Therefore, it is important to know the warning signs of a heart attack.

Warning Signs of a Heart Attack

▶ **Uncomfortable pressure, squeezing, or pain in the center of the chest that lasts for more than a few minutes**

▶ **Pain spreading to shoulders, neck, and arms**

▶ **Chest discomfort combined with lightheadedness, fainting, sweating, nausea, or shortness of breath**

Atherosclerosis

If you looked inside an old water pipe, you might find it clogged with buildup. Much less water can flow through such a pipe than through a new, clean one. Something similar can happen inside blood vessels. Fatty deposits known as *plaques* build up on the inside walls of arteries and interfere with blood flow. The disease characterized by the buildup of fatty materials on the inside walls of the arteries is called **atherosclerosis** (ATH uhr OH skluh ROH sis).

Atherosclerosis is dangerous for two reasons. First, it can reduce or stop blood flow to certain parts of the body. Second, these deposits can break free and release clots into the bloodstream. If one of these clots gets stuck in one of the coronary arteries, the result is a heart attack. If the clot lodges in the brain, a stroke results.

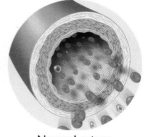

Normal artery

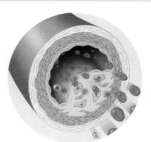

Artery with fatty buildup (Atherosclerosis)

Detecting and Treating Cardiovascular Diseases

The earlier you detect and treat a cardiovascular disease, the greater your chance of reducing the damage or danger of the disease.

Detecting Cardiovascular Diseases Doctors today can diagnose CVD earlier and more accurately than they could before. Methods to detect CVD include

▶ **Blood Pressure** To check your blood pressure, a healthcare provider wraps a cuff around your upper arm. The cuff is inflated until it is tight enough to stop bloodflow through the main artery in the arm. As air is slowly released from the cuff, the healthcare provider uses a stethoscope to listen for the heartbeat sound as blood begins to flow through the artery. He or she records the number that appears on the instrument recording the pressure. This number indicates the *systolic pressure*, the maximum blood pressure when the heart contracts.

As the cuff deflates further, the healthcare provider listens until the sound of the heartbeat disappears and the blood flows steadily through the artery. He or she records this second number. The second number, the *diastolic pressure*, indicates the blood pressure between heart contractions.

HEALTH Handbook For more information about the circulatory system, see the Express Lesson on pp. 532–535 of this text.

Analyzing DATA

Checking Blood Pressure

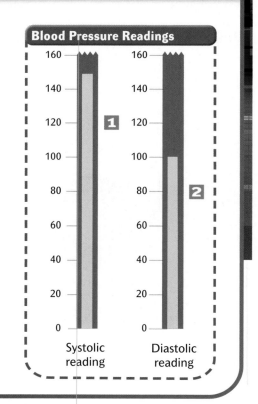

Blood pressure is measured in millimeters of mercury (mm Hg). Blood pressure is expressed as two numbers. In the diagram, the number at the end of the red bar indicates the pressure.

1 The first number measured indicates the systolic pressure. Systolic pressure is the maximum pressure when the heart contracts.

2 The second number measured indicates the diastolic pressure. Diastolic pressure is the pressure between heart contractions.

Your Turn

1. What is this person's systolic pressure?

2. What is this person's diastolic pressure?

3. **CRITICAL THINKING** Does this person have high blood pressure? If so, what can he or she do to reduce it?

4. **CRITICAL THINKING** If a woman has a blood pressure of 100/70, what is the systolic pressure? What is the diastolic pressure? Is her blood pressure low, normal, or high?

Normal blood pressure generally falls between 80/50 and 130/85 mm Hg (a unit for measuring pressure). Blood pressure over 140/90 is considered high.

▶ **Electrocardiogram** One of the most common cardiovascular tests is the *electrocardiogram*, sometimes called an *ECG* or *EKG*. An EKG measures the electrical activity of the heart. EKGs can detect damage to the heart and an irregular beat.

▶ **Ultrasound** To look at the heart in action, doctors sometimes use ultrasound, which is also used to take pictures of babies in the womb. Doctors can see the pumping of the heart and the action of the heart valves.

▶ **Angiography** Angiography (AN jee AHG ruh fee) is a test in which dye is injected into the coronary arteries. An instrument called a fluoroscope is used to see where the dye travels and to look for blockages in the coronary arteries.

Treating Cardiovascular Diseases Today, we have many choices for treating cardiovascular disease (CVD).

▶ **Diet and Exercise** Changing the diet and exercise habits of a patient is an important step in treating CVD. A low-fat, low-salt, and a low-cholesterol diet, along with light physical activity, is often prescribed to people with signs of CVD. Exercise is normally carried out under a doctor's supervision.

▶ **Medicines** Many medicines are available to treat CVDs. For example, some medicines keep the blood vessels from constricting. This helps keep blood pressure down.

▶ **Surgery** If the coronary arteries are badly clogged, doctors often perform a *coronary artery bypass operation*. Surgeons remove a length of vein from the patient and transplant it to the heart. They attach one end of the vein to the aorta and the other end to the coronary artery just below the blockage. Thus, blood can detour around the blockage and reach the heart muscle.

▶ **Angioplasty** A technique called *angioplasty* requires a doctor to insert a tube with a balloon at the tip into a blood vessel in the patient's leg. The tube and balloon are guided through vessels into the blocked artery. Once the balloon is in place, it is inflated to flatten the plaque and open the artery. Sometimes, a metal cage called a *stent* is left in the artery to prop open the artery walls.

▶ **Pacemakers** Sometimes, the heart needs help to keep beating. If the heart cannot keep a steady rhythm, surgeons may implant an artificial pacemaker in the chest. *Artificial pacemakers* are small, battery-powered electronic devices that stimulate the heart to contract.

▶ **Transplants** If the heart becomes so weak or diseased that it can't do its job, surgeons may replace it. Depending on the emergency, doctors may use artificial hearts or hearts taken from people who gave permission for their organs to be removed after their death. An operation to replace a heart is called a *heart transplant*.

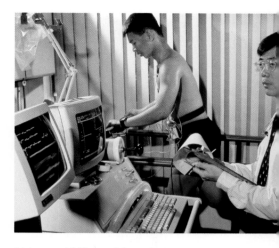

Using an EKG machine, doctors can detect damage to the heart and an irregular beat by monitoring the electrical impulses of the heart.

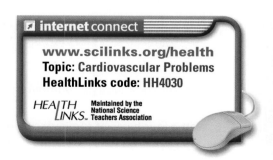

🔲 **internet** connect

www.scilinks.org/health
Topic: Cardiovascular Problems
HealthLinks code: HH4030

HEALTH LINKS™ Maintained by the National Science Teachers Association

Preventing Cardiovascular Diseases

The doctors and surgeons who treat CVD would prefer that you protect your heart and blood vessels before you get sick. Because CVD can begin as early as childhood, it is important to take steps now, such as doing the healthy activity shown in **Figure 2,** to ensure a healthy future. The following advice can help you lower your risk of CVD.

▶ **Trim the fat, and hold the salt.** Limit your consumption of saturated fats, cholesterol, and salt. Instead, eat more fruits and vegetables, lean meats, and plenty of products made from whole grains.

▶ **Keep your weight near recommended levels.** Being overweight increases your risk of CVDs. Try to keep your weight near that recommended for your height and build.

▶ **Don't smoke.** Smoking speeds up atherosclerosis and increases your risk of having a stroke or heart attack. If you don't smoke, don't start. If you do smoke, the sooner you quit, the better.

▶ **Get moving.** Regular exercise benefits your cardiovascular system in many ways. It helps you feel less stressed by daily life and is also a good way to keep your weight under control.

▶ **Watch those numbers.** Have your blood pressure and cholesterol checked regularly. If you have a family history of CVD, you should get checked now. It may be wise to start a program to control your cholesterol, even this early.

▶ **Relax.** Stress, feelings of aggression, hostility, and anger have been shown to increase the risk of CVD. The increase in risk may be due to the physical effects of stress, such as raised blood pressure, or due to smoking, drinking, or poor eating—behaviors people sometimes use to deal with stress.

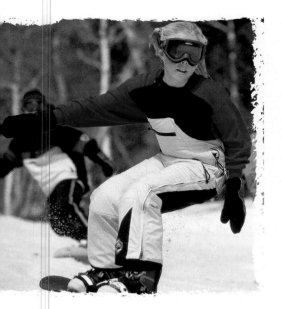

Figure 2

Exercising can help to lower your chance of developing a cardiovascular disease.

ACTIVITY *List two exercise activities that you enjoy or might enjoy doing to keep your heart healthy.*

SECTION 2

REVIEW   *Answer the following questions on a separate piece of paper.*

Using Key Terms

1. **Identify** the term for "a disease or disorder that results from progressive damage to the heart and blood vessels."

2. **Define** the term *stroke*.

3. **Name** the term for "the force that blood exerts against the inside walls of a blood vessel."

Understanding Key Ideas

4. **Describe** how lifestyle contributes to cardiovascular disease.

5. **Name** four types of cardiovascular diseases.

6. **Compare** the meaning of systolic pressure and diastolic pressure readings.

7. **Classify** each of the following as either a detection method or a treatment for cardiovascular diseases.
   a. EKG   c. angiography
   b. angioplasty   d. heart transplant

8. **LIFE SKILL** **Practicing Wellness** Identify the action that would help protect you from cardiovascular diseases.
   a. increasing salt intake c. exercising regularly
   b. smoking   d. eating a high-fat diet

Critical Thinking

9. Why do you think cardiovascular diseases are so common in the United States?

Cancer

OBJECTIVES

Describe what cancer is.

Identify three causes of cancer.

Describe four types of cancer.

Identify three ways to detect and three ways to treat cancer.

List five things you can do to lower your risk for cancer. **LIFE SKILL**

KEY TERMS

cancer a disease caused by uncontrolled cell growth

malignant tumor a mass of cells that invades and destroys healthy tissue

benign tumor an abnormal, but usually harmless cell mass

chemotherapy the use of drugs to destroy cancer cells

Every day, millions of your body's cells die. At the same time, millions of cells divide to take the place of the dying cells. Healthy cells divide at a regulated rate. Sometimes, the cells keep dividing uncontrollably. The result is a common but dangerous disease called *cancer*.

What Is Cancer?

Cancer is a disease caused by uncontrolled cell growth. More than 1 million people in the United States are diagnosed with cancer every year. Cancer is the second leading cause of death, after CVD.

Cancer begins when the way that the body normally repairs and maintains itself breaks down. To replace cells that have died or are worn out, your body makes new ones. This process is usually carefully controlled to produce only a limited number of replacement cells. Sometimes, however, these controls break down, and some cells continue to divide again and again. These out-of-control cells quickly grow in number.

Tumors As the body produces more and more of these faulty cells, they form a clump known as a *tumor*. A **malignant tumor** (muh LIG nuhnt TOO muhr) is a mass of cells that invades and destroys healthy tissue. When a tumor spreads to the surrounding tissues, it eventually damages vital organs.

Sometimes, masses of cells that aren't cancerous develop in the body. A **benign tumor** (bi NIEN TOO muhr) is an abnormal, but usually harmless cell mass. Benign tumors typically do not invade and destroy tissue and do not spread. But these tumors can grow large enough that they negatively affect the nearby tissues and must be removed.

Teens who have successfully battled cancer, as Nicole Childs has, can continue to take part in normal activities and be successful in life.

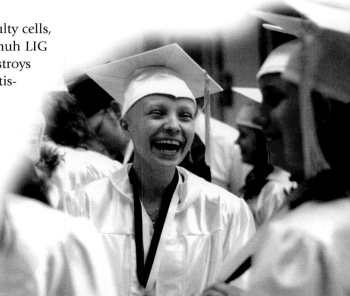

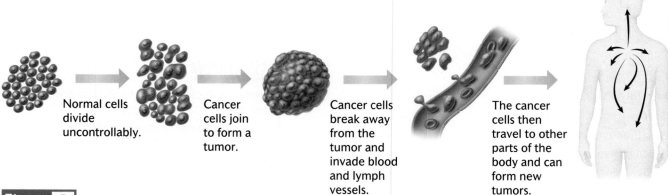

Normal cells divide uncontrollably.

Cancer cells join to form a tumor.

Cancer cells break away from the tumor and invade blood and lymph vessels.

The cancer cells then travel to other parts of the body and can form new tumors.

Figure 3

Occasionally, cells grow uncontrollably and become cancerous. Once this happens, the cancerous cells can then travel to other parts of the body.

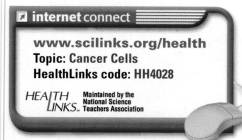

internet connect

www.scilinks.org/health
Topic: Cancer Cells
HealthLinks code: HH4028

HEALTH LINKS. Maintained by the National Science Teachers Association

Cancer Cells Are Destructive Cancer cells are very destructive to the body. They tear through and crush neighboring tissues, strangle blood vessels, and take nutrients that are needed by healthy cells. But what makes cancer especially dangerous is that the cells travel, as shown in **Figure 3.** This process is called *metastasis* (muh TAS tuh sis). The cancer cells get into the blood or lymph and move to other parts of the body. They then settle down and grow into new tumors. For example, lung cancer cells typically travel to the brain. Breast and prostate cancer cells often travel to the bones. Sometimes, the cancer cells that spread, not the original tumor, are what kill a person.

What Causes Cancer? Uncontrolled cell growth comes from damage to the genes that regulate the making of new cells. Genes that regulate cell division can become damaged in a variety of ways. A person can inherit "damaged," or mutated, genes from his or her parents. These genes make the person more likely to develop cancer than someone without those genes is. Cancer-causing agents or substances known as *carcinogens* can also be responsible for damaging genes. Some examples of carcinogens include

▶ certain viruses, such as human papilloma virus (HPV)
▶ radioactivity and ultraviolet (UV) radiation, an invisible type of energy from the sun (people are exposed to ultraviolet radiation while outside or in a tanning bed)
▶ chemicals found in tobacco smoke (for example, arsenic, benzene, and formaldehyde)
▶ asbestos (a material used to make fireproof materials, electrical insulation, and other building supplies)

All of us are exposed to some carcinogens in our daily lives. They may be in our food, water, air, or environment. However, as you'll learn later, many cancers are caused by carcinogens that you can avoid. You can control how close you come to many of these carcinogens. Choosing to work, study, and live somewhere free from these carcinogens can reduce your chance of developing cancer.

Types of Cancer

Although all kinds of cancer are the result of uncontrolled cell growth, each kind of cancer has its own characteristics. For example, cancer of the pancreas is very difficult to treat, while certain forms of skin cancer can be removed easily. **Table 1** describes several types of cancer.

Colon cancer

Table 1 Types of Cancer			
Name of cancer	What is it?	Estimated new cases each year	Estimated deaths each year
Breast	▶ cancer of the tissue and organs of the breast; more common in women but can also be found in men	205,000	40,000
Prostate	▶ cancer of the prostate, a part of the male reproductive system	189,000	30,200
Respiratory	▶ cancer of the respiratory organs, such as the lungs, larynx, and bronchus; most forms linked to the use of tobacco	183,200	161,400
Colon	▶ cancer of the colon, an organ in the digestive system	107,300	48,100
Urinary	▶ cancer of the urinary organs, such as the bladder and kidneys	90,700	24,900
Lymphoma	▶ cancer of the lymph nodes or lymph tissue	60,900	25,800
Skin	▶ cancers that affect the skin, such as basal cell carcinoma and melanoma	58,300	9,600
Leukemia (loo KEE mee uh)	▶ cancer of the tissues that produce blood; more common in males than in females	30,800	21,700
Ovarian	▶ cancer of the ovaries, a part of the female reproductive system	23,300	13,900
Nervous system	▶ cancer of the brain, spinal cord, and other parts of the nervous system	17,000	13,100
Cervical (SUHR vi kuhl)	▶ cancer of the cervix, a part of the female reproductive system	13,000	4,100

Basal cell carcinoma

Source: American Cancer Society.

Detecting and Treating Cancer

Although all cancers have similar characteristics, they differ in how they are detected, how they are treated, and how they affect the person with the cancer.

Detecting Cancer   In addition to annual medical exams, there are many ways that cancer is detected.

▶ **Self-exams** Regular self-examinations of the skin, breasts, or testicles are important. Because skin cancer is so common, watch for any new growths; a sore that doesn't heal; and for shape, size, texture, or color changes to a mole or wart.

▶ **Biopsy** A *biopsy* is a sample of tissue taken from the body that is then examined. Biopsies are commonly used to determine what type of cancer a person has and whether a tumor is malignant or benign.

▶ **X rays** An X ray of the breasts to detect tumors is called a *mammogram*. Doctors recommend regular mammograms for women over the age of 40. Computerized axial tomography (CAT scan or CT) takes multiple X rays of some part of the body, which a computer then assembles into one image.

▶ **MRI** Magnetic resonance imaging, or MRI, uses a massive magnet and a computer to gather images of the body.

▶ **Blood and DNA tests** Blood tests can detect some cancers. For example, older men are often given a prostate specific antigen (PSA) test. This test looks for a protein produced by the prostate, a small gland near the bladder. DNA tests are used to detect the likelihood of developing cancer. More tests will become available as we learn more about human genes and the ways in which cancer develops and spreads.

You and your parents should talk to your doctor about getting regular cancer-screening tests. Use the CAUTION acronym in the margin to help you remember the warning signs of cancer.

Treating Cancer   Cancer is most treatable when it is caught early. Doctors battle the disease with several weapons. Techniques used to treat cancer include the following.

▶ **Surgery** An operation can remove some tumors. Surgery is most effective when the tumor is small, has not spread, and is located where removing it will not damage surrounding tissue.

▶ **Chemotherapy Chemotherapy** (KEE moh THER uh pee) is the use of drugs to destroy cancer cells. Unfortunately, chemotherapy also kills some of the body's healthy cells. It can cause side effects such as nausea, fatigue, vomiting, and hair loss.

▶ **Radiation therapy** As you learned earlier, radiation can cause cancer. But doctors also use radiation to destroy cancer cells, an approach called *radiation therapy*. Usually, a beam of radiation is fired at the tumor from outside the body.

Warning Signs of Cancer

Change in bowel or bladder habits

A sore that doesn't heal

Unusual bleeding or discharge

Thickening or a lump anywhere in the body

Indigestion or difficulty swallowing

Obvious change in a wart or mole

Nagging cough or hoarseness

Often, doctors recommend a combination of surgery, chemotherapy, and radiation. The success of any treatment depends on the type of cancer, how long the tumor has been growing, and whether the cancer has spread to other parts of the body. One promising treatment scientists are developing is to "starve" tumors by cutting off their blood supply. Another possibility is to create a cancer "vaccine" that would stimulate the immune system to destroy cancer cells.

Living with Cancer Cancer is difficult for the person who has cancer, as well as for loved ones. A person with cancer may often be tired or weak. They may also feel down. Children with cancer are often scared, confused, and upset by medical procedures and strange surroundings.

How can you help a person who has cancer? Be patient. Offer to spend time doing quiet things, such as talking, reading, or watching TV. Many people recover from cancer and go on to lead healthy lives. So, a positive outlook during the treatment process greatly helps.

LIFE SKILL Activity

Using Community Resources

Cancer Resources in Your Community

The first step toward learning more about cancer is to use the resources in your community. Taking advantage of these resources will help you protect yourself from having cancer in the future.

1 Your doctor can help you find reliable information on cancer.

2 Find out about nonprofit organizations in your city that are devoted to cancer awareness, such as the American Cancer Society.

3 The Internet can also provide valuable resources related to cancer. But be careful when using the Internet. Although many Web sites have reliable information, some have misleading and false information.

LIFE SKILL **Using Community Resources**

1. Identify programs offered by cancer resource centers in your community.

2. What are two ways that you can promote cancer awareness in your community?

HEALTH Handbook For more information about evaluating health Web sites, see the Express Lesson on pp. 564–565 of this text.

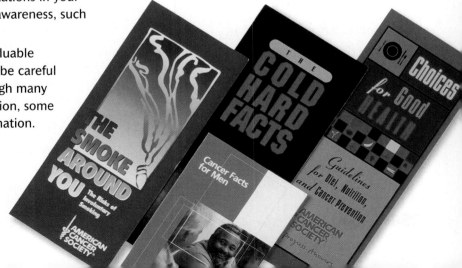

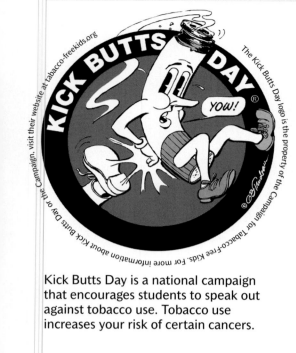

Kick Butts Day is a national campaign that encourages students to speak out against tobacco use. Tobacco use increases your risk of certain cancers.

Preventing Cancer

Taking charge of these five controllable risk factors can greatly reduce your risk of getting cancer.

1. **No butts about it: don't smoke.** Tobacco use is responsible for about one-third of the cancer deaths in the United States. People who use tobacco are prone to cancers of the mouth, throat, esophagus, pancreas, and colon. Despite what you might hear, there is no safe form of tobacco.

2. **Safeguard your skin.** Limit your exposure to the damaging UV radiation that causes skin cancer. You can do so by protecting exposed areas of skin with sunscreen and clothing, even on cloudy days. Do not sunbathe, use tanning beds, or use sunlamps.

3. **Eat your veggies, and cut the fat.** No diet can guarantee that you won't get cancer. However, people who eat large amounts of saturated fat are more likely to get cancer of the colon and rectum. Studies suggest that people who eat fruits, vegetables, and foods high in fiber have a lower risk of some cancers.

4. **Stay active, and maintain a healthy weight.** Studies have shown that regular physical activity helps protect against some types of cancers. Exercising also helps prevent obesity, another risk factor for developing cancer. Teens should get at least 60 minutes of activity daily.

5. **Get regular medical checkups.** Your doctor can answer questions you may have about cancer risk factors, preventions, and treatments. He or she will also be able to advise you on self-examinations and when to begin regular cancer screening tests.

When we make positive choices with regard to these controllable risk factors, we can work toward a healthy future for ourselves.

SECTION 3

REVIEW
Answer the following questions on a separate piece of paper.

Using Key Terms

1. **Define** the term *cancer*.

2. **Compare** a benign tumor to a malignant tumor.

3. **Define** the term *chemotherapy*.

Understanding Key Ideas

4. **Describe** how cancer cells differ from normal body cells.

5. **State** three common carcinogens.

6. **Identify** the form of cancer that has the highest death rate. (Hint: See Table 1 on p. 351.)
   a. pancreas
   b. liver
   c. lung
   d. colon

7. **Describe** three methods that doctors use to detect cancer.

8. **Describe** how chemotherapy works to treat cancer.

9. **Identify** which of the following actions would help reduce your chances of developing cancer.
   a. not smoking
   b. wearing sunscreen
   c. eating fruits
   d. all of the above

10. **LIFE SKILL** **Practicing Wellness** Identify one part of your lifestyle that you can change to decrease your chance of developing cancer.

Critical Thinking

11. Why do you think cancer is more common in some families than in others?

Living with Diabetes

OBJECTIVES

Describe the role of insulin in diabetes.

Compare type 1 and type 2 diabetes.

Identify two ways to detect and two ways to treat type 1 and type 2 diabetes.

Name two ways that you can prevent type 2 diabetes. **LIFE SKILL**

KEY TERMS

insulin a hormone that causes cells to remove glucose from the bloodstream

diabetes a disorder in which cells are unable to obtain glucose from the blood such that high blood-glucose levels result

diabetic coma a loss of consciousness that happens when there is too much blood sugar and a buildup of toxic substances in the blood

Estimates indicate that 16 million people in the United States have diabetes. Unfortunately, about 5 million people who have diabetes do not know that they have it and are not being treated for it.

What Is Diabetes?

When you eat, the nutrients in foods are broken down to provide your cells with energy. Carbohydrates are broken down to glucose which then enters your bloodstream where it can circulate to the rest of your body. Once glucose reaches the cells, it moves from the bloodstream into the cells. The cells then use the glucose for energy.

Insulin The body can't use glucose without insulin. **Insulin** is a hormone that causes cells to remove glucose from the bloodstream. Thus, insulin lowers the amount of glucose traveling free in the bloodstream. Insulin is produced by special cells in the the pancreas. When blood glucose levels are high, insulin is released into the bloodstream. When glucose levels are lower, insulin is no longer released into the bloodstream.

Insulin and Diabetes Sometimes, the pancreas doesn't produce enough insulin, or the body's cells don't respond to insulin. The result is diabetes. **Diabetes** is a disorder in which cells are unable to obtain glucose from the blood such that high blood-glucose levels result. The kidneys excrete water, resulting in increased urination and thirst. Cells then use the body's fat and protein for energy, which causes a buildup of toxic substances in the bloodstream. If this continues, a diabetic coma can result. A **diabetic coma** is a loss of consciousness that happens when there is too much blood sugar and a build up of toxic substances in the blood. Without treatment, diabetic comas can result in death.

Testing blood glucose is one way that people with diabetes can deal with their illness. Blood glucose is the amount of glucose in the blood.

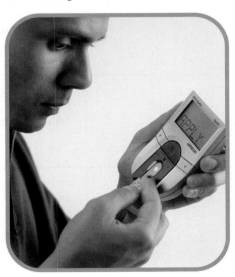

Types of Diabetes

The three most common forms of diabetes are type 1 diabetes, type 2 diabetes, and gestational diabetes. As shown in **Table 2,** each kind of diabetes has its own characteristics.

Type 1 Diabetes Type 1 diabetes accounts for only 5 to 10 percent of diabetes cases in the United States. Type 1 diabetes develops when the immune system attacks the insulin-producing cells of the pancreas. Once these cells are destroyed, the body is unable to make insulin. Scientists believe that type 1 diabetes is caused by both genetic factors and viruses.

Type 1 diabetes is sometimes called *insulin-dependent* or *juvenile diabetes.* This type of diabetes is treated with daily injections of insulin and is usually diagnosed before the age of 18. Symptoms are usually severe and develop over a short period of time. Common symptoms include increased thirst, frequent urination, fatigue, and weight loss.

Type 2 Diabetes The most common form of diabetes in the United States is type 2, sometimes called *noninsulin-dependent diabetes.* Unlike type 1 diabetes, type 2 diabetes is most common among adults who are over 40 years of age and among people who are overweight.

In type 2 diabetes, the pancreas makes insulin, but the body's cells fail to respond to it. The result is the buildup of glucose in the blood and the inability of the body to use the glucose as a source of fuel. Common symptoms of type 2 diabetes include frequent urination, unusual thirst, blurred vision, frequent infections, and slow-healing sores. These symptoms usually appear gradually.

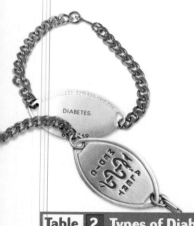

Medical alert bracelets alert medical personnel that a person, such as a diabetic, needs special care. Some warning signs of a diabetic emergency include feelings of weakness or faintness, irritability, rapid heartbeat, nausea, and drowsiness.

Table 2	Types of Diabetes		
Type of Diabetes	**What is it?**	**Symptoms**	**Treatment**
Type 1	▶ diabetes resulting from the body's inability to produce insulin	▶ increased thirst, frequent urination, fatigue, weight loss, nausea, abdominal pain, and absence of menstruation in females	▶ diet and insulin
Type 2	▶ diabetes resulting from the inability of the body's cells to respond to insulin	▶ frequent urination, increased thirst, fatigue, weight loss, blurred vision, frequent infections, and slow-healing sores	▶ diet, exercise, and occasionally insulin
Gestational	▶ diabetes that develops during pregnancy	▶ frequent urination, increased thirst, fatigue, weight loss, blurred vision, frequent infections, and slow-healing sores	▶ diet and occasionally insulin

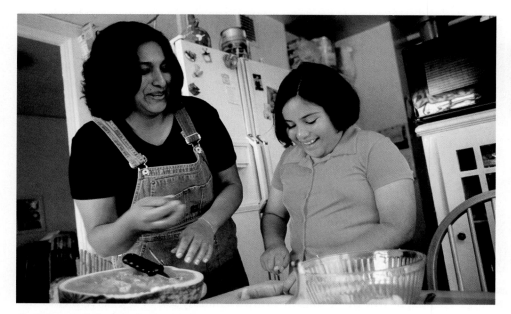

People who have, or may be at risk for, type 2 diabetes need to carefully watch their Calorie, fat, sugar, cholesterol, and fiber intake.

Gestational Diabetes Occasionally, a pregnant woman can develop diabetes near the end of her pregnancy. Usually, the diabetes goes away after the baby is born. Gestational diabetes can increase the chances of complications during the pregnancy. The symptoms are the same as those of type 2 diabetes but milder. The risk of developing gestational diabetes increases if the mother has a family history of diabetes, is obese, is over 25 years of age, or has previously given birth to a child who weighed more than 9 pounds at birth.

Detecting and Treating Diabetes

Detecting and getting medical care for diabetes as early as possible can decrease your chances of developing serious side effects.

Detecting Diabetes Early detection is important in cases of diabetes. Diabetes patients risk complications such as blindness, kidney disease, strokes, and amputations of the lower limbs. The first step in detecting diabetes is to see your doctor if you have symptoms. Your doctor will use a variety of lab tests, such as urinalysis, a glucose-tolerance test, or an insulin test to determine if you have diabetes. Once diagnosed, a person can work with his or her doctor to keep the diabetes under control. Unfortunately, there is no cure for diabetes yet.

Treating Type 1 Diabetes The goal of treatment is to keep blood-glucose levels as close to normal as possible. People who have type 1 diabetes usually must test their blood glucose several times a day. Many people who have type 1 diabetes also need several doses of insulin each day to keep their blood-glucose levels within a normal range. Most diabetics must learn to give themselves insulin injections.

Treating Type 2 Diabetes Although insulin is sometimes used to treat type 2 diabetes, more common control measures focus on diet and exercise. A healthy diet can help people with type 2 diabetes control the amount of glucose they eat and can help them control

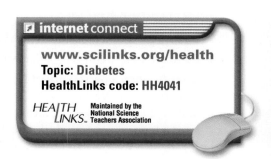

internet connect

www.scilinks.org/health
Topic: Diabetes
HealthLinks code: HH4041

HEALTH LINKS. Maintained by the National Science Teachers Association

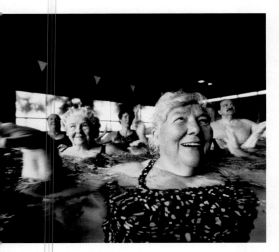

Staying active through regular exercise can help reduce your risk of developing type 2 diabetes.

their weight. Foods with sugar do not need to be avoided completely, but must be eaten in moderation. Physical activity is also important because it helps the body use more of the glucose in the blood and keeps the person's weight at a healthy level.

New Treatments Researchers are working on new treatments for diabetes. The researchers are hoping that these new treatments will help diabetics monitor their blood-glucose better, will provide new methods of delivering insulin, and will help reduce the severity of symptoms. Scientists are also working on ways to transplant insulin-producing cells into people with type 1 diabetes.

Preventing Diabetes

As in so many diseases, genes play a role in diabetes. For example, people who have diabetes in their family are at a greater risk of developing diabetes. People in certain ethnic groups, particularly African Americans, Hispanics, and Native Americans, are also at a greater risk for developing certain forms of diabetes.

There is currently no way to prevent type 1 diabetes. But exercise, a healthy diet, and insulin injections as needed can allow a person to lead a healthy life.

There are several things a person can do to reduce his or her risk of developing type 2 diabetes including:

▶ Maintain a healthy weight. Exercise regularly and eat a healthy diet. Physical activity and a healthy diet can greatly reduce the risk of developing type 2 diabetes in people who are overweight.

▶ Avoid tobacco products.

▶ Reduce the amount of stress in your life.

SECTION 4

REVIEW   *Answer the following questions on a separate piece of paper.*

Using Key Terms

1. **Name** the term for "a hormone that causes cells to remove glucose from the bloodstream."

2. **Define** the term *diabetes*.

3. **Define** the term *diabetic coma*.

Understanding Key Ideas

4. **Describe** the role of insulin in the body.

5. **Compare** type 1 and type 2 diabetes.

6. **Identify** when a person may develop gestational diabetes.
   a. as a child
   b. as a teen
   c. after age 65
   d. during pregnancy

7. **Name** three risk factors for developing type 2 diabetes.

8. **List** three symptoms that help a person detect type 1 and type 2 diabetes.

9. **Identify** which of the following is *not* a treatment for diabetes.
   a. urinalysis
   b. insulin injections
   c. healthy diet
   d. regular exercise

10. **Describe** why it is important for a person who has diabetes to eat a healthy diet.

Critical Thinking

11. Why do you think type 2 diabetes is more common in the United States than in other countries?

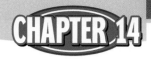

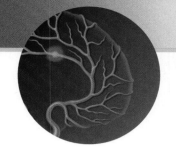

Highlights

Key Terms

The Big Picture

✔ Lifestyle diseases are caused partly by a person's lifestyle, which includes habits and behaviors.

✔ Many risk factors, some controllable and some uncontrollable, contribute to a person's chances of developing a lifestyle disease.

✔ Diet, physical activity, smoking, sun exposure, and body weight are controllable risk factors. Age, gender, ethnicity, and genes are uncontrollable factors.

✔ People who inherit a tendency for a lifestyle disease can still do a lot to reduce their chances of developing such a disease.

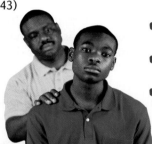

✔ A person's lifestyle influences their chances of developing cardiovascular diseases such as strokes, high blood pressure, heart attacks, and atherosclerosis.

✔ Doctors use many different methods, such as EKG, ultrasound, and angiography, to diagnose cardiovascular diseases.

✔ There are many treatment options for cardiovascular diseases including a healthy diet, exercise, medicine, and surgery.

✔ Eating sensibly, avoiding cigarettes, exercising, and having your blood pressure and cholesterol checked regularly can help prevent cardiovascular diseases.

✔ Cancer occurs when cells divide uncontrollably. Certain "damaged" genes can make a person more likely to develop cancer. Exposure to viruses, radioactivity, ultraviolet radiation, and tobacco can damage genes.

✔ There are many types of cancer. Each type has its own characteristics.

✔ Early detection and treatment of cancer can increase a person's chances of survival.

✔ Not smoking, protecting your skin from the sun, following a balanced diet, staying active, and getting regular medical checkups help reduce your chances of developing cancer.

✔ Diabetes occurs when cells are unable to obtain glucose from the blood such that high blood-glucose levels result.

✔ Type 1 diabetes is believed to be caused by an autoimmune response. Type 2 diabetes is usually the result of lifestyle choices.

✔ Although there is no cure for diabetes, lifestyle changes and medicines can often keep the disorder under control.

✔ The best way to prevent diabetes is to take control of the risk factors that you can change, such as diet, exercise, and weight.

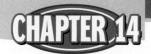

Review

Using Key Terms

atherosclerosis (345)
benign tumor (349)
blood pressure (344)
cancer (349)
cardiovascular disease
  (CVD) (343)
chemotherapy (352)

diabetes (355)
diabetic coma (355)
heart attack (345)
insulin (355)
lifestyle disease (340)
malignant tumor (349)
stroke (344)

1. For each definition below, choose the key term that best matches the definition.
   a. a disease caused by uncontrolled cell growth
   b. the force that blood exerts against the inside walls of a blood vessel
   c. an abnormal, but usually harmless cell mass
   d. a hormone that causes cells to remove glucose from the bloodstream
   e. the damage and loss of function of an area of the heart muscle

2. Explain the relationship between the key terms in each of the following pairs.
   a. *malignant tumor* and *benign tumor*
   b. *insulin* and *diabetic coma*

Understanding Key Ideas

Section 1

3. Explain why infectious diseases have become less common and why lifestyle diseases are the most common causes of death.

4. _____ are uncontrollable risk factors for lifestyle diseases.
   a. Tobacco use, gender, and age
   b. Genes, age, and gender
   c. Age, exercise level, and family history of disease
   d. Gender, exercise level, and tobacco use

5. To help prevent the development of a lifestyle disease, a person should
   a. not smoke.
   b. exercise.
   c. have a low-fat diet.
   d. All of the above

6. What two steps could you take during school to lower your risk of developing a lifestyle disease? **LIFE SKILL**

Section 2

7. How can lifestyle contribute to cardiovascular disease?

8. Which of the following is *not* a type of cardiovascular disease?
   a. stroke
   b. atherosclerosis
   c. cancer
   d. high blood pressure

9. Which of the following is *not* a treatment for cardiovascular disease?
   a. angioplasty
   b. bypass surgery
   c. heart transplant
   d. echocardiography

10. How can regular exercise reduce your chances of developing cardiovascular disease? **LIFE SKILL**

11. **CRITICAL THINKING** Smoking decreases the amount of oxygen that the blood can carry. How can this effect increase the chances that a smoker will develop cardiovascular disease?

Section 3

12. Describe what cancer is and why it is so dangerous.

13. Refer to **Table 1** on p. 351. What is the main cause of the type of cancer that results in the most deaths each year?

14. _____ is *not* a method of detecting cancer.
   a. Prostate specific antigen testing
   b. MRI
   c. Regular self-examination
   d. Chemotherapy

15. Identify three cancer treatments used today.

16. What are two ways that a person can safeguard their skin from ultraviolet radiation?

Section 4

17. What is the relationship between insulin and glucose in diabetes?

18. What are the major differences between type 1 and type 2 diabetes?

19. What are two ways to detect and two ways to treat type 1 and type 2 diabetes?

20. List two steps you can take to lower your risk of developing type 2 diabetes. **LIFE SKILL**

Interpreting Graphics

Study the figure below to answer the questions that follow.

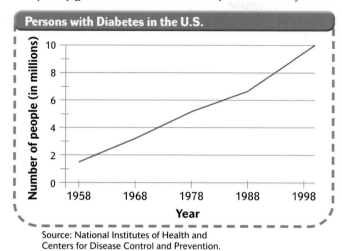

Persons with Diabetes in the U.S.

Source: National Institutes of Health and Centers for Disease Control and Prevention.

21. How many people were diagnosed with diabetes in 1978?

22. What is the difference in the number of people diagnosed with diabetes in 1988 and the number diagnosed in 1998? **MATH SKILL**

23. **CRITICAL THINKING** Why do you think diabetes has become more common since 1958?

Activities

24. **Health and You** Make a list of the uncontrollable risk factors for lifestlye diseases. Create a poster that explains how a person can reduce the health risks posed by uncontrollable risk factors.

25. **Health and Your Community** Research one of the cancers listed in **Table 1.** Prepare an informational handout that describes how to detect, treat, and prevent the cancer. **WRITING SKILL**

26. **Health and You** Research a new approach to treating cancer. Write a one page paper that describes what the approach is, how it works, and when it is expected to be available to cancer patients. **WRITING SKILL**

Action Plan

27. **LIFE SKILL** **Assessing Your Health** Establishing healthy patterns of living during adolescence reduces the risks of developing a lifestyle disease. Discuss two risk factors over which you have control. How can you reduce or eliminate these risk factors?

Standardized Test Prep

Read the passage below, and then answer the questions that follow. **READING SKILL** **WRITING SKILL**

Heart disease is the leading cause of death in the United States. Heart disease causes over 900,000 deaths per year. These deaths <u>constitute</u> 40 percent of all deaths in the United States. Twenty-five percent of deaths due to heart disease occur in people under the age of 65. Death rates for the 10-year period ending in 1985 were 30 percent less than they were for the previous 10-year period. This decline in mortality is related to improvements in heart disease risk factor levels, as well as in diagnosis and treatment.

28. In this passage, the word *constitute* means
   A propose.
   B make up.
   C follow.
   D concern.

29. What can you infer from reading this passage?
   E There are more deaths due to heart disease in the United States than there are anywhere else in the world.
   F The number of deaths due to heart disease has not changed since 1985.
   G Changes in lifestyle risk factors have decreased the number of deaths due to heart disease.
   H Nothing can be done to prevent deaths from heart disease.

30. Write a paragraph describing how changes in lifestyle could reduce the number of deaths due to heart disease in the United States.

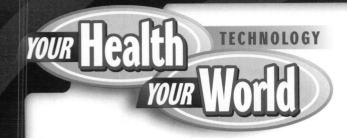

YOUR **Health** TECHNOLOGY
YOUR **World**

Every day, the newspapers are full of new discoveries in genetics, the science of heredity. How could the latest developments in genetics affect your health or the health of a family member?

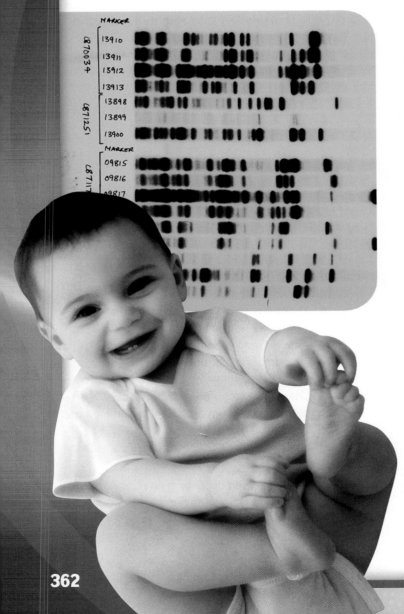

Making Sense of Genetic Technology

In 2001, scientists published a complete list of all human genes. Genes are the set of instructions found in every person's body that describe how that person's body will look, grow, and function. Many scientists have now turned their attention to figuring out what each gene does. The application of our knowledge about genes to help meet human needs is known as genetic technology.

Our Growing Knowledge of Human Genetics

Scientists are asking how our genes determine the kind of blood that we have, the way that our skin cells work, or the color of our eyes. In addition, other researchers are working hard to apply this new knowledge to detect and cure genetic disorders. There are many kinds of genetic disorders. Down syndrome, sickle cell anemia, hemophilia, cystic fibrosis, and muscular dystrophy are only a few well-known ones. In fact, more than 4,000 different human disorders are caused by errors in our genes. Someone you know might have cancer that has a genetic basis. In your lifetime, cures for cancers are likely to arise from today's research in genetic technology.

In addition to studying genetic disorders, scientists are using techniques in genetic technology in other ways. For example, scientists in pharmaceutical companies use genetic technology with bacteria to produce medicines that help humans. Doctors treat dwarfism by using human growth hormones made with the new genetic technology. Drug companies are manufacturing new vaccines, by using modern techniques. In fact, so much genetic work is being done that understanding these new developments can seem overwhelming.

Genetics and Technology

Let's look at some specific examples of the new genetic technology and see how it is affecting the world around us.

▶ **Transplanted Genes** It is possible to take a certain gene from one kind of organism, such as a human, and place it into another organism, such as a bacterium. This idea may seem strange, but the results can be remarkable. For example, a scientist can take the human gene that makes the hormone insulin out of a human cell and place it in a bacterial cell. Millions of these bacterial cells can then make pure human insulin.

Many very pure substances can be made in this way. The transfer of genes from one organism to another for medical or industrial use is called *genetic engineering*. Today genetic engineering is used to change the nature of many of our domestic plants and animals.

▶ **Genetic fingerprinting** Scientists are now able to take a sample of genetic material from a person and develop a "fingerprint" of that person's genetic makeup. The genetic material is first broken up into smaller fragments. These fragments are then placed into a gelatinous substance, and under the influence of an electric current, the pieces of genetic material are separated from one another. The way in which they separate is unique to each person. The result is a "fingerprint." Genetic fingerprinting can be used to research family trees, or to identify an adult who carries a gene that causes a genetic disorder. It can also be used as legal evidence in criminal trials.

Understanding a New Technology

As you get older, scientists will make more and more discoveries in genetics. These discoveries are likely to change the way you live. Genetic disorders, such as Tays-Sachs, sickle cell anemia, and thousands of other diseases, may be a thing of the past. The possibility of real change is awesome. For example, will you be able to ensure that your children have certain traits? Will you or your children be able to eliminate genetic diseases? Genetics is the most powerful and exciting science to affect our lives, and its effects will be more profound as the years go by. How do you make sense of so many important discoveries? Here are some suggestions:

▶ **Read the latest news about science in newspapers, in magazines, and on the Internet.** The most important discoveries will be presented here for everyone to read and understand. However, be skeptical of what you read. So many exciting discoveries are being made that it is only natural that writers and reporters will sometimes exaggerate. Use your common sense. Get information from more than one source.

▶ **Use your research skills to look up information that you don't understand.** Books and reputable Internet sites are sources you can rely on to learn more about genetic technology.

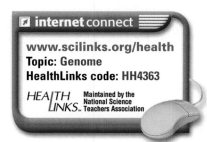

YOUR TURN

1. **Summarizing Information** Why should all citizens become informed about genetic technology and modern genetic research?

2. **Inferring Conclusions** In what ways has modern medical and genetic technology improved our lives since the days of your grandmother and grandfather?

3. **CRITICAL THINKING** Do you think that people should be allowed to choose the traits of their children by changing their children's genes? How would you go about finding the information to make your point in a discussion?

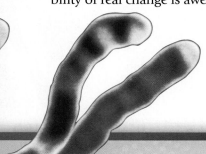

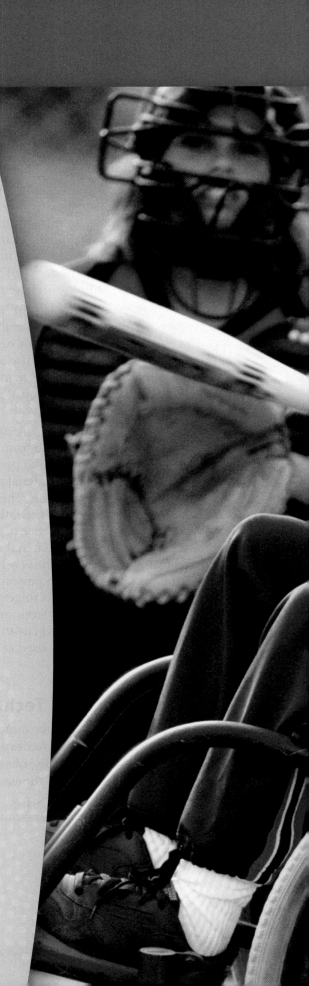

CHAPTER 15

Other Diseases and Disabilities

What's Your Health IQ?
KNOWLEDGE

Which of the statements below are true, and which are false? Check your answers on p. 642.

1. A person's chances of developing a hereditary disease are determined only by his or her genes.

2. The Human Genome Project has allowed scientists to develop new treatments for hereditary diseases.

3. Autoimmune diseases are caused by viruses that attack the immune system.

4. Allergies, asthma, and arthritis are all examples of autoimmune disorders.

5. The most common cause of disabilities involving movement is injury to the nervous system.

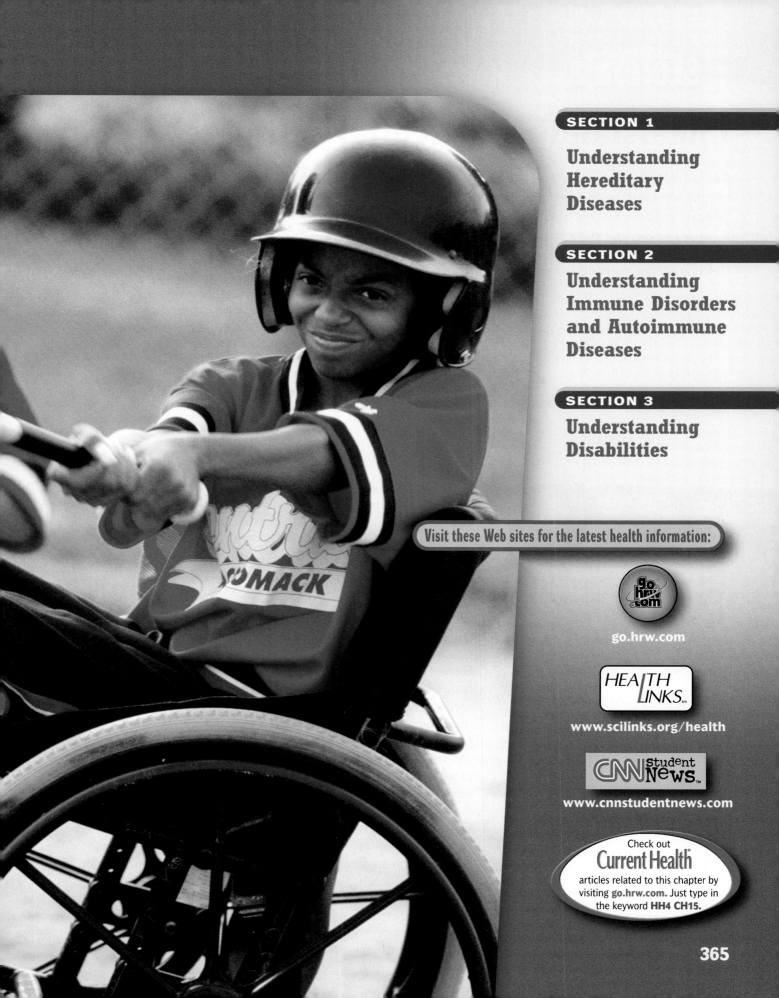

SECTION 1

Understanding Hereditary Diseases

SECTION 2

Understanding Immune Disorders and Autoimmune Diseases

SECTION 3

Understanding Disabilities

Visit these Web sites for the latest health information:

go.hrw.com

HEALTH LINKS

www.scilinks.org/health

CNN student NEWS

www.cnnstudentnews.com

Check out **Current Health** articles related to this chapter by visiting go.hrw.com. Just type in the keyword **HH4 CH15.**

Understanding Hereditary Diseases

OBJECTIVES

Identify how genes are involved in hereditary diseases.

Compare the three different types of hereditary diseases.

Summarize three ways that a person with a genetic disease can cope with the disease.

Describe a future medical treatment for hereditary diseases.

KEY TERMS

hereditary disease a disease caused by abnormal chromosomes or by defective genes inherited by a child from one or both parents

gene a segment of DNA located on a chromosome that codes for a specific hereditary trait and that is passed from parent to offspring

genetic counseling the process of informing a person or couple about their genetic makeup

Human Genome Project a research effort to determine the locations of all human genes on the chromosomes and to read the coded instructions in the genes

gene therapy a technique that places a healthy copy of a gene into the cells of a person whose copy of the gene is defective

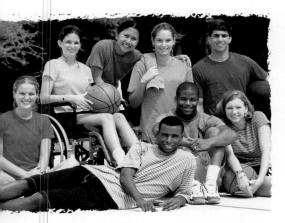

Just as hair color and height are determined by the genes that a person receives from his or her parents, so are certain diseases.

Julia has been lucky—she has had only a few colds, the flu, and chickenpox during her 16 years of life. Others in her family have had more serious diseases, such as diabetes and cancer. Julia is curious about whether she has inherited some of these diseases.

What Are Hereditary Diseases?

Unlike infectious diseases, hereditary diseases aren't caused by pathogens. Instead, **hereditary diseases** are diseases caused by abnormal chromosomes or by defective genes inherited from one or both parents.

Genes **Genes** are segments of DNA located on a chromosome that code for a specific hereditary trait. Genes are passed from parent to offspring. The genes that you inherited from your parents determine many of your characteristics. For example, whether you have blue or brown eyes is determined by your genes. The color of your hair is determined by your genes. Together, your genes tell your body how to grow, develop, and function throughout life. Your genes also determine your chances of developing certain diseases—hereditary diseases.

Genes and Hereditary Diseases How are genes involved in hereditary diseases? Occasionally, the instructions that a gene is carrying contain an error. When a gene carries incorrect instructions, this is called a *mutation*. Sometimes, a mutation can have a harmful effect on the person. In hereditary diseases, a mutation can cause a disease or increase a person's chances of getting a disease.

Types of Hereditary Diseases

Hereditary diseases can result from a mutation on one gene, on several genes, or from changes to an entire chromosome where the genes are found. Thus, hereditary diseases are sometimes classified as single-gene, complex, or chromosomal diseases.

Single-Gene Diseases Single-gene diseases occur when 1 gene out of the 30,000 to 40,000 genes in the body has a harmful mutation. The severity of the illness depends on what instructions the gene normally carries. **Table 1** summarizes the symptoms and treatments for several single-gene diseases.

Huntington's disease is an example of a disease caused by one defective gene. When people with Huntington's disease reach the age of 35 to 40, cells in their brain begin to die. Over time, their movements become jerky and uncontrollable, their personality changes, and their mental abilities deteriorate. Huntington's disease is always fatal.

Another example of a single-gene disease is *sickle cell anemia.* Sickle cell anemia occurs when the body makes a faulty version of *hemoglobin,* the protein that carries oxygen to your cells. Hemoglobin is found in red blood cells. As shown in **Figure 1,** the red blood cells of someone with sickle cell anemia have an abnormal shape. These cells tend to clog up small blood vessels, cutting off blood flow to some tissues.

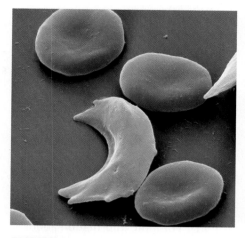

Figure 1

Normal red blood cells have a circular, biconcave shape. In sickle cell anemia, the red blood cells have an abnormal, sickle shape, making it difficult for the cells to carry oxygen to the body.

Table 1 Single-Gene Diseases

Disease	Description	Symptoms	Treatment
Huntington's disease	▶ inherited disease that leads to the degeneration of brain cells	▶ involuntary movements, mood swings, depression, irritability, and inability to remember facts	▶ no cure; medicines to help control symptoms, such as emotional and movement problems
Sickle cell anemia	▶ inherited blood disease in which the body produces defective hemoglobin	▶ fatigue, paleness, shortness of breath, pain, infections, and stroke	▶ no cure; medicine to treat pain; blood transfusions
Hemophilia	▶ inherited blood disease in which the body produces little of or none of the blood proteins necessary for clotting	▶ severe bruising, excessive bleeding after a simple cut, hemorrhaging (internal bleeding), chronic joint disease, and joint pain	▶ no cure; blood transfusions; blood-clotting proteins
Cystic fibrosis	▶ inherited disease of the body's mucous glands; primarily affects the respiratory and digestive systems of children and young adults	▶ difficulty breathing, cough, accumulation of mucus in the intestines and lungs, infections, and weight loss	▶ no cure; medicines to treat symptoms, such as difficulty breathing and infections

Sickle cell anemia is the most common genetic disease among African Americans. This disease affects about 1 in 500 African Americans. Although sickle cell anemia isn't curable, with medical care people who have the disease usually live into their 50s.

Cystic fibrosis is another single-gene disease. It affects nearly 30,000 people in the United States. Cystic fibrosis causes large amounts of thick mucus to clog the lungs, the pancreas, and the liver. This buildup of mucus leads to malnutrition, breathing difficulties, and infections that can damage the lungs. Although there is currently no cure for cystic fibrosis, scientists are developing new treatments, such as gene therapy to help reduce the effects of this disease.

Complex Diseases In complex diseases, more than one gene influences the onset of the disease. Lifestyle behaviors also contribute to a person's chance of developing a complex disease. Cardiovascular diseases (strokes, heart attacks, high blood pressure, and atherosclerosis), type 2 diabetes, and cancer are examples of complex diseases. Many genes influence whether you get these diseases.

Is there anything you can do about complex diseases? Yes! Because you have control over your lifestyle, you can help lower your risk of developing a complex disease by making healthy lifestyle choices. Eating healthy foods and exercising regularly are two good ways to reduce your chances of developing a complex disease.

Chromosomal Diseases Genes are located on chromosomes. Humans normally have 23 pairs of chromosomes inside each of their cells (except for sperm and egg cells). Sometimes, a disease can occur when a person inherits the wrong number of chromosomes or when one of the chromosomes is incomplete. Because each chromosome carries a large number of genes, chromosomal diseases are usually fatal.

The most common chromosomal disease in the United States is *Down syndrome.* Down syndrome, also called Trisomy 21, occurs when a person inherits an extra copy of the 21st chromosome. People who suffer from Down syndrome often have varying degrees of mental retardation and difficulties with physical development. Down syndrome is typically not fatal.

Coping with Hereditary Diseases

Coping with a hereditary disease can be difficult. There are several things you can do if you or someone in your family has a hereditary disease.

1. **Genetic counseling** A genetic counselor is a specialist in human genetics. **Genetic counseling** is the process of informing a person or couple about their genetic makeup. As shown in **Figure 2,** the genetic counselor can study a family's chromosomes and medical history and explain the risks of passing on a hereditary disease to a child. Genetic counselors also provide information to help people accept a diagnosis and cope with a genetic disease.

TOPIC link For more information about diabetes, see Chapter 14.

Figure 2

A genetic counselor can help potential parents understand the chances of passing on a hereditary disease to their child. Genetic counselors often examine each parent's chromosomes.

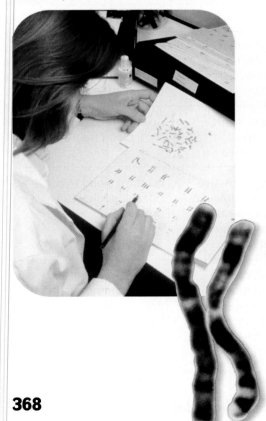

2. **Personal health records** Most of us can't remember all the details of our medical history, but this information is important for our doctors. You should keep your records up to date. Get copies of your health records if you change doctors.

It's also important to know what illnesses your relatives have experienced. Try to collect information on what hereditary diseases your relatives had, when these diseases appeared, and what your deceased relatives died from.

3. **Health information** Read the latest information about the hereditary disease. This will help you know what to expect and how to help a person with a specific hereditary disease. Knowing about the hereditary disease is a good first step in helping yourself or another person cope.

Future Medical Treatment for Hereditary Diseases

We know a lot more about human genes than we did in the past. This information is currently being used in treating hereditary diseases and developing treatments for the future.

Human Genome Project Scientists are trying to learn what all of our genes do and how they affect the development of diseases like cancer, heart disease, and diabetes. One major advancement in this research was the completion of the Human Genome Project. The **Human Genome Project** was a research effort to determine the locations of all human genes on the chromosomes and to read the coded instructions in the genes. The collection of all of our genes make up our *genome*. You can think of the genome as an instruction manual for human beings. The project was completed in 2003.

With the genetic information gathered from the Human Genome Project, scientists hope to treat hereditary diseases in different ways, including

▶ designing powerful drugs that target a particular hereditary disease

▶ making drugs to prevent diseases

▶ improving **gene therapy,** a technique that places a healthy copy of a gene into the cells of a person whose copy of the gene is defective

▶ creating genetic tests that can tell you which hereditary diseases you might develop in your lifetime

With the information from genetic tests, you can take steps early in life to head off the disease. For example, for heart diseases, these steps may include eating a diet low in saturated fats, exercising regularly, or controlling your weight.

MAKING GREAT DECISIONS Imagine that your friend's father has just been diagnosed with Huntington's disease. There's a 50 percent chance that your friend has the defective gene too. She can know for sure by getting a genetic test that requires only a sample of blood. The problem is that there is no treatment or cure for Huntington's disease. However, even if she does have the faulty gene, she may not start to get sick for 10 years or even longer. Should she get tested?

Write on a separate piece of paper the advice you would give your friend. Remember to use the decision-making steps.

G ive thought to the problem.
R eview your choices.
E valuate the consequences of each choice.
A ssess and choose the best choice.
T hink it over afterward.

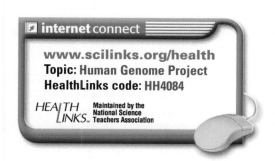

internet connect

www.scilinks.org/health
Topic: Human Genome Project
HealthLinks code: HH4084

HEALTH LINKS Maintained by the National Science Teachers Association

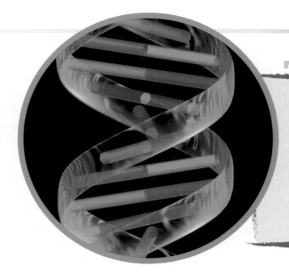

Positive Uses of Genetic Information

▶ **improved diagnosis of disease**
▶ **gene therapies**
▶ **vaccines incorporated into foods**
▶ **customized drugs for specific diseases**
▶ **improved ability to predict genetic diseases**
▶ **help in studying our past**

DNA molecules like this one are what make up our genes, the coded instructions for building our bodies.

Gene Therapy   Scientists are improving their ability to treat hereditary diseases by gene therapy. They are inserting working genes to cancel the effects of defective genes. Getting a gene into the body and making it work has been very difficult, but some diseases have been treated in this way. In the future, scientists hope to use gene therapy to insert missing genes or to replace the faulty genes that cause cystic fibrosis, sickle cell anemia, and other hereditary diseases.

Concerns About Genetic Information   Our growing knowledge of human genes raises concerns about how the information will be used. Some people worry that insurance companies might discriminate against people based on results of genetic tests. This is called *genetic discrimination*. Another worry is that genetic techniques might be abused to change characteristics such as eye color, height, or intelligence. In the next few years, society will be trying to decide what kinds of genetic changes are acceptable. The issue of genetic information may raise some troubling questions, but this new information is expected to help save many lives.

SECTION 1

REVIEW   *Answer the following questions on a separate piece of paper.*

Using Key Terms

1. **Define** the term *hereditary disease.*
2. **Compare** the terms *gene* and *gene therapy.*
3. **Define** the term *Human Genome Project.*

Understanding Key Ideas

4. **Summarize** how genes are involved in hereditary diseases.
5. **Classify** each of the following as a single-gene disease or a complex disease.
   a. hemophilia   c. cystic fibrosis
   b. diabetes   d. cancer

6. **Compare** three types of hereditary diseases.
7. **State** three ways that people can cope with a genetic disease.
8. **Identify** two ways information from the Human Genome Project may help treat hereditary diseases in the future.

Critical Thinking

9. What are two ways that society could deal with future concerns about genetic information?
10. Imagine you are a scientist working on the Human Genome Project. What would you say to news reporters about your research? **LIFE SKILL**

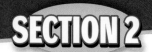

SECTION 2

Understanding Immune Disorders and Autoimmune Diseases

OBJECTIVES

Compare immune disorders and autoimmune diseases.

Describe two types of immune disorders.

Describe two types of autoimmune diseases.

Summarize how people can cope with immune disorders and autoimmune diseases.

KEY TERMS

autoimmune disease a disease in which the immune system attacks the cells of the body that the immune system normally protects

allergy a reaction by the body's immune system to a harmless substance

asthma a disorder that causes the airways that carry air into the lungs to become narrow and to become clogged with mucus

arthritis inflammation of the joints

multiple sclerosis (MS) an autoimmune disease in which the body mistakenly attacks myelin, the fatty insulation on nerves in the brain and spinal cord

magine that your body begins to destroy its own cells. Even though this idea sounds far fetched, many common diseases occur when the immune system does just this.

What Are Immune Disorders and Autoimmune Diseases?

Your immune system is made up of special cells that protect your body from disease. These cells are constantly patrolling your blood and tissues. When an immune system cell does not recognize an object as part of the body, it attacks the foreign particle. Your immune system guards you from viruses, bacteria, foreign substances, and cancer cells.

Immune Disorders If the immune system does not function properly, the result is an immune disorder. Some immune disorders are relatively mild; others can be life threatening. Examples of immune disorders include allergies, asthma, human immunodeficiency virus (HIV), and severe combined immunodeficiency disease (SCID).

Autoimmune Diseases In people with **autoimmune diseases,** the immune system attacks the cells of the body that the immune system normally protects. Depending on the cells that are destroyed, these attacks can result in many conditions. For example, rheumatoid arthritis is caused when the immune system attacks the joints. In multiple sclerosis, the immune system attacks myelin, the fatty insulation of nerves in the brain and spinal cord.

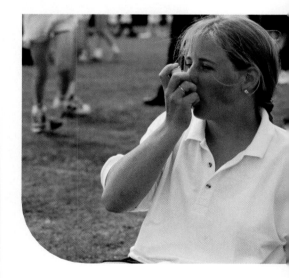

Preventive medications are one way that many people are able to control immune disorders such as asthma.

Types of Immune Disorders

When immune system cells encounter a foreign particle, they send out chemical signals that cause the body to react. Usually, this reaction helps the immune system fight disease. Sometimes, however, the reaction causes more problems than the foreign particle would.

Allergies   An **allergy** is a reaction by the body's immune system to a harmless substance. A long list of things, including foods, dust, plant pollen, and animals, can cause allergic reactions. Do you sneeze when a cat comes around? Do your eyes itch and water when you go outside on a spring day? If so, you may have an allergy.

When inhaled substances, such as the pollen grains shown in **Figure 3,** cause an allergic attack, a person may experience a runny nose, sneezing, and itchy, watery eyes. Allergies to foods or certain drugs can sometimes cause *hives,* itchy swellings on the skin. Most allergies are a nuisance. But some people have extreme and life-threatening reactions to allergies. Their blood pressure falls, and the tubes carrying air into the lungs constrict, making it difficult to breathe.

One way to prevent allergic symptoms is to avoid things that cause a reaction. Some ways you can help reduce allergic symptoms include
- ▶ avoiding substances that you are allergic to
- ▶ washing sheets and blankets weekly
- ▶ cleaning bathrooms and kitchens to avoid molds

Avoiding allergenic substances is not always possible. Some people use over-the-counter drugs called *antihistamines*. Antihistamines work to suppress the symptoms of an allergy. A doctor can also prescribe a series of injections containing gradually larger doses of the substance to which the person is allergic. Over the course of 2 or 3 years, the person's sensitivity to the substance declines.

Asthma   **Asthma** is a disorder that causes the airways that carry air into the lungs to become narrow and to become clogged with mucus. This causes shortness of breath, wheezing, and coughing. The airways, called *bronchioles*, are shown in **Figure 4.** The bronchioles are covered with rings of muscle that adjust the width of the tubes. This allows your lungs to take in more or less air. For example, the width of the airways increase when you excercise.

Occasionally, the muscles covering the airways overreact to substances in the air, causing the airways to narrow. These airways can be too sensitive and tighten in response to things like dust, cigarette smoke, stress, exercise, foods, and pollution. The result is an asthma attack. During an asthma attack, the lining of these air passages may also swell and become inflamed, making breathing difficult.

When the tubes narrow, drawing a breath is very hard. Asthmatics often explain that breathing during an asthma attack is like trying to breathe through a straw. Other symptoms of asthma are coughing, wheezing, and chest tightness. Asthma attacks are very serious. Some attacks can even be life threatening. More than 5,000 people die from asthma each year.

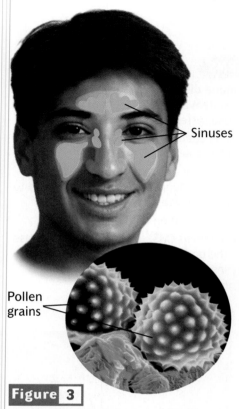

Sinuses

Pollen grains

Figure 3

Sinuses are hollow areas in the skull that open into the nasal cavity. When allergens, such as pollen grains, enter the sinuses, they can trigger an allergic reaction.

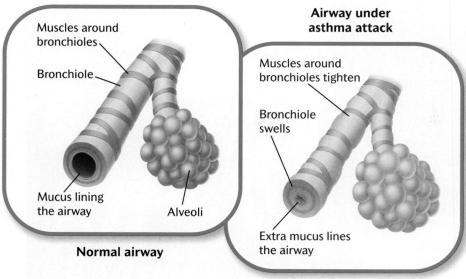

Airway under asthma attack

Muscles around bronchioles

Bronchiole

Muscles around bronchioles tighten

Bronchiole swells

Mucus lining the airway

Alveoli

Extra mucus lines the airway

Normal airway

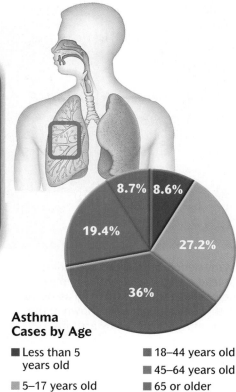

8.7%   8.6%

19.4%

27.2%

36%

Asthma Cases by Age

- Less than 5 years old
- 5–17 years old
- 18–44 years old
- 45–64 years old
- 65 or older

Source: American Lung Association.

Figure 4

An asthma attack occurs when the muscles that encircle the airways of the lung (bronchioles) constrict, making it difficult to breathe.

ACTIVITY *Why do you think there are so many cases of asthma in 5- to 7-year-olds?*

People can often prevent asthma attacks by avoiding the substances that irritate their lungs. Two kinds of drugs are also available to relieve asthma symptoms. Long-term control drugs are taken every day to soothe the airways. It is important that people with asthma take these drugs every day. For emergencies, asthmatics also have quick-relief drugs that, when inhaled, open the airways. These treatments have made it easier for people with asthma to lead normal, active lives. Moderate exercise can also strengthen the lungs of people who suffer from asthma.

Types of Autoimmune Diseases

When a person's immune system attacks the cells of the body it is meant to protect, the person has an autoimmune disease. There may be several factors that start the immune attack. An infection caused by pathogens with molecules similar to the body's own cells may cause the immune system to attack the cells in the body. If an infection enters a body tissue that is usually not patrolled by immune cells, the tissue may be attacked as well.

Arthritis   Your joints move smoothly because the ends of the bones are covered with a smooth layer of cartilage that allows the bones to glide across one another. When this layer of cartilage is damaged, moving the bones and joints becomes difficult and painful. The result is **arthritis,** or inflammation of the joints. Arthritis is one of the most common joint diseases in the United States. There are two main kinds of arthritis: rheumatoid arthritis and osteoarthritis.

The disease known as *rheumatoid arthritis* is an autoimmune disease. For unknown reasons, the immune system begins to destroy the lining of the joints. The joints swell, become painful, and may become stiff or unable to move. This stiffness may be worse in the morning, just after waking, or after being inactive. Eventually, the bones of the joints may begin to deteriorate.

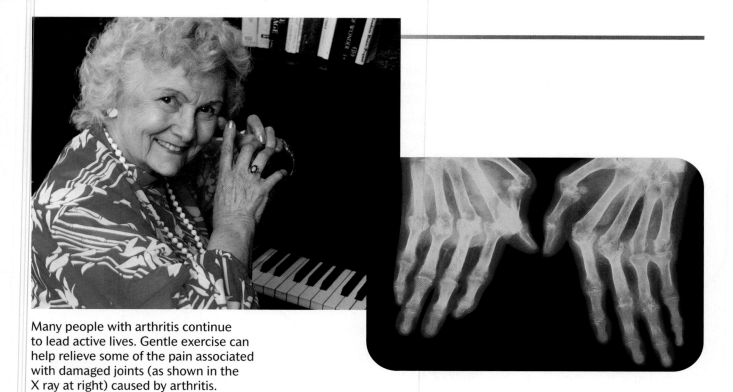

Many people with arthritis continue to lead active lives. Gentle exercise can help relieve some of the pain associated with damaged joints (as shown in the X ray at right) caused by arthritis.

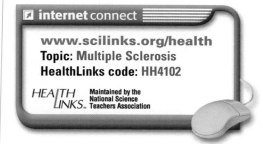

Osteoarthritis is different from rheumatoid arthritis in that it is not an autoimmune disease. Instead, with osteoarthritis, the joints of the skeleton begin to wear out as a person grows older. This is similar to the way that a hinge on a car door will wear out if it is opened and closed enough times. The cartilage inside a joint begins to deteriorate, and movement, or even changes in the weather, can cause intense pain. The joint can swell, distort, or even develop bony knobs.

A plan that mixes medications, rest, and gentle exercise can help treat moderate forms of rheumatoid arthritis and osteoarthritis. Severe damage to a vital joint, such as the hip or knee, however, may require surgery to install a replacement joint made from plastic, metal, or porcelain. Drugs are also being developed to help reduce inflammation of the joints and to slow or stop joint damage.

Multiple Sclerosis   Just like the power lines that carry electricity to your home, the nerves that carry impulses through the body are covered by a layer of insulation that speeds up nerve signals. The autoimmune disease known as **multiple sclerosis (MS)** occurs when the body attacks myelin, the fatty insulation on nerves in the brain and spinal cord. This damage causes the transmission of nerve impulses to slow down or stop.

Multiple sclerosis is twice as common in women as in men and usually strikes young adults. It can be hard to diagnose. Symptoms include blurred vision, tingling or burning sensations, weakness, numbness, mental problems, unsteadiness, slurred speech, or loss of bladder control. The symptoms of multiple sclerosis usually come and go. Months and sometimes years may pass between episodes. However, the disease usually gets worse over time and may eventually interfere with vision, balance, and walking. Patients may eventually become paralyzed. In some cases, the disease can be fatal.

Although there is currently no cure for multiple sclerosis, many drugs and treatments can ease the symptoms and slow the deterioration of the nerves. Drugs such as steroids can reduce the length and severity of attacks. New drugs are currently being developed.

Coping with Immune Disorders and Autoimmune Diseases

Understanding immune disorders and autoimmune diseases can help you treat people with these types of diseases with compassion and respect. If you are diagnosed with an immune or autoimmune disease, be sure to do the following:

▶ **Understand your disorder and your doctor's treatment plan.** Ask questions, especially about the changes and symptoms you can expect to encounter. Learn about the side effects of medications and medical tests. Be aware of all aspects of your condition.

▶ **Follow the treatment plan designed by your physician.** Play an active role in determining your treatment plan. Do not be afraid to get a second or third opinion. Once you and your family are satisfied that the treatment is right for you, follow it.

▶ **Let your doctor know if a new symptom is occurring.** New symptoms can signal important changes in your disorder. It is very important to discuss any changes in your condition with your doctor. This is the only way to find out what the change might mean and how it might be treated.

▶ **Be honest with your doctor.** You hurt only yourself if you are not honest with your physician. A doctor cannot give you good advice without accurate information. Your health is too important to leave anything out.

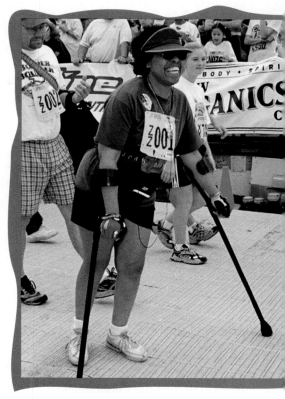

People with multiple sclerosis, such as Sharon Jodoin, can enjoy physical activities. Being active helps maintain their health.

SECTION 2

REVIEW *Answer the following questions on a separate piece of paper.*

Using Key Terms

1. **Define** the term *autoimmune disease*.

2. **Compare** *allergy* and *asthma*.

3. **Identify** the term for "inflammation of the joints."

Understanding Key Ideas

4. **Differentiate** between immune disorders and autoimmune diseases.

5. **Describe** two different types of immune disorders.

6. **Summarize** how common substances can trigger allergic reactions.

7. **Compare** the causes of rheumatoid arthritis and multiple sclerosis.

8. **Identify** the disease in which the body mistakenly attacks the fatty insulation on nerves in the brain and spinal cord.
   a. allergies
   b. asthma
   c. arthritis
   d. multiple sclerosis

9. **State** three ways that a person can better manage his or her autoimmune disease.

Critical Thinking

10. **Identify** how people with allergies or asthma can reduce the allergens in their homes.

Understanding Disabilities

OBJECTIVES

List three myths about disabilities.

Describe three different types of disabilities.

Identify two ways people cope with disabilities.

Identify one way that you can help create a positive environment for people with disabilities. **LIFE SKILL**

KEY TERMS

disability a physical or mental impairment or deficiency that interferes with a person's normal activity

tinnitus a buzzing, ringing, or whistling sound in one or both ears that occurs even when no sound is present

Americans with Disabilities Act (ADA) wide-ranging legislation intended to make American society more accessible to people who have disabilities

People in many different careers, such as artist Chuck Close, have been able to excel despite their disabilities. Chuck Close was partially paralyzed by a blood clot in his spinal cord.

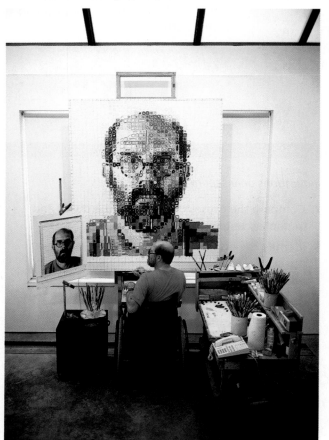

In the past, people with disabilities were often discriminated against. They were believed to be unable to hold jobs or participate in other activities. Today, however, attitudes in society are changing as many people with disabilities are succeeding in all areas of life, despite their disabilities.

What Are Disabilities?

Disabilities are physical or mental impairments or deficiencies that interfere with a person's normal activity. Disabilities can take many forms, including forms that involve vision, hearing, and movement.

Myths About Disabilities Over the years, there have been many myths about people who have disabilities. For example, one myth is that people with disabilities prefer to be around only other people with disabilities. Another common myth is that people with disabilities always need help. In reality, many people with disabilities live independantly and are part of mainstream society.

Actors living with disabilities, such as Christopher Reeve and Michael J. Fox, help obtain funding for research to treat disabilities and bring special concerns to the attention of lawmakers and the public. People with disabilities also work as congressmen, artists, lawyers, doctors, and in many other careers. Limits caused by disabilities do not limit a person's ability to achieve their goals.

Educating others about the different types of disabilities is an effective way to help eliminate such myths and to build a positive atmosphere for all members of society.

Types of Disabilities

Disabilities are typically classified according to the body function that is affected by the disability. For example, disabilities involving vision include all disabilities that affect a person's ability to see. Although there are a variety of disabilities, the severity of the disabilities in each category can range from moderate to severe. Moderate disabilities may only slightly affect a person's ability to do everyday activities. Severe disabilities can sometimes require that a person have constant medical attention.

Disabilities Involving Vision When people think of disabilities involving vision, they usually think of people who are completely blind. Although there are about 1.3 million Americans who are legally blind, there are nearly 10 million Americans with impaired vision. Thus, there are many people in the United States with disabilities involving vision who are not completely blind.

Accidents, diabetes, glaucoma, and macular degeneration account for most blindness in the United States. For example, in a condition

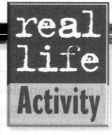

real life Activity

UNDERSTANDING DISABILITIES

LIFE SKILL
Coping

Materials

✔ bandana

Procedure

1. **Choose** two paths through the classroom. Make sure that the paths do not cross.

2. **Form** teams, with two people in each team.

3. **Choose** one team member to be blindfolded and one team member to be his or her guide.

4. **Tie** the bandana so that it completely covers the eyes of the "blind" team member so that he or she cannot see.

5. **Line up,** two teams at a time, at the beginning of each path.

6. **Guide** the blindfolded person through the path.

7. **Switch** roles, and repeat the activity.

Conclusions

1. **Summarizing Results** What did it feel like to walk through the classroom without any sense of sight?

2. **Summarizing Results** What challenges did you face when leading the person who was blindfolded?

3. **Predicting Outcomes** What changes could you make in your classroom to make it easier for a person with a vision disability to move around?

4. **CRITICAL THINKING** Other than moving around, what other daily activities might pose a problem for people who are blind?

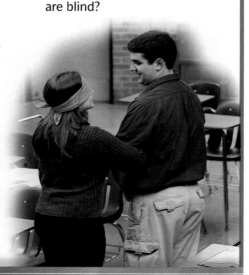

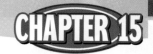

Review

Understanding Key Terms

allergy (372)
Americans with Disabilities Act (ADA) (380)
arthritis (373)
asthma (372)
autoimmune disease (371)
disability (376)
gene (366)
gene therapy (370)
genetic counseling (368)
hereditary disease (366)
Human Genome Project (369)
multiple sclerosis (MS) (374)
tinnitus (378)

1. For each definition below, choose the key term that best matches the definition.
   a. a buzzing, ringing, or whistling sound in one or both ears that occurs even when no sound is present
   b. inflammation of the joints
   c. a technique that places a healthy copy of a gene into the cells of a person whose copy of the gene is defective
   d. a reaction by the body's immune system to a harmless substance
   e. the process of informing a person or couple about their genetic makeup
   f. a research effort to determine the locations of all human genes on the chromosomes and read the coded instructions in the genes

2. Explain the relationship between the key terms in each of the following pairs.
   a. *genes* and *hereditary disease*
   b. *disability* and *Americans with Disabilities Act*
   c. *autoimmune disease* and *multiple sclerosis*

Understanding Key Ideas

Section 1

3. Describe how genes are involved in hereditary diseases.

4. A person's eye color is determined by his or her
   a. age.   c. gender.
   b. genes.   d. All of the above

5. Describe one example of each of the three types of hereditary diseases.

6. Identify how keeping personal health records can help a person cope with hereditary diseases.

7. Describe how gene therapy might help people who have cystic fibrosis.

8. **CRITICAL THINKING** Explain why couples who are even distantly related might have a greater chance of having a child with a hereditary disease.

Section 2

9. What is the difference between immune disorders and autoimmune diseases?

10. Which of the following is an immune system disorder?
    a. multiple sclerosis   c. allergies
    b. rheumatoid arthritis d. all of the above

11. Describe two treatments for asthma.

12. Which of the following is an autoimmune disease?
    a. multiple sclerosis   c. osteoarthritis
    b. flu   d. cardiovascular disease

13. What are three symptoms of multiple sclerosis?

14. How can asking questions of their doctors help people cope with their autoimmune diseases?

Section 3

15. State the reason it is important to know the difference between myths and truth about disabilities.

16. Describe three ways that people with uncorrectable vision problems can cope with their disability.

17. State the most common cause of hearing loss in children.

18. Compare the two different levels of paralysis.

19. Identify ways that you can help create a positive environment for people living with disabilities.

20. **CRITICAL THINKING** Why might a misconception that recovery cannot occur after a spinal cord injury prevent a person from maximizing his or her potential for recovery?

Interpreting Graphics

Study the figure below to answer the questions that follow.

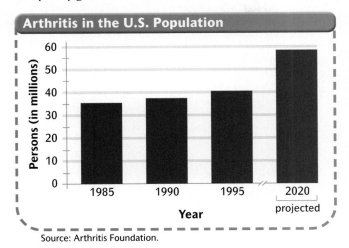

Arthritis in the U.S. Population

Persons (in millions) vs Year (1985, 1990, 1995, 2020 projected)

Source: Arthritis Foundation.

21. How many people in the United States had arthritis in 1985?

22. How many more people are expected to have arthritis in 2020 as compared to 1985? **MATH SKILL**

23. **CRITICAL THINKING** Why do you think the number of people diagnosed with arthritis is expected to rise so dramatically from 1995 to 2020?

Activities

24. **Health and Your Family** Research the diseases that are common in your family. What hereditary diseases have been the cause of death for members of your family?

25. **Health and Your Community** Research several facilities in your community that are designed to help people who have disabilities. Create a poster detailing the different ways one of these facilities helps these people.

26. **Health and You** Research a new approach to treating hereditary diseases that has come from the Human Genome Project. Write a one-page paper describing the treatment and the way it works. **WRITING SKILL** **READING SKILL**

Action Plan

27. **LIFE SKILL** **Communicating Effectively** In the past, myths have led to many misconceptions about people with disabilities. Write one page summarizing how you could help eliminate these myths and help people better understand disabilities. **WRITING SKILL**

Standardized Test Prep

Read the passage below, and then answer the questions that follow. **READING SKILL** **WRITING SKILL**

Sickle cell anemia affects millions of people throughout the world. The majority of these people have ancestors who came from Africa. In order for people to receive proper treatment for this disease, early diagnosis is critical. Approximately 40 U.S. states now perform a blood test to detect <u>faulty</u> versions of hemoglobin on all newborn infants. Hemoglobin is the protein in red blood cells that carries oxygen. If a child is found to have the disease, treatments begin immediately. Although there is currently no cure for sickle cell anemia, treatments can help control the side effects.

28. In this passage, the word *faulty* means
   A important.   **C** unnecessary.
   B defective.   **D** preferred.

29. What can you infer from reading this passage?
   E There are more deaths due to sickle cell anemia in the United States than anywhere else in the world.
   F Having ancestors from Africa increases a person's chances of developing sickle cell anemia.
   G Researchers expect a cure for sickle cell anemia very soon.
   H Blood tests for sickle cell anemia are inaccurate.

30. Write a paragraph describing how early diagnosis of sickle cell anemia could affect a person's life. **WRITING SKILL**

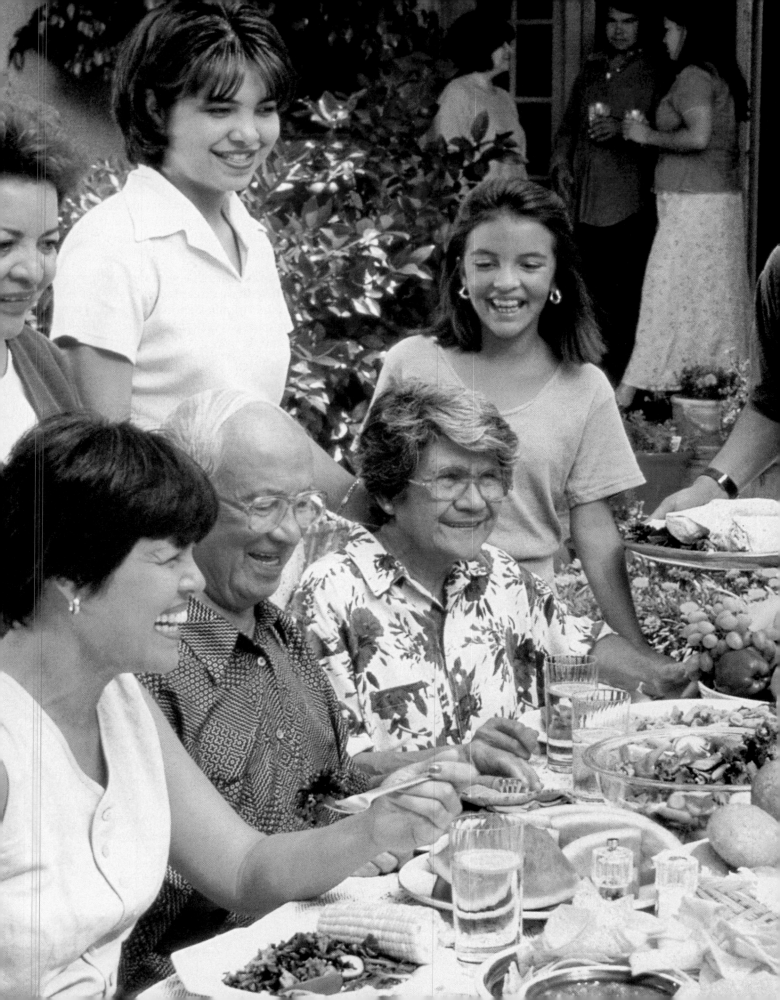

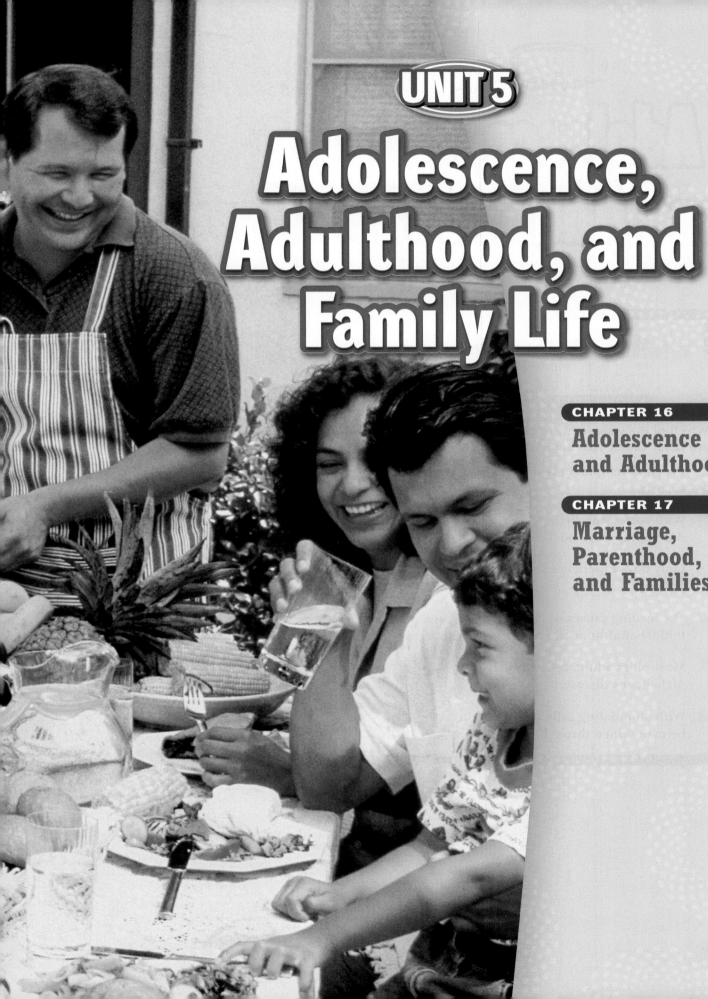

UNIT 5
Adolescence, Adulthood, and Family Life

CHAPTER 16

Adolescence and Adulthood

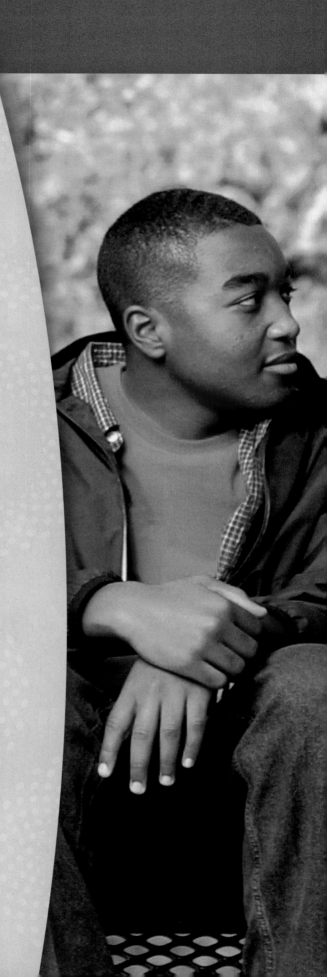

What's Your Health IQ?

KNOWLEDGE

Which of the statements below are true, and which are false? Check your answers on p. 642.

1. Breast development is the first sign of puberty in girls.

2. With successful dieting, a girl can avoid developing extra body fat.

3. Only boys experience voice changes during puberty.

4. The leading causes of death in young and middle adulthood are cancer and heart disease.

5. Most older adults eventually develop Alzheimer's disease.

6. With stimulating activities, mental capacity can be maintained throughout adulthood.

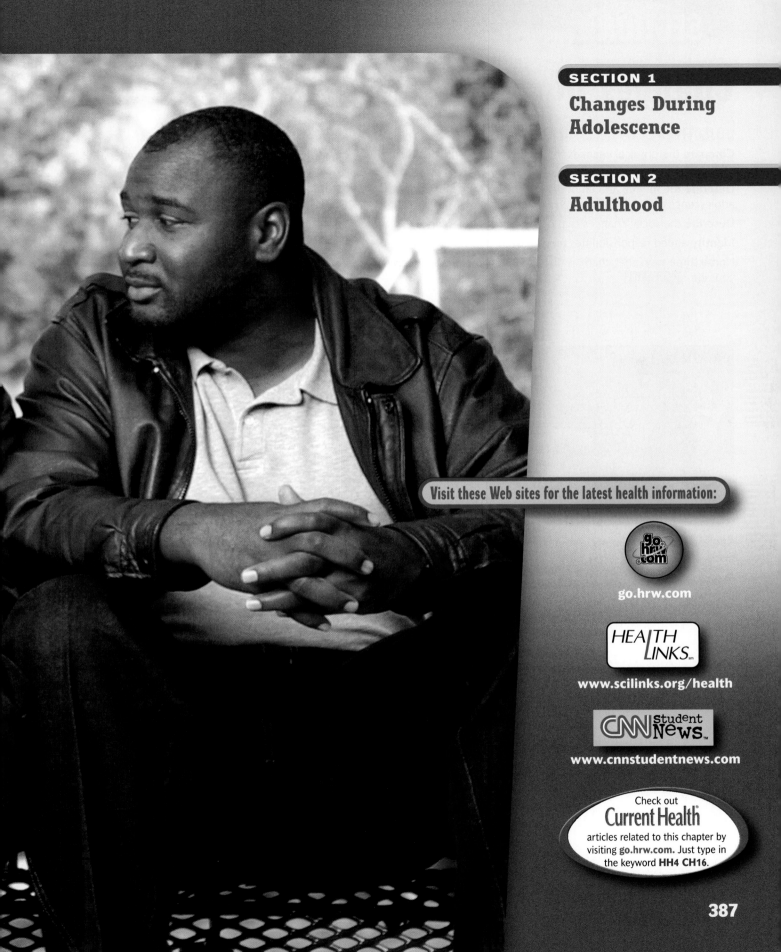

Visit these Web sites for the latest health information:

go.hrw.com

HEALTH LINKS℠

www.scilinks.org/health

CNN Student News™

www.cnnstudentnews.com

Check out
Current Health
articles related to this chapter by
visiting go.hrw.com. Just type in
the keyword **HH4 CH16**.

Changes During Adolescence

OBJECTIVES

Compare the physical changes that occur in boys and girls during adolescence.

Describe the mental and emotional changes that occur during adolescence.

Describe the social changes that occur during adolescence.

Identify added responsibilities teens have during adolescence.

Name three ways that changes during adolescence have affected your life. **LIFE SKILL**

KEY TERMS

adolescence the period of time between the start of puberty and full maturation

puberty the period of human development during which people become able to produce children

hormone a chemical substance made and released in one part of the body that causes a change in another part of the body

testes the male reproductive structures that make sperm and produce the male hormone testosterone

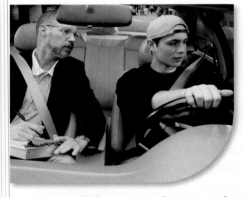

Adolescence brings many changes and responsibilities.

Franco was both excited and nervous about his driving test. He had always looked forward to the day when he would get his driver's license. Now, though, he was beginning to realize all of the responsibilities that come with driving a car. He thought to himself, Am I ready for this?

Physical Changes

Franco's worries about the changes in his life are common to many teens during adolescence. **Adolescence** is the period of time between puberty and full maturation. It is a time of change—changing body, changing emotions, changing mental abilities, and changing social life. All these changes can cause teens to feel awkward and unsure of themselves. Knowing as much as possible about the changes that are taking place helps adolescents realize that these changes are normal.

The beginning of adolescence is typically marked by the onset of puberty. **Puberty** is the period of human development during which people become able to produce children. Puberty begins when specific hormones are released. **Hormones** are chemical substances made and released in one part of the body that cause a change in another part of the body. The changes typical of puberty start when the female and male reproductive organs begin to release hormones. The male hormone is called *testosterone*. The female hormones are called *estrogen* and *progesterone*.

Physical Changes in Both Girls and Boys Most girls start puberty between 8 and 14 years of age. Boys usually begin puberty later, between 10 and 16 years of age. While some changes are common to both girls and boys, many of the changes are unique to each sex, as shown in **Figure 1.** Some of the changes that both girls and boys can expect to experience include facial acne, growth spurts, and an increase in muscle strength. Also, girls experience voice changes, just as boys do.

Physical Changes in Girls

Girls experience many changes during puberty, all of which occur at different times for different girls. As girls reach puberty, they naturally develop more body fat than boys do. The fat is needed for normal development during puberty. Hormones cause the hip bones to widen and fat to be deposited around the hips. Fat is also used for development of the breasts. Shortly after development of the breasts, hair begins to appear under the arms and in the pubic area. These changes are typically followed by a growth spurt.

Menarche, or the start of menstruation, begins when estrogen and progesterone levels begin to rise. The average age for menarche is 12 years old, although the age range for menarche varies widely. Girls should remember that these physical changes are a natural and healthy part of puberty.

Physical Changes in Boys

As testosterone levels rise in boys, the first physical change seen is an increase in the size of the testes. The **testes** are the male reproductive structures that make sperm and produce the male hormone testosterone. Afterwards, hair begins to appear under the arms and in the pubic and facial areas. At this time, many people notice that the voice deepens. A growth spurt usually occurs toward the end of puberty. Because growth spurts occur earlier

HEALTH Handbook For more information about skin care, see the Express Lesson on pp. 566–569 of this text.

Figure 1

As boys and girls go through puberty, they experience many changes. The most obvious are the physical changes.

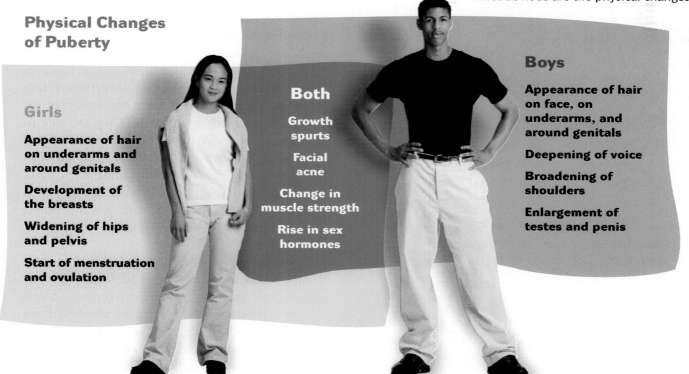

Physical Changes of Puberty

Girls

Appearance of hair on underarms and around genitals

Development of the breasts

Widening of hips and pelvis

Start of menstruation and ovulation

Both

Growth spurts

Facial acne

Change in muscle strength

Rise in sex hormones

Boys

Appearance of hair on face, on underarms, and around genitals

Deepening of voice

Broadening of shoulders

Enlargement of testes and penis

in puberty for girls than for boys, girls are usually taller than boys during these first years of puberty. Boys develop larger, stronger muscles throughout puberty.

Because puberty is a time of dramatic change, the body needs special attention during this period. Increases in height and weight mean that the body has greater nutritional needs. Adolescence is a good time to set healthy diet and exercise habits that can be continued throughout adulthood.

Mental and Emotional Changes

While physical changes during puberty are easily seen, mental and emotional changes may not be as noticeable. Coping with mental and emotional changes can be difficult because they are felt by the person but are not visible to others. Mental changes are changes that occur in the thinking process. These changes happen because the brain is still developing. Emotional changes occur as teens learn to cope with all of the changes that occur during adolescence.

A New Way of Thinking Intellectually, teens undergo enormous changes. During early adolescence, boys and girls process information in a simple way. Situations are usually seen from only one side without considering the other person's point of view.

During the middle adolescent period, teens often believe that nothing bad will ever happen to them. For example, teens believe that others may get into accidents but that they themselves will not. They may think this way because the brain is still maturing.

As adolescence progresses, teens can learn to think in a more sophisticated and complex manner. They are able to understand that actions taken today can have consequences the following day or in 10 years. They are able to reason more effectively, compare options, and make logical, mature decisions. They are also able to view situations from another person's perspective. This development helps teens become more compassionate toward others and greatly improves their relationships.

A New Way of Feeling Emotional changes may be the toughest part of adolescence. Many new feelings arise, particularly during adolescence. These new feelings come not only from changes in thinking but also from differences in the way teens see themselves. The new feelings also come when adolescents are treated

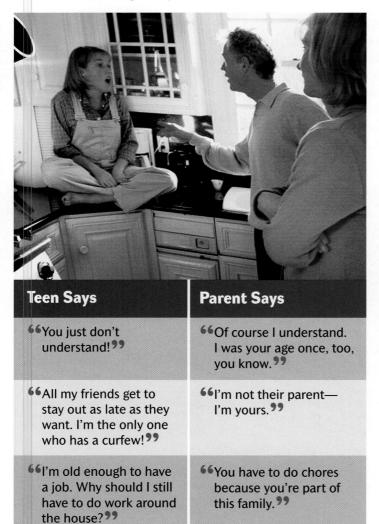

Figure 2

Most adolescents feel that their parents don't understand them. Hang on, because these feelings will pass.

Teen Says	Parent Says
"You just don't understand!"	"Of course I understand. I was your age once, too, you know."
"All my friends get to stay out as late as they want. I'm the only one who has a curfew!"	"I'm not their parent— I'm yours."
"I'm old enough to have a job. Why should I still have to do work around the house?"	"You have to do chores because you're part of this family."

differently by friends and parents. Both boys and girls may find that their feelings get hurt more easily than they did before. Sometimes, these new feelings can cause teens to feel alone, insecure, and confused. These feelings are common during adolescence.

A New Desire for Independence Anger, loneliness, and even depression can be common during adolescence. Many of these feelings come from the teen's desire to become more independent. Frustration and confusion about how to become independent can sometimes seem overwhelming, as seen in **Figure 2.** These feelings arise mostly because up to this point teens have been dependent on other people.

The process of leaving dependence behind and forming a new identity is complex and sometimes scary. Teens may desire independence but feel dependent. These conflicting emotions exist together because the processes of leaving some emotions behind and getting new ones occur at the same time. Having conflicting emotions is healthy and normal. If prolonged periods of sadness or anxiety become too overwhelming, seeking help from a parent, school counselor, or doctor is important.

 TOPIC link For more information about dealing with conflict, see Chapter 3.

LIFE SKILL Activity

Communicating Effectively

Communicating Effectively with Your Parents

Conflict with parents can be frustrating, but you can learn to resolve it. Consider the following situation.

John was tired when he came home from school. He put off cleaning his room until later. When John's mom came home, his room was a mess and he was watching TV. She started to yell at him. John ran to his room and yelled back, "You never give me a chance to get things done." John's mom called him disrespectful and lazy. John felt that his mom just did not understand.

Follow these guidelines to help you communicate more effectively with your parents and others.

1 Vent frustration and anger in a healthy way. Call a friend, or write about how you feel. Even when you are angry, hurting others, their stuff, or yourself is not an appropriate response.

2 Assess what happened. How were you right or wrong? How were your parents right or wrong?

3 Take action to resolve the conflict. Go to your parents, and apologize. Express how you felt during the argument.

4 Listen to your parents' side, and try to understand their point of view. Chances are that they are right in some way and are frustrated, too.

5 Plan with your parents to avoid conflict in the future. Ask for ways that you can show them that they can trust you.

LIFE SKILL Communicating Effectively

Write down two ways that John could have resolved the conflict with his mother. Then, write down two ways that John could build trust with his mother. **WRITING SKILL**

"All my friends are allowed to…"
"YOU NEVER…"
"You just don't understand…"
"Things were different when you were young…"

Dealing with New Feelings Learning how to deal with new, strong feelings is an important part of becoming a mature teenager. Along with these new feelings comes a greater desire to act on them. Controlling these desires is a serious challenge during adolescence. For example, when we are mad, we may want to express our anger by yelling. Feeling anger can be healthy, but yelling because one is angry is immature. Emotional maturity means learning to handle those strong feelings in an emotionally healthy way.

Controlling Your Emotions Sometimes mental, emotional, or sexual emotions during adolescence can feel so strong that some teens believe that they do not have control over what they do. This belief is not true. Teens are very capable of learning to feel intense emotions and not act on them. Successfully separating feelings from behaviors makes a teen truly more mature and independent.

Social Changes

What is most important in our lives is not necessarily how many clothes we own or how much money we have in the bank. Our relationships with people are what matter most. Social changes refer to those changes that occur within the relationships in a teen's life. These relationships may be intimate ones with family or they may be more impersonal ones, such as with a boss at work. During adolescence, relationships change because mental, emotional, and physical changes are happening all at once. Parents, teachers, and siblings begin to respond differently to an adolescent because, in a sense, a new person is evolving in their presence.

Increased Expectations As you mature, you may find that your parents expect more from you. And hopefully, you will find that your expectations of yourself increase as well. Evaluating these expectations and discussing which are negotiable and which are not are important for teens. It is normal for curfew, chores, and dating rules to change. It is also important to talk to parents about these expectations and to be willing to negotiate with your parents about them.

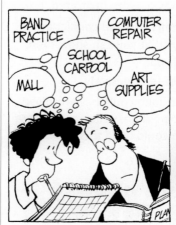 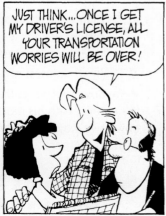 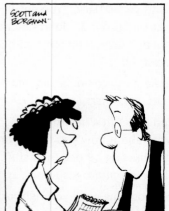 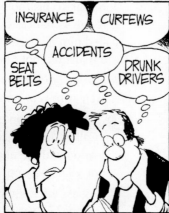

ZITS reprinted with special permission of King Features Syndicate, Inc.

Teens must also expect that some rules will be nonnegotiable, because everyone lives with some fixed rules. For example, no matter how old a person is, stopping at red traffic lights and abiding by other community rules are required. Social maturity means understanding, accepting, and living by each negotiable and nonnegotiable rule.

Changing Relationships Your relationships with your friends also change and become increasingly important during adolescence. As a teen, you may find yourself wanting to spend more time with friends than with family. Your changing relationships with your friends can be stressful for parents, too. Parents may feel hurt that their teen prefers spending more time with their friends than with them. Or parents may worry that their teenager is engaging in friendships that are unhealthy.

Evaluating Your Relationships Friendships can be difficult to assess during the teen years because emotions run high and can change quickly. Teens must take a hard look at their friendships and decide whether the friendships are good for them. You can evaluate your friendships by asking the following questions:

▶ Does this friendship bring out the best in me, or does it discourage me?

▶ Does the friendship make me a stronger or a weaker person?

▶ Does this person respect me and allow me to share my opinions and beliefs, or does this person insist that I conform to his or her ways?

A healthy friendship is one in which each person encourages the other. If the answers to the questions above indicate that a relationship is unhealthy, then the problems in the relationship must be addressed to resolve them. If they can't be resolved, then you must have the strength to end the relationship.

A teen's desire to be accepted can be very strong. Teens usually look to friends to find acceptance. But sometimes this strategy doesn't work. Take teen cliques, for example. *Cliques* are small, exclusive groups of friends that are judgmental of both their friends and others. Cliques can be painful to those on the outside, who may feel rejected. Gangs are another example of groups that can cause more harm than good.

Increased Responsibilities Independence is really about taking responsibility for one's feelings, thoughts, and behaviors. If a teen is to mature into an independent adult, taking responsibility in the teen's relationships at home is the best place to begin. As a teen's feelings and thoughts about his or her parents and siblings change, the teen's responsibilities toward them also change. Teens must start to communicate in a more mature manner, which entails listening well, allowing others to talk, and respectfully considering others' feelings and ideas. Good communication skills can also help to strengthen relationships with others. Some examples of

Evaluating Changing Relationships

1 Ask questions. Is this a healthy friendship? Is this friendship allowing me to grow?

2 Take charge. You can now think more like an adult, so decide on positive changes you can make to improve your relationships.

3 Get tough. Some of your friendships may become unhealthy. If you have difficulty breaking those relationships off, ask a good friend or teacher to help you.

4 Commit yourself to improving. You'll make some mistakes in your relationships, but you will learn from your mistakes.

MAKING GREAT DECISIONS

Your best friend is 16 years old, and she is at a sleepover with eight other girls. At midnight, a good friend of hers sneaks over to the house, taps on the bedroom window, and asks her to a party at his friend's house. No parents are at the party. She tells her friend that she doesn't want to go because she doesn't feel right sneaking out. The others at the slumber party ask her to drive them to the party. What should she do?

Write on a separate piece of paper the advice you would give your best friend. Remember to use the decision-making steps.

Give thought to the problem.

Review your choices.

Evaluate the consequences of each choice.

Assess and choose the best choice.

Think it over afterward.

how you can take more responsibility in relationships at home include

- ▶ showing concern for how people are feeling by asking how they are doing
- ▶ listening to another's tone of voice, ideas, and opinions. If the person sounds tired or sad, ask what you can do to help
- ▶ looking for ways to encourage other people and support them with kind words

As teens begin to take on more responsibility, they will find that those around them will trust them more. Teens often complain that parents don't trust them, but trust is something that has to be demonstrated and earned. Teens must look for opportunities to show their trustworthiness.

Working Outside the Home The teen years often bring the first opportunity for a paid job outside of the home. This experience is exciting but requires maturity and responsibility. Employers expect workers to perform to the best of their ability. The consequences of a job poorly done can range from receiving a pay cut to being fired. A teen who hasn't been responsible around the house will likely have many problems at work. Teens must realize that in families and in the world at large, many rules exist. Some rules are negotiable, but many are not. Thus, the demand for teens to act mature, to dress appropriately and to have good hygiene habits is greater than ever on the job. Teens can behave maturely by understanding the expectations of their boss and following through with commitments.

SECTION 1

REVIEW   *Answer the following questions on a separate piece of paper.*

Using Key Terms

1. **Compare** the terms *adolescence* and *puberty*.

2. **Identify** three hormones that contribute to the start of puberty.

3. **Describe** the role of the testes in physical development.

Understanding Key Ideas

4. **Identify** a change that is common to boys and girls during puberty.
   a. broadening of the shoulders
   b. widening of hips and pelvis
   c. facial acne
   d. facial hair

5. **Describe** how teens' ways of thinking change during puberty.

6. **Describe** three ways that teens can take on more responsibility at home.

7. **State** three ways that teens can be more mature while working outside the home.

Critical Thinking

8. **LIFE SKILL** **Practicing Wellness** Identify ways that you can tell if a relationship is healthy. Discuss what you can do if the relationship isn't healthy.

9. **LIFE SKILL** **Coping** State three changes that you have experienced during adolescence. Then, identify two ways to cope with these changes.

Adulthood

OBJECTIVES

Describe the changes that occur during young adulthood.

Identify the opportunities middle adulthood offers.

Name three concerns that an older adult might have.

List behaviors that promote healthy aging.

State three ways in which you can help an older adult you know lead a healthy life. **LIFE SKILL**

D o you ever dream of the day when you will be completely independent? When you'll own your own car? Independence comes with many responsibilities. Knowing what is expected of adults will allow you to start now to prepare yourself for adulthood.

Young Adulthood

Even though Americans are considered legal adults at the age of 18, a person who is 18 is still technically a teenager. Young adulthood is considered to be the period of adulthood between the ages of 21 and 35. This period is full of changes, challenges, and decisions.

Physical Changes During young adulthood, the growth rate of adults begins to slow down. As young adults' bodies begin to mature, they also enter a time of peak physical health. Many young adults take advantage of their health by playing sports or taking part in outdoor activities.

Mental and Emotional Changes With the changing emotions of the teen years behind, many young adults experience a sense of settling. Many of the conflicting feelings that occur during adolescence disappear and allow young adults to feel better about life. They enjoy the independence from their family but continue developing close relationships. Young adults begin to relate to their parents on an adult level. Keeping in touch with family is one way to adjust to the separation young adults may feel.

Intellectually, young adults think more abstractly. They can more consistently make mature, responsible choices. All of these changes give young adults a clearer sense of their identity: who they are, what they want from friendships, and what job they want to have.

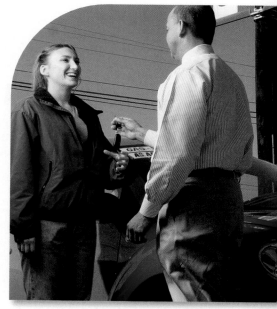

Along with the increased responsibilities of young adulthood come many rewards.

Social Changes Many young adults choose to marry and start a family during this time in their life. Before entering into such strong commitments, one must know oneself well—one's skills, values, strengths, weaknesses, and beliefs.

Commitment in relationships is very important. Some young adults choose to remain single. Others are afraid to marry. One reason may be that they have never seen a positive relationship. As a result, they may wonder if their marriage will fall apart. It is important that they know that they *can* make their marriage work. Seeking advice from older adults who have successful marriages is helpful.

Financial Concerns One exciting aspect of young adulthood is that you can start working toward your dream job. You might get a job or continue your education. You make decisions about the things you thought, planned, and prepared for as an adolescent. Young adults enjoy financial independence and freedom, perhaps for the first time in their lives. They are responsible for earning and spending their own money. While such independence can be scary, it can also be exciting. With this financial freedom comes the ability to choose where to work, where to live, and what car to buy.

real life Activity

CALCULATING A BUDGET

LIFE SKILL
Setting Goals

Materials

✔ paper
✔ calculator
✔ list of salaries and monthly expenses

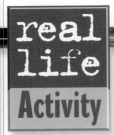

Week	1	2	3
Housing	$300		
Food	$100		
Transportation	$100		
Entertainment	$50		
Total	$550		

Procedure

1. **Divide** into groups of three students. Each group should be assigned a salary and given a list of monthly expenses.

2. **Divide** your salary by 12 to calculate your monthly allowance.

3. **Calculate** how much money you need per month for each expense category.

4. **Analyze** with your partners how much money you need in total. Divide the monthly salary accordingly. Some categories will need more money than others.

5. **Decide** as a group which categories are more important than others.

Conclusions

1. **Calculating Data** What is your group's monthly salary? **MATH SKILL**

2. **Calculating Data** How much money do you need per month for each expense category? **MATH SKILL**

3. **Summarizing Results** Does your salary meet the needs of your budget? Discuss ways to help your budget meet your salary.

4. **CRITICAL THINKING** For most jobs, the higher the education level, the higher the salary. Discuss the decisions that you can make now to affect your future job. How will you carry out those decisions?

Maintaining Wellness Young adults face many of the same health risks as adolescents. The No. 1 cause of death in people between the ages of 15 and 24 is unintentional injuries. Auto accidents, many of which involve alcohol, account for most of these accidents. The second and third leading causes of death are homicide and suicide, respectively.

Young adults who smoke, drink, and fail to exercise may feel healthy for a number of years and believe that these habits aren't harmful. But later in life, the ill effects of these bad habits appear. Suddenly, it may be too late to reverse the effects of bad habits. Because patterns developed during young adulthood affect your life later on, it is important to develop healthy habits during this time.

Middle Adulthood

We often hear the teen years described as being the best years of life. In fact, for many adults, this is not true. Middle adulthood, the period between 35 and 65 years of age, can prove to be "the best years" for many reasons.

Physical Changes The body goes through many changes during middle adulthood. Middle age used to be seen as a time when your body would start to slow down. Fortunately, with changes in attitude, diet, and physical exercise, adults have enjoyed greater physical stamina. Muscle tone and strength naturally begin to diminish, but with regular, moderate exercise, they can be maintained.

Women typically begin menopause between the ages of 50 and 55. **Menopause** is the period of time in a woman's life when the woman stops ovulating and menstruating. As a woman's estrogen and progesterone levels fall, the body's reproductive capacity begins to slow down. After menopause, women no longer menstruate or ovulate (produce eggs). Changes that accompany menopause may include hot flashes, a decrease in breast size, anxiety, and sometimes depression. Lower levels of estrogen put women at risk for osteoporosis, or thinning of the bones. Taking supplemental calcium and exercising can decrease the risk of developing osteoporosis.

Men also experience many physical changes during middle adulthood. Just as women experience a decline in their ability to reproduce, so do males. As men age, their sex hormone and sperm production gradually decrease.

Mental and Emotional Changes Many middle-aged adults begin to accept their mortality as they see friends and loved ones die. They reflect on these changes and begin to evaluate their lives. A healthy mind will see mistakes made, accept them,

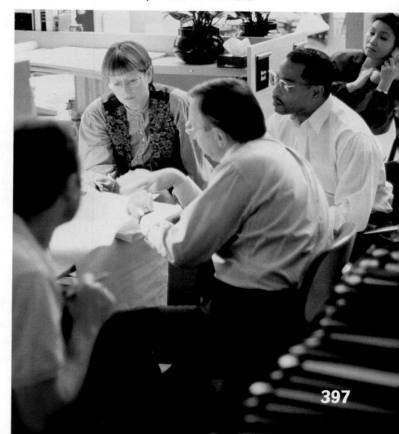

Many rewards accompany the added responsibilities of middle adulthood, such as a rewarding career and friendships with co-workers.

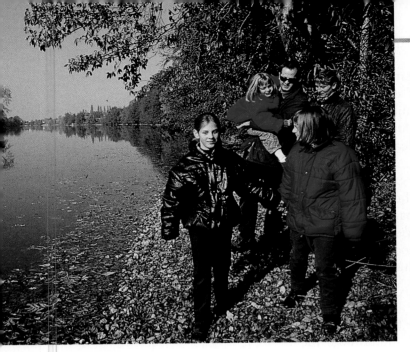

Midlife years are the best years of life for many people. Many are able to enjoy and focus on their families and job.

and move forward by trying to learn and change. Accepting the passage of time brings maturity. Satisfaction is gained from reflecting on the birth and growth of children, job accomplishments, and healthy relationships. A healthy, mature mind can accept changes and look forward to the later parts of life with hopeful anticipation.

Occasionally, an adult may experience a midlife crisis. A **midlife crisis** is the sense of uncertainty about one's identity and values that some people experience in midlife. If someone experiences a midlife crisis, it usually begins in the person's forties. Adults may feel that their life is slipping away and that they are losing their youth. Thus, they try to hold onto that youth rather than accept their maturation. They may make dramatic changes in their life, such as taking a new job, in an effort to feel better about themselves. However, such changes do not solve their problem because they do not deal with the root of the problem, which is fear of accepting the loss of their youth. Many middle-aged adults experience psychological changes. These changes are healthy and normal.

Social Changes   Adults in this stage often enjoy clearer identity formation—they know who they are. By the time adults reach the middle years, they are able to positively focus on their family and their job. They understand their role in each area and make choices accordingly. They guide their family through changes in life and take on leadership roles in child-rearing and in their job. Stresses do arise. When handled in a healthy manner, though, these stresses can mature a person and deepen one emotionally and intellectually.

Financial Concerns   Most adults learn to accept more responsibility during middle adulthood because other people depend on them for financial and emotional support. As with any responsibility, there are pleasures in addition to the strains. Some adults experience immense satisfaction from providing for others. These greater financial needs can also bring on greater stress.

The effects of stress can be serious, and adults must learn to cope. But for some people, the stress may get overwhelming. Health problems from stress can erupt. Such problems may include depression, ulcers, high blood pressure, or heart disease. Mental health deeply affects physical health during these years, and caring for both aspects of health is very important.

Maintaining Wellness   The leading cause of death during middle adulthood is cancer. Cancer is followed closely by heart disease as a cause of death. Adults can reduce their risks of cancer and heart disease by exercising, not smoking, and eating a low-fat diet to prevent high blood cholesterol. Many young adults do not feel the effects of eating a poor diet, smoking or chewing tobacco, not exercising, and being overweight. As these young adults grow older, however, they may begin to experience the ill effects of these habits.

Receiving yearly medical care from a physician is very important for preventing and treating problems. For example, one may have high blood pressure or cancer and not know it. To ensure good health, both women and men need regular medical exams from a physician.

Older Adulthood

The population of older adults (those 65 years of age and older) in the United States has grown rapidly during the past decade. This trend is predicted to continue well into the new century. Some reasons for this trend are improved understanding of nutrition, exercise, and disease prevention as well as advances in medical care. Sadly, our cultural attitudes have encouraged young people to view older adults as uninformed, unproductive, and unable to enjoy life. In reality, older adults may enjoy experiences that are not possible in the early or middle adult years. Descriptions of this and other stages of adulthood can be seen in **Table 1.**

Physical Changes As adults move into older adulthood, they continue the aging process. As they age, they may find that their ability to recover from illnesses or injuries is not as quick as before. In addition, the effects of years of unhealthy habits started during adolescence may become evident during this time of life. For example, smoking-related lung cancer and obesity-related diabetes are two common concerns for older adults.

Mental and Emotional Changes Most older adults are more emotionally stable than they were earlier in life. This stability is a natural consequence of maturity. They have endured hardships such as the death of a close friend, spouse, or family member. Many come to terms with the meaning of life—what is important and what is not. Young adults can learn much from older adults.

Table	1	Stages of Adulthood	
Age	Stage	Description	
21–35	young adulthood	This period of life is marked by a first career job, marriage, children, and financial independence.	
35–65	middle adulthood	Greater financial security, satisfaction with a growing family, and emotional maturity mark this time of life.	
65 and older	older adulthood	Wisdom accumulated from a variety of life experiences marks this stage. Loneliness and isolation can be serious problems.	

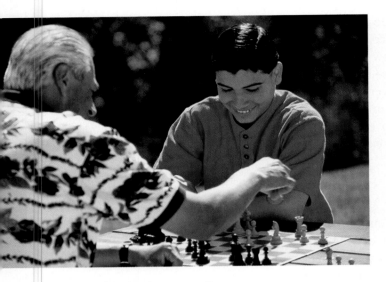

Ways to Interact with Older Adults

1 Visit them. Sit and listen to them. Ask them what they would do in certain situations. Ask for their opinion.

2 Offer to do simple household chores. They'll love having you around while you get work done that perhaps they can't do.

3 Bring them food. Bake cookies, and deliver them personally. Ask if they need groceries, and then get them.

internet connect

www.scilinks.org/health
Topic: Alzheimer's Disease
HealthLinks code: HH4009

HEALTH LINKS. Maintained by the National Science Teachers Association

Despite the extensive life experiences they have had, older adults are not immune from many of the same mental problems that are possible in the earlier years. Depression, anxiety, or loneliness may also plague the elderly. Younger family members must be alert for signs of such problems in older family members. The younger family members too can benefit from helping older loved ones. Such help could be as simple as an occasional visit or phone call. If we take time to listen to older adults, we find that many of their feelings are similar to ours—whether we are a teen or a middle-aged adult.

Many younger adults believe that older adults lose their intelligence and wisdom to age and disease. This belief is not true for most older adults. For example, Alzheimer's disease occurs in only a small percentage of the population of adults between the ages of 65 and 80. **Alzheimer's disease** is a disease in which one gradually loses mental capacities and the ability to carry out daily activities.

Alzheimer's disease affects the brain and usually progresses slowly. A person with this disease first begins losing short-term memory and then long-term memory. Sometimes the patient forgets where he or she is. Sometimes the patient does not recognize loved ones. Alzheimer's is an emotionally painful disease to both the patient and the family.

Social Changes   Many adults look forward to retirement after age 65. Leaving a career of many years can be enjoyable but also stressful. Any major lifestyle change is hard. Adapting to retirement usually requires time. Adapting may take a few weeks or even months. Believe it or not, when an adult has focused for many years on a career, shifting that focus onto an enjoyable hobby or recreation can be difficult. Most people eventually come to appreciate the freedoms and free time retirement offers.

Financial Concerns   Older adults who do decide to work less or retire may find that their financial situation has changed. Although taking advantage of this time period by enjoying such activities as traveling and visiting family members is important, planning ahead is also important. Some adults may require expensive healthcare. In some cases, they may even have to face moving into a retirement home and losing their independence.

Maintaining Wellness   Health problems that the elderly face are similar to those of middle-aged adults. Cancer and heart disease are the leading causes of illness in older adults. So, maintaining healthy habits is very important for older adults. There is no reason that age alone should make a person less productive in society or prohibit him or her from fully enjoying life.

"All old people get Alzheimer's, so I don't want to get old."	Only 2 percent of people aged 65 to 80 get Alzheimer's disease.
"The teen years are always the best years of life."	The teen years can be difficult. Often, people feel more settled and satisfied with relationships and life later in adulthood.
"Most older people are sickly and are unable to take care of themselves."	The majority of older people are fairly healthy and self-sufficient.
"Older people should stop exercising and get a lot of rest."	Exercise at any age strengthens heart and lung function. Older people can benefit from exercising as much as anyone else.

Healthy Aging

When we look at the big picture of life from adolescence to older adulthood, we see the health risks shift from accidents and injuries to illnesses such as heart disease and various forms of cancer. We can see the importance of establishing healthy patterns of behavior early in adolescence to reduce serious health risks during the teen years as well as later in life. As a teen, you may rarely think of how eating, exercising, and risk-taking affect your health later in life. The truth is that healthy changes in your behavior during these critical years are extremely important to your health in older adulthood.

Common Concerns During Aging Building a positive attitude about each stage of life can ensure that a person will care for his or her health. Having a positive outlook is important because mental health and physical health affect each other. For example, physical exercise can reduce psychological depression by increasing the circulation of certain brain chemicals.

One of the tragic myths of aging is that as we age, we lose our intellectual sharpness and our ability to enjoy life and be productive. The truth is that advancing age brings greater wisdom and, in many ways, an ability to enjoy life more than we did during early adulthood. As adults mature, however, they must keep their minds stimulated. This can be accomplished through active work, such as reading, listening to music, and talking to others, rather than passively watching television and movies.

Many emotional challenges arise throughout adulthood. Loneliness, depression, or various stages of grief occur as we move through difficult life experiences, such as the death of friends, the death of a spouse, or perhaps divorce. It is very important for adults to pay attention to their feelings and moods and to seek help from loved ones.

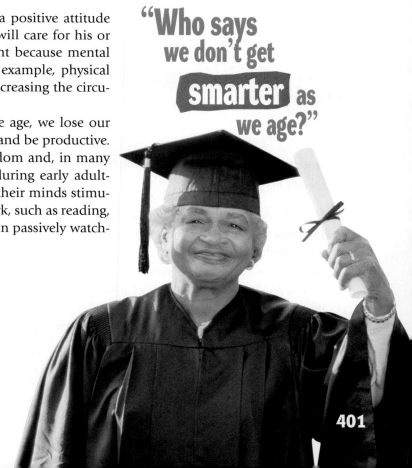

"Who says we don't get smarter as we age?"

401

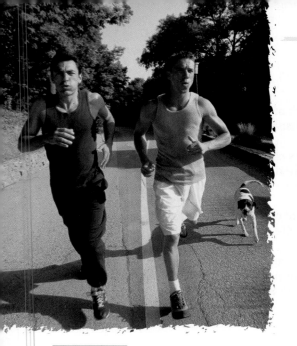

Tips for Healthy Aging The average length of time an individual is expected to live, or **life expectancy,** has risen dramatically since 1960. Most men and women who live to be 65 can also expect to live until age 80. Scientists predict that the greatest increase in population over the next few decades will occur in people over the age of 85. Thus, making certain that older adults are independent, healthy, mentally keen, and productive is important.

The most important habits to form during adolescence and early adulthood are those that keep us physically healthier, as seen in **Figure 3.**

▶ Establishing regular exercise can actually help us live longer. Regular exercise improves quality of life and may prevent premature death and disease.

▶ Even the simple measure of not smoking can dramatically reduce the risks of developing heart disease, cancer, and other diseases.

▶ Not drinking alcohol also decreases the risk of death by car accidents, alcoholism, and liver disease.

▶ Maintaining a healthy weight helps to prevent diabetes later in life.

▶ Lowering salt intake and keeping total Calories at a level at which normal weight for height is maintained are important to a person's health as they age.

The development from adolescence to adulthood is a miraculous journey, and life can get better with each passing year. Growing older is a privilege and process worthy of our respect and care. We should not reject the process but should look forward to and enjoy every part of this journey.

Figure 3

Regular exercise is one way to maintain your health now and in the future.

ACTIVITY *What is one form of exercise you can start now?*

SECTION 2

REVIEW   *Answer the following questions on a separate piece of paper.*

Using Key Terms

1. **Describe** the symptoms of Alzheimer's disease.
2. **Define** *life expectancy.*

Understanding Key Ideas

3. **Describe** how emotions change during young adulthood.
4. **Identify** the leading cause of death in young adults, and describe actions they can take to reduce the risk of dying during this period.
5. **Describe** three changes that you might face during middle adulthood.
6. **State** the leading causes of illness in older adults.

7. **State** whether our culture portrays older adults as having less intelligence. Explain why this portrayal is true or why it isn't true.
8. **LIFE SKILL** **Practicing Wellness** State three ways that you can help an older adult to lead a healthier life.
9. **LIFE SKILL** **Practicing Wellness** Identify four habits that you can begin today to improve the quality of your life in 10 years.

Critical Thinking

10. Some people describe the teen years and young adulthood as the "best years of life." Do you agree or disagree? Why?

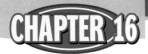

Highlights

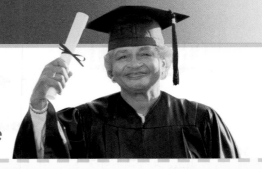

Key Terms

The Big Picture

adolescence (388)
puberty (388)
hormone (388)
testes (389)

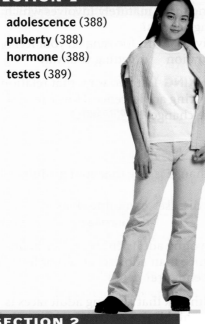

✔ Changes in hormone levels mark the beginning of puberty.

✔ Puberty involves many physical changes, some of which are unique to boys and girls.

✔ As teens mature, they begin to think in a more complex and sophisticated manner.

✔ Adolescence is a process of gradually accepting more responsibility for one's behaviors, thoughts, and feelings.

✔ Mental maturity allows adolescents to see life from another person's viewpoint, not simply from their own. This maturity helps them respect others.

✔ During adolescence, teens' relationships change as more is expected from them.

✔ Working outside the home requires a high level of maturity and commitment on the part of the teen.

menopause (397)
midlife crisis (398)
Alzheimer's disease (400)
life expectancy (402)

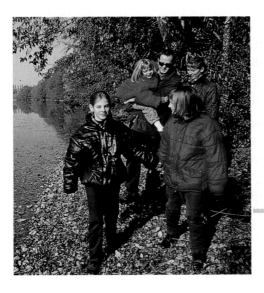

✔ Moving from young adulthood into older adulthood involves many mental, physical, and emotional changes.

✔ Young adulthood is a time marked by increased independence.

✔ Young adults can exert great influence over all areas of their health and can reduce their risk of developing diseases by making healthy lifestyle choices.

✔ During middle adulthood, the different aspects of adults' lives become more stable. This stability allows for greater focus on their job and family.

✔ With the increased financial responsibilities of middle adulthood also comes satisfaction from providing for others.

✔ Keeping physically, mentally, and socially active can ensure that older adulthood is an enjoyable time marked by good health.

✔ The older adult years can be a time of great satisfaction, productivity, and wisdom. Aging is a natural process that should be viewed positively.

Coming of Age

What does it mean to be an adult? In answering this question, scientists and social scientists look at cultures all over the world to find what we have in common. One thing most cultures share is some sort of ritual marking the transition from childhood or adolescence to adulthood. The rituals associated with this transition are called *rites-of-passage* or *coming-of-age ceremonies*.

Almost every society has a ritual to mark the transition from childhood to adulthood. Some coming-of-age rituals are quite informal, while others are ceremonial.

Rites of Passage

Think about your own life. What incidents do we use to mark your maturity? When does our society say to you, "Now you are an adult with its rights and responsibilities"? Some of our rituals are informal. For example, obtaining a driver's license has great significance to many teenagers. Voting at 18 gives you the rights and responsibilities of a political voice. Turning 21 gives you new rights and responsibilities. More-formal rites of passage may include your school's most formal dance.

Many religions have a very formal coming-of-age rite called confirmation. In the Catholic Church, for example, a bishop places his hands on a young person's head to signify that they have received the wisdom to make their own decisions about faith.

Coming of Age Around the World

All over the world, people just like you engage in rites of passage. Although some of these rites may seem unusual, each has the same kind of significance that the various ways our society marks the transition to adulthood do.

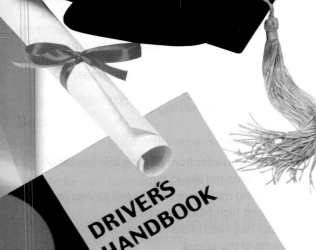

▶ **Maasai** As part of elaborate coming-of-age ceremonies, Maasai boys from the African nation of Kenya go to live in *manyattas,* camps built by adult women of the society. Adult women also chaperone the girls who live in the camp. Boys practice ancient rituals, including using spears and wielding shields, to become *morans* (warriors).

▶ **Mexico** When a girl reaches 15 years of age, many people mark that milestone with a rite of passage called a *quinceañera*. A girl of 15 arrives at a thanksgiving mass in a traditional white or pastel Mexican dress full of frills. Her friends, who act as attendants, may accompany the girl. After mass, there may be a birthday party, at which a dance with the girl's favorite boy highlights the festivities.

▶ **Navaho Nation** When a Navaho girl comes of age, she participates in a traditional ceremony called *Kinaalda*. This ceremony lasts for 4 days. It is based on a cycle of songs called the *Blessing Way*. The ritual ends on the fourth day with a traditional campfire in which the girl bakes a special corn cake to symbolize her acceptance of the hard work that comes with adulthood.

▶ **Judaism** Many coming-of-age rituals are religious in nature. When a young boy of the Jewish faith makes a transition into manhood, he is part of a ceremony called a *bar mitzvah*. This ceremony takes place around his 13th birthday. The ceremony takes place in a day, but learning about the Jewish faith may take months or years of preparation. Girls participate in a *bat mitzvah*. Both terms mean "commandment age" and signify that one has become an adult of the faith.

▶ **Japan** Coming of age in Japan takes on a national significance. *Seijin-no-hi*—"Coming of Age Day"—takes place every year on January 15 in Japan. This day is set aside to honor anyone who has turned 20 during the past year. Twenty is a significant legal age in Japan, too. People can vote, and other options become open to them. The day often begins with athletic events or town celebrations. People who are 20 dress up and go out with their friends for a night on the town.

One thing that characterizes all of these rituals is the society's enthusiasm for children. Although the message that one is becoming an adult is serious, the rites and rituals themselves can be exciting and show that the adults accept the youth as one of their own.

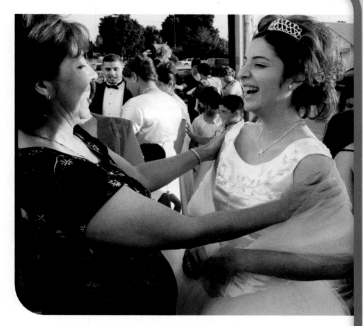

The quinceañera celebrates this teen's entry into young adulthood.

YOUR TURN

1. **Summarizing Information** Why does almost every society have coming-of-age rituals and rites?

2. **Interpreting Information** Research one culture, and write a paragraph about how that culture marks the transition from childhood to adulthood.

3. **CRITICAL THINKING** How do you think that coming-of-age rituals in your society help you focus on your rights and responsibilities?

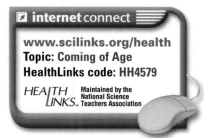

■ **internet** connect

www.scilinks.org/health
Topic: Coming of Age
HealthLinks code: HH4579

HEALTH LINKS. Maintained by the National Science Teachers Association

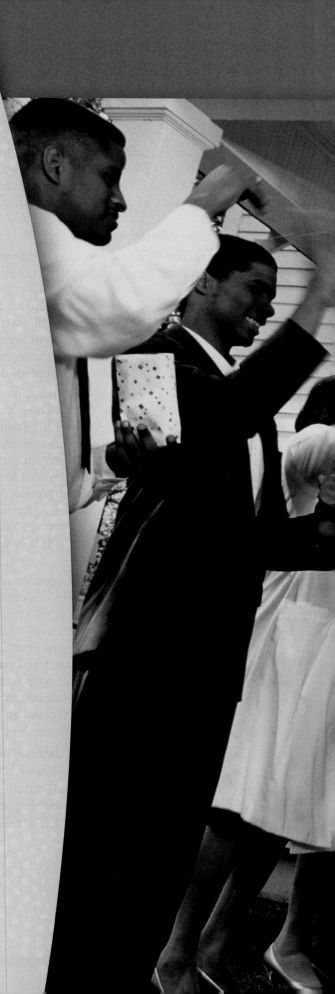

CHAPTER 17

Marriage, Parenthood, and Families

What's Your Health IQ?
KNOWLEDGE

Which of the statements below are true, and which are false? Check your answers on p. 642.

1. In healthy marriages, the spouses try to meet each other's needs.

2. The serious emotional consequences of divorce are felt only by the couple divorcing.

3. A spouse should depend on his or her partner to solve all conflict in the marriage.

4. A parent's behavior affects how his or her children feel about themselves.

5. An increasing number of single fathers are raising their children.

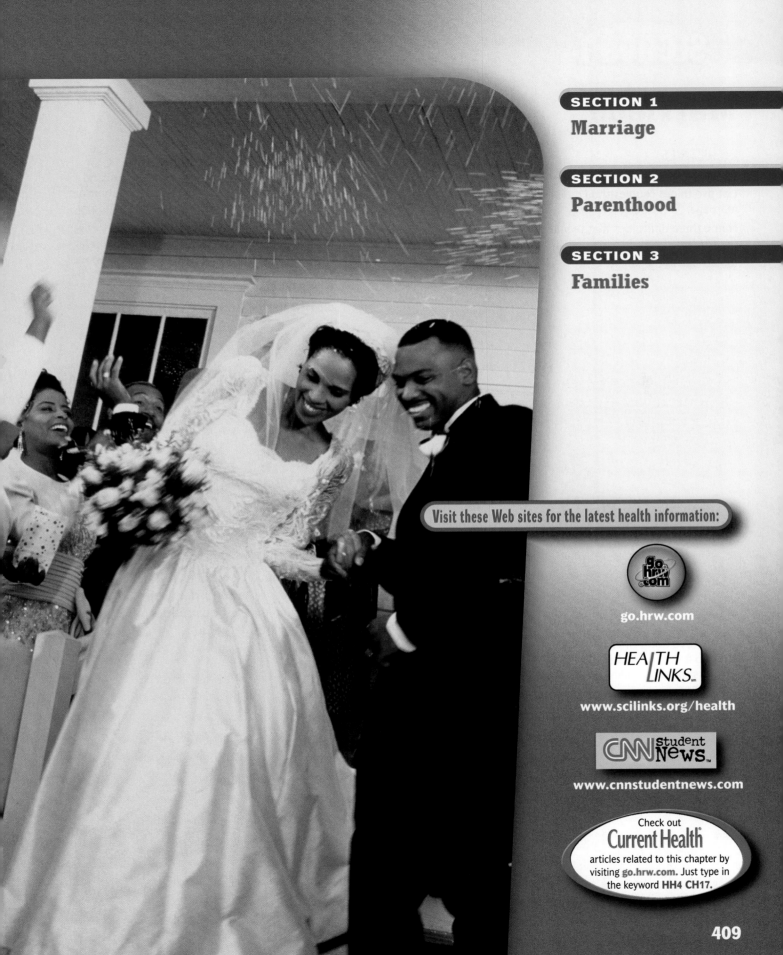

SECTION 1

Marriage

SECTION 2

Parenthood

SECTION 3

Families

Visit these Web sites for the latest health information:

go.hrw.com

HEALTH LINKS.

www.scilinks.org/health

CNN student News.

www.cnnstudentnews.com

Check out
Current Health
articles related to this chapter by
visiting **go.hrw.com**. Just type in
the keyword **HH4 CH17.**

409

Marriage

OBJECTIVES

Describe the responsibilities of married partners.

List five things couples should discuss if they are considering marriage.

Name three difficulties that teenagers who are married may face.

Identify four ways in which a teen can cope with a divorce or remarriage in the family.

Two halves of one whole. The resting place for deep friendship. The blending of souls. All of these phrases have been used to describe marriage. But marriages do not form easily. Marriages are created by the strength of loving actions, commitment, compromise, and emotional intimacy.

Healthy Marriages: Working Together

You have probably observed many married couples. Have you noticed how the interactions of each couple differ? A **marriage** is a lifelong union between a husband and a wife, who develop an intimate relationship. Deciding whether to marry is one of the most serious decisions a person can make. Marriage can provide great rewards for both partners, such as deep friendship, emotional intimacy, and children. Knowing the responsibilities of a healthy marriage can help you prepare for this decision.

Mature love takes time to develop. To develop a serious relationship, the partners must be willing to learn about each other.

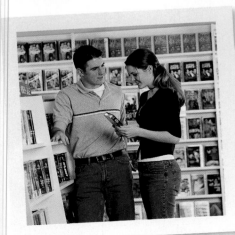
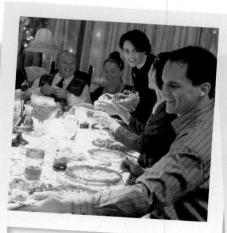
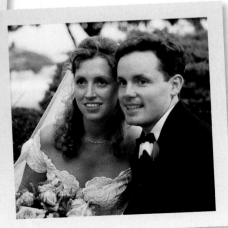

Responsibilities of Marriage A healthy marriage requires that both partners work together to meet each other's needs. Other responsibilities for each partner include the following:

▶ **Love** In a healthy marriage, spouses show their love for each other through actions and do not depend solely on feelings of love. Feelings of love change over time. Sometimes, couples may not feel the same intensity of love they felt when they were first married. However, if the spouses are patient and work together, they can regain feelings of love and support. Often, a couple's love grows deeper and stronger after the couple has worked through a hard time.

▶ **Commitment** A *commitment* is an agreement or pledge to do something. In a healthy marriage, spouses make a commitment to work through their differences, remain faithful to one another, and to make their relationship work. Commitment in marriage requires that both partners be willing to change themselves for the good of the couple. A person cannot change his or her spouse's habits; the person can change only his or her own.

▶ **Compromise** Compromise is essential in a healthy marriage. Compromise in marriage means not always getting your way and sometimes giving up what you want. Each partner must prioritize needs and desires and then discuss these priorities with his or her spouse. Although compromise requires sacrifice, both partners benefit from the stronger relationship that compromise brings.

▶ **Emotional intimacy** Intimacy, or familiarity with each other, is important in a healthy marriage. **Emotional intimacy** is the state of being emotionally connected to another person. The most common way for a couple to develop emotional intimacy is through good communication. Each partner is responsible for expressing feelings in a truthful, loving way if the relationship is to grow.

A person can have a healthy marriage even if he or she has not seen an example of one. Those who have not seen a healthy marriage need to know that a healthy marriage is possible for them through loving actions, commitment, compromise, and emotional intimacy.

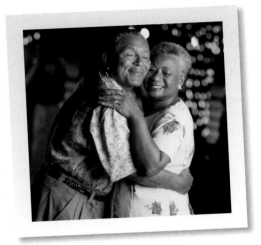

Benefits of Marriage

▶ **Emotional and physical intimacy**

▶ **Companionship and deep friendship**

▶ **Financial support system**

▶ **Greater emotional stability**

Engagement: Developing Your Relationships

Developing emotional maturity is an important part of the engagement period. **Emotional maturity** is the ability to assess a relationship or situation and to act according to what is best for oneself and for the other person in the relationship. It is important for the couple to make sure that the relationship is built on mature love, not on *infatuation,* or exaggerated feelings of passion. In mature love, each partner tolerates and accepts the other person's flaws. With emotional maturity you can better determine what is needed to improve a relationship and to allow it to grow.

TOPIC link For more information about relationships, see Chapter 19.

Discussing Important Issues Using the engagement period to talk about the commitment ahead is essential to building a strong relationship. Talking seriously can be difficult because each person feels intense love and is eager to marry. Each partner must ask some important questions and gain advice from others to make the best decisions possible. During the engagement period, couples should discuss issues such as the following:

▶ What are our values and beliefs?
▶ Should we have children?
▶ How will we handle conflict between family members?
▶ Should both of us work outside of the home?
▶ Where should we live?
▶ What are our economic expectations?

Couples should come to agreement on these issues to clearly understand each person's desires and goals.

Premarital Education Classes Premarital education classes can help couples openly discuss their goals and expectations of marriage. Major differences may surface, and a counselor can help the couple decide if those differences can or cannot be resolved. If they cannot be resolved, couples may decide to break the engagement. Other good reasons to break an engagement include physical or emotional abuse or alcohol and drug abuse.

Teen Marriages

The teen years are a time of dramatic changes. As a teen, you leave behind old ways of thinking and behaving and emerge as a more grown up person. Your interests and concerns will be different from those you had when you were younger.

When teens marry, changes in thinking and behavior are not yet complete. Thus, the spouse a teenager chooses may be different from the spouse the teen would choose later in life.

When teens marry, they must cope with many stresses in addition to their physical and emotional changes. The stresses of teen marriages include

▶ independence from parents and family
▶ financial worries
▶ changes in relationships with close friends
▶ interaction with in-laws
▶ concern for a spouse's emotional and physical well-being
▶ possible parenthood

Many married teens also put education plans on hold. They are financially unable to meet the expenses of marriage and tuition. Delaying education can cause resentment and can keep a person from reaching his or her potential.

Some teenagers are unable to mentally, physically, and intellectually mature into adulthood while married. Those who can successfully mature into adulthood while married have a lot of help from parents or other adults.

"We never thought being married could be so hard."

Divorce and Remarriage

Unfortunately, not all marriages are successful. When a marriage has trouble, sometimes the couple tries *separating*, or living apart for awhile. If one or both partners decide that the marriage is over, they may seek a *divorce*. A **divorce** is a legal end to a marriage. Going through a divorce is often difficult not only for the adults, but also for the other family members. Everyone in the family must adjust to the new situation.

Reasons for Divorce Many times, divorce seems like the best solution to an unhappy marriage. Problems such as abuse and addiction are often grounds for divorce. But marriages end in divorce for many other reasons including emotional immaturity, marital unfaithfulness, conflicts with family, and selfishness. Additional reasons for divorce include the following:

▶ **Communication problems** Breakdown in good communication is a common cause of divorce. If a couple fails to communicate well, anger may accumulate over the years. The spouses may then turn away from each other emotionally and refuse to openly communicate.

▶ **Unfulfilled expectations** Lack of fulfilled expectations accounts for other divorces. One partner may enter marriage hoping that life will become different or that his or her spouse can be changed as time passes. These expectations are unrealistic. Partners should enter marriage with the understanding that marriage will not solve life's problems and that one person cannot change the habits of another.

▶ **Different financial habits and goals** Differences in financial habits can also lead spouses to divorce. Before and during marriage, it is important to discuss finances, to make a budget, and to figure out how each partner will stay within the budget.

Impact of Divorce on Teens Numerous losses occur in a teen's life after divorce. Some teens experience a change in the relationship with their parents. Others feel the financial stress of a divorce. Many teens face other emotional stresses. For example, some teens may experience feelings of abandonment. Others may feel angry at themselves for not having been able to change the situation.

Many of these feelings are hard to identify when experiencing them. Counseling can help a teen understand these feelings better. The tips listed in **Figure 1** can help teens cope with divorce.

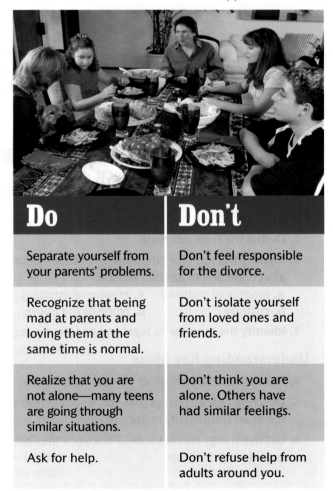

Figure 1

A divorce or remarriage in the family can be difficult. A few tips for coping with these situations appear below.

Do	Don't
Separate yourself from your parents' problems.	Don't feel responsible for the divorce.
Recognize that being mad at parents and loving them at the same time is normal.	Don't isolate yourself from loved ones and friends.
Realize that you are not alone—many teens are going through similar situations.	Don't think you are alone. Others have had similar feelings.
Ask for help.	Don't refuse help from adults around you.

Families

OBJECTIVES

Discuss why family relationships are important.

Describe different types of families

Name the characteristics of healthy families.

State four ways to cope with family problems.

List three ways that you could help make your family healthier. **LIFE SKILL**

H ave you ever noticed how many different types of families there are? Although families may have different structures, the relationships between family members are the most important part of all families.

Family Relationships Are Important

For most people, the relationships they have with their mother, father, sister, brother, aunts, grandparents, or other family members are sources of much joy and love. Family relationships teach us how to love and what being loved is like. They teach us who we are, who we want to be, and what feeling accepted or rejected is like.

Family relationships are powerful because they influence our emotions and help shape our character, either positively or negatively. Think about your own experiences with your family. Families provide for the emotional and physical needs of their members. Families help family members develop their individual identities. Families also instill moral values.

Families Need Time Because our families are so important, it makes sense for us to put energy into our family relationships. Unfortunately, not all of us do so. We sometimes spend more time concentrating on friendships, schoolwork, or athletic pursuits because doing these things is easier. As you mature, it is important to refocus on family relationships and take responsibility for working harder on them. This is particularly true if your family relationships are troubled or strained.

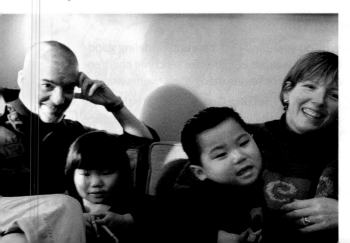

Regardless of the makeup of a family, the relationships between family members are the most important part of the family.

Types of Families

Helene's family is made up of her mother and her brother. Joe's family is made up of his parents and a grandmother. The members that make up a family of today may be different from those of families in years past. Children in a family are referred to as **siblings,** or brothers or sisters related to another brother or sister by blood, the marriage of the individual's parents, or adoption. Today, there are many different types of families.

Nuclear Families The most traditional family structure is the nuclear family. A **nuclear family** consists of a family in which a mother, a father, and one or more biological or adopted children live together.

Blended Families Over the past few decades, family structures have changed for many reasons, including an increase in the number of divorces. A blended family may result if a divorced or widowed parent chooses to remarry. *Blended families* are made up of the biological mother or father, a step-parent, and the children of one or both parents. The parents may decide to have children together. The parent who is not a child's biological parent is known as a *step-parent*.

Single-Parent Families Some families consist of a single mother and her children or a single father and his children. This type of family is a *single-parent family*. Single-parent families can occur if the parent was divorced, never married, or widowed. Most single-parent families are headed by a mother. But, in recent years, an increasing number of single fathers are raising their children.

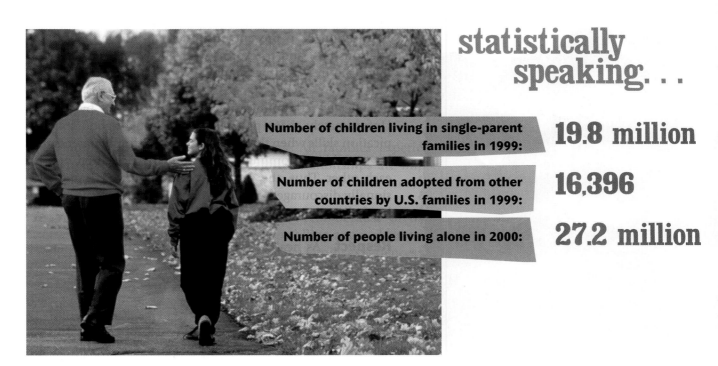

statistically speaking. . .

Number of children living in single-parent families in 1999: **19.8 million**

Number of children adopted from other countries by U.S. families in 1999: **16,396**

Number of people living alone in 2000: **27.2 million**

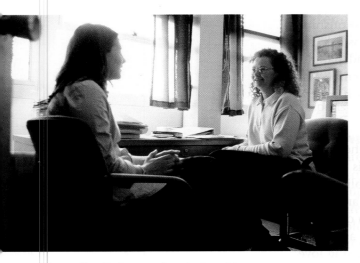

If your family is experiencing problems, help can be found. Find someone you trust who is willing and available to listen.

While the strategy for coping with each family problem may differ according to the problem, some methods are better than others. One good way to deal with your emotions is to communicate them to people you trust. In a situation like divorce, you might want to spend time talking with your friends, especially those who have also had a divorce in their family. Also, trusted adults, such as a grandparent, aunt, uncle, school guidance counselor, teacher, or religious leader, can sometimes give you some of the emotional support that you may be missing.

Another thing you could do is get involved in a new hobby or sport. Find something that absorbs your interest and takes your mind off problems that you cannot solve.

Family Counseling Family counseling is sometimes necessary to help a family improve its relationships. **Family counseling** involves counseling discussions that are led by a third party to resolve conflict among family members.

Family counselors can give another perspective, help family members see each other's point of view in a positive way, and help to evaluate the family's problems. But the real work comes from the family members themselves. If a family needs counseling, it is more helpful if the entire family receives counseling. But if that is not possible, one family member should not hesitate to go by himself or herself.

Good family relationships are important to your emotional and physical well-being. Although it is often difficult to confront family problems and take action, by staying encouraged and not giving up you can be a part of the solution to the problem. The rewards are worth the effort!

SECTION 3

REVIEW
Answer the following questions on a separate piece of paper.

Using Key Terms

1. **Define** the term *nuclear family*.

2. **Identify** the term for "the people who are outside the nuclear family but related to the nuclear family, such as aunts, uncles, grandparents and, cousins."

3. **Define** the term *family counseling*.

Understanding Key Ideas

4. **Identify** two reasons that family relationships are important.

5. **Compare** three types of families.

6. **Identify** which one of the following is *not* a characteristic of a healthy family.
   a. commitment   c. love
   b. selfishness   d. good communication

7. **LIFE SKILL** **Coping** List four ways you can cope with problems in your family.

Critical Thinking

8. How would you help your family if a parent was recently diagnosed with cancer?

9. **LIFE SKILL** **Coping** Identify a problem a family might face and outline how a teen might work to resolve the problem.

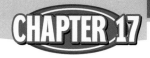

Highlights

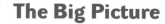

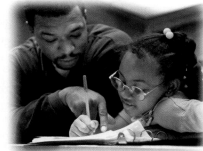

Key Terms

marriage (410)
emotional intimacy (411)
emotional maturity (411)
divorce (413)

parental responsibility (415)
discipline (416)

sibling (419)
nuclear family (419)
extended family (420)
family counseling (422)

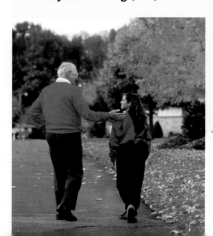

The Big Picture

✔ Love, commitment, compromise, and communication are essential to developing a healthy marriage.

✔ Couples should use the engagement period to ask questions and make decisions about the commitment of marriage.

✔ Teen marriages are often extremely difficult because the teen years involve many dramatic changes.

✔ Lack of communication, unfulfilled expectations, and different financial goals are common causes of divorce.

✔ Although parental divorce and remarriage affect many teens, it is important for teens to accept the situation, avoid blaming themselves, and to use healthy strategies to cope with their feelings.

✔ Parenting requires commitment, love, discipline, and support.

✔ Parents are responsible for the physical and emotional needs of their children from before birth through the teen years.

✔ Discipline provides guidance for children.

✔ It is important for parents to be supportive of their children, especially during the teen years.

✔ Because children learn from their parents, parents' behavior greatly affects children.

✔ Families provide guidance and support, help develop family members' identities, and instill moral values.

✔ As family structures have changed over the past few decades, many more children now live in different types of families including blended, single-parent, extended, adoptive, and foster families.

✔ Healthy family relationships are developed through effective communication, respect, commitment, and love.

✔ It is important that all family members try to work together to solve family problems.

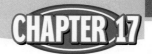

Review

Understanding Key Terms

discipline (416)

divorce (413)

emotional intimacy (411)

emotional maturity (411)

extended family (420)

family counseling (422)

marriage (410)

nuclear family (419)

parental responsibility (415)

sibling (419)

1. For each definition below, choose the key term that best matches the definition.
   a. the people who are outside the nuclear family but are related to the nuclear family, such as aunts, uncles, grandparents, and cousins
   b. counseling discussions that are led by a third party to resolve conflict among family members
   c. a brother or sister related to another brother or sister by biology, marriage, or adoption
   d. teaching a child through correction, direction, rules, and reinforcement
   e. the duty of a parent to provide for the physical, financial, mental, and emotional needs of a child

2. Explain the relationship between the key terms in each of the following pairs.
   a. *divorce* and *marriage*
   b. *emotional maturity* and *emotional intimacy*

Understanding Key Ideas

Section 1

3. Name two responsibilities of partners in a healthy marriage.

4. The benefits of marriage include
   a. deep friendship.   c. emotional intimacy.
   b. financial stability.   d. All of the above

5. What is the purpose of premarital education classes?

6. Why is it important for individuals in a relationship to have realistic expectations of each other?

7. Explain why it is difficult for teen marriages to succeed.

8. Many marriages fail because of
   a. poor communication.
   b. lack of commitment.
   c. emotional immaturity.
   d. All of the above

9. Name four ways in which a teen can cope with a divorce or remarriage in the family.

10. **CRITICAL THINKING** Write one paragraph explaining why you think compromise plays such an important role in the success of a marriage. **WRITING SKILL**

Section 2

11. Describe what is meant by the term *parental responsibility*.

12. The responsibilities of parents begin
    a. before their child's birth.
    b. when their child can walk.
    c. after their child is born.
    d. during their child's teen years.

13. Describe the responsibilities of a parent.

14. **CRITICAL THINKING** Describe traits a person should work on before becoming a parent.

15. **CRITICAL THINKING** Write two paragraphs on why you think parents' behaviors have such a great effect on their children throughout the children's lives. **WRITING SKILL**

Section 3

16. What are two important things that family relationships teach us?

17. Compare two different family structures.

18. List qualities that are necessary for a healthy family.

19. Explain how family counseling might help families experiencing conflict.

20. **CRITICAL THINKING** List three ways you could help make your family relationships healthier. **LIFE SKILL**

Interpreting Graphics

Study the figure below to answer the questions that follow.

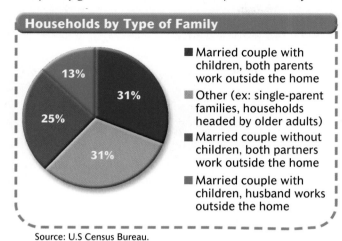

Households by Type of Family

- 31% — Married couple with children, both parents work outside the home
- 31% — Other (ex: single-parent families, households headed by older adults)
- 25% — Married couple without children, both partners work outside the home
- 13% — Married couple with children, husband works outside the home

Source: U.S Census Bureau.

21. What percentage of households are made up of married couples who have children and in which both parents work outside the home?

22. CRITICAL THINKING Why do you think the households made up of married couples who have children and in which only the husband works outside the home is the smallest category?

Activities

23. Health and Your Community Imagine you are a counselor advising a man and a woman who are engaged to be married in 3 months. Write three questions that you feel will help them decide if their marriage will be healthy. State why these questions are important. **WRITING SKILL**

24. Health and Your Community Choose a television program that portrays a marriage, and watch the program. Answer the following questions about the program: How is marriage portrayed? Do you agree or disagree with the show's portrayal of marriage? Support your answers.

25. Health and You Write five positive character traits that you possess and that you believe will make you a good parent. Then, explain why each trait is important to good parenting. **WRITING SKILL**

Action Plan

26. LIFE SKILL Coping It is important for families to develop problem-solving skills. Devise a plan for a family to work out its problems.

Standardized Test Prep

Read the passage below, and then answer the questions that follow. **READING SKILL** **WRITING SKILL**

Since Anne and Collin were married, Anne has wanted to move back to her home state. When they had a son, Anne went back to work to help pay bills. She loved her job, but Collin wanted her to stay home with the baby. One day, Collin told Anne that he had received a promotion. Anne knew the promotion meant they wouldn't move and that Collin might want her to quit her job. Both Anne and Collin told each other what they wanted. Then, each decided to <u>relent</u>. Collin took his promotion. They did not move back to Anne's home state. However, Anne requested a flexible work schedule and was able to keep her job.

27. In this passage, the word *relent* means to
A resist.
B state your desires clearly.
C give way under pressure.
D insist on something.

28. What can you infer from reading this passage?
E Marriage requires that spouses consider each other's needs.
F Marriage always interferes with your career plans.
G Parenthood reduces one's chances of promotion.
H The reason that most couples stay married is that they live close to their families.

29. Write a paragraph that compares the benefits of working through difficulties in marriage.

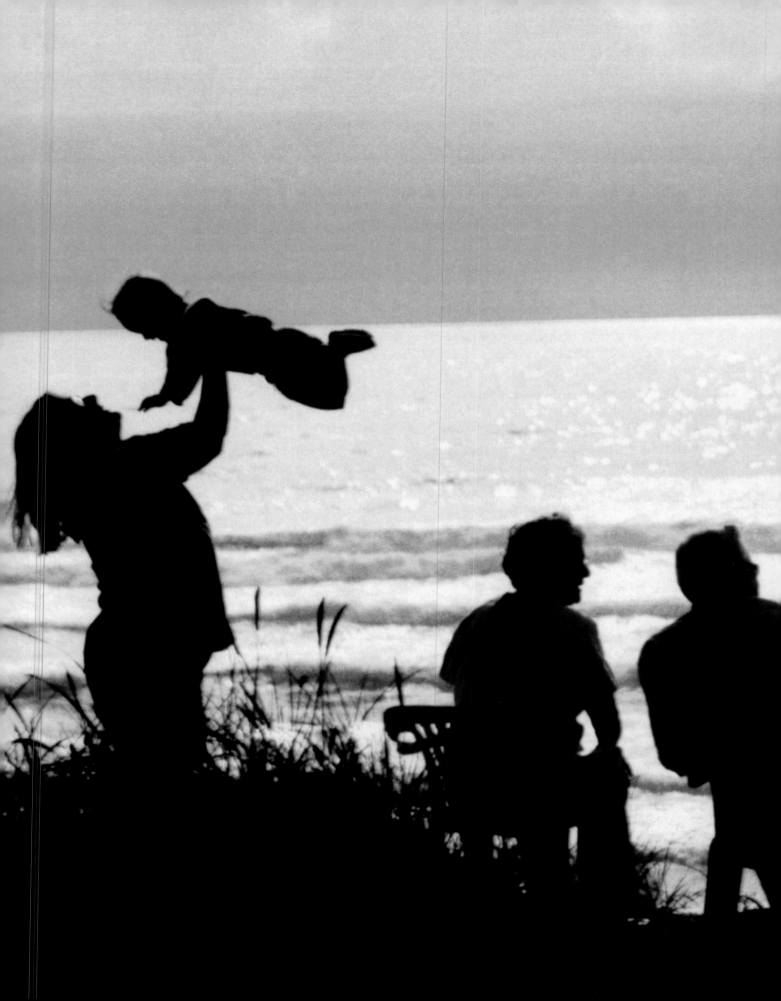

UNIT 6
Reproductive Health

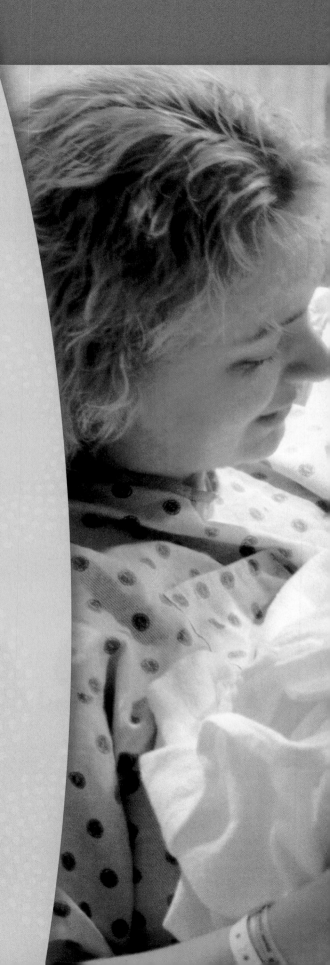

CHAPTER 18

Reproduction, Pregnancy, and Development

What's Your Health IQ?
KNOWLEDGE

Which of the statements below are true, and which are false? Check your answers on p. 642.

1. Sperm are made in the vas deferens.

2. Both sperm and urine travel through a man's urethra, although not at the same time.

3. Testicular cancer is most common among men who are over the age of 50.

4. Estrogen is the primary hormone in males.

5. Eggs are made in the ovaries.

6. The uterus is the organ in which a fetus develops.

7. A woman produces several eggs every month.

8. Fertilization of the egg usually occurs in the fallopian tubes.

9. By the end of the sixth month of pregnancy, all the baby's major body structures are formed.

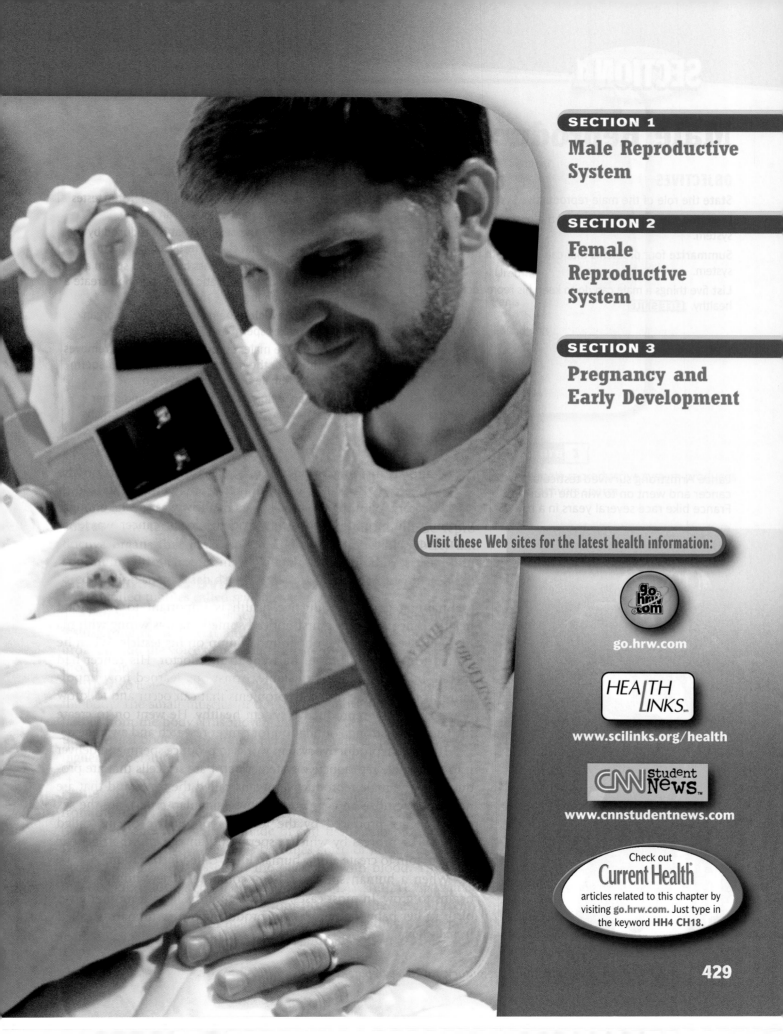

Visit these Web sites for the latest health information:

go.hrw.com

HEALTH LINKS.

www.scilinks.org/health

CNN Student News.

www.cnnstudentnews.com

Check out **Current Health** articles related to this chapter by visiting go.hrw.com. Just type in the keyword HH4 CH18.

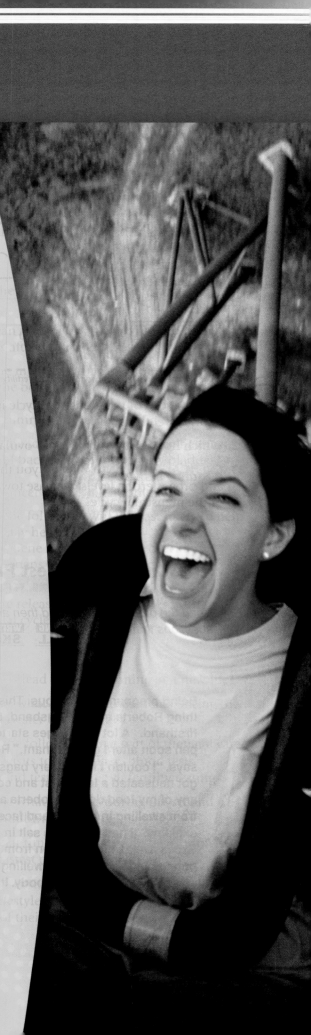

CHAPTER 19

Building Responsible Relationships

What's Your Health IQ?
KNOWLEDGE

Which of the statements below are true, and which are false? Check your answers on p. 642.

1. Differences in values and personality don't really matter when choosing a dating partner.

2. There's really nothing a teen can do to avoid the pressures to become sexually active.

3. The majority of high school students have never had sexual intercourse.

4. Many teens who have had sex wish they'd waited.

5. Taking drugs or drinking alcohol can lead to unwanted sexual activity.

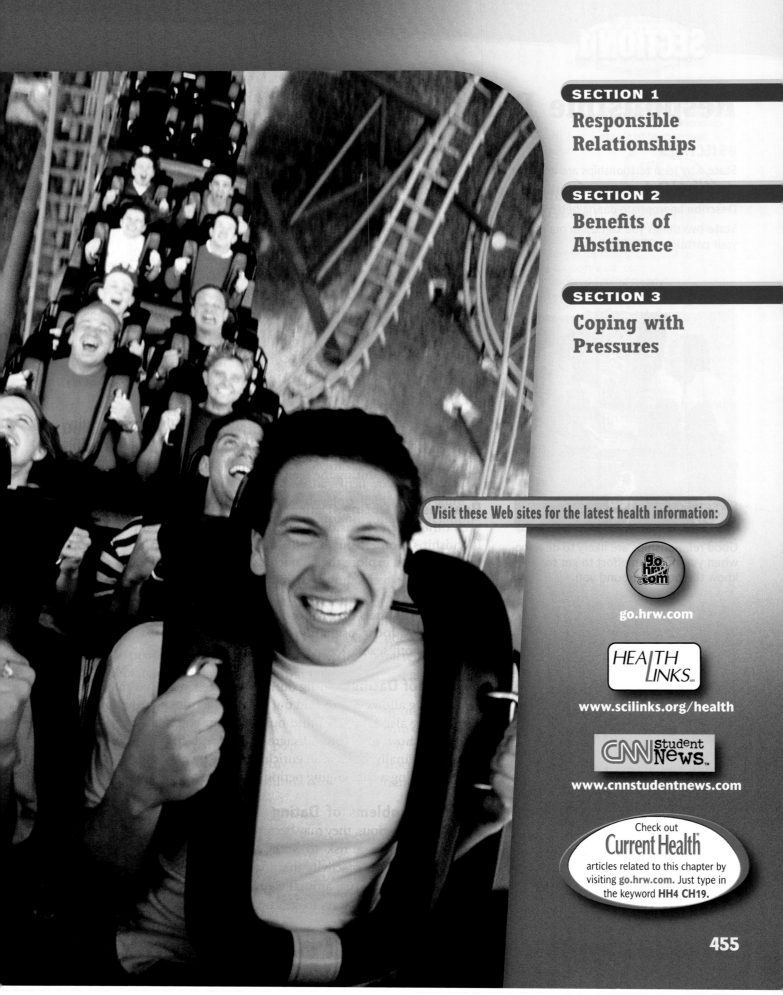

Visit these Web sites for the latest health information:

go.hrw.com

HEALTH LINKS

www.scilinks.org/health

CNN student News

www.cnnstudentnews.com

Check out
Current Health
articles related to this chapter by
visiting **go.hrw.com**. Just type in
the keyword **HH4 CH19.**

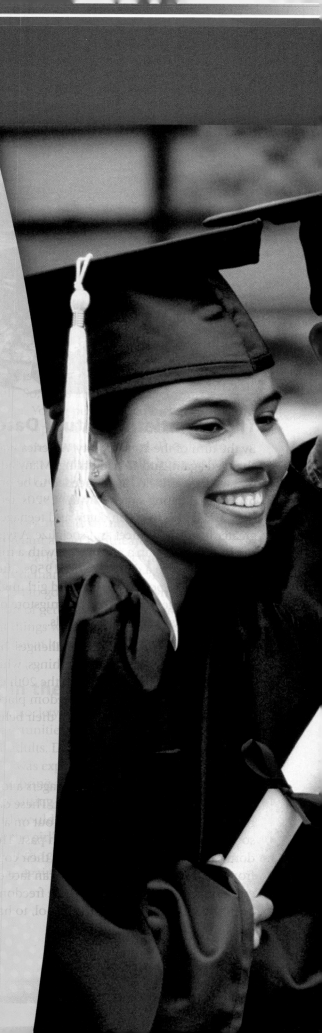

CHAPTER 20

Risks of Adolescent Sexual Activity

What's Your Health IQ?
KNOWLEDGE

Which of the statements below are true, and which are false? Check your answers on p. 642.

1. Only about one-third of pregnant teenagers ever complete high school.

2. Most teen mothers eventually marry the father of their child.

3. Teen parents usually must interrupt their education to work.

4. Babies born to teen mothers are more likely to suffer health problems.

5. There is no effective way to prevent all of the risks of teen sexual activity.

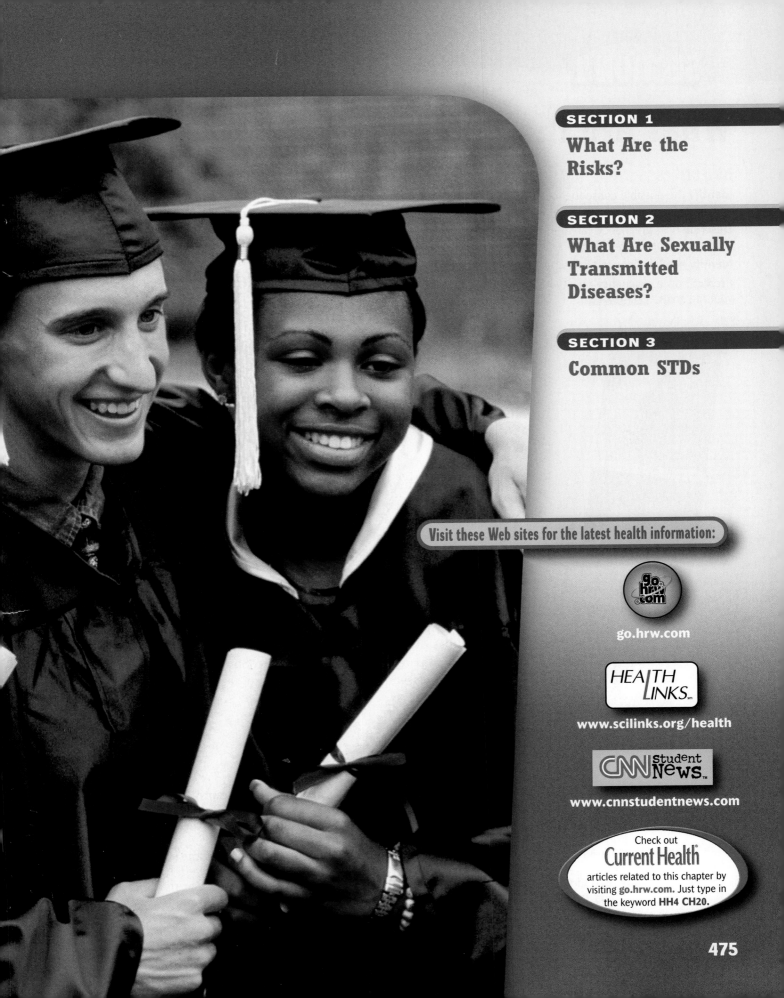

Visit these Web sites for the latest health information:

go.hrw.com

HEALTH LINKS.

www.scilinks.org/health

CNN student News.

www.cnnstudentnews.com

Check out **Current Health**® articles related to this chapter by visiting go.hrw.com. Just type in the keyword **HH4 CH20.**

What Are the Risks?

OBJECTIVES

Identify the possible consequences, especially for teens, of sexual activity before marriage.

Describe how pregnancy can affect the lives of teen parents and babies of teens.

Identify how abstinence eliminates the risks of teen sexual activity.

Predict how a pregnancy now (yours or your partner's) would affect your life goals. **LIFE SKILL**

KEY TERMS

sexually transmitted disease (STD) an infectious disease that is spread by sexual contact

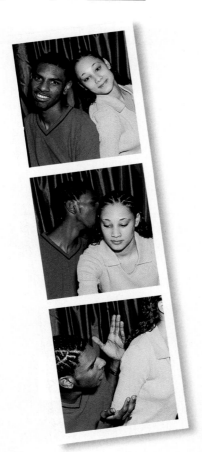

Sex is not a game, and neither is having a baby or a sexually transmitted disease. Yet many teens ignore the risks of teenage sexual activity. Ignoring the risks won't make the consequences go away.

Risks of Teen Sexual Activity

Although many teens don't want to admit it, a sexually active teen faces many risks. These risks include emotional and social consequences, such as feeling troubled about lying to one's parents. Many teens lose self-esteem and self-respect when they go against their own values and religious beliefs. Other serious consequences can include

- ▶ unplanned pregnancy
- ▶ **sexually transmitted diseases (STDs),** infectious diseases that are spread by sexual contact, such as HIV/AIDS

In spite of the risks, many teens have not thought about the realities of teenage sexual activity. Knowing the realities helps teens to be prepared when situations arise. Shown below are just some of the beliefs—and the realities—about teen sexual activity and its consequences.

Beliefs VS. Reality

"If I have a baby, I'll be the center of attention."	Few teenagers want to constantly be around a baby.
"He won't leave me if I'm pregnant with his baby."	Teen pregnancy adds stress to a teen relationship.
"I can't get pregnant the first time I have sex."	You CAN get pregnant the first time you have sex.
"Jan is a really nice girl. She'd never have a sexually transmitted disease (STD)."	All sexually active individuals are at risk of catching an STD regardless of their background.

Teen Pregnancy

Many teenage pregnancies occur because teens think, "It won't happen to me." But in fact it does happen to between 800,000 and 900,000 female teenagers each year. This means that 1 in 10 female teenagers gets pregnant each year. One in 5 sexually active female teenagers gets pregnant each year. Four in 10 of all girls become pregnant at least once before they reach the age of 20. With so many teen girls getting pregnant, it is not surprising to find out that the teen birth rate in the United States is very high. In fact, both the teen pregnancy rate and the teen birth rate are among the highest of any industrialized nation in the western world. The majority of these pregnant young women are not married.

Teen pregnancies are hard on the mother's health. The bones and muscles of teenagers are not ready for the physical stresses of pregnancy. Teenagers are still developing physically. Pregnant teens must eat well and get adequate medical care in order to stay healthy and to increase their chances of delivering a healthy baby. Otherwise, both the mother and the baby can have health problems.

> One in five sexually active female teenagers gets pregnant each year.

real life Activity

CHARTING YOUR COURSE

LIFE SKILL
Setting Goals

Materials

✔ 8 1/2 in. x 11 in. sheet of paper
✔ pencil
✔ ruler

Procedure

1. **Draw** a line lengthwise across the paper to represent your life.

2. **Draw** marks every inch along the line.

3. **Write** "0" at the left end of the line to show your birth. Label the first mark "10 years." Label each mark after that in 10-year increments (20 years, 30 years, etc.).

4. **Use** an X to mark the point that shows your current age.

5. **Draw** marks at four points that represent important events in your life. Label each mark with a descriptive phrase, such as "Moved to California."

6. **Draw** marks at four points that represent events that you hope will take place in the future. Label each mark with a descriptive phrase, such as "Buy a car."

Conclusions

1. **Summarizing Results** What future events did you mark?

2. **Predicting Outcomes** What things could change the expected events of your future?

3. **Predicting Outcomes** How might becoming a single teen parent change the expected events of your future?

4. **CRITICAL THINKING** What short-term goals do you need in order to reach each of the expected events of your future?

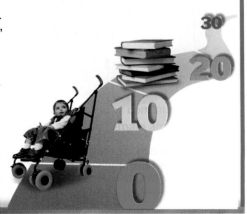

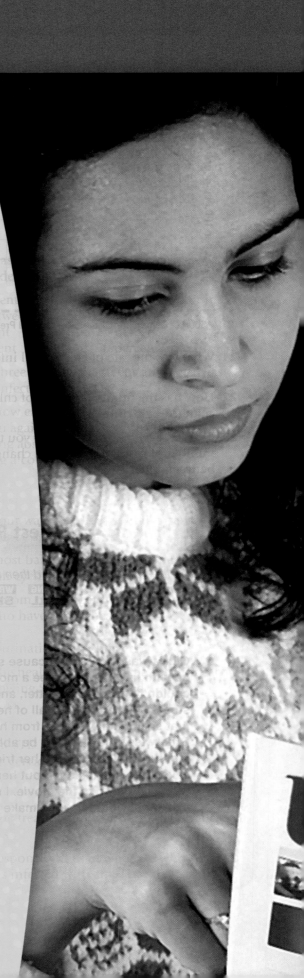

CHAPTER 21

HIV and AIDS

What's Your Health IQ?
KNOWLEDGE

Which of the statements below are true, and which are false? Check your answers on p. 642.

1. Even young and healthy people are at risk of becoming infected with HIV.

2. You cannot tell if a person is infected with HIV just by looking at him or her.

3. You can get HIV after shaking hands with a person infected with HIV.

4. If you drink from a water fountain after a person infected with HIV has, you are at risk of becoming infected with HIV.

5. You cannot become infected with HIV by using a toilet after a person infected with HIV has used it.

6. You are not at risk of becoming infected with HIV by kissing the cheek of a person infected with HIV.

7. If you donate blood at the blood bank, you are at risk of becoming infected with HIV.

8. Most people who are infected with HIV know they are infected and will warn others that they are infected.

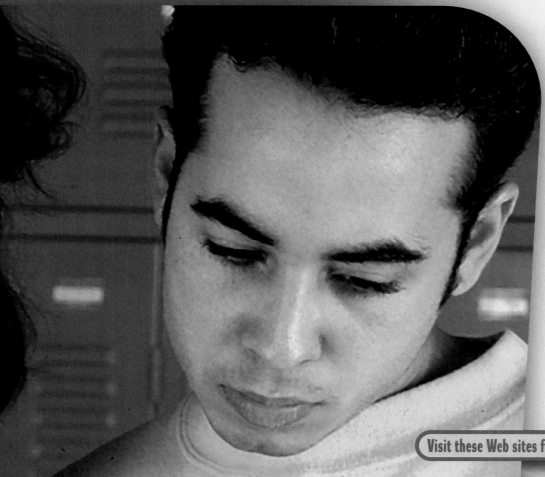

Visit these Web sites for the latest health information:

go.hrw.com

www.scilinks.org/health

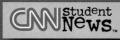

www.cnnstudentnews.com

Check out
Current Health®
articles related to this chapter by
visiting go.hrw.com. Just type in
the keyword **HH4 CH21**.

HIV and AIDS Today

OBJECTIVES

Distinguish between an HIV infection and AIDS.

Name the three areas in the world that have the greatest number of people living with HIV/AIDS.

Compare the number of people in the United States living with HIV infection to the number of people in the United States living with AIDS.

Summarize why teens are one of the fastest-growing groups infected with HIV.

KEY TERMS

human immunodeficiency virus (HIV) the virus that primarily infects cells of the immune system and that causes AIDS

acquired immune deficiency syndrome (AIDS) the disease that is caused by HIV infection, which weakens the immune system

pandemic a disease that spreads quickly through human populations all over the world

Every day, about 110 Americans are infected with HIV. Three million people died from AIDS in 2000. Currently, there is no cure for AIDS. Do you know how to help fight against the spread of HIV and AIDS?

What Are HIV and AIDS?

HIV and AIDS are different. **Human immunodeficiency virus (HIV)** is the virus that primarily infects cells of the immune system and that causes AIDS. **Acquired immune deficiency syndrome (AIDS)** is the disease that is caused by HIV infection, which weakens the immune system.

HIV infection is an infection in which HIV has entered the blood and is multiplying in a person's body cells. HIV specifically infects cells of the immune system. HIV eventually destroys the body's ability to fight off infection. After someone is infected with HIV, the virus

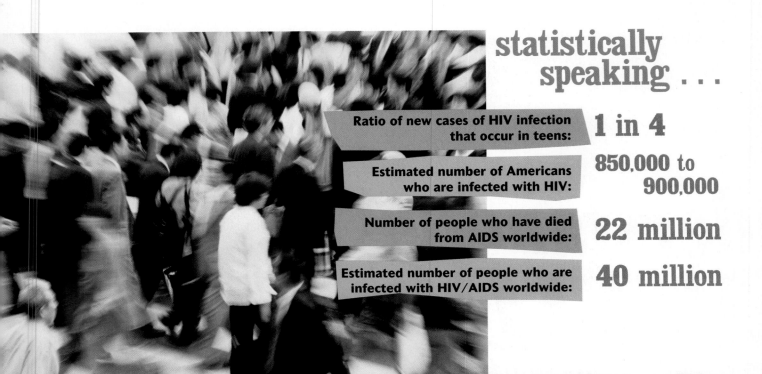

statistically speaking . . .

Ratio of new cases of HIV infection that occur in teens:	**1 in 4**
Estimated number of Americans who are infected with HIV:	**850,000 to 900,000**
Number of people who have died from AIDS worldwide:	**22 million**
Estimated number of people who are infected with HIV/AIDS worldwide:	**40 million**

starts making new copies of itself inside the immune system cells. The new copies of the virus destroy the cells they infect. The copies of the virus are then released into the bloodstream and enter other immune system cells. The destructive cycle then continues.

Getting AIDS Being infected with HIV doesn't mean the person has AIDS. A person is said to have AIDS when the virus has destroyed many immune system cells and has badly damaged the immune system. It usually takes 5 to 10 years for a person who is infected with HIV to develop AIDS if the person has not received treatment. People with AIDS cannot fight off illnesses that a healthy person's immune system could easily defeat. AIDS patients suffer from and often die from these illnesses.

There is still no cure for AIDS. Once the virus infects a person's body, there is no way to remove the virus. Most people with HIV infection eventually develop AIDS. So, learning about HIV and AIDS and protecting yourself from being infected are very important.

HIV Around the World

AIDS is a **pandemic,** a disease that spreads quickly through human populations all over the world. More than 20 million people throughout the world have died from AIDS in the last 20 years.

HIV was first discovered in the United States in the early 1980s. Most scientists think that HIV came from central Africa. The virus spread very quickly from Africa to other regions and countries. HIV is still spreading rapidly in many parts of the world, including Asia and Eastern Europe (especially in the Russian Federation). However, the hardest hit area is Africa. AIDS is now the leading cause of death in sub-Saharan Africa. To get an idea of how widespread HIV and AIDS are in the world, look at the statistics in **Figure 1.**

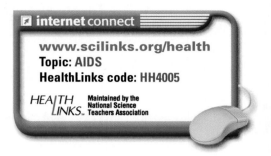

www.scilinks.org/health
Topic: AIDS
HealthLinks code: HH4005

HEALTH LINKS. Maintained by the National Science Teachers Association

Figure 1

These statistics show that AIDS has spread through populations around the world.

ACTIVITY *If the population size of North America is 316 million, what percentage of the* **MATH SKILL** *population is infected with HIV/AIDS?*

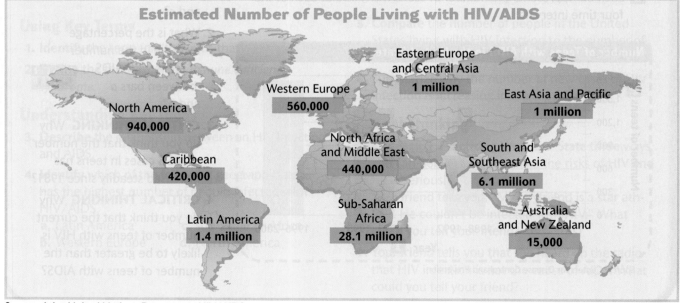

Estimated Number of People Living with HIV/AIDS

Eastern Europe and Central Asia
1 million

Western Europe
560,000

East Asia and Pacific
1 million

North America
940,000

North Africa and Middle East
440,000

South and Southeast Asia
6.1 million

Caribbean
420,000

Latin America
1.4 million

Sub-Saharan Africa
28.1 million

Australia and New Zealand
15,000

Source: Joint United Nations Program on HIV/AIDS.

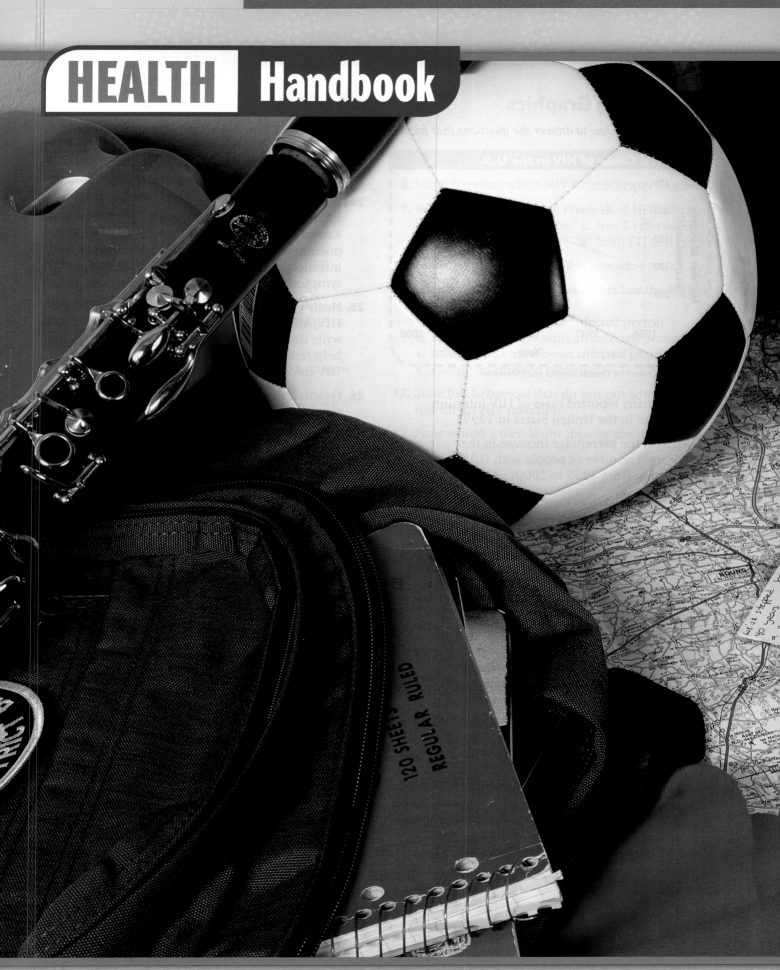

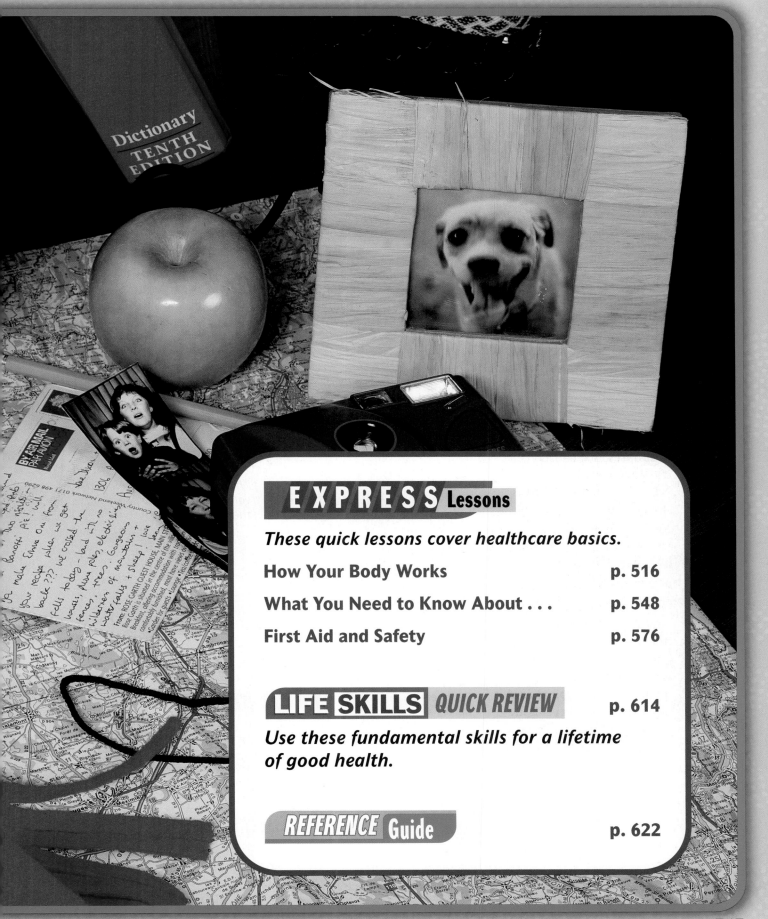

EXPRESS Lessons

These quick lessons cover healthcare basics.

Use these fundamental skills for a lifetime of good health.

Nervous System

The nervous system is your body's control center and communications network.

What does the nervous system do?

The nervous system works with the endocrine system to control how your body works and to help your body respond to changes in its surroundings. Messages picked up from inside and outside of the body cause the nervous system to create signals. These signals coordinate the body's thoughts, senses, movements, balance, and many automatic responses. Specialized cells, called **neurons,** receive and send the signals. Neurons form all the tissues of the nervous system.

What are the parts of the nervous system?

The brain, the spinal cord, and many nerves make up the nervous system. **Nerves** are bundles of tissue that carry signals from one place to another. The **spinal cord** is the column of nerve tissue that runs through the backbone. The nervous system is divided into two main parts.

The brain and spinal cord make up the **central nervous system (CNS).** The nerves that connect the brain and spinal cord to other parts of the body make up the **peripheral nervous system (PNS).**

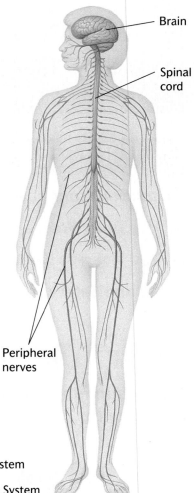

Brain

Spinal cord

Peripheral nerves

■ Central Nervous System

■ Peripheral Nervous System

How do the parts of the nervous system work together?

Some nerves of the PNS gather messages from inside and outside the body and carry signals to the CNS. The CNS interprets the incoming signals. If a response is needed, the CNS sends signals back to the muscles and the organs of the body through other nerves of the PNS. The signals from the CNS cause a response.

The nervous system enables these volleyball players to coordinate their movements.

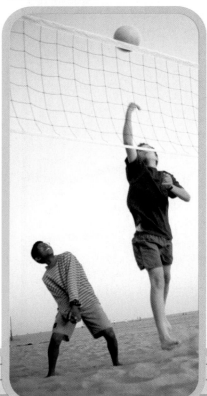

What do neurons look like?

A neuron has three parts. The central part of a neuron is the *cell body*. Branches from the cell body, called *dendrites*, receive signals. A long extension of the cell body, called an *axon*, carries signals to the next cell. One nerve cell meets another at a synapse. A **synapse** is a tiny space across which nerve impulses pass from one neuron to the next. The ends of axons release chemicals called **neurotransmitters** which move across the *synaptic cleft* and bind to receptors on the surface of the next cell. When the chemicals bind, they pass a signal on to the next cell.

How does the nervous system work?

Sensory receptors detect messages for the nervous system and create signals. Examples of these receptors are the taste buds and the receptors for touch, smell, temperature, and light. **Sensory nerves** are nerves that carry the signals from the sense organs toward the CNS, where they are processed or relayed. **Motor nerves** are nerves that carry signals from the brain or the spinal cord to the muscles and glands. These nerves cause the body to respond.

The nervous system responds in two basic ways. Some of the responses by the nervous system are voluntary, which means that you can make them happen. These responses include moving your arms and legs to walk or run and turning your head to look in a particular direction. Other responses are involuntary, or automatic. They happen whether you think about them or not. For example, shivering when you're cold and pulling your hand away from a very hot object are involuntary responses. Reflexes and the control of internal body organs are involuntary.

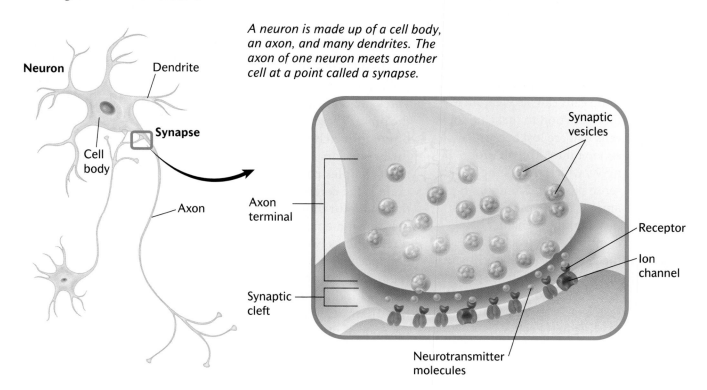

A neuron is made up of a cell body, an axon, and many dendrites. The axon of one neuron meets another cell at a point called a synapse.

Neuron

Dendrite

Synapse

Cell body

Axon

Axon terminal

Synaptic cleft

Synaptic vesicles

Receptor

Ion channel

Neurotransmitter molecules

Nervous System *continued*

Do nerves grow back after an injury?

Doctors once thought that injured nerves could not heal or be repaired. But recent studies now show that some nerve tissue can be repaired or can heal to some degree. Sensory and motor nerves can heal completely, but the process is very slow. Spinal nerves have also shown the ability to grow, but they generally do not grow well enough to repair significant damage. This is why spinal cord injuries and the resulting paralysis are often permanent.

Researchers are studying the nature of the spinal cord and spinal nerves to determine why they do not heal. Nerves of the brain can heal somewhat. Some types of brain cells can also rearrange their function to make up for cells that are lost because of severe injury. The olfactory nerve, which creates the sense of smell, is unique among all nerves. It is able to heal rapidly, even after being completely severed. The mechanism for this healing is not yet known. Intense study is underway to unlock the secret and pass this ability on to other nerve cells.

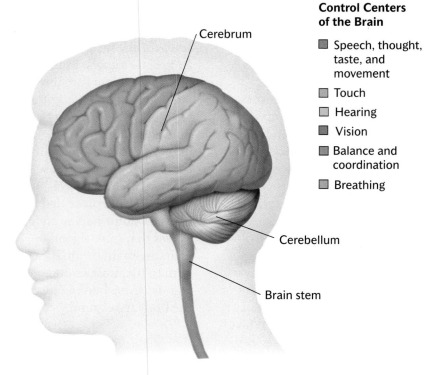

Cerebrum

Control Centers of the Brain

- Speech, thought, taste, and movement
- Touch
- Hearing
- Vision
- Balance and coordination
- Breathing

Cerebellum

Brain stem

What do the parts of the brain do?

The **brain** is the main control center for the body. Three major areas make up the brain. These are the cerebrum, the cerebellum, and the brain stem. The largest, most complex part of the brain is the **cerebrum.** It is the center for thought, imagination, and emotions. The cerebrum has two halves, or *hemispheres*. Each half has four lobes that act as control centers for different activities. These activities include the control of movement and the processing of signals that create vision, hearing, taste, and touch.

The **cerebellum** is the part of the brain that controls balance and posture. It also smooths out movement that requires fine coordination.

The **brain stem** is the part of the brian that guides signals coming from the spinal cord to other parts of the brain. There are three parts to the brain stem. The *pons* is the wider area just below the cerebrum. The *midbrain* is above the pons. Below the pons, the brain stem narrows into the *medulla oblongata*. The medulla oblongata helps control many automatic actions such as heartbeat, breathing, digestion, swallowing, vomiting, sneezing, and coughing.

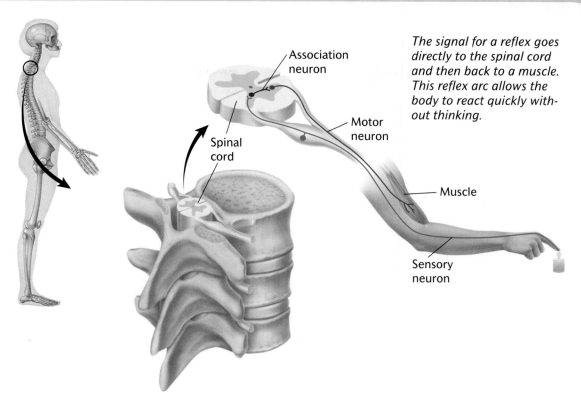

Association neuron

Spinal cord

Motor neuron

Muscle

Sensory neuron

The signal for a reflex goes directly to the spinal cord and then back to a muscle. This reflex arc allows the body to react quickly without thinking.

How does the brain send messages to the body?

The spinal cord is the major line of communication between the brain and the body. It is a cylinder of nerve tissue about 18 in. long and about as thick as your index finger. The bones of the spine, the spinal fluid, and three layers of tissue surround and protect the spinal cord. **Spinal nerves** are nerves that branch from the spinal cord and that go to the brain and to the tissues of the body. Unfortunately, despite all its protection, the spinal cord is still delicate and subject to injury.

How do reflexes work?

A **reflex** is an involuntary response that enables the body to react immediately to a stimulus, such as a possible injury. Some reflexes involve the brain, but many do not. Many reflexes, such as the reaction to intense pain, result from signals that travel to the spinal cord through one or more sensory nerves. The signals move to association neurons in the spinal cord and then to a motor nerve. The motor nerve returns a signal that causes you to pull away from the source of the pain.

EXPRESS Lesson REVIEW

1. Summarize the functions of the central nervous system and the peripheral nervous system.
2. Explain how the signals carried by nerves pass from one neuron to the next.
3. Describe the functions of the cerebrum, the cerebellum, and the brain stem.
4. **CRITICAL THINKING** If all nerves could be made to heal rapidly, what groups of people might benefit?

Vision and Hearing

Your vision and hearing enable you to sense the world around you.

How do we see?

Your eyes and brain enable you to see. The **eye** is the sense organ that gathers and focuses light and that generates signals that are sent to the brain. Light that enters the eye falls on the retina. The **retina** is the light-sensitive inner layer of the eye. Two basic types of cells that respond to light—rods and cones—are found in the retina. *Rods*, which produce black-and-white vision, receive dim light and detect shape and motion. *Cones*, which produce color vision, receive bright light and sharpen your vision.

Rods and cones respond to light by creating nerve signals. These signals leave the eye by the *optic nerve*, which extends from the back of the eye to the area of the brain that processes sight. Your brain interprets the nerve signals created in response to light, which enables you to see the object the light came from.

What is the blind spot?

The *blind spot* is the place where the optic nerve meets the retina. There are no photoreceptors in this area of the retina. So, any image that forms on the blind spot cannot be seen.

Do you see only in black and white if you are colorblind?

No, people who are colorblind see some colors. Three different types of cones collect three basic colors of light—red, green, and blue. A person who is colorblind has a deficiency, but not a total lack, of cones that detect one or more of these basic colors of light.

How does the eye focus?

Light rays enter the eye through the *lens*, which changes shape to focus the light on the retina. It is interesting to note that images form upside down on the retina. The brain corrects the images, and thus we see things right side up.

What happens when you're nearsighted?

If you are nearsighted, your eyes are elongated from front to back. This causes distant objects to focus in front of the retina rather than on it. As a result, distant objects look fuzzy. Images of nearby objects are still in focus on the retina. This condition is called *myopia*.

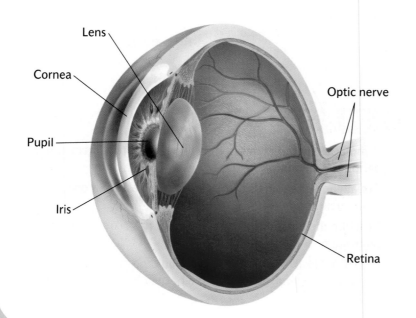

Lens
Cornea
Pupil
Iris
Optic nerve
Retina

How do we hear?

Your ears and your brain enable you to hear. The **ear** is the sense organ that functions in hearing and balance. The *outer ear* gathers in vibrations that cause sound and directs them to the eardrum. The **eardrum** is a membrane that transmits sound waves from the outer ear to the middle ear. Sound vibrations cause the eardrum to vibrate. The *middle ear* has three tiny bones—the hammer, the anvil, and the stirrup—that transmit vibrations from the eardrum to the inner ear. The bones also increase the force of vibrations.

The *inner ear* contains the fluid-filled semicircular canals and the cochlea. The **cochlea** is a coiled, fluid-filled tube. Tiny hairs in the cochlea are the receptors for sound. Signals created by the receptors go through the *auditory nerve* from the cochlea to the temporal lobe of the brain. There, the brain interprets the signals as different sounds.

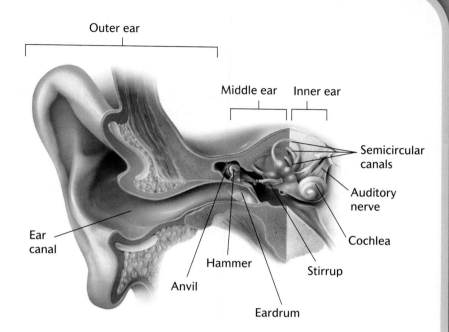

Outer ear

Middle ear   Inner ear

Semicircular canals

Auditory nerve

Ear canal

Cochlea

Hammer

Stirrup

Anvil

Eardrum

What part of the ear controls balance?

Movement of the sensory receptors in the inner ear controls balance. Some of the receptors detect gravity and changes in speed. Receptors in the semicircular canals detect rotational motions, such as spinning.

Why do ears pop in an airplane?

A tube called the **eustachian tube** connects the middle ear to the throat. The eustachian tubes maintain equal air pressure on both sides of your eardrums. Air pressure is much lower at high altitudes, where airplanes fly. You do not usually notice any changes in air pressure as you slowly gain altitude. But when you experience a rapid change from high altitude to low altitude, the air pressure on your eardrums increases suddenly. This causes the eardrums to be pushed inward, impairing your hearing temporarily. When the pressure on both sides of an eardrum is equalized, the eardrum moves back to its normal position. As a result, you hear a popping sound, and normal hearing is restored.

EXPRESS Lesson REVIEW

1. List and describe the two basic types of light receptors in the retina of the eye.
2. Explain what causes a person to be nearsighted.
3. List in order the series of structures through which sound vibrations pass in the ear.
4. **LIFE SKILL** **Practicing Wellness** Research several causes of deafness. What can a hearing person do to protect himself or herself from hearing loss?

Male Reproductive System

The male reproductive system makes male reproductive cells and hormones that cause male characteristics to appear.

What does the male reproductive system do?

The male reproductive system makes sperm and delivers them to the female reproductive system. **Sperm** are the sex cells that are made by males and that are needed to fertilize an egg.

Where are sperm made?

Sperm are made in **testes (testicles),** the male reproductive organs that also make testosterone. Inside the testes, there are tightly coiled tubes called *seminiferous tubules*, which make sperm. About 100 million sperm are made each day! The testes must be kept cooler than normal body temperature. Sperm made at high temperatures are defective and cannot fertilize eggs. The testes, therefore, are not inside the body cavity but outside of it. Testes are found in a skin-covered sac called the **scrotum.** The scrotum contracts and relaxes to make the testes move closer to or farther from the body. When the testes are away from the body, sperm stay cooler.

What do sperm look like?

Sperm are the smallest cells in the human body. Each mature sperm is made up of three basic parts: a head, a midpiece, and a tail. The head contains substances that help the sperm enter an egg. The head also holds half the genetic information required to start a new life. The midpiece of the sperm contains structures that make the energy needed for the long trip through the female reproductive system. The tail is made of proteins that help the sperm move.

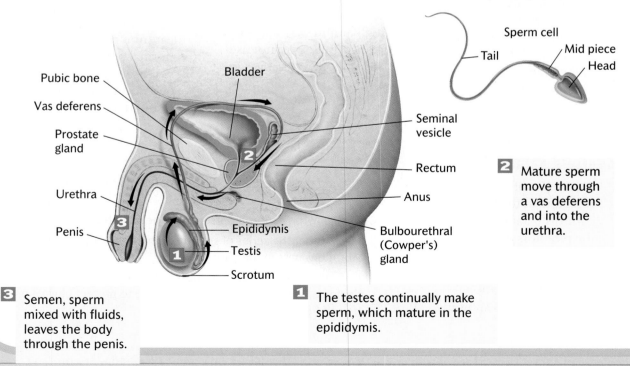

Sperm cell
Tail
Mid piece
Head

Pubic bone
Vas deferens
Prostate gland
Urethra
Penis
Bladder
Seminal vesicle
Rectum
Anus
Bulbourethral (Cowper's) gland
Epididymis
Testis
Scrotum

2 Mature sperm move through a vas deferens and into the urethra.

3 Semen, sperm mixed with fluids, leaves the body through the penis.

1 The testes continually make sperm, which mature in the epididymis.

What happens to sperm once they are made?

Once sperm are made, they move into a coiled tube called the *epididymis*. Here, immature sperm take 2 to 10 days to fully mature. The mature sperm then travel into another tube, called the *vas deferens*. The sperm are stored here until they leave the body or are reabsorbed.

How do sperm survive the long travel?

As sperm move through the body, several organs add fluids to the sperm. These organs are the *seminal vesicles*, the *bulbourethral glands* (Cowper's glands), and the prostate gland. The **prostate gland** is a gland in males that adds fluids that nourish and protect sperm when the sperm are in the female body. Sperm and the added fluids make up *semen*.

How do sperm leave the body?

Sperm leave the body during ejaculation via the *urethra*, a tube that passes through the penis. The **penis** is the organ that removes urine from the male body and that can deliver sperm to the female reproductive system. A flap in the urethra prevents urine and semen from going through the penis at the same time.

What does testosterone do?

Testosterone is the male hormone made by the testes. It causes many of the changes that happen when males reach *puberty*, or sexual maturity. For example, the shoulders get wider, the muscles get larger, hair grows on the face and other parts of the body, and the voice deepens. At this time, testosterone also causes the body to start making sperm.

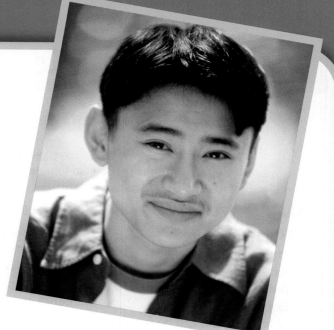

The male hormone testosterone causes masculine characteristics (such as a mustache) to appear.

EXPRESS Lesson REVIEW

1. Identify the locations where sperm are made and where they mature.

2. List the three main parts of a sperm.

3. List the components of semen.

4. **LIFE SKILL** **Practicing Wellness** Prostate cancer is one of the leading causes of cancer in men. Read more about the prostate gland. What are other problems that can affect the prostate?

EXPRESS Lesson

Female Reproductive System

The female reproductive system makes female reproductive cells and hormones that cause female characteristics to appear.

What does the female reproductive system do?

The female reproductive system makes eggs and gives them a place to develop. **Eggs,** or *ova*, are the sex cells of females and can be fertilized by sperm. When an egg and a sperm join, a new life begins. Organs of the female reproductive system nurture and protect developing humans. Parts of the system also make female hormones, which cause young girls to develop breasts and other features of women. The female hormones also help eggs to mature and prepare the body for pregnancy.

Where are eggs made?

Eggs are made in ovaries. The **ovaries** are the female reproductive organs that produce eggs and the hormones estrogen and progesterone. Girls already have all their eggs at birth. On average, there are about two million! But the eggs are immature. The eggs begin to mature when a girl reaches *puberty*. One egg matures about every 28 days. The process by which the ovaries release mature eggs is called **ovulation.**

Where are eggs fertilized?

Eggs are fertilized in the fallopian tubes. A **fallopian tube** is a female reproductive organ that connects an ovary to the uterus. After a mature egg is released, it moves into one of the fallopian tubes. The ends of these tubes do not really touch the ovaries. Tiny hairs around the opening of a fallopian tube draw an egg into the tube. If there are sperm in the tubes, a sperm may fuse with the egg and fertilize it.

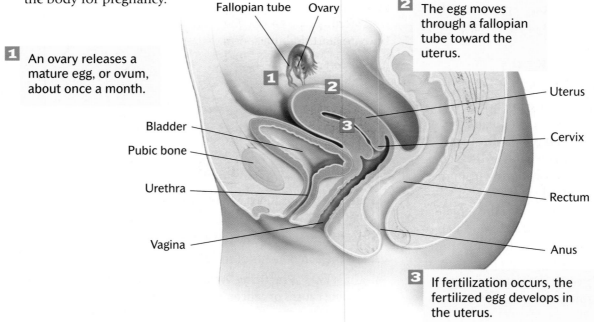

1 An ovary releases a mature egg, or ovum, about once a month.

2 The egg moves through a fallopian tube toward the uterus.

Fallopian tube   Ovary

Uterus

Bladder

Cervix

Pubic bone

Urethra

Rectum

Vagina

Anus

3 If fertilization occurs, the fertilized egg develops in the uterus.

Where do fertilized eggs develop?

Fertilized eggs develop in the **uterus,** which is a muscular organ about the size of a fist. The **cervix** is the narrow base of the uterus. As an egg matures, the lining of the uterus, or the **endometrium,** thickens. Many tiny blood vessels feed this lining. These blood vessels will bring food and oxygen to a growing baby and will carry away its wastes. This exchange happens via the **placenta,** a blood vessel–rich tissue that forms in a mother's uterus.

When a baby is ready to be born, the cervix expands to allow the baby to pass into the vagina. The **vagina** is the reproductive organ that connects the uterus to the outside of the body.

What happens if an egg isn't fertilized?

If an egg is not fertilized, the blood vessels in the endometrium break down. Blood and tissue that built up in the uterus flow out of the body through the vagina in a process called **menstruation.**

What happens during the menstrual cycle?

The **menstrual cycle** is a monthly series of hormone-controlled changes that mature an egg and prepare the uterus for pregnancy.

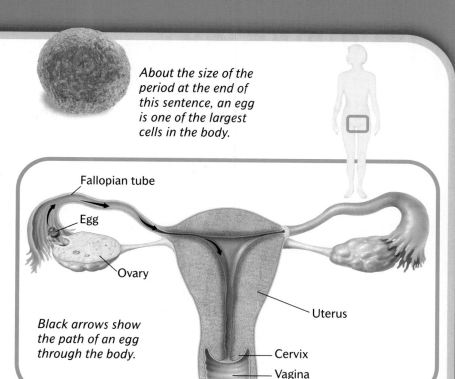

About the size of the period at the end of this sentence, an egg is one of the largest cells in the body.

Fallopian tube

Egg

Ovary

Black arrows show the path of an egg through the body.

Uterus

Cervix

Vagina

Days 1–5 Menstruation begins. Blood and the lining of the uterus (the menstrual fluid) flow out of the body.

Days 6–14 The hormone estrogen helps prepare the body for pregnancy. The hormones FSH and LH cause an egg to mature in an ovary. As the egg matures, the endometrium thickens. Ovulation occurs on about day 14.

Days 15–28 The hormone progesterone helps maintain the lining of the uterus as the uterus waits for a fertilized egg. Hormone levels remain fairly steady for several days. If a fertilized egg has not attached to the wall of the uterus by about day 28, hormone changes cause the blood vessels in the uterine lining to break down.

EXPRESS Lesson REVIEW

1. List the functions of the female reproductive system.
2. Describe the pathway an egg takes after it is released from an ovary.
3. Summarize the steps of the menstrual cycle.
4. **LIFE SKILL** **Evaluating Media Messages** Some products claim to be able to treat premenstrual syndrome (PMS). After reading more about PMS, discuss whether you think these drugs are likely to be effective.

EXPRESS Lesson

Skeletal System

Your skeletal system gives your body shape and support, provides protection for vital organs, and produces blood cells.

What does the skeletal system do?

The skeletal system gives your body the shape it has. Without bones, you would be a shapeless blob pooled on the floor. The **skeleton** is a framework of bones that support the muscles and organs and protect the inner organs. Bones also serve as points to which the muscles attach and create body movement. Inside some bones, there is a soft tissue that makes new blood cells.

How do bones grow?

At birth, the skeletal system is soft and made mostly of *cartilage*. As a child grows, bone tissue begins to replace the cartilage. At the end of long bones is a band of cartilage called the *epiphysis*, or growth plate. Cartilage that will be replaced by bone tissue grows here. When a person reaches full height, the cartilage stops growing. At this point, bone tissue has completely replaced the cartilage, except at the very tips of the bones in the joints.

What is the "soft spot" on a baby's head?

The bones of an infant's skull are not fully developed. Areas of soft cartilage called *fontanels* separate the bones. These "soft spots" allow the skull bones to move as a baby passes through the birth canal. After birth, the skull bones grow until the soft cartilage is completely replaced. The joints where the skull bones meet are called *sutures*. Some fontanels close up within two months after birth. But the one at the top of the head takes about a year to close completely.

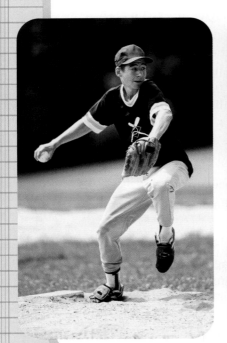
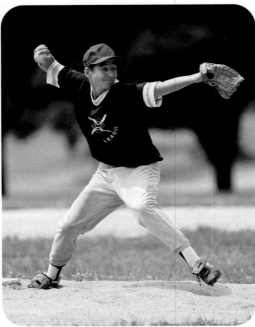

Understanding how the bones act as levers can help a baseball pitcher learn how to throw the ball faster and harder.

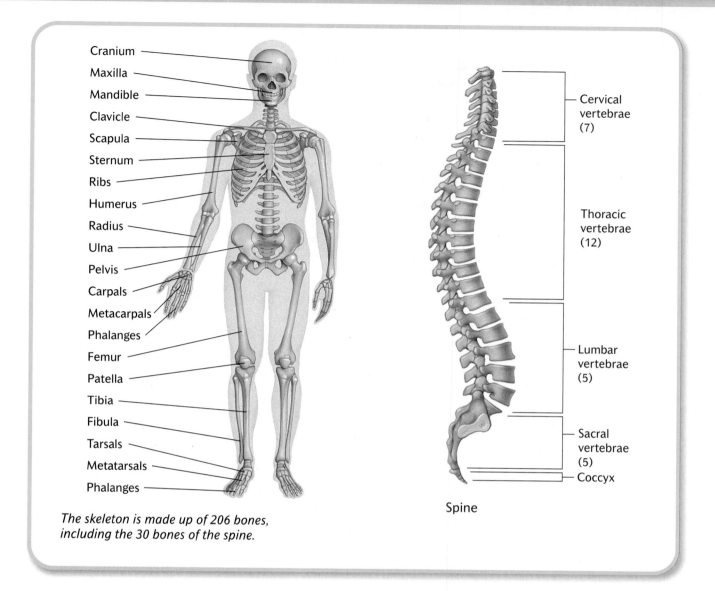

Cranium
Maxilla
Mandible
Clavicle
Scapula
Sternum
Ribs
Humerus
Radius
Ulna
Pelvis
Carpals
Metacarpals
Phalanges
Femur
Patella
Tibia
Fibula
Tarsals
Metatarsals
Phalanges

Cervical vertebrae (7)
Thoracic vertebrae (12)
Lumbar vertebrae (5)
Sacral vertebrae (5)
Coccyx

Spine

The skeleton is made up of 206 bones, including the 30 bones of the spine.

How many bones do we have?

Your skeleton has 206 bones and has two main parts. The *axial skeleton* is made up of the skull, the spinal column, the rib cage, and the sternum. These central bones work together to protect vital organs. The bones of the skull, for example, surround and protect the brain. The *appendicular skeleton* is made up of 126 bones. These bones form the frame to which the muscles are attached.

Are mature bones alive?

Bone is very much alive. Cells called *osteoblasts* form new bone continuously. This allows bones to heal when they are broken. Lumps of new bone may also form on parts of bones that are repeatedly stressed.

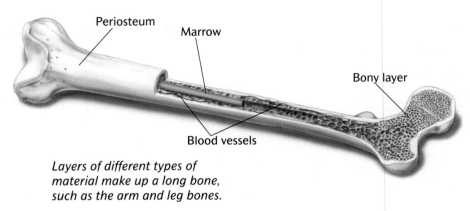

Periosteum

Marrow

Bony layer

Blood vessels

Layers of different types of material make up a long bone, such as the arm and leg bones.

How do broken bones heal?

The human femur (upper leg bone) is stronger than a bar of iron of the same weight. Even so, bones sometimes break. When a bone breaks, the outer layer tears, causing severe pain and some bleeding. Blood clots form inside the break and seal both sides. Next, white blood cells come and clean out fragments of broken bone and dead cells. Fibrous strands of cartilage begin to fill in the fracture and bridge the gap between the two sides. The final step in the healing process occurs when compact bone replaces the cartilage.

What are bones made of?

Bones generally have three layers. The top layer, called the *periosteum*, is a tough membrane that forms a smooth seal over the surface of a bone. This layer has many nerves and blood vessels that transport food and oxygen to the inner layers of the bone. The second layer, called the *bony layer*, consists of the white, hard substance that gives bones their great strength. The bony layer is not just a solid mass of calcium but is made up of many tiny cells that are surrounded by rings of calcium. At the center of many bones, there is a layer of soft tissue called **bone marrow.** The bone marrow is one of the key places that the body makes new blood cells.

How are bones held together?

Muscles, tendons, and ligaments hold bones together. Two or more bones meet at places in the body called **joints. Ligaments,** which are tough bands of tissue, hold the ends of bones together at joints. **Tendons** are cords of connective tissue that attach muscles to bones. Muscles and tendons attach to the bones on either side of a joint, holding the joint together tightly.

Is it bad to crack my knuckles?

No, the popping or cracking sound made by some joints is very normal. Pulling on a joint creates a vacuum inside the joint. This vacuum causes tiny air bubbles in the joint fluid to burst. The result is a "pop" or a "crack" that you can hear. Popping joints is not clearly linked to getting **arthritis,** a painful inflammation of the joints.

What keeps joints from scraping?

Joints that move contain a very slippery liquid called *synovial fluid.* The pads of cartilage that serve as shock absorbers at the ends of bones also help bones glide smoothly across each other.

Do all joints move?

No, some joints are fixed, such as the ones between the bones in the skull. A *fixed joint* does not allow any movement.

Other joints, such as the *semimovable joints* between the *vertebrae* in the spine, allow only a small amount of movement. Several different kinds of joints allow the body to move in different ways. The simplest is the *hinge joint*. This is the type found in your elbows and knees. There, bones attach to each other in such a way that the joint can bend only back and forth.

One more flexible type of joint is the *ball-and-socket joint*. This is the type of joint found in your hips and shoulders. On one bone, a knoblike piece, or ball, sticks out. On the other bone or set of bones, there is a cup that the ball fits into. The ball is free to rotate inside the cup in almost any direction. The first two vertebrae allow your head to rotate right and left. This is called a *pivot joint*. Pivot joints in the elbow enable the forearms to rotate back and forth, as well. The last type of joint allows movement in all ways except rotation. The wrists and ankles are of this type, called an *ellipsoidal joint*.

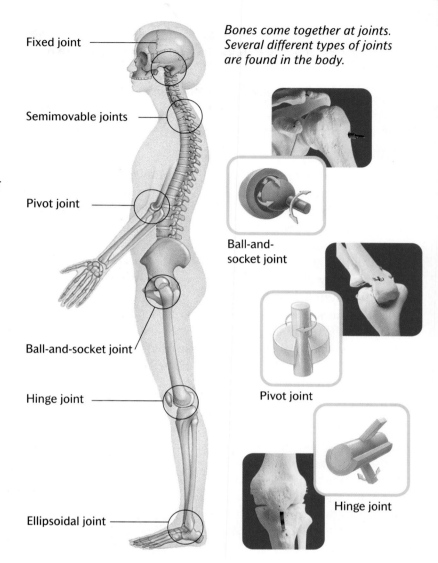

Fixed joint

Semimovable joints

Pivot joint

Ball-and-socket joint

Hinge joint

Ellipsoidal joint

Bones come together at joints. Several different types of joints are found in the body.

Ball-and-socket joint

Pivot joint

Hinge joint

EXPRESS Lesson REVIEW

1. Name the three layers found in most bones, and identify the function of each.
2. Describe how bones grow.
3. List three types of joints.
4. **LIFE SKILL** **Practicing Wellness** Your bones store calcium for your body. If you do not get enough calcium from your diet, calcium will be taken from your bones for use where it is needed. Research the roles of calcium in the body, the sources of calcium in your diet, and the consequences that may result for your skeletal system if you eat a diet that is deficient in calcium.

EXPRESS Lesson

Muscular System

Your muscular system moves all your moving parts.

What does the muscular system do?

The muscular system accounts for all of the ways that the parts of the body move. This includes actions such as running, eating, breathing, digesting food, and pumping blood. The muscular system also helps protect your joints and helps create the heat that keeps your body warm.

What are muscles made of?

Bundles of special cells called *fibers* make up the muscles. Muscle fibers have long strands of proteins that are able to contract. Paired strands of these proteins latch together like the two parts of an extension ladder. When muscle fibers contract, one half of each protein ladder moves up along the other half. This makes the protein ladders, and thus the whole muscle, shorten.

Are all muscles the same?

There are three types of muscle tissue in the body. *Skeletal muscle*, or striated (striped) muscle, is the type that you can move voluntarily. *Smooth muscle* causes the involuntary movements of the eyelids, internal organs, and blood vessels. *Cardiac muscle* is a special kind of involuntary, striated muscle found only in the walls of the heart.

How do muscles move the body?

Muscles move the body by pulling on bones that meet at joints. Muscles are connected to the bones by tendons. Muscles at a movable joint either pull the joint into a bent position or pull it straight. Muscles usually work in pairs, one on either side of the joint. When one contracts, the other relaxes.

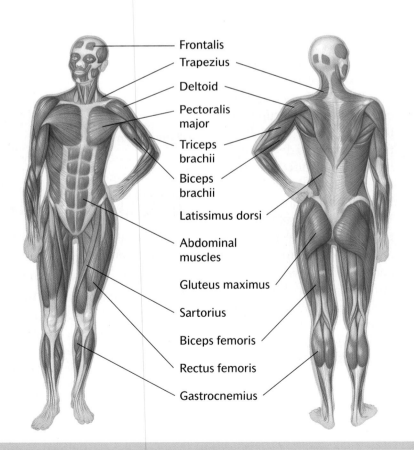

- Frontalis
- Trapezius
- Deltoid
- Pectoralis major
- Triceps brachii
- Biceps brachii
- Latissimus dorsi
- Abdominal muscles
- Gluteus maximus
- Sartorius
- Biceps femoris
- Rectus femoris
- Gastrocnemius

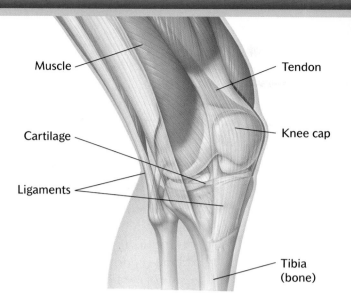

Muscle

Tendon

Cartilage

Knee cap

Ligaments

Tibia
(bone)

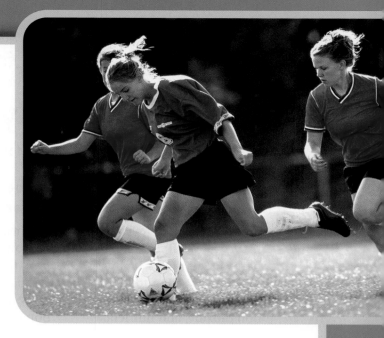

Muscles help hold bones together in joints such as the knee. Strong muscles help prevent knee injuries in soccer players and other athletes.

What causes muscles to get bigger when you exercise?

When you exercise a muscle by lifting something heavy, the muscle fibers in the muscle contract. Repeated strong contractions cause the muscle fibers and the muscle itself to grow in diameter and strength. In contrast, moderate contractions, such as those that result from walking, do not increase the diameter of a muscle as much. However, repeated moderate exercise greatly increases a muscle's endurance by enabling it to obtain more oxygen.

Why do muscles get tired?

Your muscles need oxygen in order to produce the energy needed for contracting. Muscles that are working very hard use up all the oxygen at hand. When this happens, less energy is available for creating contractions, which makes you feel weak or tired. But if you're running from a tiger, you can't quit just because your muscles run out of oxygen.

In order for muscles to keep working without oxygen, a process that makes the chemical *lactic acid* provides a small amount of energy. Unfortunately, lactic acid is poisonous to cells. Muscle cells need extra oxygen to get rid of lactic acid before they can make more energy. The extra oxygen needed to return conditions to normal is called an *oxygen debt*. Only time and rest can erase an oxygen debt.

EXPRESS Lesson REVIEW

1. Identify the components of muscle tissue.
2. Name the tissue that connects muscle to bone.
3. Explain how the process that causes muscle tiredness can be reversed.
4. **LIFE SKILL** **Practicing Wellness** In the past, people thought that they couldn't build muscle without going into an oxygen debt. Think about how muscles increase in size, and explain why this belief is not true.

Circulatory System

Your circulatory system is your body's internal transport system.

What does the circulatory system do?

The circulatory system moves blood all through the body. **Blood** is a tissue that is made up of cells and fluid and that carries oxygen, carbon dioxide, and nutrients in the body. Blood flows inside of tubes called **blood vessels.** The **heart** is the organ that pumps the blood through the body.

Is blood really red and blue?

Hemoglobin is the oxygen-carrying pigment in the blood. Hemoglobin is bright red when oxygen is attached to it. Blood is very dark red when the hemoglobin in it does not carry oxygen. Some veins are close enough to the surface of your skin to be seen. These veins appear to be blue because different colors of light reach different depths in the skin. Red light penetrates farther into the body than other colors of light. Blue light, however, does not go very far before being reflected back by the veins. This makes the veins look blue. Arteries are usually so deep that they cannot be seen.

How does the heart work?

The heart beats constantly without rest. With every beat, the heart pushes blood through the vessels of the body. Blood that carries carbon dioxide returns from the body and enters the right atrium of the heart.

An **atrium** is a chamber of the heart that receives blood from the body. The blood in the right atrium is pushed through an *A-V valve* (atrioventricular valve) into the right ventricle. A **ventricle** is one of the two large, muscular chambers that pump blood out of the heart. The right ventricle squeezes blood out of the heart and pushes it toward the lungs. There, carbon dioxide is exchanged for oxygen.

Oxygen-rich blood comes back to the heart at the left atrium. The blood in the left atrium is pushed through an A-V valve into the left ventricle. From there, blood is pushed out to all parts of the body.

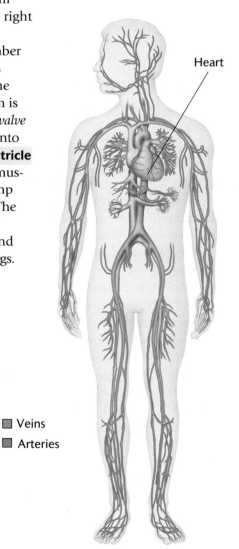

Heart

■ Veins
■ Arteries

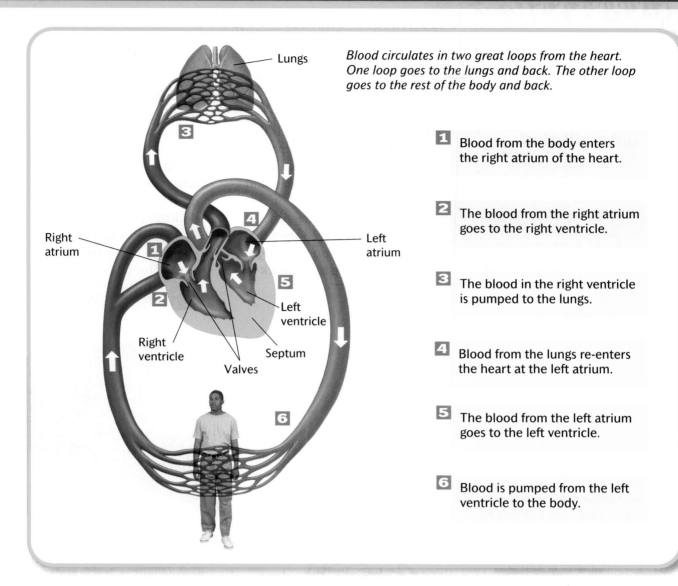

Lungs

Blood circulates in two great loops from the heart. One loop goes to the lungs and back. The other loop goes to the rest of the body and back.

Right atrium

Left atrium

Right ventricle

Left ventricle

Septum

Valves

1 Blood from the body enters the right atrium of the heart.

2 The blood from the right atrium goes to the right ventricle.

3 The blood in the right ventricle is pumped to the lungs.

4 Blood from the lungs re-enters the heart at the left atrium.

5 The blood from the left atrium goes to the left ventricle.

6 Blood is pumped from the left ventricle to the body.

What makes the heart beat?

The heartbeat is a rhythmic contraction of the heart. Signals that begin at the top of the heart cause the heartbeat. A group of cells at the top of the right atrium, called the **cardiac pacemaker,** starts a signal. This group of cells is also called the *S-A node* (sinoatrial node). First, the signal causes the atria to contract. Then, the signal goes down through the heart to another group of cells near the bottom of the septum between the two atria. This group of cells, the *A-V node* (atrioventricular node), passes the signal along to the ventricles. As a result, the ventricles contract a split second after the atria.

What causes the sound of a heartbeat?

As it beats, the heart makes two distinct sounds that are caused by the closing of the valves in the heart. The closing of the A-V valves makes the first sound, or S1. The closing of the valves that allow blood from the ventricles to enter the arteries that leave the heart makes the second sound, or S2.

EXPRESS Lesson

Respiratory System

Your respiratory system brings oxygen in and lets carbon dioxide out of the body.

What does the respiratory system do?

The respiratory system brings life-giving oxygen into the body. It also helps the body get rid of carbon dioxide, a waste product made by cells. The process of bringing in oxygen and getting rid of carbon dioxide is called *respiration*. The **lungs** are the main organs of gas exchange in the respiratory system.

What path does air take as it enters my body?

Air enters the body through the mouth and *nasal cavities*. The air is warmed and moistened so it does not dry out the delicate lung tissue. Air then flows into the *pharynx*, or *throat*. At the base of the pharynx is the *larynx*, or voice box, where the vocal cords are located. Attached to the voice box is the **trachea,** or windpipe, which carries air to the lungs. Rings of cartilage strengthen the trachea and protect it from injury and collapse.

The trachea branches into two tubes. Each tube, called a **bronchus,** sends air to a lung. In the lungs, the bronchi branch many times into smaller and smaller tubes. The smallest of these tubes is called a **bronchiole.** At the end of each bronchiole is a cluster of thin-walled air sacs. Each air sac, called an **alveolus,** is a site for gas exchange. Capillaries around each alveolus pick up oxygen and get rid of carbon dioxide.

How does oxygen get into my blood?

Oxygen molecules naturally move from the alveoli, where oxygen is more plentiful, into the capillaries, where there is less oxygen. Alveoli and the capillaries around them have very thin walls that gases easily move through. Red blood cells pick up the oxygen molecules and release carbon dioxide.

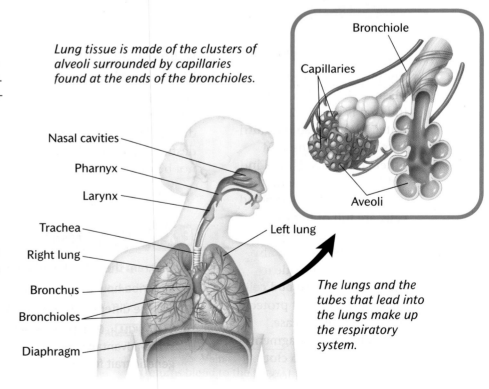

Lung tissue is made of the clusters of alveoli surrounded by capillaries found at the ends of the bronchioles.

Nasal cavities
Pharynx
Larynx
Trachea
Right lung
Bronchus
Bronchioles
Diaphragm

Left lung

Bronchiole
Capillaries
Aveoli

The lungs and the tubes that lead into the lungs make up the respiratory system.

What makes air flow into and out of my lungs?

Movement of the rib muscles and the diaphragm pull air into the lungs and push air out. The **diaphragm** is a sheet of muscle that separates the chest cavity, which holds the lungs and heart, from the abdominal cavity, which holds the digestive system. When you breathe in, the diaphragm contracts and moves downward. The rib muscles contract and pull the chest wall up and outward. This causes air to rush in and fill the lungs. When the diaphragm and rib muscles relax, the diaphragm bows upward and the chest cavity becomes smaller, forcing air back out of the lungs.

What controls how fast I breathe?

Breathing rate is controlled by centers in the brain stem that detect carbon dioxide in the blood. Because carbon dioxide is toxic to tissues, it must not build up in the blood. When the amount of carbon dioxide in the blood rises, the breathing center in the brain stem signals the diaphragm to contract more often. So, you breathe faster. The reverse happens when the amount of carbon dioxide in the blood drops.

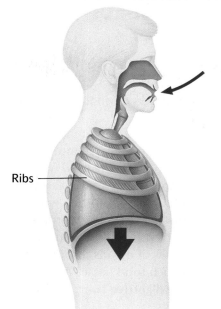

When you breathe in, your diaphragm moves down, and your chest cavity gets larger.

Ribs

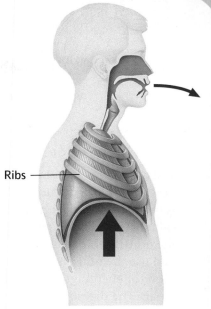

When you breathe out, your diaphragm moves up, and your chest cavity gets smaller.

Ribs

Why does the respiratory system make mucus?

Mucus is a thick, slimy fluid that coats the lining of organs and glands. Mucus lines the bronchi, trachea, and nasal passages. It serves two purposes. First, it adds moisture to the air entering the lungs. Second, it traps particles and bacteria that might otherwise clog the tiny bronchioles or cause infection in the lungs.

What causes hiccups?

Hiccups are tiny spasms of the diaphragm. We do not know for certain what causes the diaphragm to spasm. Irritation of the diaphragm is one possibility. Many studies have been done to try to find guaranteed cures for the hiccups.

EXPRESS Lesson REVIEW

1. Trace the path of air through the lungs.
2. Name the region of the airway that contains the voice box.
3. Identify the small tubes that attach to alveoli.
4. **LIFE SKILL** **Practicing Wellness** When you run, your body automatically starts breathing faster. What causes this increase in breathing rate?

Digestive System

Your digestive system breaks down food into the nutrients your body needs.

What does the digestive system do?

The digestive system breaks down food into the things it is made of. This process is called *digestion*. As a result, the body is able to absorb and use the nutrients in food for energy, growth, and repair. The digestive system also eliminates undigested food from the body.

How are teeth involved in digestion?

Teeth begin the process of digestion. They break food down into smaller pieces that can be swallowed. Teeth also help mix food with saliva, which has an enzyme that begins to break down starch. **Enzymes** are proteins or other types of molecules that help chemical processes happen in living things.

What path does food take in the body?

Food taken in by the mouth is chewed and swallowed. The food then moves down through the long, straight tube called the **esophagus** and into the stomach. From there, it passes through the small intestine.

Finally, food moves through the large intestine. From there, the food moves into the **rectum,** the last part of the large intestine where undigested waste is stored until it leaves the body. This series of organs through which food passes is called the **digestive tract.**

How does food move through the digestive tract?

Waves of rhythmic motion, called *peristalsis,* run through the walls of organs in the digestive tract. These waves gently push food through the digestive tract.

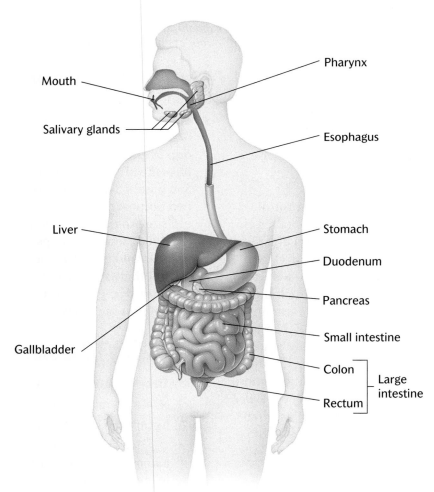

Mouth

Salivary glands

Pharynx

Esophagus

Liver

Stomach

Duodenum

Pancreas

Small intestine

Gallbladder

Colon

Rectum

Large intestine

What happens as food moves from the stomach to the colon?

In the *stomach,* a strong acid and powerful enzymes mix with the food. These chemicals kill bacteria that can be harmful and begin to break down proteins. A mixture of partly digested food and stomach enzymes, called *chyme,* results.

Digestion continues in the *small intestine,* which also absorbs nutrients from digested food. Secretions from the liver and pancreas finish breaking down carbohydrates, fats, and proteins. The lining of the small intestine has millions of tiny, fingerlike projections, called villi. Capillaries in the villi take up nutrients as the digested food works its way to the *large intestine.*

The major part of the large intestine is called the **colon.** There, bacteria that live on the undigested food make important vitamins, such as vitamins A, B_6, and K, for the body. The vitamins, along with water and minerals, are taken from undigested food before the waste is removed from the body.

What do the liver and pancreas do?

The liver and pancreas are important to digestion but are not part of the digestive tract. Chemicals secreted by the *liver* help with the digestion of fats in the small intestine. Your body also depends on the liver in other ways. The liver stores energy reserves, iron, and vitamins A, D, and B_{12}. The liver also takes chemical wastes and poisons from the blood and breaks them down. Enzymes secreted by the *pancreas* break down carbohydrates and proteins in the small intestine. The pancreas also produces *insulin,* which regulates blood-sugar levels.

Why doesn't stomach acid burn the stomach?

The acid in your stomach is strong enough to "dissolve" metal. Luckily, the lining of the stomach secretes a coat of mucus that protects the wall of the stomach.

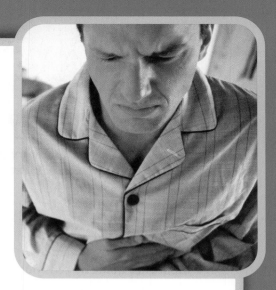

The uncomfortable feeling of heartburn results when stomach acid leaks into the esophagus.

Mucus is a thick, slimy fluid that coats the lining of organs and glands. Without a coat of mucus, the stomach would digest itself. Sometimes, stomach acid leaks into the esophagus, which does not have a protective lining of mucus. The result is *GERD* (gastroesophageal reflux disorder), or *acid reflux.* **Heartburn** is the pain that is caused by GERD and has nothing to do with the heart.

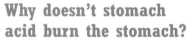

EXPRESS Lesson **REVIEW**

1. Name the process that moves food through the digestive tract.
2. List the major organs of the digestive tract, and describe what each organ does.
3. Describe the functions of the liver and the pancreas.
4. **LIFE SKILL** **Practicing Wellness** When a person has cirrhosis of the liver, the healthy liver tissue turns to scar tissue and stops working. Look up some of the problems that can arise if a person's liver is not working properly.

Excretory System

Your excretory system removes harmful wastes from your body and maintains the body's water and salt balance.

What does the excretory system do?

The excretory system takes the wastes made by cells out of the blood and moves the wastes out of the body. It also keeps up the body's proper salt content, water content, blood pressure, and acid-base balance. The **kidneys** are the main organs of the excretory system. They filter about 1,200 mL of blood per minute. The lungs and the skin are also part of the excretory system. Carbon dioxide is excreted by the lungs. Many substances are excreted by the skin through the *sweat glands*.

How do the kidneys work?

The kidneys filter all of your blood about 10 times every day. A kidney has millions of tiny blood filtering units called **nephrons.** Blood with wastes is brought to the kidneys by *renal arteries.* Each nephron takes water, salts, minerals, and cell wastes out of the blood. If wastes were released from your body at this stage, you would lose too much water.

Before wastes leave a kidney, capillaries in the kidney reclaim about 99 percent of the water removed by the nephrons. The concentrated liquid waste that leaves the kidney is called **urine.** *Renal veins* carry filtered blood back to the heart.

What is the urinary tract?

The *urinary tract* is the path taken by urine as it exits the body. A tube called a *ureter* takes urine from each kidney to the urinary bladder. The **urinary bladder** is the hollow, muscular sac that stores urine until there is enough to release. Another tube, called the *urethra,* leads from the urinary bladder to the outside of the body.

Lungs
The lungs excrete carbon dioxide and water vapor in exhaled air.

Kidneys
The kidneys excrete nitrogen wastes, salts, water, and other substances in urine.

Skin
The skin excretes water, salts, small amounts of nitrogen wastes, and other substances in sweat.

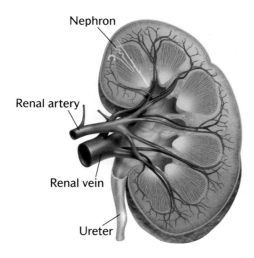

Nephron

Renal artery

Renal vein

Ureter

Inside the kidney, filtering units called nephrons *filter wastes from the blood.*

Drinking several glasses of water daily replaces the water lost as the kidneys, skin, and lungs do their work. Not drinking enough water can lead to dehydration and the buildup of toxins in the body.

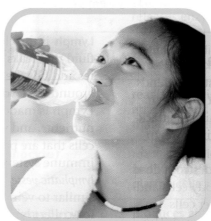

What is urine made of?

Urine is mostly water mixed with things your body needs to get rid of. These things include minerals such as sodium, calcium, and potassium and cellular wastes such as ammonia, urea, and uric acid. Urine may also contain bacteria that have been killed by the immune system and dead blood cells that must be removed.

How much urine can the bladder hold?

On average, the bladder can hold about 600 mL of urine. You feel the need to urinate at about 200–300 mL. At 600 mL, holding the urine becomes painful. With more than 1,000 mL, the bladder may become dangerously swollen.

How does the body control urination?

Two circular muscles control the flow of urine out of the bladder. Adults have voluntary control of these muscles and can hold or release urine at will. Stretching of the bladder triggers a reflex that gives you the urge to urinate. Stress and illness can interfere with the voluntary control of urination. Loss of voluntary control of urination is called **incontinence.**

What can happen if you are unable to urinate?

If a person is unable to urinate, for example because of spinal cord injury, his or her bladder can become too stretched to hold its shape. If the bladder is emptied too suddenly, there is a risk that it will collapse. If the bladder is not emptied, stress on the body can raise the person's blood pressure. If the problem is not resolved, this condition can lead to a *stroke.*

EXPRESS Lesson REVIEW

1. Name the structures that filter blood in the kidneys.
2. List the parts of the urinary tract.
3. Describe how urine is made in the kidneys.
4. **LIFE SKILL** **Setting Goals** Drinking plenty of water can help you keep your urinary tract healthy. Make a chart to monitor your water-drinking habits. Set a goal to drink six to eight glasses of water a day, and evaluate your progress.

Immune System continued

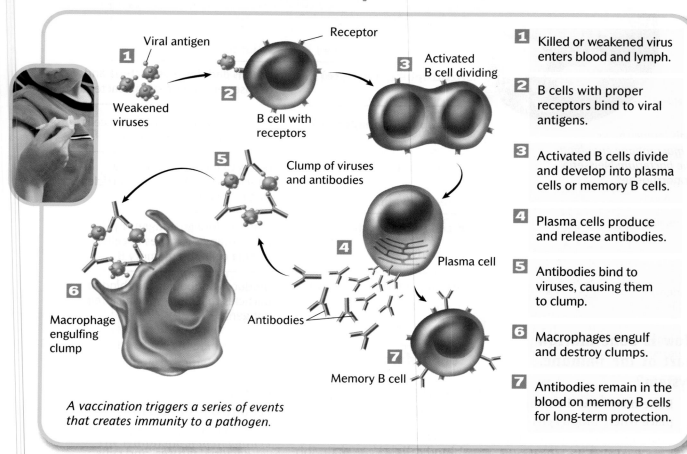

1 Viral antigen

Weakened viruses

Receptor

2 B cell with receptors

3 Activated B cell dividing

5 Clump of viruses and antibodies

4 Plasma cell

6 Macrophage engulfing clump

Antibodies

7 Memory B cell

1 Killed or weakened virus enters blood and lymph.

2 B cells with proper receptors bind to viral antigens.

3 Activated B cells divide and develop into plasma cells or memory B cells.

4 Plasma cells produce and release antibodies.

5 Antibodies bind to viruses, causing them to clump.

6 Macrophages engulf and destroy clumps.

7 Antibodies remain in the blood on memory B cells for long-term protection.

A vaccination triggers a series of events that creates immunity to a pathogen.

How do antibodies fight disease?

Antibodies are proteins the immune system makes in response to specific antigens. White blood cells that are exposed to a bacterium or to a virus make antibodies that can attach only to that bacterium or virus. In this way, antibodies stop bacteria and viruses from invading body cells and keep them in the bloodstream. This process gives white blood cells time to locate and destroy these disease-causing agents.

Can the immune system work against you?

Yes, your immune system will attack a transplanted organ if it carries antigens that differ from your own.

An **autoimmune disease** is one in which the immune system attacks the cells of the body that the immune system normally protects.

EXPRESS Lesson REVIEW

1. Describe three body parts that help the immune system.
2. List the types of white blood cells.
3. Explain how the immune system identifies invaders.
4. **LIFE SKILL** **Practicing Wellness** Does your immune system respond to stress? Keep a calendar and a journal. Write in advance all the tests, reports, projects, and extracurricular activities that you have coming up for a month. In your journal, keep track of how you feel each day. Are there any patterns?

Endocrine System

Your endocrine system regulates your growth, development, and body chemistry.

What does the endocrine system do?

The endocrine system works with the nervous system to coordinate and regulate the body. Hormones do the work of the endocrine system. **Hormones** are chemicals that are made and released in one part of the body and cause a change in another part of the body. Organs that release hormones are called **endocrine glands.**

How is the endocrine system different from the nervous system?

The nervous system reacts instantly to a stimulus but has a short-lived effect. The endocrine system responds more slowly and has a longer-lasting effect. Both nerves and chemical messengers carry signals in the nervous system. These signals affect only certain parts of the body. But only hormones carry signals for the endocrine system. The chemical messengers in the nervous system work only at the gaps between nerve cells. Carried by blood, hormones can spread all over the body and can affect many organs.

How do hormones work?

Hormones work by binding to receptors either outside or inside a cell. Each kind of hormone molecule has a shape that fits only certain receptors. Each organ has cells with receptors for certain kinds of hormones. When a hormone binds to a receptor on a cell, the cell reacts. The result depends on the kind of hormone and the organ the cell is in.

What are the endocrine glands?

Several different endocrine glands are scattered about your body. They are the pituitary gland, the thyroid gland, parathyroid glands, adrenal glands, gonads, the pancreas, the thymus gland, and the pineal gland. The table on the next page shows the hormones and functions of each endocrine gland.

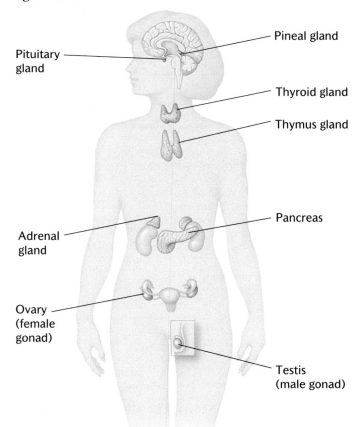

Pituitary gland

Pineal gland

Thyroid gland

Thymus gland

Adrenal gland

Pancreas

Ovary (female gonad)

Testis (male gonad)

Endocrine System *continued*

Glands of the Endocrine System

Gland	Hormone	Function
Pituitary (anterior)	human growth hormone (HGH) thyroid stimulating hormone (TSH) adrenocorticotropic hormone (ACTH) follicle stimulating hormone (FSH) luteinizing hormone (LH) prolactin	regulates growth directs thyroid gland directs adrenal glands directs reproductive organs directs reproductive organs stimulates production of breast milk
Pituitary (posterior)	antidiuretic hormone (ADH) oxytocin	regulates amount of water released by the kidneys stimulates uterine contractions and breast-milk flow
Thyroid	thyroxine	regulates metabolism, body-heat production, and bone growth
Adrenal (medulla)	epinephrine, norepinephrine	stimulate "fight-or-flight" response
Adrenal (cortex)	cortisol aldosterone	regulates carbohydrate and protein metabolism maintains salt and water balance
Pancreas	glucagon, insulin	regulate blood-sugar level
Parathyroid	parathyroid hormone (PTH)	regulates blood-calcium level
Thymus	thymosin	influences maturation of some immune system cells
Pineal	melatonin	controls internal clock and sleep rhythm
Gonads	estrogen, progesterone, testosterone	stimulate development of sex characteristics, affect egg and sperm formation, and control reproductive cycles

Do all diabetics have to take insulin?

No, usually only type 1 diabetics have to take insulin injections. Type 2 diabetics control their blood-sugar level with oral medications, diet, and exercise. Most diabetics have type 2 diabetes, which normally develops after the age of 40. Low blood sugar, or *hypoglycemia,* is also related to insulin and is more common in teens. A high-carbohydrate diet can stimulate the release of too much insulin, which causes the body to use blood sugar too quickly. Low blood sugar makes you feel weak and interferes with your ability to think.

Is it true that everyone has both male and female hormones?

We used to think that only men had male hormones and that only women had female hormones. Now we know that both men and women have both kinds of sex hormones but in different amounts. The male hormone *testosterone* governs the changes in boys as they mature. In women, the "male" hormone causes the normal growth of body hair. The female hormones *estrogen* and *progesterone* govern the changes in girls. In men, the "female" hormones help keep body fat at a safe level.

What determines how tall I am?

Nutrition and other environmental factors affect growth, but genes ultimately determine how tall you are. Genes act by causing the body to make hormones. *Human growth hormone* (*HGH*) is the main hormone that promotes growth in children. HGH is made by the pituitary gland. *Dwarfism* is an inherited trait that results from the underproduction of HGH. *Gigantism* is an inherited trait that results from the overproduction of HGH.

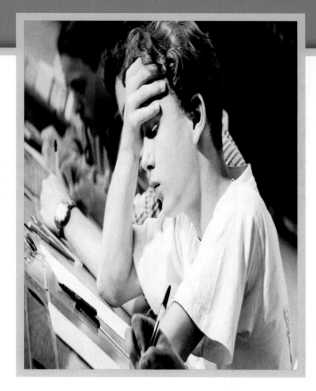

An event such as taking a test causes stress. Your body responds to this stress in the same way that it responds to fear.

What is the "fight-or-flight" response?

Your body responds to stressful situations by getting ready to either fight or run away to protect itself. This "fight-or-flight" response is directed in part by two hormones made by the adrenal glands. **Epinephrine** (EP uh NEF rin) is one of the hormones released by the body in times of stress. Epinephrine is also known as adrenaline. Norepinephrine is another hormone released in times of stress. These stress hormones raise your heart rate, blood pressure, and breathing rate and slow your digestion. As a result, more blood flows to your muscles, bringing them plenty of oxygen—just in case you have to run for your life!

EXPRESS Lesson REVIEW

1. Compare the endocrine system and the nervous system.
2. List three glands of the endocrine system.
3. Describe the way that hormones work.
4. **LIFE SKILL** **Evaluating Media Messages** A new trend in athletic training involves using human growth hormone (HGH) to increase muscle growth. After researching the topic, explain whether you think this is a safe practice.

Environment and Your Health

There was a big meeting tonight at Daniel's school. The community wanted to discuss what to do about the recent news that the water supply might be contaminated. What's the big deal, thought Daniel.

Why should I care about the environment?

The **environment** is the living and nonliving things that surround an organism. The environment includes plants, animals, air, water, and land. Your health and the health of your community is affected by your environment. If the environment in which you live is unhealthy, the chances increase that your health and the health of your community will suffer.

What makes an environment healthy?

A healthy environment is one in which the air is clean, the water is clear, and the land is fertile. It is one in which there is plenty of food for all the inhabitants. A healthy environment is free of pollutants and wastes that can make water, air, and land unsafe for living things. A healthy environment is a balanced environment.

Why are ecosystems important to our health?

An **ecosystem** is a community of living things and the nonliving parts of the community's environment. The living and nonliving parts of an ecosystem interact and depend on each other. If one part of an ecosystem is damaged, the whole ecosystem could become unhealthy. We depend on the ecosystem we live in to produce the resources we need to survive. We can be healthy only if our ecosystem is healthy.

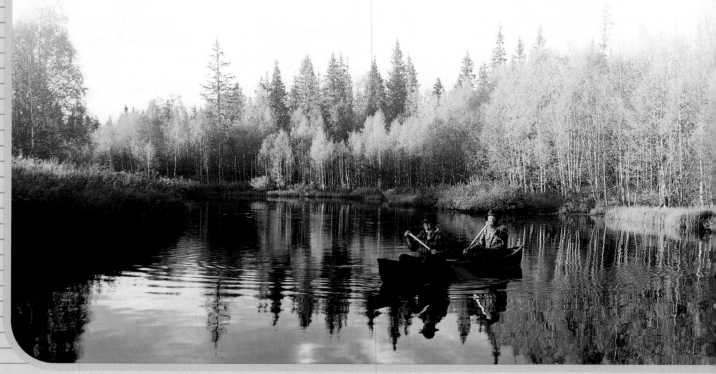

How can pollution be harmful?

Pollution can harm your ecosystem and thus, your health in several ways, as shown in the table. For example, many chemical pollutants such as smog can cause respiratory problems and eye irritation.

Gases produced by the burning of fossil fuels can react with water vapor in the air and produce acid rain. **Acid rain** is any precipitation that has a below-normal pH (acidic).

Chlorofluorocarbons (CFCs) are pollutants released by certain coolants and aerosol sprays. Chloro-fluorocarbons are another type of pollution that can harm your health. CFCs can increase your risk of skin cancer. CFCs move into the Earth's upper atmosphere and destroy ozone. *Ozone* is a gas in the upper atmosphere that reduces the amount of ultraviolet radiation from the sun. **Ultraviolet (UV) radiation** is radiation in sunlight that is responsible for tanning and burning skin. Excessive exposure to UV increases your risk of skin cancer and premature aging of the skin. The ozone is beneficial because it absorbs harmful UV radiation.

Pollution and Your Health

Pollutants	Effects on your health
Water pollutants	
Sewage	breeds pathogens that cause hepatitis, cholera, typhoid fever, and amebic dysentery
Pesticides	cause brain and nerve disorders, birth defects, and cancer
Fertilizers	cause damage to ecosystems and death of fish
Mercury and other metals	cause brain damage, mental retardation, nerve disorders, kidney disorders, paralysis, and loss of vision
Indoor and outdoor air pollutants	
Smog and other gases	cause or worsen respiratory illnesses such as asthma
Carbon monoxide	prevents red blood cells from carrying oxygen; causes weakness, loss of consciousness, or death
Cigarette smoke	causes lung cancer, asthma, emphysema, and sudden infant death syndrome (SIDS)
Radiation	causes sunburn, glaucoma, and cancer
Noise	causes hearing damage
Soil pollutants	
Acid rain	causes lower soil fertility, damages vegetation and buildings, and causes famine
Radon	causes cancer
Pesticides and herbicides	cause brain disorders and nerve disorders, birth defects, and cancer

What is conservation?

A *resource* is a material that can be used to meet a need. **Conservation** is the wise use and protection of natural resources. To protect our health and improve our environment, we need to conserve several specific resources in the environment.

▶ **Water** Fresh, clean water is needed for us to live; to keep clean; to grow, prepare, and process our food; and to make items we use.

▶ **Air** To live, we need certain gases that are in the air. For example, we need oxygen in order to get energy from our food. Carbon dioxide is used by plants to make food. Ozone, in the upper atmosphere, reduces the amount of UV radiation from the sun.

▶ **Minerals** We need minerals such as phosphorus, calcium, and sodium to carry out our bodies' activities. We get minerals from the plants and animals we eat and from our drinking water.

▶ **Food** Our bodies need energy in order to live. We get nutrients for energy from plants and animals.

▶ **Land** All living things need a certain amount of land in order to live. Land also provides a growing space for trees. Trees provide food for animals, shelter from the weather, and oxygen.

Why should we conserve natural resources?

Conserving our natural resources helps ensure that resources will be available in the future. A natural resource that can be replaced over a short period of time is called a **renewable resource.** Trees and crops are renewable resources.

Nonrenewable resources are natural resources that can be used up faster than they can be replenished naturally. Oil and natural gas are examples of nonrenewable resources.

Some renewable resources can also be used up too quickly to be replaced. Resources such as fresh water, topsoil, timber, and ocean fish must be conserved.

How does overpopulation affect our health and environment?

The point at which a population is too large to be supported by the available resources is called **overpopulation.** Earth's human population has been increasing rapidly. Overpopulation can lead to many problems.

Low food supplies Overpopulation makes it difficult to find and produce enough food to support the community. Famine is common in overpopulated areas.

Polluted water Polluted water from bathing, washing, and dumping wastes is a frequent result of overpopulation. Drinking, swimming, and bathing in polluted water spread disease.

Poverty, poor sanitation, and disease These problems are common in overpopulated parts of the world.

Overuse of the land and resources In order to feed, clothe, and shelter a growing population, we must use more natural resources. Nonrenewable resources can become depleted because of overuse, which results from supplying a large population.

Deforestation Many countries do not have enough farmland to feed their populations. Populations in tropical areas have little clear land for farming. **Deforestation** is the clearing of trees from natural forests to make space for crops or development. When crops are grown on soil from tropical forests, the nutrients in the soil are depleted quickly. More forest must be cleared for people to continue farming.

Overfishing Overpopulation can also lead to overfishing. Because oceans do not belong to any one country, regulating the amount of fishing in oceans is difficult. Our government places limits on the fishing industry in the United States to preserve species. However, not all countries do the same.

How does our government protect our environment?

One approach to protecting our environment has been to make pollution more expensive by placing a tax on it. The gasoline tax is a good example of such a tax. A second approach has been to pass laws. The United States has many laws aimed at protecting the environment.

▶ The Clean Air Act of 1970 limits the release of pollutants into the environment and sets safe levels of several air pollutants.

▶ The Clean Water Act of 1972 limits the release of sewage and chemicals into water in the United States.

The U.S. Environmental Protection Agency (EPA) is the agency that sets and enforces the standards established by these laws.

Who else protects the environment?

A number of local, national, and international organizations also work to protect the environment. Members of these organizations talk to lawmakers, raise money to help preserve land, and publish educational material to teach people about the importance of protecting the environment.

How can you help improve the environment?

▶ **Recycle or reuse products. Recycling** is reusing materials from used products to make new products.

▶ **Conserve electricity and water.** Take showers instead of baths, water lawns in the evenings to prevent evaporation, and fix leaky faucets.

▶ **Become involved in a local environmental issue.** Support recycling and conservation projects in your school. Join or start a group that keeps litter off school and neighborhood lawns.

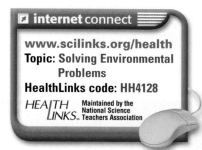

internet connect

www.scilinks.org/health
Topic: Solving Environmental Problems
HealthLinks code: HH4128

HEALTH LINKS Maintained by the National Science Teachers Association

EXPRESS Lesson REVIEW

1. What do living things need from their environment to live a healthy life?

2. How do pollution and overpopulation affect an ecosystem?

3. **CRITICAL THINKING** What are three ways you can help reduce each of the following: water pollution, air pollution, and soil pollution?

4. **LIFE SKILL** **Using Community Resources** Describe how you can plan a school or community effort to improve the environment around your school.

Public Health

Nurse García was concerned. Another patient came into the Emergency Room with nausea, vomiting, and diarrhea. It could be food poisoning, she thought. This patient was the seventh one in 2 days with these symptoms. She worried that this could be the beginning of an epidemic.

Why is public health important?

Public health is the practice of protecting and improving the health of people in a community. Because the people living in a community interact with one another, they affect each other's health and well-being.

The public health system is important in fighting infectious diseases and preventing other health problems, many of which are related to people's behaviors.

Infectious diseases can spread rapidly through a community and cause many people to become ill. This unexpected increase in illness is called an **outbreak.** The cause of an outbreak must be identified and treated quickly to keep the disease from becoming an epidemic. An **epidemic** is the occurrence of more cases of a disease than expected.

Noninfectious diseases are caused by genetic, environmental, or behavioral factors. Noninfectious diseases often affect a community because the people in the community have many behavioral and environmental factors in common. Noninfectious diseases are harder to eliminate because their treatment requires an improvement in the environment or a change in people's lifestyle.

Why do epidemics spread?

A **high-risk population** is any group of people who have an increased chance of getting a disease. Epidemics can spread quickly through certain high-risk populations.

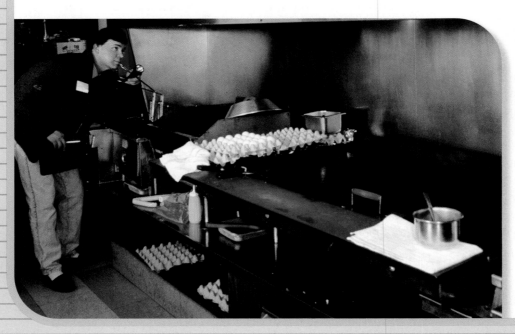

Restaurant inspections by public health workers help to ensure our food is safe.

Populations that have a high risk of developing an epidemic include the following:

▶ **Populations with poor sanitation** Sanitation is the practice of providing sewage disposal and treatment, solid waste disposal, clean drinking water, and clean living and working conditions. Bacteria breed in wastes and unsanitary water, which easily spreads disease.

▶ **Populations with poor nutrition** Poor nutrition makes it difficult for the body to fight disease.

▶ **Populations with low rates of immunization** Many diseases have been controlled through immunization. Unfortunately, there are many populations that do not have access to supplies for immunization.

▶ **Populations with overcrowding** Overcrowding is the condition in which there are too many inhabitants in an area to live healthily.

Public Health Agencies

Agency	Function
Centers for Disease Control and Prevention (CDC)	works with state health departments to monitor health trends, detect health problems, and control epidemics
Food and Drug Administration (FDA)	works to ensure that food and medicines are safe, healthy, and effective
National Institutes of Health (NIH)	directs and promotes research on prevention, diagnosis, and treatment of disease
Substance Abuse and Mental Health Services Administration (SAMHSA)	researches problems related to alcohol, drug abuse, and mental health issues
World Health Organization (WHO)	works to control AIDS worldwide, monitors emerging infections, such as Ebola and Hanta virus, and administers childhood immunizations in many countries
United Nations Children's Fund (UNICEF)	assists children with healthcare, nutrition, education, and sanitation

What public health concerns do we have in the United States?

Cardiovascular disease, cancer, stroke, and respiratory diseases are leading causes of death in the United States. These diseases threaten public health because the behaviors that can lead to them are common among many members of the community. These are **lifestyle diseases**—diseases that are caused partly by unhealthy behaviors and partly by other factors. Preventing infectious diseases is also a major concern.

What do public health agencies do?

Public health agencies at several levels of government help protect public health.

Local and state health departments These agencies protect the health of the community in many ways. They regulate community food and water supplies, help prevent infectious and lifestyle diseases, work to control epidemics, educate the public to improve personal and community health, and keep health statistics to watch for trends in illness or injury.

Public Health *(continued)*

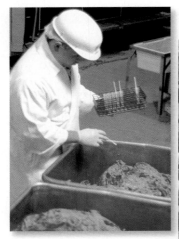

The Food and Drug Administration (FDA) works to ensure the food we eat is safe.

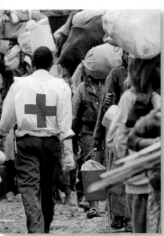

The Red Cross works to help those in need around the world.

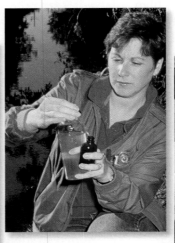

Government laws and regulations help prevent our water from being contaminated.

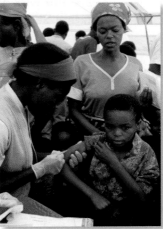

Health clinics offer immunizations to help keep children healthy and diseases under control.

National health agencies
These agencies set broad public health objectives; regulate food and drug production; fight epidemics; organize, fund, and conduct research to find cures for diseases; regulate healthy work practices; and sponsor programs that help people stay healthy.

International health agencies International health agencies such as the World Health Organization (WHO) work to fight global health problems. Some of the issues they address include poor nutrition, lack of basic medical care, poor sanitation, lack of clean water supplies, natural disasters, and disease.

How do private health organizations affect public health?

Private organizations also provide important public health support around the world. The International Red Cross, for example, provides food, clothing, temporary shelter, and medical care to people affected by wars, other acts of aggression, and natural disasters.

Many other private organizations work to solve public health problems. Usually, they focus on a specific group in the population or a specific disease. Private organizations depend on donations and volunteers to fund their work.

How do public health policies affect public health?

Public health policies are based on laws designed to protect citizens and promote the health of a community. Examples of these policies are as follows:

▶ **Laws and programs that promote mass immunization** All states have laws that require children to be immunized before they can attend public schools. These laws and programs have been very effective in eliminating diseases such as smallpox and polio and controlling other diseases such as measles and whooping cough.

Goals of Healthy People 2010

- ► Reduce the number of deaths from heart disease.
- ► Reduce the number of deaths from cancer.
- ► Reduce the number of deaths from AIDS.
- ► Reduce the percentage of overweight people.
- ► Increase the percentage of people who exercise regularly.

- ► Reduce the percentage of adolescents who smoke cigarettes.
- ► Reduce the number of children exposed to cigarette smoke.
- ► Reduce the number of women who smoke while pregnant.
- ► Reduce the number of deaths from car accidents.
- ► Reduce the number of deaths from drunk driving.

► **Waste disposal laws** Laws regulating waste disposal and dumping prevent an increase in rat, mice, and insect populations, which spread disease.

► **Standards for sanitation and health and safety practices** Safe standards for food preparation, seat belt use, and blood-alcohol concentrations are public health policies. The Occupational Safety and Health Administration (OSHA) is a federal agency that sets safety standards in the workplace.

► **Requirements for medical licensing** Doctors must have a license to practice medicine in the United States. Licensing ensures that doctors have the knowledge and training to provide medical treatment for a community.

What is Healthy People 2010?

Healthy People 2010 is a set of health objectives established by the U.S. Department of Health and Human Servies for improving the nation's health by 2010. These objectives are goals based on risk factors for diseases that are at least partly preventable.

Eliminating risk factors usually requires significant changes in personal habits, such as eating, smoking, and exercising. The benefits from making these changes are improvements in both personal and public health.

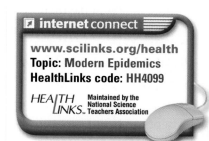

internet connect

www.scilinks.org/health
Topic: Modern Epidemics
HealthLinks code: HH4099

HEALTH
LINKS. Maintained by the National Science Teachers Association

EXPRESS Lesson REVIEW

1. What kinds of factors increase the risk of an epidemic spreading throughout a population?

2. Summarize the functions of local, state, and national public health agencies.

3. **LIFE SKILL** **Using Community Resources** You recently noticed that the water in your school has an unpleasant taste and smell. What could you do to start an investigation of the cause?

4. **LIFE SKILL** **Practicing Wellness** Name two behaviors you can change today to reach one or more of the Healthy People 2010 goals.

EXPRESS Lesson

Selecting Healthcare Services

After spending the weekend hiking with his friends, Isaac woke up Monday morning to find his legs covered with red, itchy bumps. His mom opened the phone book to look for a doctor and discovered three pages of listings for doctors. How could they choose which doctor to see?

How do I select a healthcare provider?

Selecting a healthcare provider usually begins with choosing a primary care physician. A **primary care physician (PCP)** is a family doctor who handles general medical care. This doctor is the first one you see when you have a health concern. If your parents plan to use insurance to pay for your visit, your doctor must be able to accept payment from your insurance company.

What kind of healthcare provider can I choose?

There are several different types of healthcare providers from which to choose:

▶ **Doctor of medicine (M.D.)** An M.D. is a physician who is trained in the diagnosis and treatment of disease.

▶ **Doctor of osteopathy (D.O.)** A D.O. is a doctor who has the same training as an M.D. but also specializes in the care of the muscular and skeletal system.

▶ **Physician's assistant (PA)** A PA carries out medical procedures under the supervision of a physician. In rural areas, physician's assistants have become very popular providers of healthcare.

▶ **Nurse practitioner (NP)** An NP is a registered nurse who has additional training and expertise in certain medical practices.

Depending on your needs, you and your parents may choose any of these kinds of medical professionals.

What is a specialist?

If your primary care physician encounters a complex or serious condition or a condition that he or she cannot identify or treat, he or she will send you to a specialist for an accurate diagnosis. A *specialist* is a doctor who studies and becomes an expert in one specific area of medicine. A specialist will have extensive knowledge of a certain body part or illness. The process of sending a patient from one healthcare provider to another is called a *referral*.

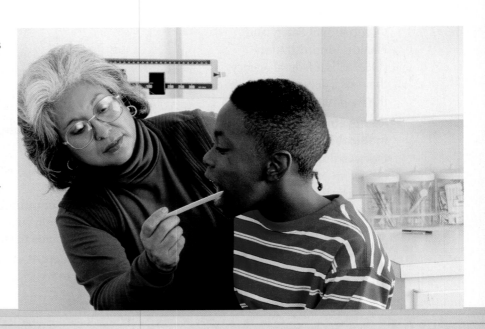

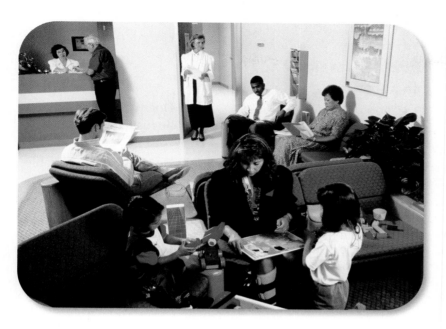

How do I know my doctor is qualified?

You and your parents should check your healthcare provider's qualifications. According to the law, your doctor must be licensed. It is illegal for a doctor to practice medicine without a license in the United States. It is a good idea to choose a doctor who is board certified. This means that the doctor has passed special tests given by a physician's association to verify his or her skill and knowledge.

You may also want to talk with other medical professionals to find out who they would recommend. Family and friends can also help by telling you what they like or don't like about their doctors.

How do I prepare for my visit to the doctor?

Patients meet doctors through get-acquainted visits or during the first checkup. At that time you'll meet the doctor's office staff. The staff will schedule appointments and answer questions about insurance and referrals.

Find out from the office staff how the doctor's practice operates. Will a nurse obtain routine medical information from you? Are sick patients separated from well patients while waiting to see the doctor? Do several doctors share patient care responsibilities? Are there specific hours to speak to the doctor by phone? How are emergencies handled during evening and weekend hours?

Making out a fact sheet like the one on the next page will help you prepare for your visit. Your list should include the following:

▶ your basic medical history

▶ any medications you are taking

▶ any allergies you have, especially if you have an allergy to a medicine

▶ a list of questions you want to ask your doctor

▶ the reason for your visit

Questions to ask:

Choosing a Doctor

▶ Is this doctor a member of your insurance plan?

▶ Where did this doctor attend medical school?

▶ How long has this doctor been practicing medicine?

▶ Is this doctor recommended by people you respect?

▶ Does this doctor communicate in a way that you understand?

▶ Do you feel comfortable with this doctor?

▶ Are this doctor's office hours and location convenient?

▶ Are the prices fair and reasonable?

▶ How long do you have to wait for an appointment?

▶ How long do you usually wait in the doctor's office?

Selecting Healthcare Services (continued)

How do I make sure I understand my doctor?

When speaking with your doctor, make sure your doctor explains your illness so that you understand the problem and the recommended treatment plan. If your doctor's advice is unclear, you may not be able to follow the treatment plan.

Ask your doctor to clarify anything you do not understand about your visit. If your doctor is in a hurry to see another patient, something important may be overlooked.

Make sure your doctor takes the time to answer your questions. You must feel comfortable and confident with your doctor.

How do I evaluate my doctor?

Choose a few of these questions to ask your family physician. Discuss his or her answers with your parents, and decide as a family whether you are happy with your doctor or would like to choose another.

▶ How long do you have to wait for an appointment?

▶ How long do you have to wait in the waiting room?

▶ Does your doctor seem to be rushed when seeing you?

▶ Do you feel comfortable asking your doctor questions?

▶ Does your doctor explain the diagnosis and treatment clearly?

HEALTHCARE PROVIDER VISIT FACT SHEET

Date: _____ Healthcare Provider: _____

1. Reason(s) for seeing doctor: _____
   _____

2. Symptoms and when they started: _____
   _____

3. Current medicines and dosage: _____
   _____

4. Family health history: _____
   _____

5. Allergies: _____

6. Recommended treatment: _____
   _____

7. Cost of treatment: _____
   _____

8. Other treatment options: _____
   _____

9. Questions and concerns: _____
   _____

What are a patient's rights?

Every patient has the right and responsibility to

▶ receive accurate, easily understood information

▶ receive assistance in making informed healthcare decisions

▶ have a choice of healthcare providers

▶ have access to emergency health services when and where the need arises

▶ participate in all health-related decisions

▶ make wishes about healthcare known, such as being an organ donor

▶ receive considerate, respectful care

▶ not be discriminated against in the delivery of healthcare services

▶ have confidential communication with healthcare providers

▶ have a fair and efficient process for resolving complaints or disagreements

What should I do if my doctor is too busy to see me?

Many times the healthcare providers are very busy. If your doctor has to rush through your evaluation to hurry on to the next patient, you may not feel that you're getting the best care. Feeling rushed may also keep you from asking questions and making sure you understand your doctor's advice and treatment. When you choose your primary care physician, make sure your doctor has enough time to spend with you. You and your parents may need to visit with several doctors before choosing one who will be your primary care physician.

What types of patient care are available?

Inpatient care is medical care that requires a person to stay in a hospital for more than a day. **Outpatient care** is medical care that requires a person to stay in the hospital only during his or her treatment. **Home healthcare services** are medical services, treatment, or equipment provided for the patient in his or her home.

WORDS TO KNOW

primary care physician (PCP) a family or personal doctor you visit when you have a healthcare concern

specialist a healthcare provider trained to treat a specific medical condition or area of the body

referral a written recommendation from your PCP to see a specialist

inpatient care medical care that requires an extended hospital stay

outpatient care medical care that requires a hospital stay only during treatment

home healthcare services medical care that is provided at the patient's home

internet connect

www.scilinks.org/health
Topic: Consumer Protection and Education
HealthLinks code: HH4037

HEALTH LINKS™ Maintained by the National Science Teachers Association

EXPRESS Lesson REVIEW

1. **LIFE SKILL** **Being a Wise Consumer** If you were dissatisfied with your healthcare provider, what steps could you take to find a new provider you would be happy with?

2. Explain why a patient might need a referral.

3. **LIFE SKILL** **Communicating Effectively** What information should you take to the doctor with you if you have a health problem? What are three questions you could prepare to ask your doctor?

Financing Your Healthcare

A visit to the emergency room can cost from 150 dollars to several thousand dollars. Very few people can afford to pay medical bills without any help. Having health insurance can help you afford medical costs.

What does health insurance actually do?

Many healthcare services are too expensive for people to afford on their own. Health insurance allows people to pay a set amount of money each month in exchange for protection against large medical bills. If you were ever to have an accident or become seriously ill, health insurance would help you pay your medical bills.

How do I get health insurance?

There are two ways people can get health insurance in the United States. One way is through work. Many companies offer insurance as a benefit to their employees by paying all or part of the cost. Other people purchase their own health insurance.

What kind of health insurance is available?

The three major types of health insurance plans are
▶ fee-for-service plans
▶ managed-care plans
▶ government-assisted health plans

What is a fee-for-service plan?

Fee-for-service insurance plans are traditional insurance plans, in which the patient must pay a premium and a deductible. A **premium** is a monthly fee for insurance. A **deductible** is the amount that the subscriber must pay before an insurance company begins paying for medical services. Fee-for-service plans can be expensive, but patients are free to choose any healthcare provider they wish to see.

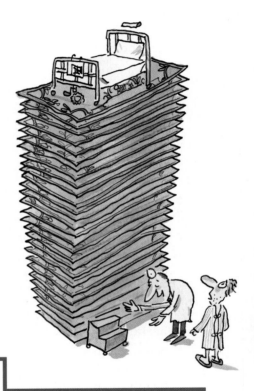

Questions to ask:

Choosing Health Insurance

▶ Can I afford this insurance?
▶ Do I have to pay a deductible? How much is the deductible?
▶ Do I have to pay a copayment? How much is the copayment?
▶ Do I get hospital, surgical, medical, and prescription benefits?
▶ Can I visit any doctor, or do I have to choose from a list of doctors?
▶ If I have a preexisting condition, is the condition covered?

▶ How much does going to the emergency room cost?
▶ What conditions or services are excluded?
▶ Is part of the cost of insurance covered by my job or parent's job?
▶ Can I get a cheaper rate by belonging to a group of subscribers?
▶ Can I continue my insurance if I lose my job?
▶ Can I cancel my insurance if I need to?

What are managed-care plans?

Managed-care plans are plans in which an insurance company makes a contract with a group of doctors. These doctors provide care and services at a lower fee to patients who have this insurance. Usually, the patient pays a yearly (or monthly) premium and a copayment for each doctor visit. A copayment is the amount that the patient pays each time medical care is received. Managed-care plans are generally less expensive than other types of insurance, but patients have a limited choice of providers.

What is an HMO?

A **health maintenance organization (HMO)** is a managed-care plan in which patients must use a doctor who contracts with the insurance company. If the patient uses a doctor who is not part of this contract, the insurance company will not pay for the services. The only exception is in the case of an emergency.

What is a PPO?

A **preferred provider organization (PPO)** allows the patient to see a doctor who does not contract with the insurance company. The patient pays a higher fee to do this.

What happens if you can't afford health insurance?

Local health departments provide many health services, including information, immunizations, and HIV/AIDS testing and counseling, either free or for a very small fee. The Children's Health Insurance Program (CHIP) provides health insurance in most states for children who are not covered by insurance. This program helps ensure that all children receive quality healthcare.

What is government-assisted healthcare?

Medicare and Medicaid are healthcare programs provided by the government. **Medicare** is a healthcare program for people who are 65 years old or older and for younger individuals who are disabled. **Medicaid** is a healthcare program for people who are on welfare, have dependent children, or are elderly, blind, or disabled.

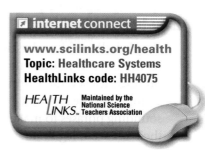

EXPRESS Lesson REVIEW

1. Describe three types of health insurance.
2. List three groups of people who can receive healthcare through Medicaid.
3. **LIFE SKILL** **Being a Wise Consumer** Your family has been offered a fantastic deal on a traditional health insurance policy. What questions should you ask the insurance agent before purchasing the policy?

Evaluating Health Web Sites

If a health Web site claimed that fluorescent lightbulbs are scientifically proven to cause pink eye, would you believe that claim? Probably not. Sorting out accurate health information on the Internet can be confusing if you don't know what to look for.

How can you tell if a health Web site is reliable?

Anyone can give health information or sell health-care products through the Internet. Some Web sites may seem very reliable and may be full of health advice that sounds very convincing. Some Web sites may sell healthcare products by giving information that sounds scientific.

To determine if a health Web site is reliable, assess the following features.

Author Who sponsored or created the Web site? Be careful if you cannot tell who the author is. Is the author qualified to publish health information? Health information is generally more reliable if it comes from a medical professional. Does the author objectively present health information? Be wary if the author is trying to sell a product.

Information Is the information outdated? When was the Web site last updated? Information more than a year old may not be accurate. Is the health Web site trying to inform or advertise? Web sites that are providing reliable information usually have links to other reliable Web sites.

Web sites that sell products based on only the testimony of people who used the product are often fraudulent. This fact may seem strange. However, there is no way to prove that any of the people listed ever actually used the product.

References The Web site should provide the reader with complete references. Make sure the references are from science journals or U.S. government publications.

Questions to ask:

Identifying Fraudulent Health Web Sites

▶ Is the Web site designed primarily to promote or sell a product?

▶ Is the purpose of the Web site unclear?

▶ Does the Web site give health advice without identifying a source of information?

▶ Does the Web site use evidence based mostly on the testimony of users?

▶ Does the Web site have a lot of "pop-up" advertising?

▶ Are you required to open a membership and give your credit card number?

▶ Were you linked to the Web site by unsolicited e-mail?

▶ Does the Web site promise free trial offers?

▶ Does the Web site send e-mail that says you were referred to them by an unidentified friend?

▶ Is the content of the Web site outdated?

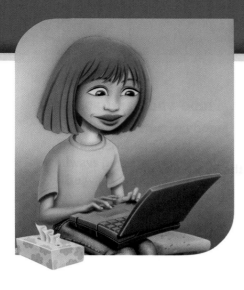

Which health Web sites can I trust?

Health information that you can trust is provided by government agencies such as

▶ the National Institutes of Health (NIH)

▶ the Centers for Disease Control and Prevention (CDC)

▶ the Food and Drug Administration (FDA)

Health information found on educational Web sites sponsored by universities is also probably trustworthy.

Is there any group that monitors health Web sites?

The **Health on the Net (HON) Foundation** is an organization of Web sites that agree to follow a code of ethics regarding health information. The *HONcode* lists rules that its member Web sites must follow regarding the health information they provide, which include the following:

▶ The Web sites must offer health advice from trained health professionals unless a clear statement is made that the advice is from a nonmedical individual or organization.

▶ The Web sites are required to honor doctor-patient confidentiality.

▶ The Web sites are required to provide information about who wrote the text and paid for the Web site.

▶ Any claims relating to a specific treament or commercial product or service must be supported with scientific evidence.

A complete list of *HONcode* rules can be found at the HON Foundation Web site. Web sites that are members of the Health On the Net Foundation are allowed to add a symbol to their Web site so that readers know they follow *HONcode* rules.

What else can I do to make sure health Web sites are providing reliable information?

Other ways that you can evaluate health Web sites include the following:

▶ Always cross-check information between several reliable Web sites.

▶ Do plenty of research before you believe anything as fact.

▶ Check with your parents, your doctor, or your pharmacist before you try any health recommendations from a Web site.

EXPRESS Lesson REVIEW

1. List three health Web sites that would be likely to have accurate information.

2. List five signs that a health Web site is not a reliable source of information.

3. **LIFE SKILL** **Being a Wise Consumer** Explain why a health Web site that is selling a product might not offer accurate information.

Caring for Your Skin *(continued)*

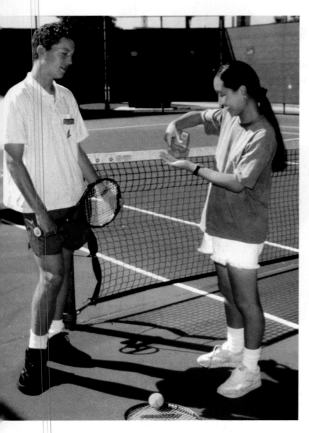

If I tan easily, do I still need sunscreen?

Melanin is the body's natural protection against UV radiation. The skin produces more melanin when it is exposed to the sun. However, melanin can't completely block the sun's UV rays. Prolonged exposure to the sun will lead to sunburn in even the darkest-skinned people. Sunburns can lead to skin cancer and premature aging of the skin. So, even if you tan easily, you should still use sunscreen.

What causes sunburns?

Ultraviolet radiation is divided into two types, UVA and UVB rays. Both types of radiation are found in sunlight. UVB rays cause sunburn when you spend too much time outside. If a burn is not too severe, the skin will be red but will not have blisters. Aloe vera gel or cool, wet cloths can soothe the burn until the skin has healed. If your sunburn causes blistering or affects your vision, you should see a doctor right away.

Are all sunscreens the same?

Everyone should use some form of sunscreen when spending prolonged time outside. For most people, a sun protection factor (SPF) of 30 or more will prevent burning for about 1.5 hours. Babies and people who have pale skin should use an SPF of 45 or more.

Are tanning beds safe?

Even though UVA rays do not cause sunburn, they are not safe. The UVA radiation, which is used in commercial tanning beds, penetrates deeper into the skin than UVB rays do. This kind of radiation damages DNA and has been linked to some types of skin cancer.

What causes skin cancer?

Skin cancer can be caused by several factors, including genetics and UV radiation. The most common types of skin cancer are carcinomas (KAHR suh NOH muhz). *Carcinomas* are masses of cells that begin in the skin or layers that line organs. Carcinomas originate in skin cells that do not produce pigments. If they are detected early, carcinomas can be treated. In its early stages, a carcinoma may look like a wart.

A small percentage of skin cancers are caused by mutations that occur in pigment-producing skin cells. These cancers are called melanomas (MEL uh NOH muhz). *Melanomas* are cancerous tumors that begin in the cells that produce melanin. Melanomas may spread quickly to other parts of the body. A melanoma often looks like a mole with an unusual color and shape.

You can reduce the risk of skin cancer by avoiding overexposure to both natural and artificial UV radiation. Use sunscreens and wear long sleeves and a hat when exposed to the sun for an extended period of time.

Are tattoos and body piercings safe?

Tattoos and body piercings have become very popular forms of decoration. However, because tattooing and body piercing involve puncturing the skin, they can pose health risks. Diseases such as hepatitis and AIDS are spread easily through needles. Using sterile practices can help reduce the risk of contracting such a disease. A tattoo or piercing artist should

▶ wash his or her hands for 15 to 20 seconds with an antibacterial solution before and after each session

▶ wear protective latex or vinyl gloves at all times during the procedure

▶ use individual sterile needle packets and materials (which should be opened in front of the client)

▶ have a machine for sterilizing equipment on site

▶ properly dispose of contaminated materials after each session (needles should be discarded in biohazard containers)

▶ provide adequate information for proper care of tattoo or piercing

What other problems can piercing and tattooing cause?

Some body parts are more prone to infection than others. The upper ear is mostly cartilage and has little blood flow. If bacteria enter here, it is difficult for the body to fight the infection.

The navel is also very prone to infection. This area heals slowly and is constantly rubbed by clothing. Piercing in areas that have naturally high bacteria counts, such as the tongue and nose, can cause severe infections.

Tattoos can also become infected if not cared for properly. Infected tattoos are very painful.

Some people develop large scars as a result of piercings and tattoos. These large, raised scars are called *keloids*.

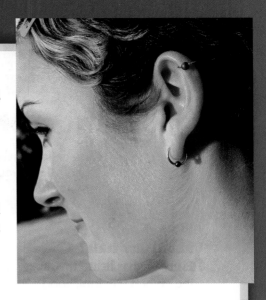

What if I change my mind about a piercing or tattoo?

Most holes from body piercing will eventually close if left alone. However, it is easier to get a tattoo than to remove one. Laser removal is expensive, very painful, and causes scarring. Be sure to carefully consider the dangers and consequences before doing anything permanent to your body.

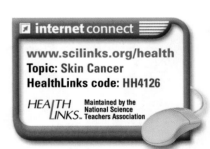

internet connect

www.scilinks.org/health
Topic: Skin Cancer
HealthLinks code: HH4126

HEALTH LINKS. Maintained by the National Science Teachers Association

EXPRESS Lesson REVIEW

1. What should you do to get rid of acne?

2. How can you protect yourself from overexposure to the sun?

3. **LIFE SKILL** **Being a Wise Consumer** Check the phone book for tattoo artists. How many advertise that they comply with the U.S. Environmental Protection Agency (EPA) standards?

Dental Care

Have you ever noticed that a model's teeth are always perfect? Models spend lots of money on dental work to improve their teeth. But if you take care of your teeth now, you can have beautiful teeth without spending a lot of money.

What are the parts of a tooth?

A tooth can be divided into three parts—the visible part, called the *crown*, the *neck* of the tooth just below the gum line, and the *root* below the gum line. The root holds the tooth in the jaw.

A tooth also has three layers. Enamel, the outermost layer, protects the crown and is the hardest substance in the body. The middle layer is cementum—a thin, bone-like layer that covers and protects the root. The innermost layer is dentin—a hard tissue that makes up most of the tooth and surrounds the pulp. The pulp is the living center of the tooth and contains nerves and blood vessels.

How do I whiten my teeth?

Certain substances, such as coffee, tea, and tobacco stain the enamel of teeth. Dentists use special bleaches to remove stains from teeth. Some over-the-counter products claim to remove these stains. Consult a dentist to make sure any product you use is safe for your teeth.

What causes cavities?

If you don't brush your teeth after you eat, bacteria that live in your mouth will digest food stuck to your teeth. The mixture of food particles, saliva, and bacteria on the tooth is called **plaque.** If plaque is not removed by brushing and flossing, it will harden into tartar. Tartar must be removed at a dentist's office.

Both plaque and tartar are slightly acidic. The acid irritates the gums and slowly dissolves the hard surfaces of the teeth. This process is called **tooth decay.** Eventually, the acid from tartar will eat through the dentin and into the pulp of the tooth.

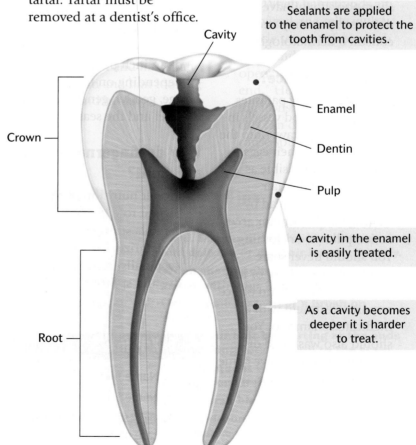

Sealants are applied to the enamel to protect the tooth from cavities.

Cavity

Crown

Root

Enamel

Dentin

Pulp

A cavity in the enamel is easily treated.

As a cavity becomes deeper it is harder to treat.

The hole in the tooth produced by tooth decay is called a **cavity.** When decay reaches the pulp, the pulp becomes infected with bacteria. Because the pulp contains nerves, cavities can be painful.

How are cavities treated?

Dentists can put a plastic sealant on teeth to keep acids from damaging the enamel. If a cavity is treated early, a dentist can clean the hole and fill it with metal or other hard substances to prevent further decay.

When a cavity reaches the pulp, the dentist must drill into the pulp of the tooth to remove the infection caused by a cavity. This procedure is called a **root canal.** If the infection is too deep for a root canal to be effective, the tooth must be removed.

What is gum disease?

Bacteria on the teeth can irritate and infect the gums, which can lead to gingivitis. **Gingivitis** is a condition in which the gums become red and infected and begin to pull away from the teeth. Once you have gingivitis, more bacteria can fill the pockets between the teeth and gums. If gingivitis is not treated, the tooth will become loose and will eventually fall out.

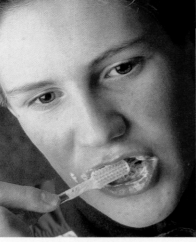
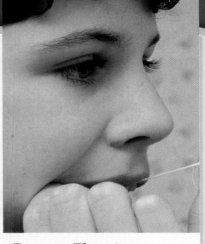

Proper Brushing Technique

▶ **Place the toothbrush at a 45-degree angle to your gums.**

▶ **Gently, brush teeth in short strokes away from the gum.**

▶ **Brush the outer, inner, and top surfaces of your teeth.**

▶ **Brush your tongue.**

▶ **Rinse your mouth with water.**

Proper Flossing Technique

▶ **Use about 18 inches of dental floss.**

▶ **Wind the ends of the floss around your middle fingers.**

▶ **Gently, insert the floss between two teeth.**

▶ **Rub the side of the tooth with the floss.**

▶ **Repeat steps 1 through 4 on the rest of your teeth.**

▶ **Rinse your mouth with water.**

What other problems can teeth have?

Tobacco use, chronic infections, and poor oral hygiene increase a person's chances of developing oral cancer. Oral cancer must be surgically removed. If it is not removed, it could spread to other parts of the body.

How can I protect my teeth?

You can easily prevent bad breath, cavities, and gum disease. Follow the guidelines listed to brush and floss your teeth after every meal. Eat a balanced diet. Avoid food high in sugar or acid and foods that stick to your teeth. Get dental checkups twice a year.

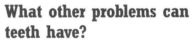

EXPRESS Lesson REVIEW

1. Describe the process that leads to a cavity.

2. Explain why gingivitis can cause you to lose a tooth.

3. **LIFE SKILL** **Practicing Wellness** List three things you can do that will help prevent tooth decay.

EXPRESS Lesson

Protecting Your Hearing and Vision

After the rock concert, Julie's ears were ringing. "That's how you know you were at a good concert!" Julie shouted. "I'm not so sure about that," said her best friend, "I heard loud music can make you deaf."

Can loud music make me lose my hearing?

The ears are delicate and sensitive organs. Unfortunately, they have no way to shut out loud noises. Sounds above a certain level can permanently damage the ear. That's why you must protect your hearing.

How can I tell if I've damaged my hearing?

By the time teens become young adults, many have already suffered some degree of hearing loss. After the ears have been exposed to loud noise, the ears may ring and words may seem muffled. The effect usually disappears in a day or two, but damage from noise adds up over time. A buzzing, ringing, or whistling sound in one or both ears that occurs even when no sound is present is called **tinnitus** (ti NIET es). Some people are born with tinnitus; others may develop it as a result of damage to hearing.

How loud is too loud?

Sound is measured in units called **decibels** (DES uh BUHLZ). The abbreviation for decibels is dB.

The faintest sound a person can hear is 0 decibels. Prolonged exposure to noise above 70 decibels may begin to damage hearing. Serious damage occurs if a person is exposed to sounds above 120 decibels. Sounds of 140 decibels or more can cause pain. Sounds of 180 decibels or more cause immediate and irreversible hearing loss.

The length of time you are exposed to sounds is also important. For example, listening to loud music for a couple of hours is just as damaging as hearing a much louder sound for a short time.

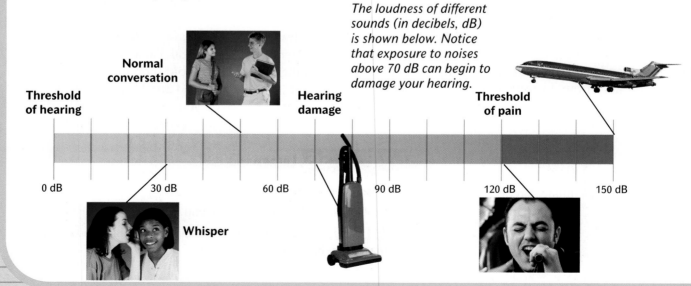

The loudness of different sounds (in decibels, dB) is shown below. Notice that exposure to noises above 70 dB can begin to damage your hearing.

Threshold of hearing

Normal conversation

Hearing damage

Threshold of pain

0 dB   30 dB   60 dB   90 dB   120 dB   150 dB

Whisper

How can I protect my hearing?

Following these tips can help you make sure you can enjoy a good concert for many years to come.

▶ Keep your ears clean. Use a soft cotton swab to remove dirt and wax.

▶ Do not push a cotton swab into your ear canal.

▶ Never use a pencil or sharp object to clean your ear.

▶ Protect your ears from the cold to prevent frostbite and inner ear infections.

▶ Avoid loud noises and keep volume low when using headphones.

▶ Have your hearing checked once a year.

Can using a computer damage my eyes?

Reading in dim light or from a computer screen cannot damage your eyes. However, these activities do cause temporary eye strain. Part of the reason for the strain is that people engaging in these activities do not blink as often as they usually would. Not blinking enough can cause the eyes to feel dry and irritated. Refresh your eyes by taking frequent breaks to blink. Look up from your work, and focus on distant objects to relieve eye strain.

How can I protect my vision?

Follow these tips to keep your eyes as healthy as possible.

▶ Be sure to eat a healthful diet rich in dark green and orange vegetables.

▶ Take regular breaks when you are reading or using the computer. Focus your eyes on distant objects.

▶ If you have glasses or contacts, wear them. Trying to focus without your corrective lenses will strain your eyes.

▶ Choose sunglasses that block 90 to 100 percent of UVA and UVB radiation (the two types of ultraviolet radiation from the sun).

▶ Any time you're working with chemicals or power tools, be sure to wear safety goggles.

▶ Sit at least 5 feet from the television.

▶ Use a room light and a reading lamp to reduce glare.

▶ Because infections can be spread by your hands, avoid touching or rubbing your eyes unless your hands have been washed with soap and water.

▶ To avoid infection, do not share contacts or contact solutions.

▶ Visit your eye doctor once a year.

What should I do if I hurt my eyes?

Even the best protection can't ensure you'll never injure your eyes. Any injury to the eye should be treated seriously. Often, the eye may seem fine at first, but symptoms of vision loss may begin to appear later. If you experience any eye injury, you must see a doctor immediately. Eye injuries can be treated, but only if you get professional medical help.

EXPRESS Lesson REVIEW

1. Name five things you can do to protect your vision.

2. According to the figure on the pervious page, what noises fall within the range of 120 to 140 dB?

3. **LIFE SKILL** **Practicing Wellness** What activities do you do that may put your eyes at risk for injury? What can you do to decrease this risk?

4. **LIFE SKILL** **Assessing Your Health** What noises are you exposed to in your daily life that could possibly damage your hearing?

EXPRESS Lesson

Responding to a Medical Emergency

Sam was riding his bike along a trail near a campground. He suddenly came upon someone who was unconscious and bleeding. What should he do?

What should I do if I encounter a medical emergency?

Quickly survey the scene for hazards that might harm you or the victim. Call out to bystanders for help. Determine how many people (if there is more than one victim) are injured or ill. Ask each person, "Are you OK?" If a person does not respond, you or a bystander should immediately call for medical help.

Check for life-threatening injuries. Then ask, "May I touch you?" Do not touch the person without consent.

If there is no response, you have implied consent to help. Try to determine the cause of the injuries or illness to tell medical personnel when they arrive. Check to see if the victim has a medical-alert necklace or bracelet.

What medical conditions should I look for?

If needed and if you can do so safely, give life-saving first aid and then obtain medical help if you have not already done so. If the person might have a head or spinal injury, do not allow the head or neck to move. Remain with the person until help arrives.

How do I know whether to go for help if I am alone with a victim?

A person needs medical attention if he or she is not alert, is not aware of the surroundings, and does not respond to questions.

If you can get to a phone or to others and return within 3 minutes, then go for help. If not, stay with the victim, check for life-threatening injuries, and give life-saving first aid.

After these measures, if the victim remains unresponsive or needs medical attention, you must decide whether it is better to go for help or to stay. Consider factors such as the following:

▶ how long it might be before someone finds you

▶ whether the person will survive if you leave

▶ whether the person will survive if you do not obtain medical help

Do not risk your own safety.

Steps to Take

When You Encounter a Medical Emergency

1 Look for hazards and remove them.

2 Determine the cause of injury or nature of illness.

3 Determine the number of victims.

4 If the victim is unresponsive, seek medical help.

5 If the victim is responsive, obtain consent to touch him or her.

6 Check the ABCs (Airway, Breathing, Circulation).

7 Give first aid for life-threatening conditions.

8 Seek medical help if not done previously.

9 Stay with the victim until help arrives.

*Do not risk your own safety in order to rescue or provide first aid to another person. For more information on these and other topics, see the Express Lessons on pp. 576–613.

How to Check the ABCs of Life-Threatening Conditions in an Unresponsive Person

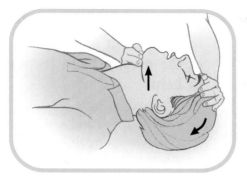

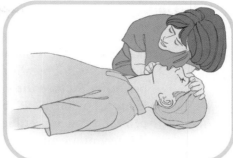

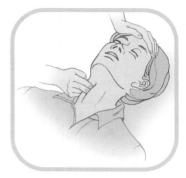

A **_Airway_**—*Open the airway by tilting the head back and lifting the chin. Make sure the tongue is not blocking the airway.*

B **_Breathing_**—*Look for movement of the chest. Listen and feel for air movement by placing your ear and then your cheek at the mouth and nose of the victim.*

C **_Carotid Pulse_**—*Place your index and middle fingers into the groove of the neck next to the voice box to feel the cartoid artery pulse.*

What can I do to aid the victim until help arrives?

To aid the victim, you must know what is wrong. First, check the **ABCs.** ABC is an acronym to remind you to check three important vital signs during an emergency. The **A** reminds you to check whether or not a person's **a**irway is obstructed (blocked). The **B** reminds you to check if the person is **b**reathing. The **C** reminds you to check the person's **c**artoid pulse.

How do I check if a person's airway is obstructed?

If a person is talking or crying, his or her airway is open. If the person cannot talk but is alert and aware, he or she might have an obstructed airway. In this case, administering abdominal thrusts (the Heimlich maneuver) may clear the airway. **(See the Express Lesson "Choking" on p. 586.)**

If the person is unresponsive and does not appear to have a spinal injury, place the victim face up. Open the airway by tilting the head back and lifting the chin. If the victim appears to have a spinal injury, ask others to help you roll the victim so that no twisting of the body occurs. Lift the victim's lower jaw without tilting the head. Remove any visible object or vomit from the mouth.

How do I determine if the victim is breathing?

Always ask the victim, "Are you all right?" If there is no response or if he or she is breathing less than 8 times per minute or more than 24 times per minute or is having trouble breathing, seek medical assistance.

To detect breathing in an unresponsive person, look for movement of the chest. Then, listen and feel for air movement by placing first your ear and then your cheek at the mouth and nose of the victim. If the victim is not breathing, keep the airway open and provide rescue breathing. **(See the Express Lesson "Rescue Breathing" on p. 580.)**

Responding to a Medical Emergency *continued*

How do I check for circulation?

To check circulation, check the victim's carotid pulse. The **carotid pulse** is the pulse felt at the carotid arteries, the major arteries of the neck. A carotid artery runs along each side of the voice box (Adam's apple). Take the carotid pulse by placing your index and middle fingers into the groove of the neck next to the voice box. Do not use your thumb; it has a pulse of its own. Do not take the pulse on both sides at the same time, as it can cut off blood flow to the brain.

What if there is no pulse?

If the victim has no pulse, has no other signs of circulation, and is not breathing, perform CPR **(see the Express Lesson "CPR" on p. 582)** if you are certified in this technique and call for medical assistance. If you are not certified to perform CPR, call for medical assistance immediately, and then remain with the victim until help arrives.

Can I be held responsible for the death or injuries of the person I am trying to help?

Good Samaritan laws have been designed and enacted to encourage people to help others in an emergency. These laws vary from state to state. Generally, if you provide help during an emergency, you are protected from lawsuits if you obtain consent, act in good faith, are not paid, use reasonable skill and care, are not negligent (careless), and do not abandon the person.

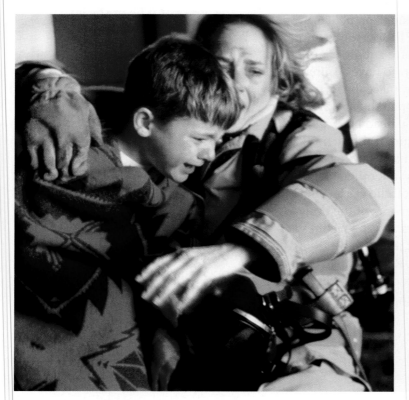

Shock can be a life-threatening event if not treated properly.

Symptoms of Shock

A person experiencing shock may

▶ appear anxious, restless, or combative

▶ be lethargic, difficult to arouse, or unconscious

▶ have pale, cold, and "clammy" skin

▶ become nauseated and vomit

▶ experience increased pulse and respiration rates

▶ have a bluish tinge to his or her skin

▶ be thirsty

▶ have dilated (enlarged) pupils

What is shock, and when do people usually experience it?

Many types of trauma can cause a person to go into shock, which can be life threatening. **Shock** is a condition in which some body organs are not getting enough oxygenated blood. Shock may occur when the heart is not pumping properly, when a considerable amount of blood is lost from the body because of hemorrhaging, dehydration, or a systemic infection, or when the nervous system is damaged because of injury or drugs. Significant injuries usually cause shock, so automatically treat injured victims for shock.

What should you do if someone is in shock?

▶ First, check the ABCs and treat a victim for any injuries you know how to.
▶ Lay the victim on his or her back.
▶ Raise the legs 8 to 12 inches.
▶ Cover the victim with blankets, coats, or other coverings.
▶ Call for medical assistance.
▶ Do not give the victim anything to eat or drink.

How should you treat someone for shock if he or she has head or spinal injuries or is having trouble breathing?

If the victim has head injuries, assume the neck and spine are also affected. If the victim has spinal injuries, do not raise the head or feet. Place victims with breathing difficulties, chest injuries, eye injuries, or a heart attack in a half-sitting position. This position will help breathing.

How should you treat an unconscious person for shock?

If a shock victim becomes unconscious, lay the person on his or her left side. To do this, move to the victim's left side and outstretch his or her left arm. Bend the right arm, placing the back of the right hand on the left cheek. Roll the victim toward you by pulling on the far knee.

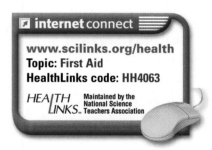

internet connect

www.scilinks.org/health
Topic: First Aid
HealthLinks code: HH4063

HEALTH LINKS™ Maintained by the National Science Teachers Association

EXPRESS Lesson REVIEW

1. List the steps you should take when encountering an emergency medical situation.

2. If you were alone with an accident victim, how would you determine whether to stay and help the victim or go for help?

3. Describe the steps you should follow to help someone in shock.

4. **LIFE SKILL** **Communicating Effectively** Imagine that you found someone who was injured in an accident. A bystander has gone to seek help. What questions would you ask the victim if he or she is responsive? What would you tell emergency medical help if he or she is unresponsive?

Rescue Breathing

Naveen saw flames coming from David's house. Then he saw David stumble from the house and collapse on the lawn. David wasn't breathing. David needed Naveen's help quickly!

What is rescue breathing?

Rescue breathing is an emergency technique in which a rescuer gives air to someone who is not breathing. To perform rescue breathing, a person blows air into a victim's lungs to give him or her oxygen. You may hear rescue breathing referred to as *artificial respiration* or *"mouth to mouth."*

How do I know if a person has stopped breathing?

In responding to a medical emergency, you will need to determine if a person has stopped breathing by checking the person's ABCs (airway, breathing, and carotid pulse). To determine if a person has stopped breathing, **see the Express Lesson "Responding to a Medical Emergency" on p. 576.** If the victim is not breathing, keep the airway open and provide rescue breathing.

How do I help an adult who has stopped breathing?

Follow these steps to help an adult:

Tilt Head Be certain that the head is properly tilted by gently pressing the victim's forehead back with one hand while raising the chin with the other.

If the person appears to have a spinal injury, do not tilt the head. Instead, lift the jaw by placing your palms on the victim's cheekbones and lifting the jaw with your fingers.

Administer Breath Now that the airway is open, pinch the victim's nostrils closed, and seal your mouth around the mouth of the victim. Blow gently into the victim's mouth for 2 seconds and watch for the chest to rise. Unpinch the nostrils, and remove your mouth so that the victim can "exhale." Watch for the chest to fall, listen for air sounds, and feel for a flow of air from the victim's mouth and nose.

Performing Rescue Breathing on an Adult

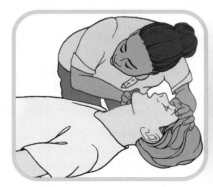

If the person does not have a spinal injury, tilt the head back and raise the chin.

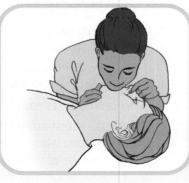

Administer breath as described above.

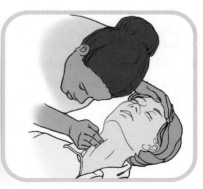

Check for pulse and signs of breathing.

If the chest rose and fell, give another rescue breath. If not, retilt the head and check the mouth and nose seals; try another rescue breath.

If air is still not entering the victim's lungs, check the head tilt, check for an airway obstruction, and administer abdominal thrusts. **(See the Express Lesson "Choking" on p. 586.)** Then try rescue breathing again.

Check for Signs of Breathing
After two successful rescue breaths (chest rises and falls), look, listen, and feel for signs of breathing. Also, check the victim's pulse. If the victim is still not breathing, give rescue breaths once every 5 seconds.

How do I help a young child or infant who has stopped breathing?

Rescue breathing for a young child ages 1 to 8 years or for an infant is performed as for an adult, with these exceptions:

▶ First, tilt the head of a child less than the head of an adult, and the head of an infant less than the head of a child.

▶ Second, in the case of an infant, seal your mouth around its mouth and nose.

▶ Third, each rescue breath should last only 1 second rather than the 2 seconds for an adult. CAUTION: blow slowly and gently, using only enough air to make the chest rise.

Performing Rescue Breathing on a Young Child

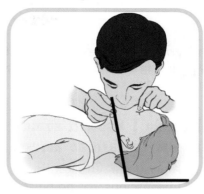 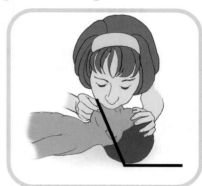

To position a child for opening of the airway, tilt the child's head less than you would tilt an adult's. Blow gently once every three seconds. Each rescue breath should last only one second.

To position an infant for opening of airway, tilt the infant's head less than you would a child's. Blow gently once every three seconds for only one second. You should seal your mouth around the infant's mouth and nose.

▶ Fourth, breathe into the victim once every 3 seconds, rather than the once every 5 seconds for adults.

How do I know when to stop rescue breathing?

After performing rescue breathing for 1 minute, look, listen, and feel for signs of breathing. If the victim is breathing on his or her own, stop rescue breath-

ing. If not, continue rescue breathing until the victim is breathing on his or her own or until medical help arrives.

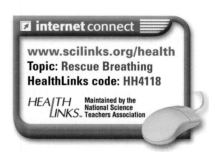

internet connect

www.scilinks.org/health
Topic: Rescue Breathing
HealthLinks code: HH4118

HEALTH LINKS. Maintained by the National Science Teachers Association

EXPRESS Lesson REVIEW

1. What is rescue breathing?

2. When is rescue breathing used?

3. Compare rescue breathing in adults with rescue breathing in young children and infants.

4. **LIFE SKILL** **Practicing Wellness** In a short paragraph, describe two situations that may cause a person to stop breathing.

EXPRESS Lesson

CPR

Nigel's grandfather grabbed his chest and fell to the floor. Nigel thought that his grandfather was having a heart attack and that his heart may have stopped. Panicked, he didn't know what to do.

What is CPR?

CPR stands for **cardiopulmonary** (heart-lung) **resuscitation. CPR** is a life-saving technique that combines rescue breathing and chest compressions. During CPR, the rescuer performs the job of the heart, artificially pumping blood to the body. The pumping provides oxygen to the lungs.

What is the difference between a heart attack and cardiac arrest?

A heart attack is the damage and loss of function of an area of the heart muscle. A heart attack occurs when part of the heart muscle does not receive enough oxygen as a result of insufficient blood flow. As the heart muscle dies, it may trigger the heart to stop beating, a condition known as cardiac arrest. Other causes of cardiac arrest include stroke (an attack of weakness or paralysis that occurs when blood flow to the brain is interrupted), severe injuries, electrical shock, drug overdose, chest trauma, drowning, and suffocation.

How do I know if someone is in cardiac arrest?

A person in cardiac arrest is unconscious, has no pulse (a throbbing that can be felt in certain arteries as the blood rushes through), and has no signs of circulation. Therefore, victims who are alert and responsive are not in cardiac arrest.

If a victim is unresponsive, quickly look for signs of circulation, which include pinkness of the nail beds and warm skin. If the nail beds or skin are blue-gray, or if the skin is cool, circulation may be poor or may have stopped. Next, turn the victim face up and check the carotid pulse. The **carotid pulse** is felt at the carotid arteries, the major arteries of the neck. One carotid runs along each side of the voice box (Adam's apple). Take the carotid pulse by placing your index and middle fingers into the groove of the neck next to the voice box. Do not use your thumb; it has a pulse of its own. Do not take the pulse on both sides at the same time.

What should I do if a person is in cardiac arrest?

A victim can die from cardiac arrest in minutes. Therefore, get medical help immediately for an adult, or after 1 minute of CPR for a child or infant.

Perform CPR only if you are certified in this technique. CPR is a technique that cannot successfully be learned from a book. Any training that you might receive in CPR or any other emergency procedure will help you perform competently and effectively in case of an emergency situation.

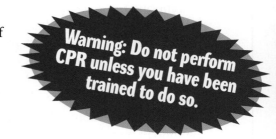

Warning: Do not perform CPR unless you have been trained to do so.

How do I give CPR to an adult?

Only give CPR to a victim in cardiac arrest and only if you are certified to perform this technique. To perform CPR on an adult, do the following steps:

1. **Open and clear the airway.** Do this by tilting the head back and lifting the chin. Remove any objects or vomit blocking the throat.
2. **Give two slow rescue breaths.** Be sure to pinch the nostrils and seal your mouth around the victim's mouth.

Watch for the chest to rise, and then unpinch the nostrils and remove your mouth to allow the victim to "exhale." **(See the Express Lesson "Rescue Breathing" on p. 580.)**
3. **Perform chest compressions.** Place the heel of one hand in the center of the victim's chest between the nipples, and place the heel of the other hand on the back of the first. Depress the chest 1 1/2 to 2 inches. Give 15 chest compressions at a rate of about 5 every 3 seconds. After 15 chest compressions, repeat cycle steps 2 and 3.

4. **Check for signs of circulation and breathing.** After 4 cycles of compressions and breaths (about 1 minute), check the carotid pulse and other signs of circulation and breathing.

If the victim still has no pulse, continue with cycles of compression and breathing, rechecking the signs of circulation every few minutes. Continue until medical help arrives or until you are unable to continue.

Giving CPR to an Adult

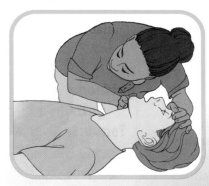

1 Open and clear the airway.

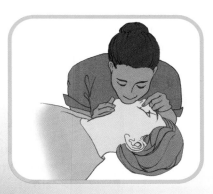

2 Give two slow rescue breaths.

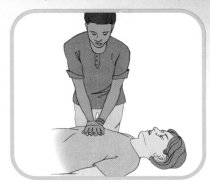

3 Perform chest compressions.

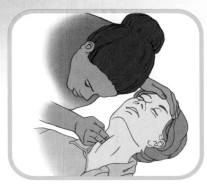

4 Check for signs of circulation and breathing.

EXPRESS Lesson

Choking

Elisa and Carlos were having lunch when Elisa suddenly stopped talking, looked scared, and put her hands up to her throat. Carlos wasn't sure what to do.

How do I know if someone is choking?

Choking occurs when the windpipe is partly or completely blocked. A choking person usually grabs his or her throat, the universal sign of choking. As the victim coughs, wheezes, and gags, his or her face turns red. A choking person cannot breathe or talk. The face of this person will turn bluish.

How do I help a person who is choking?

If a person eight years of age or older is choking, conscious, and can speak, ask him or her to try to cough up the object. After a few minutes, seek medical help if the person is unsuccessful.

If the victim cannot cough, speak, or breathe, or if a victim's ability to breathe decreases, use abdominal thrusts immediately. **Abdominal thrusts** (also known as the **Heimlich maneuver**) are the act of applying pressure to a choking person's stomach to force an object out of the throat.

To give abdominal thrusts, stand behind the victim,

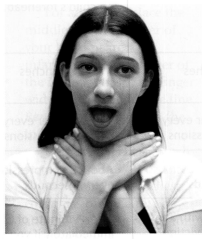

The universal sign for choking will let people know you are choking when you are unable to speak.

facing his or her back. Position a fist just above the navel (bellybutton). Grab your fist with your other hand. Quickly and forcefully press inward and upward with your fist (not your arms).

With a pregnant or obese person, give chest thrusts like abdominal thrusts but position your fist in the center of the chest. Continue thrusts until the object is dislodged or until the victim becomes unconscious because of a lack of oxygen.

For a child between the ages of 1 and 8 years, kneel behind the child to administer abdominal thrusts.

What should I do if the choking person becomes unconscious?

If the victim becomes unconscious, lower him or her to the floor. Send someone for medical help immediately. Open the victim's mouth and look for the object blocking the airway. If you see it, try to remove it with your finger. Try to administer rescue breathing. **(See the Express Lesson "Rescue Breathing" on p. 580.)** Or if you are certified in CPR, give CPR if needed. **(See the Express Lesson "CPR" on p. 582.)** Each time you give a breath, first look for an object in the throat and try to remove it with your finger.

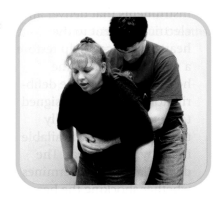

Knowing how to administer abdominal thrusts (Heimlich Maneuver) could help save a life.

How do I help an infant who is choking?

If an infant (child under 1 year) suddenly has trouble breathing, suspect choking. If the infant is coughing, allow the coughing for a few min-utes. If the object is not coughed up, seek medical help right away.

If the infant cannot breathe, is wheezing, or starts to turn blue, you must administer chest thrusts and back blows immediately. Turn the infant face down. With the infant's head lower than the rest of the body, use the heel of your hand to give five forceful back blows. Turn the infant face up, reversing the procedure for turning the infant face down. Place your middle and ring finger in the center of the infant's chest, one finger width below the nipple line. While holding the infant's head lower than his or her chest, give five chest thrusts. Continue giving back blows then chest thrusts until the object becomes dislodged or until the infant becomes unconscious.

If the infant loses con-sciousness, send someone for medical help immediately. Attempt rescue breaths or CPR if there is no pulse (if you are certified). **(See the Express Lesson "CPR" on p. 582.)**

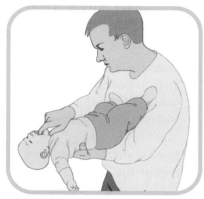

Try to clear the infant's airway.

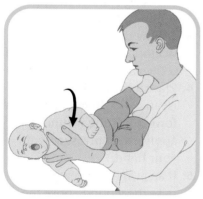

Turn the infant face down.

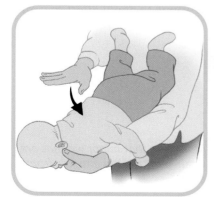

Administer back blows.

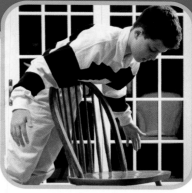

If you are choking and are alone, lean over a chair and press your abdomen upward and inward.

What should I do if I am choking and alone?

If you are alone, are choking, and cannot cough up the object blocking your airway, self-administer abdominal thrusts. Place your fist just above your navel. Cover your fist with your other hand and thrust upward and inward. If a chair, table, or other firm object is available, lean over the back of the chair or edge of the object and swiftly press your abdomen upward and inward.

🔲 internet connect 📶

www.scilinks.org/health
Topic: Choking
HealthLinks code: HH4032

HEALTH LINKS™ Maintained by the National Science Teachers Association

EXPRESS Lesson REVIEW

1. Describe the steps you should follow to help a choking adult who becomes unconscious while you are giving him or her abdominal thrusts.

2. What should you do if you are alone and choking?

3. **LIFE SKILL Communicating Effectively** Compare the steps you should follow when helping a choking adult with those you should follow when helping a choking infant.

EXPRESS Lesson

Wounds and Bleeding

Stopping severe bleeding can save a person's life. Rapid blood loss can lead to shock and even death.

What are the different types of wounds?

A **wound** is a break or tear in the soft tissues of the body. An open wound breaks the surface of the skin. Open wounds, such as cuts, result in **external bleeding,** or bleeding at the body surface. A *closed wound* does not break the surface of the skin. Closed wounds, such as bruises, result in **internal bleeding,** or bleeding within the body.

How should I care for a minor wound?

Minor wounds usually stop bleeding by themselves after a few minutes. If not, follow these steps:

1. Wash your hands, and put on disposable gloves if you have them.
2. Place a sterile or clean cloth on the wound and apply direct pressure.
3. After the bleeding has stopped, rinse the wound with water and use a clean cloth and mild soap to gently wash the wound. Rinse with water again, and pat dry.

4. If you cannot remove all the debris, dirt, or grit from a wound with gentle washing, seek medical help. You may apply an antibacterial ointment to the wound.
5. Cover the wound with a sterile or clean *dressing* (a protective covering), and secure it with a *bandage* (something used to hold the dressing in place). Change the dressing at least once a day, keeping the wound clean and dry. If the wound becomes tender, swollen, and red, it may be infected. Seek medical help.

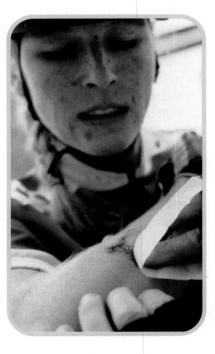

Make sure that minor wounds are washed until clean and free from debris.

How should I care for a person who has a serious wound with severe bleeding?

1. Seek medical help immediately, if possible. Protect yourself from the blood by wearing disposable gloves or other protection.
2. Lay the victim down, and elevate the feet and legs. If the bleeding is from a head wound, place the victim in a reclining (half-seated) position.
3. Follow the blood to find the wound. Expose the wound if it is covered with clothing.
4. Place a dressing, such as a clean cloth, handkerchief, or towel, over the wound, and apply direct pressure with your hand.
5. If an arm or leg is wounded, raise the wound above the level of the heart, and continue to apply direct pressure.

6. If bleeding continues, apply pressure at a pressure point. A *pressure point* is a place where an artery near the skin's surface lies over a bone. Using your hand to press the artery against the bone reduces blood flow. Use the pressure point that lies between the heart and the wound.

7. When the bleeding stops, release the pressure point and secure the dressing with a bandage. Do not remove any dressings. Place new dressings on top of the blood-soaked ones. Victims with puncture wounds (those made with blunt or pointed instruments) may need a tetanus booster (an injection that prevents tetanus, otherwise known as "lockjaw").

How do I recognize internal bleeding?

You may not be able to see internal bleeding unless it is near the surface of the skin, as in a bruise. If a person has blood coming from the ears, nose, mouth, or eyes or if the victim is coughing up or vomiting blood, he or she is likely to be bleeding internally. Lay the person down and raise the legs 8 to 12 inches unless he or she has a head injury. If the person has a head injury, put him or her in a reclining position. Lay a vomiting person on his or her left side. Cover the victim for warmth, and seek medical help immediately, as this may be a life-threatening condition.

○ pressure points

Pressure Points

To stop severe bleeding, apply pressure to a pressure point between the heart and wound. If there is more than one pressure point between the heart and wound, apply pressure to the pressure point nearest the wound, if this will not traumatize the wound or the victim.

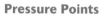

E X P R E S S **Lesson REVIEW**

1. Describe how to clean a minor wound.

2. Where do you apply pressure to stop bleeding?

3. **LIFE SKILL** **Practicing Wellness** List the steps you would take to stop bleeding in a severe wound.

Heat- and Cold-Related Emergencies

People who spend time outside in either extreme heat or extreme cold have special concerns regarding their health.

What is hyperthermia?

Hyperthermia is a condition in which the body's internal temperature is higher than normal. It occurs in two stages—heat exhaustion and heatstroke.

What is heat exhaustion?

Heat exhaustion is a condition in which the body becomes heated to a higher temperature than normal. Heat exhaustion can occur when people exercise or work in a hot, humid place where body fluids are lost through heavy sweating. Heat exhaustion may result in a mild form of shock.

Symptoms The physical symptoms of heat exhaustion include cold, moist skin, normal or below-normal body temperature, headache, nausea, and extreme fatigue.

Treatment People experiencing heat exhaustion need to have their bodies cooled. The victim should be moved to a shady place or an air-conditioned room. Cool the victim by removing his or her clothes and applying cool, wet towels. A fan will help speed up the cooling process. Give the victim something cool (not cold) to drink, about half of a glass of cool water every 15 minutes. Observe the victim closely for changes in his or her condition. Seek medical attention if the person's condition does not change. A person suffering from heat exhaustion left untreated may suffer heatstroke.

What is Heatstroke?

Heatstroke is a condition in which the body loses its ability to cool itself by sweating because the victim has become dehydrated.

Symptoms The symptoms of heatstroke include hot, dry skin; higher than normal body temperature; rapid pulse; rapid, shallow breathing; and possible loss of consciousness.

Treatment Because heatstroke is life-threatening, seek emergency medical help immediately. If there are no emergency facilities nearby, move the person to a cool place, and try to cool the body rapidly. The victim can be cooled by immersing him or her in a cool (not cold) bath or by the methods for cooling a heat exhaustion victim. If the person is vomiting or unconscious, do not give him or her water or food. Seek medical attention as soon as possible.

Keeping oneself hydrated is the best way to prevent heat exhaustion and heatstroke.

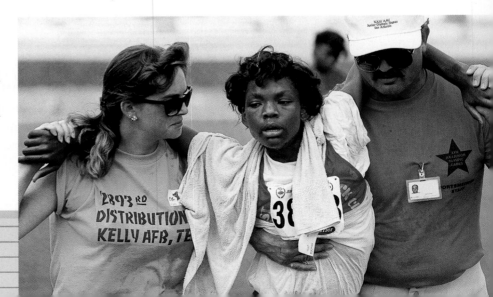

How can I prevent heat exhaustion and heat-stroke?

Heat exhaustion and heat-stroke can best be prevented by drinking 6 to 8 ounces of water at least 10 times a day when you are active in warm, humid weather.

What is frostbite?

Frostbite is a condition in which body tissues become frozen. Ice forms within the tissues and cuts off circulation to the area. Frostbite can involve the skin and much deeper tissues.

Symptoms Symptoms of frostbite include a change in the skin color to white, gray, or blue. The part of the body that has been frostbitten may feel numb. When warmth is restored to the body part affected, the pain can be severe.

Treatment Warmth must be restored to the affected part of the body. Do not rub the area; rubbing can cause damage to the tissue. Handle the areas gently. Remove wet or tight clothing. Cover the affected area with a dry, sterile dressing. If you are unable to get medical attention immediately, warm the affected area slowly in warm (not hot) water. Bandage the body part loosely with gauze and seek medical attention as soon as possible.

What is hypothermia?

Hypothermia is a condition in which the internal body temperature becomes dangerously low because the body loses heat faster than it can generate heat. When hypothermia occurs, the brain loses its ability to function at cold body temperatures, and body systems shut down. Hypothermia is usually associated with cold weather, but can also occur in windy or rainy weather when the body becomes cold and can't warm itself.

Symptoms Symptoms of hypothermia include stiff muscles, shivering, weakness, dizziness, cold skin, and slow breathing and heart rate.

Treatment To treat a person experiencing hypothermia, first remove any wet clothing and then wrap the person in blankets, towels, or newspapers. Offer warm food or drink. Do not try to heat the body with hot drinks, hot water, or electric blankets.

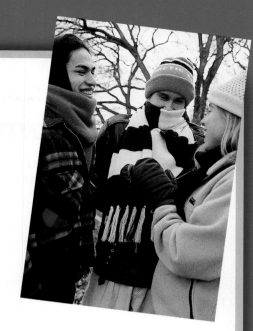

Seek medical attention as soon as possible.

How can I prevent frostbite and hypothermia?

Frostbite and hypothermia can best be prevented by wearing several layers of warm clothing and a warm hat. Also, going inside frequently to warm oneself will help prevent frostbite and hypothermia.

EXPRESS Lesson REVIEW

1. How can you tell if someone is suffering from heat exhaustion or heatstroke?
2. What should you do to treat someone with heatstroke?
3. **LIFE SKILL** **Practicing Wellness** Describe what you would do to prevent frostbite and hypothermia if you were going to be out in cold weather for a long period of time.

Bone, Joint, and Muscle Injuries

Bill injured his arm while he and Tim were mountain biking. Tim wasn't sure whether or not he should splint Bill's arm.

What are fractures?

A **fracture** is a crack or break in a bone. In a *closed fracture,* the skin is unbroken. In an *open fracture,* the skin is broken and bone ends may stick out from the skin. An open fracture has the obvious signs of the wound and visible bones. Signs and symptoms of a closed fracture include one or more of the following: pain and tenderness, loss of function, deformity, unnatural movement, swelling, bruising, and a grating sensation or sound. An X ray usually determines with certainty whether a bone is fractured.

How do you treat a fracture?

Check for bleeding and call for medical help. Splint the area of the fracture. A **splint** is a device used to stabilize (hold secure) a body part. Stabilizing a fracture will help reduce pain, prevent further damage to tissues surrounding the fracture, and reduce bleeding and swelling.

Splint the area in the position it was found. Cover any open wounds with a clean, dry dressing, and apply the splint, placing padding between the splint and the body. Be certain that the splint is long enough to extend beyond the joint above and the joint below the fracture. (joints are places where two bones meet.)

Things you can use to make a splint include heavy cardboard, rolled newspapers, or even an adjacent body part (for example, you can tape two fingers or two legs together).

Tie the splint or self-splint to the body tightly enough to prevent movement but not so tightly as to cut off circulation. When possible, place splints on both sides of the injured part.

What is a dislocation?

A **dislocation** is an injury in which a bone has been forced out of its normal position in a joint. Usually the joint is swollen and looks deformed. A dislocation is usually painful, and the dislocated joint may be "locked" in position. Splint a dislocation as you would a bone fracture, and seek medical help.

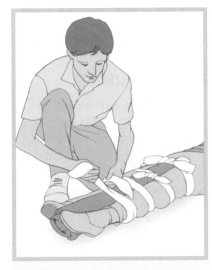

How to Apply a Splint

▶ Find materials to make a splint.

▶ Hold the splint close to the injured area.

▶ Place padding between the splint and the body.

▶ Use extra padding in body hollows and around deformities.

▶ Be sure that the splint extends beyond the joint above and the joint below the fracture.

▶ Tie the splint comfortably to the body.

What are the differences between sprains and strains?

A **sprain** is an injury in which the ligaments in a joint are stretched too far or torn. Ligaments are bands of connective tissue that hold bones to bones. A **strain** is an injury in which a muscle or tendon has been stretched too far or torn. Tendons are bands of connective tissue that hold muscles to bones.

What should you do to treat injuries to bones, joints, and muscles?

Use the RICE technique:
Rest—don't use the injured area
Ice—use an ice pack or cold pack on the injured area to reduce swelling
Compression—wrap the injured area with an elastic bandage to prevent movement and swelling
Elevation—raise the injured area above heart level when lying or sitting down

How do you know if someone has a neck or spinal injury?

A person with spinal injuries may have no obvious signs and symptoms. However, some signs and symptoms of spinal injuries are swelling and bruising at the site of the injury; numbness, tingling, or a loss of feeling in the arms and legs; inability to move the arms or legs; pain; difficulty breathing, and shock. If the victim was injured in a way that is likely to have caused a neck or spinal injury, assume that such an injury exists.

How do you treat an injury to the neck or spine?

An injury to the bones of the neck or spine can damage the spinal cord and the nerves that branch out from the spine. Therefore, do not move a person that may have a neck or spinal injury. Get medical help immediately. If the person must be moved, steady and support the head and neck by holding it in the position in which you find it. Keep your arms steady by placing them on your thighs, or place heavy objects on either side of the head. Steady and support the victim's feet as well.

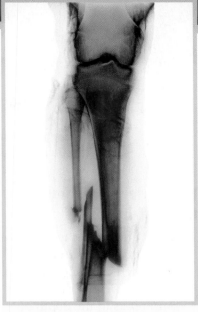

How To Care For Fractures and Dislocations

▶ Check for bleeding. Cover open wounds with a clean, dry dressing.
▶ Seek medical help.
▶ Stabilize the fracture or dislocation with a splint.

internet connect

www.scilinks.org/health
Topic: Joints and Muscles in the Body
HealthLinks code: HH4090

HEALTH LINKS™ Maintained by the National Science Teachers Association

EXPRESS Lesson REVIEW

1. Explain the difference between a fracture, a dislocation, a strain, and a sprain.

2. What danger exists in moving a person with a neck or spinal injury?

3. **LIFE SKILL** **Practicing Wellness** Make a list of things in your home that could be used for splints. Identify objects of various sizes.

Burns

Recognizing burns and giving proper, immediate burn treatment will reduce tissue damage and relieve pain.

What are the different types of burns?

Burns are injuries to the skin and other tissues caused by heat, chemicals, electricity, or radiation. The degree of a burn refers to the depth of tissue damage.

▶ **First-degree burns** are burns that affect only the outer layer of the skin and look pink. First-degree burns include minor sunburns and burns caused by a very short exposure to intense heat, such as an explosion. First-degree burns take about 3 to 6 days to heal, and they heal without scarring.

▶ **Second-degree burns** are burns that extend into the inner skin layer and are red, swollen, and blistered. Second-degree burns are caused by brief exposures to flashes of intense heat, such as spilling hot liquid on yourself or grabbing a curling iron by the heated end. Second-degree burns usually take less than 3 weeks to heal. Deeper second-degree burns may take longer to heal. Scarring is possible if the wounds are not treated properly.

Recognizing and Treating Burns

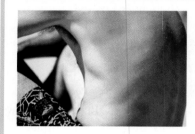

1st degree burn

Treatment
▶ Apply cool water until the pain stops.
▶ Apply moisturizing lotion.

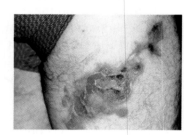

2nd degree burn

Treatment
▶ Apply cool water until the pain stops.
▶ Apply antibacterial ointment.
▶ If burn is severe, seek medical attention.

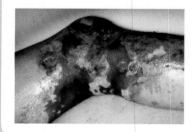

3rd degree burn

Treatment
▶ Cover with a clean, dry cloth.
▶ Treat victim for shock (raise feet if safe; cover with blanket)
▶ Seek medical attention immediately.

▶ **Third-degree burns** are full-thickness burns. They penetrate all skin layers as well as tissue beneath the skin. These burns appear pearly white, tan colored, or charred. Third-degree burns are caused by extended exposure to steam or fire or to immersion in scalding water.

There is usually no immediate pain because of damage done to underlying nerves, but there is severe pain later. A skin graft must be performed if healing is to occur. Some scarring is inevitable, and these burns can take months to heal.

What should I do if I or someone else receives a burn?

For first- and second-degree burns, cool the burn immediately. Do this by immersing the burn in cool water, pouring cool water over the burn, or covering the burn with a clean, cool, wet cloth. Cool the burn until it is pain free both in and out of water.

You may apply a moisturizing ointment to a first-degree burn. It may be appropriate to apply an antibiotic cream to a second-degree burn.

For third-degree burns, cover the burn with a clean cloth. (Do not cool the burn.) Treat the victim for possible shock.

What are the major sources of burns?

There are three major sources of burns. The source of the burn will influence how it should be treated.

1. **Thermal burns** Thermal burns are caused by contact with open flames, hot liquids or surfaces, or other sources of high heat.
2. **Chemical burns** Contact with certain chemicals can burn the skin.
3. **Electrical burns** Direct exposure to electricity can also cause burns.

Do I treat thermal, chemical, and electrical burns in the same way?

No. For thermal burns, remove the victim from the heat source and cool the burn with water. Check for bleeding and for shock, and seek professional medical attention immediately.

Chemical burns caused by liquid chemicals should be flushed with large amounts of cool water to remove the chemical from the body. For chemical burns caused by dry or powdered chemicals, brush the chemical off of the skin with a clean cloth. Water may activate a dry chemical and cause more damage than has already occurred.

For electrical burns involving an appliance, shut off the current to the house. Be sure the area is safe before approaching. Cool the burn with cool water. Check the victim's breathing, and stop any bleeding. Treat for shock if necessary, and seek professional medical attention immediately.

Special Considerations for Burns

▶ **Obtain medical attention immediately for severe second-degree burns, third-degree burns, chemical burns, or electrical burns.**

▶ **Seek medical attention for severe sunburns.**

▶ **Never apply ointment or cream to a severe burn.**

▶ **Never try to remove clothing that is stuck to a burn wound.**

▶ **Always treat burns on the face, hands, and feet as severe, and seek prompt medical attention.**

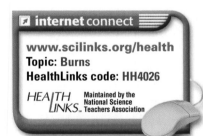

internet connect

www.scilinks.org/health
Topic: Burns
HealthLinks code: HH4026

HEALTH LINKS. Maintained by the National Science Teachers Association

EXPRESS Lesson REVIEW

1. Differentiate between the first, second, and third degree burns.
2. What is the first thing you should do to treat first- and second-degree burns?
3. **LIFE SKILL** **Practicing Wellness** List three ways that you can prevent thermal, chemical, and electrical burns in your home.

Poisons

In 2000, over 2 million poisonings were reported by poison control centers in the United States. Nearly all poisonings happen in the home, and over half occur among young children.

What are the different types of poisoning?

A **poison** is a substance that can cause illness or death when taken into the body. Poisons can be swallowed (ingested), inhaled, absorbed through the skin by contact, or can occur as a result of being bitten or stung by an insect or animal. The table shows these types of poisonings.

What are the signs of poisoning?

Suspect poisoning whenever someone becomes ill suddenly and for no apparent reason. Search for clues, such as chemical odors, leftover food, or suspicious containers. Any poisoning victim may lose consciousness and have trouble breathing, but other signs and symptoms depend on the poison and how it entered the body.

Signs and symptoms of ingested poisons include nausea, vomiting, abdominal cramps, diarrhea, discoloration of the lips, burns in and around the mouth, and an odor on the breath.

Signs and symptoms of inhaled poisons include breathing difficulty, coughing, chest pain, headache, and dizziness.

Signs and symptoms of contact poisons include reddening of the skin, blisters, swelling, and burns. Poisons injected through the skin usually irritate the spot where they were injected.

Types of Poisoning and Their Possible Sources

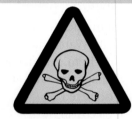

Inhalation

Possible Sources
▶ paints   ▶ gasoline
▶ solvents   ▶ glue
▶ toxic gases

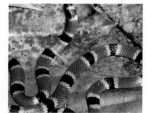

Bites and stings

Possible Sources
▶ bites from spiders, snakes, etc.   ▶ stings from wasps, bees, hornets, and scorpions

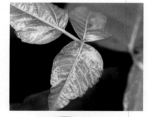

Contact

Possible Sources
▶ chemicals   ▶ plants

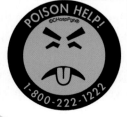

POISON HELP!
©CHospPgh®
1-800-222-1222

Ingestion

Possible Sources
▶ medications   ▶ chemicals
▶ household products   ▶ certain plants

What should I do if someone has been poisoned?

Poisoning is a medical emergency. You should call 911 immediately, then call the **Poison Control Center** in your area, or the American Association of Poison Control Centers at 1-800-222-1222. Staff there can judge the seriousness of the poisoning and provide advice.

If you suspect inhaled poisoning, move the victim away from the poison and into fresh air immediately. Seek medical help promptly if the victim is unconscious. Take the container of the suspected poison along with you to the emergency room to aid the staff in treating the poisoning. Check the victim's ABCs. **(See the Express Lesson "Responding to a Medical Emergency" on p. 576).**

If you need to give rescue breaths or administer CPR (if you are certified in this technique), be certain that no poison is on the victim's mouth. **(See the Express Lesson "CPR" on p. 582.)** If so, hold the victim's mouth closed, seal your mouth around the victim's nose, and provide rescue breaths through the nose. Open the victim's mouth to allow him or her to "exhale." **(See the Express Lesson "Rescue Breathing" on p. 580).**

How can I prevent poisonings from occurring in my home?

There are many areas of the home where poisonings can occur. Taking precautions can help stop poisonings from occurring. In households with small children, install child-safety latches on all cabinets and drawers containing harmful products.

Kitchen Keep products in original containers and out of reach of children. This includes detergents and other cleaning products.

Bathroom Keep all medications in their original, child-proof containers. Discard all old medications. Keep all medications, cosmetics, petrochemical-based lotions, and grooming products out of reach of children.

Garage Keep all products in their original containers with their original labels. Lock up all harmful products, or at least place them out of reach of children. This includes gasoline and other products for your car, solvents, and pesticides.

The best way to avoid an accidental poisoning is to avoid exposure to sources of poison.

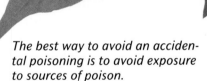
internet connect

www.scilinks.org/health
Topic: Poisons
HealthLinks code: HH4114

HEALTH LINKS. Maintained by the National Science Teachers Association

EXPRESS Lesson REVIEW

1. Find the number of the poison control center in your area. Post this number at home and at school.

2. List the steps you should follow to help an individual who appears to have been poisoned.

3. **LIFE SKILL** **Practicing Wellness** Make a list of things in your home that may be considered poisons and where they are located. What can be done to keep these items from small children? Check your responses with information you obtain from the poison control center.

Motor Vehicle Safety

Brittany read the headlines: "Automobile accidents are the leading cause of death for 15- to 20-year-olds." She wondered what she could do to drive more safely.

What factor contributes most often to automobile accidents?

The factor that contributes most often to automobile accidents is driver behavior. Unsafe driving behavior may be due to a lack of driving skills or due to inexperience behind the wheel. Therefore, it is important for young drivers to take a driver education course and to gain driving experience with a skilled driver in the car. Additionally, driving behaviors that should be avoided include speeding, aggressiveness, impaired driving, and distractions such as cell phones and adjusting stereos.

Speeding The greater the speed of a car, the longer it takes to stop. Therefore, driving more slowly helps a driver avoid crashes because he or she can stop more quickly. Although many automobile accidents occur at low speeds, these accidents are more likely to result only in injuries or property damage. Accidents occurring at 45 miles per hour (mph) or faster are more likely to result in death than those occurring under 45 mph.

Aggressiveness Aggressive drivers not only speed but also tend to tailgate, make frequent or unsafe lane changes, disregard traffic signals, fail to signal when changing lanes or making turns, and fail to yield the right of way. These behaviors are all unsafe driving practices. They increase the chances of having an automobile accident.

Impaired Driving Alcohol, other drugs, and sleepiness can impair driving abilities. The chances of being involved in a car crash and the seriousness of a crash increase with alcohol involvement. Additionally, drivers who have been drinking are less likely to use seat belts. Wearing seat belts cuts the risk of dying in car crashes in half. Young people are also at risk for drowsy-driving crashes. Drivers aged 29 years and younger are involved in nearly two-thirds of all drowsy-driving crashes.

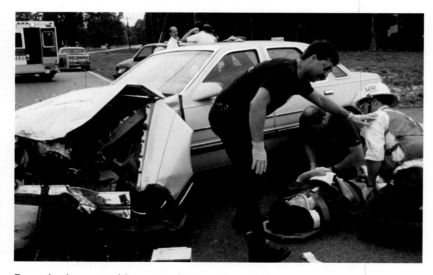

Even single car accidents can be very devastating.

What does it mean to be a "defensive driver"?

A *defensive driver* practices behaviors that help avoid car crashes. Follow these steps to be a defensive driver:

▶ Do not drive while under the influence of alcohol or other drugs that may impair your reflexes, judgment, and ability to stay awake.

▶ Avoid fatigue by getting plenty of rest. On long drives, stop at least once every three hours and rotate drivers.

▶ Stay far behind the car in front of you. Leave at least 1 car length for every 10 mph you are traveling. When roads are wet, snowy, or icy, leave more room.

▶ Drive within posted speed limits, and slow down during poor weather. Use your directional signals when making turns and changing lanes. Obey all traffic laws.

▶ Continually monitor the road for pedestrians, cyclists, stopped vehicles, or other persons or obstacles. Be aware of the space around you to determine where you could move if a person or obstacle suddenly appeared.

▶ Be a courteous driver. If someone else makes unwanted gestures or unsafe driving maneuvers near you, avoid that driver. Do not engage in unsafe driving practices for revenge.

What else can I do to keep myself and others safe when I am driving?

1. **Maintain your vehicle properly.** Complete maintenance and safety checks as suggested by the manufacturer. Be certain that your tires are appropriate for the weather conditions in your area.

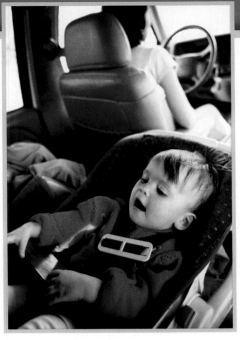

All persons traveling in a vehicle should use proper safety restraints.

2. **Insist that all passengers in your vehicle wear seat belts.** Put children under 12 years in the back seat, away from air bags. Use child safety seats according to manufacturer's instructions. Persons in the front seat should sit back 10 inches from air bags.

3. **Plan your route.** Be sure that you are familiar with maps and directions in order to avoid confusion. For long trips, tell others what your route is and when you plan to depart and arrive.

4. **Have necessary emergency and first-aid equipment in the car.** See the list "Things You Should Carry in Your Car."

Things You Should Carry in Your Car

In all types of weather:

▶ Flashlight
▶ Jumper cables
▶ Warning devices
▶ First-aid Kit
▶ Cell phone

In addition, in cold and snowy conditions:

▶ Shovel
▶ Ice scraper/snow brush
▶ Sand, kitty litter, or traction mats
▶ Blanket(s)

In addition, for long trips:

▶ Water
▶ Food
▶ Medications, if needed

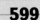

Are there any unique safety concerns for driving a motorcycle?

Yes, a motorcycle provides no protection for its driver or passenger, unlike a car. A motorcyclist has no vehicle surrounding him or her, no air bag, and no seat belts.

If a motorcycle crashes, the persons on the motorcycle are ejected. Therefore, motorcyclists should wear

▶ protective clothing, including a properly designed helmet and eye protection

▶ a leather or heavy denim jacket

▶ long pants and gloves

▶ sturdy low-heeled boots that extend above the ankles.

Motorcycles are also less visible than cars. Motorcyclists can increase their visibility by wearing brightly colored clothing and applying reflective material to their motorcycles and helmets. Also, motorcyclists should have their vehicle lights on when operating the motorcycle, even in the daylight.

Along with following the defensive driving tips mentioned previously, motorcyclists should be particularly watchful at intersections, where most motorcycle-automobile collisions occur.

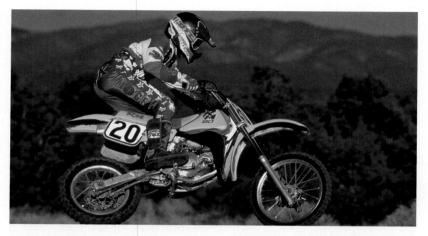

Motor Vehicle Safety

▶ Operate the vehicle only if you are skilled and experienced and have a required license.

▶ Operate the vehicle at reasonable speeds.

▶ Operate the vehicle in a courteous and defensive manner, not in an aggressive manner.

▶ Do not operate the vehicle while drowsy or under the influence of alcohol or other drugs.

▶ Wear protective clothing, headgear, and footgear when operating open vehicles.

▶ Be certain that your vehicle is in proper working condition.

What can I do to be safer on a motorcycle?

Additionally, many of the causes of motorcycle crashes are linked to the driver's inexperience or inability to handle the vehicle properly. Therefore, motorcyclists should attend motorcycle training courses prior to obtaining their motorcycle licenses.

What safety precautions should I take when operating recreational vehicles?

Before using any recreational vehicle, such as a snowmobile, mini-bike, personal watercraft, or all-terrain vehicle, be sure that it is in top-notch mechanical condition. If your vehicle is small, use a safety flag to help others see you.

Wear protective clothing appropriate for the weather and the vehicle, and check weather reports before you leave. When riding any of these vehicles, wear a helmet with goggles or a face shield to protect yourself from flying debris, such as twigs, stones, and ice chips. Avoid trailing clothing, such as a long scarf, which can get caught in vehicle parts.

What do I need to know about the terrain I will drive over?

If you are unfamiliar with the terrain over which you'll be riding, discuss its characteristics with someone who has traveled it. If you are riding over frozen lakes, ponds, or streams, be sure that the ice is thick enough to support your weight and that of your vehicle. On a personal watercraft, it is important to know where tree stumps or other obstacles may lie hidden in the water. Always ride with another person; never ride alone.

As with the operation of other types of vehicles, do not operate recreational vehicles while under the influence of alcohol or drugs or while drowsy. And before you drive a recreational vehicle, receive instruction from an experienced driver.

Are there any general rules for driving that apply to all motor vehicles?

Yes, some rules that apply when driving any type of motor vehicle are as follows:

▶ **Don't eat while you are driving.** You can't pay full attention to the road when you are trying to handle food. If you have something to drink, make sure you have a proper cup holder and a cup that has a lid.

▶ **Don't wear headphones.** It is difficult to hear what is going on around you in traffic even if you have the volume turned down low.

▶ **Don't talk on the phone while you are driving.** If you need to talk on the phone, pull over to a safe area on the side of the road or into a rest stop.

▶ **Don't look down, even for a second.** If you drop something on the floor, pull over to a safe area on the side of the road to pick it up, or do without it until you stop.

▶ **Don't try to tend to children in the back seat while you are driving.** Again, pull over to a safe area and tend to the children.

▶ **Don't drive if your vision is obstructed.** If it is raining too hard to be able to see, pull over to a safe area and wait for the rain to subside. Turn your hazard lights on if you pull over to the side of the road so that you will be visible to other drivers.

Your windshield may become covered with bugs, pollen, dirt, or other things that can obstruct your vision.

Clean your windshield each time you put gas in your car, and carry some window cleaner and paper towels along in your car for emergencies.

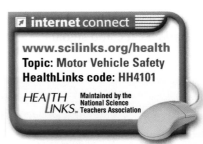

internet connect
www.scilinks.org/health
Topic: Motor Vehicle Safety
HealthLinks code: HH4101
HEALTH LINKS Maintained by the National Science Teachers Association

---

EXPRESS Lesson REVIEW

1. List and describe three unsafe driver behaviors.
2. List three things you should do to protect yourself while operating a small, open vehicle that you would not have to do while driving a car. Explain.
3. **LIFE SKILL** **Making GREAT Decisions** While driving on the highway, a passing motorist makes an angry gesture toward you because you are driving 5 mph below the speed limit. How should you respond?

Home and Workplace Safety

Because most people spend their days at home or work, it is no surprise that many unintentional injuries occur in these places.

What are the most common types of unintentional injuries in the home?

The most common types of unintentional injuries in the home are electrocution, suffocation, and injuries from fires and falls. **Electrocution** is a fatal injury caused by electricity entering the body and destroying vital tissues. **Suffocation** is a fatal injury caused by an inability to breathe when the nose and mouth are blocked or when the body becomes oxygen-deficient.

What can I do to help prevent unintentional injuries in my home?

Preventing Injuries from Fires First, prevent fires from occurring. Never leave the stove unattended when cooking. Be sure that portable heaters are 3 feet from anything that can burn, and never leave them on when you go out or go to bed. Keep matches and lighters away from children. Unplug and repair any electrical appliance that has an unusual smell, and do not overload electrical outlets.

Second, plan your escape route from every room in the house and where everyone will meet outside. If your clothes catch fire when you are escaping, stop, drop, and roll. Crawl out of the house to avoid breathing smoke and poisonous gases. Install smoke detectors on every floor of your home, test them periodically, and change the batteries once a year.

Preventing Injuries from Falls About 40 percent of fall-related deaths occur in the home. Some of the things you can do to help prevent falls include installing handrails on stairways; getting rid of clutter on stairs and floors; keeping lamp, extension, telephone, and other cords out of walkways; and refinishing slippery surfaces.

Preventing Suffocation This type of unintentional injury occurs most frequently with infants and small children. To lower the risk, be sure that infant bedding is safe. Use a firm, flat mattress that fits the crib snugly. Do not use pillows and comforters. Additionally, make sure that no places exist that a small child

could enter, become trapped, and suffocate, such as a lidded toy chest, an old refrigerator, or an unlocked car trunk. And finally, keep all plastic bags out of the reach of infants and small children.

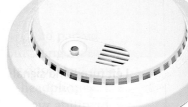

Test your fire detectors regularly.

Unplug all appliances that are near water.

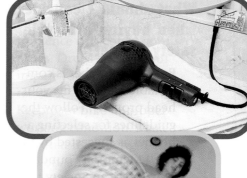

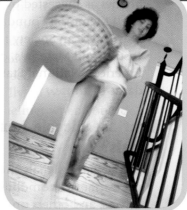

Clean up clutter on stairs and floors.

Preventing Electrocution

One aid to preventing electrocution is the ground fault circuit interrupter (GFCI). A GFCI turns off electricity before electrocution can occur. Install and test GFCI outlets or plug-ins in places where both water and electricity are used, such as kitchens and bathrooms. When small electrical appliances are not in use, unplug them. And never reach into water to get an appliance unless it is unplugged. If small children are in the house, cover unused electrical outlets with child-safety plugs. Finally, do not remove the grounding pin (third prong) from power tools or other electrical items. Instead, use a three-prong adapter to connect a three-prong plug to a two-hole outlet.

What are the most common types of unintentional injuries in the workplace?

The most common types of unintentional injuries in the workplace are the result of a travel-related accident. Workers are also injured from falls, from fires and explosions, by exposure to harmful substances, and by contact with equipment or electricity.

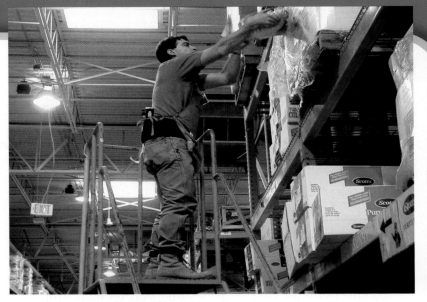
Every workplace has its own safety concerns.

What responsibilities do employers have regarding safety in the workplace?

The **Occupational Safety and Health Administration (OSHA)** is a government agency created to prevent work-related injuries, illness, and death. Since the creation of OSHA in 1970, work-related injuries have dropped by 40 percent and work-related deaths have been cut in half. Employers must obey OSHA regulations, properly train workers, and provide appropriate safety gear.

What responsibilities do employees have regarding safety in the workplace?

Employees are expected to follow OSHA and employer health and safety guidelines. They are expected to wear or use the protective equipment given them, report hazardous conditions, and report and seek treatment for job-related injuries or illnesses.

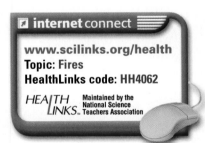

🖳 **internet** connect 〓

www.scilinks.org/health
Topic: Fires
HealthLinks code: HH4062

HEALTH LINKS™ Maintained by the National Science Teachers Association

EXPRESS Lesson REVIEW

1. What safety concerns are particularly relevant in homes with small children?

2. **LIFE SKILL** **Communicating Effectively** Describe what you would do if you saw a co-worker committing serious safety violations at work.

EXPRESS Lesson

Gun Safety Awareness

While Ashley was jogging along a path in the woods, she spotted a gun among the leaves under a tree. The gun scared her, and she wasn't sure what she should do.

What should I do if I find a gun?

If you find a gun, do NOT touch it. Also, do not disturb anything in the area surrounding it. Along with being unsafe to handle, the gun may be evidence in a crime. Other things in the area may provide evidence as well. Note landmarks so that you can lead the police to the location. Leave the area and call the police, or have a responsible adult call the police.

Where can I enroll in a gun safety class?

There are many groups throughout the country that offer courses in firearm safety as well as many other courses. These firearm safety courses explain how different types of firearms operate and how to handle and store them safely. To find firearm safety classes in your area, contact your local wildlife conservation office or local law enforcement agency.

What are safe ways to store guns?

Firearms should be stored so that unauthorized persons, such as children, cannot use them. First, firearms should be stored separately from their ammunition. Second, firearms should be stored in a locked gun case, gun cabinet, or safe. Unloaded guns may be stored with a locking safety cable or a **trigger lock,** a device that helps prevent a gun from being fired. However, even with these safety devices, a firearm can sometimes still be fired, so always be cautious.

How do I increase my safety while walking in the woods during hunting season?

Try to avoid walking in hunting areas during hunting season. If you must, carry a whistle. If you hear shots, blow the whistle until the hunter acknowledges your presence and leaves the area. Avoid being mistaken for game by wearing bright colors, such as blaze orange or fluorescent yellow.

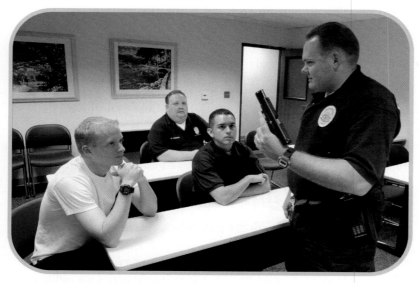

Always respect firearms, and take a firearm safety course.

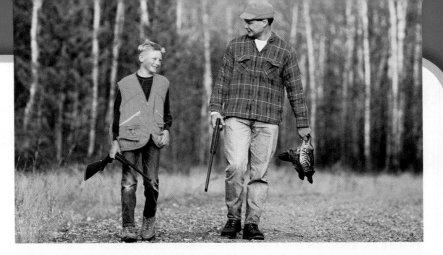

In the movies and on TV, I see people fire guns into the air. Is that safe?

No. A bullet fired upward will come down. It could severely wound someone on its descent. This is especially dangerous in urban areas and in crowds.

I inherited a gun from my grandfather. Is it safe to shoot?

You cannot know whether a used gun from any source is safe to shoot. The gun could misfire, causing severe injury. Always take a used gun to a reputable gunsmith who can determine its safety and make any repairs that may be necessary.

Why do I need to wear ear and eye protection when firing a gun?

Exposure to gunfire can cause hearing damage or loss if proper ear protection is not worn. Different types of hearing protection devices can be purchased at sporting goods and drug stores. Additionally, guns can emit debris and hot gas when fired. These substances can cause eye injury without the protection of proper shooting glasses.

Firearm Safety Awareness

Mishaps with guns can be avoided by following some basic safety rules, which include the following:

▶ Never point a loaded or unloaded gun at anything you do not want to shoot.

▶ When handling a gun, always point the barrel in a safe direction.

▶ Keep the safety on until you are ready to shoot.

▶ Keep firearms and ammunition stored separately under lock and key and away from children.

▶ Know how to use a firearm safely; enroll in a firearm safety course.

▶ Wear eye and ear protection when shooting.

▶ Keep a record of firearm serial and model numbers stored in a secure place.

▶ Know and obey all gun laws for your state.

▶ Make sure you are aware of what lies in front of and beyond your target.

▶ Never use alcohol or other drugs prior to or when shooting.

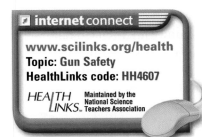

internet connect

www.scilinks.org/health
Topic: Gun Safety
HealthLinks code: HH4607

HEALTH LINKS Maintained by the National Science Teachers Association

EXPRESS Lesson REVIEW

1. Describe a safe way to store a gun.
2. List four rules for the safe use of firearms.
3. **LIFE SKILL** **Using Community Resources** Speak with a policeman, a judge, or another official in your community to find out about local gun laws.

Safety in Weather Disasters

Every year about 800 tornadoes occur in the United States. Knowing what to do in tornadoes or other hazardous weather conditions could mean the difference between life and death.

What is meant by the terms hazardous weather and natural disaster?

Weather is the state of the atmosphere at a particular place and time. It includes factors such as temperature, cloudiness, sunshine, wind, and precipitation. **Hazardous weather** is dangerous weather that causes concerns for safety. It puts property and human life in peril. Hazardous weather may result in a natural disaster. A **natural disaster** is a natural event that causes widespread injury, death, and property damage. An example of a natural disaster produced by weather is the severe flooding of a city. An example of a nonweather-related natural disaster is widespread destruction resulting from an earthquake.

What should I do to remain safe from lightning?

Lightning is caused when there is a separation of different charges. For cloud-to-ground lightning, the ground has an excess of positive charges, and clouds usually have negative charges. Just as a spark can jump from your finger to a doorknob to reunite separate charges, a lightning bolt can result.

A lightning bolt can strike when a storm is approaching, during a storm, and after a storm has passed. If you can hear thunder, you are close enough to be struck by lightning.

To reduce your risk of being struck by lightning, avoid being

▶ the tallest thing in the area (as in standing in an open field) or near the tallest thing, such as a lone tree

▶ near metal things, such as metal fences or buildings

▶ in a small, open structure, such as a baseball dugout or a gazebo

▶ near water

Seek shelter inside a large, enclosed structure or inside a car or school bus. When inside, avoid water and conductive substances. Therefore, do not use the phone, put any part of your body in water, or touch metal doors or window frames during a storm.

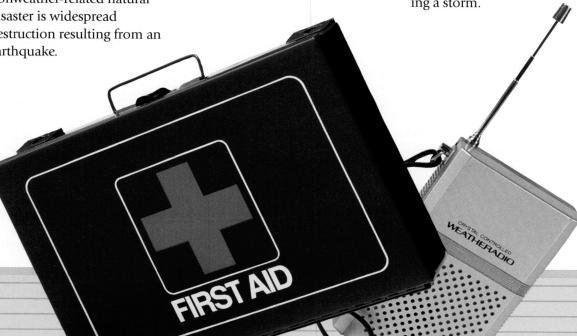

How do I know if a tornado is likely to strike?

A tornado is a violently rotating funnel-shaped column of air associated with a thunderstorm. The National Weather Service (NWS) issues a *tornado watch* when tornadoes are possible in an area. The NWS issues a *tornado warning* when a tornado has been sighted or indicated by weather radar. However, a tornado may develop quickly, without warning. Or you may not hear the warning. Therefore, look for these tornado signs: dark, greenish sky; large hail; and a loud roar. You may or may not be able to see the tornado.

What safety measures should I take if a tornado is likely to strike?

If a tornado warning has been issued or you see signs of a coming tornado, go immediately to an underground shelter, a basement, or a small interior room without windows on the lowest floor. Stay away from windows and corners. If you are in a mobile home, leave it and seek shelter in a nonmobile building. If you are in a car, seek shelter in a building if possible. Otherwise, get out of the car and lie in a ditch or other low area, covering your neck and head with your arms.

What do I need to know about safety and hurricanes?

A hurricane is a type of storm that forms over tropical areas of oceans. However, it can move inland along the coastline.

In the United States, hurricane season runs from June through November. In a hurricane, rain is heavy and winds blow greater than 75 miles per hour.

A *hurricane watch* means hurricane conditions are possible within 36 hours.

A *hurricane warning* means hurricane conditions are expected within 24 hours.

If you live in or visit hurricane-prone areas, be sure to prepare an evacuation plan prior to hurricane watches or warnings.

If a hurricane watch or warning has been issued, bring in all outdoor items that could be blown by the wind. If a hurricane warning has been issued, listen to the radio or television for evacuation instructions.

Close hurricane shutters or board windows from the outside with plywood. If you do not have to evacuate, stay indoors and away from windows.

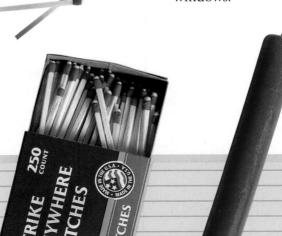

Items Needed During Any Weather Emergency

- ▶ weather radio or other battery-powered radio or television
- ▶ battery-powered lights and flashlights
- ▶ candles and dry matches
- ▶ extra batteries
- ▶ gallon of water per person per day for at least 3 days
- ▶ first-aid kit
- ▶ medicines family members might need
- ▶ blankets and/or sleeping bags
- ▶ canned food and a manual can opener

Safety in Weather Disasters *continued*

What should you do in case of a blizzard?

A blizzard is a heavy snowstorm with high winds and dangerous wind chill. If you live in or visit an area prone to severe winter weather, be sure that each family member has a warm coat and hat, insulated gloves or mittens, and water-resistant boots. Add extra blankets to your weather emergency items (see list).

A *winter storm watch* means a winter storm is possible in your area. A *winter storm warning* (or *blizzard warning*) means that a winter storm (or blizzard) is headed for your area.

If a winter storm watch is issued, listen to the radio or television for updates, and note any change in weather conditions. If a winter storm warning is issued, stay indoors if possible, wear layers warm of clothing and cover your nose and mouth if you go outside, and avoid travel by car. If you do travel by car, keep emergency items in the trunk, tell someone when you are leaving and where you are going, and carry a cell phone to call for help should you get stuck.

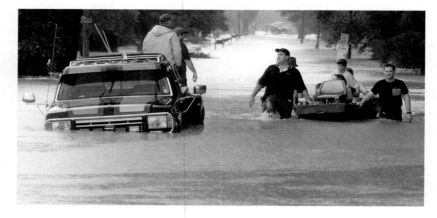

What do you need to know about safety and floods?

Floods occur when water accumulates faster than the soil can absorb it or rivers can carry it away. If you live in a flood-prone area, add raingear to your weather emergency items (see list). During periods of heavy or prolonged rain, listen to the radio or television for flood information. A *flood watch* means a flood is possible.

A *flood warning* means flooding is already occurring or will occur soon.

If you live in or visit flood-prone areas, be sure to prepare an evacuation plan prior to flood watches or warnings. Check for flash flooding (sudden flooding) in your area. When a flood warning is issued, evacuate immediately. Move to higher ground. If your car stalls in rising water, abandon it and walk or climb to higher ground.

EXPRESS Lesson REVIEW

1. Make a list of at least seven things that you and your family should have ready in case of a weather-related emergency.
2. What should you do if you think that a tornado might be approaching?
3. **LIFE SKILL** **Using Community Resources** Find out how to get emergency weather information in your community.
4. For which types of weather-related emergencies should you have a pre-planned evacuation route and destination?
5. In general, what is the difference between a weather-related watch and a warning?
6. What is the best course of action to avoid being struck by lightning?

EXPRESS Lesson

Recreational Safety

Recreational activities are meant to be fun, relaxing, and good exercise. However, many people are injured each year during these activities because they fail to follow a few safety precautions.

What should I know about safety and water sports?

Water sports include swimming, diving, and watercraft sports. To be safe while swimming, do the following:

▶ Always swim with a buddy.

▶ Do not swim in unknown waters or where "no swimming" or other swimming warning signs are posted.

▶ Do not swim outdoors when an electrical storm is approaching.

▶ Avoid swimming in frigid water; it could cause your body temperature to drop.

▶ Avoid running and horseplay near water. Slips and falls can cause serious injury.

▶ Never throw anyone into a pool headfirst.

▶ Wear a life jacket and swim in shallow water if you are just learning to swim.

▶ Learn drownproofing, a survival floating technique.

▶ Do not swim while under the influence of alcohol or other drugs.

▶ Never dive into water that may be shallow or have concealed hazards, such as tree stumps or rocks.

Four Stages of Drownproofing

1 Relax while you float with your face in the water, and dangle your arms and legs freely.

2 After a few seconds, slowly raise your arms, separate your legs, raise your head so your mouth is out of the water, and exhale.

3 Slowly press your arms down, bring your legs together, and raise your head well out of the water. Take a big slow breath.

4 Slowly relax your body to the natural floating position.

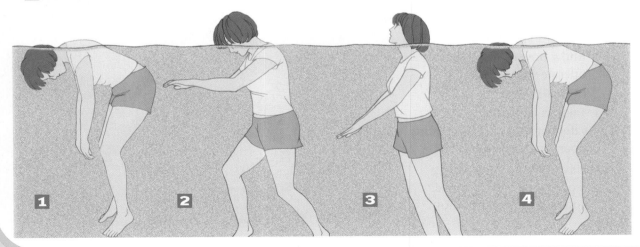

Recreational Safety *continued*

What should I know about diving into water?

There are certain things you need to consider before diving into water. To be safe while diving, dive only into water you are certain is deep enough and free of obstructions. In pools, the water must be a minimum of six feet deep for a dive.

If you swim and dive in natural bodies of water, remember that water levels may change. Therefore, walk into the water first, and check water depth. Also check for hidden objects in the diving area. Do not dive in unfamiliar waters.

What should I know about operating personal watercraft?

Here are some general safety tips for persons operating watercraft, such as motorboats, personal watercraft, canoes, and kayaks.

▶ Make sure that the watercraft is working properly.

▶ Know how to navigate and operate your watercraft properly.

▶ Take an approved water safety or boating class before operating any watercraft.

▶ Have all safety equipment required by law on board and in working condition.

▶ Always wear a life jacket, and be sure that it fits properly.

▶ Tell a friend or relative where you will be.

▶ If you are in a motorized boat, maintain a safe speed at all times.

▶ Be alert for changing weather conditions, and head to shore if conditions look threatening.

▶ Always scan the waterway in the front and on the sides of you, giving a wide berth to other watercraft.

▶ Obey federal and state boating laws and laws applying to other types of watercraft.

▶ Never operate a watercraft while under the influence of alcohol or other drugs.

How can I keep myself safe when playing sports?

There are a few general safety tips to keep in mind to play any sport safely. Always make sure to warm up before and cool down after your activities. Warming up helps your muscles to extend easily, your joints to be more flexible, and your heart and breathing rates to increase gradually. Cooling down slows your heart rate, relaxes your muscles, and helps your body recover from the stress of the physical activity. Warming up and cooling down may reduce the likelihood of injuries.

Wearing the proper safety gear when doing any sport is essential.

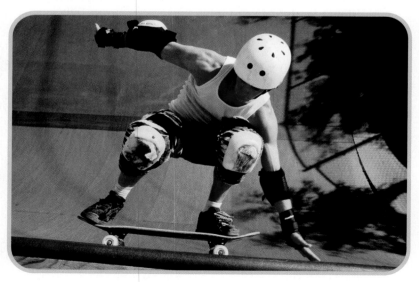

Another general safety rule for sports activities is to wear the proper safety equipment. Many sports, such as biking, football, ice hockey, and skateboarding, require helmets. A helmet that fits well touches your head all around, is comfortably snug but not tight, and should not move more than an inch in any direction. Other types of safety equipment are specific to the sport, such as knee pads and elbow pads for skateboarding, riding scooters, and inline skating.

What should I know about safety in the wilderness?

If you will be hiking or camping in the wilderness, it is essential to have proper training. Take an approved wilderness-survival and first-aid course to learn how to handle serious emergencies. Plan your trip carefully. Know the trail conditions and weather forecasts before you set out. Bring water with you but also know the water availability and quality where you will be.

Leave detailed plans of your trip with a responsible adult, including when you will return. Bring a cell phone, emergency numbers, and a weather radio with you, and carry a whistle and a small mirror for emergency use. Always have a map of

Containing a campfire is important to your safety as well as preserving the surroundings

the area and a compass. Bring the proper camping equipment for the terrain and weather conditions. Wear sturdy hiking boots and appropriate hiking clothes along with sunscreen, insect repellent, sunglasses, and a hat. Additionally, carry extra food and water, a flashlight with extra batteries, a first-aid kit, a fire starter, and matches.

Learn to build, maintain, and extinguish campfires so that they do not pose a forest fire danger. Some tips include the following:

▶ Check that fires are permitted where you will be camping.

▶ Clear an area 3 feet wide of dead leaves and debris around the site of the fire.

▶ Do not build fires under overhanging tree branches.

▶ Find an area shielded from strong winds.

▶ Never leave the fire unattended.

▶ Extinguish a campfire with water or dirt.

▶ Before you leave the area, feel for heat from the fire. Be certain that it is out and completely cool.

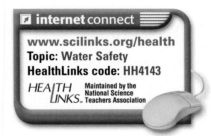

internet connect
www.scilinks.org/health
Topic: Water Safety
HealthLinks code: HH4143
HEALTH LINKS. Maintained by the National Science Teachers Association

EXPRESS Lesson REVIEW

1. List the basic safety guidelines you should observe while playing sports.

2. What are some things that should cause you to cancel an activity involving a watercraft?

3. **LIFE SKILL** **Practicing Wellness** Choose your favorite recreational activity. Discuss things that can affect your safety doing this activity, such as the weather.

4. John and his family own a cottage at a lake. John likes to run the length of the pier and dive into the water as soon as they arrive. Why is this unsafe to do?

The 10 Skills for a Healthy Life

Some people have the skills needed for working with computers. Others have the skills for playing music or sports. There are also skills that are needed for leading a healthy life.

What is a healthy life?

A healthy life is a life where the components of health—physical, emotional, social, mental, spiritual and environmental—are in balance. Leading a healthy life requires some skills that are easily learned. The 10 skills for a healthy life are called life skills. **Life skills** are tools for building a healthy life. You will find these life skills throughout this textbook and be able to use them throughout your life. The life skills are identified by this icon:

LIFE SKILL

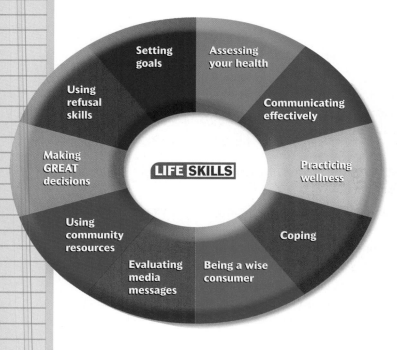

How does each of the 10 life skills help me to lead a healthy life?

LIFE SKILL **Assessing Your Health** This life skill requires that you evaluate the actions and behaviors that affect your health. Learning the things that have negative effects on your health and avoiding them is very important.

LIFE SKILL **Communicating Effectively** This life skill is important in dealing with family, friends, teachers, and anyone else you encounter throughout the day. Communicating effectively will help you to get your point across and avoid misunderstandings with others. You will also learn listening skills. Being able to listen to someone is as important as being able to express yourself.

LIFE SKILL **Practicing Wellness** This life skill will help you practice healthy behaviors, maintain good health, and avoid sickness. You can do this by doing such things as getting enough sleep, choosing nutritious foods, and avoiding risky behaviors.

LIFE SKILL **Coping** Coping means dealing with troubles or problems in an effective way. Things don't always go the way that we would like them to. Accepting this fact is important to your overall health. This life skill will help you deal with emotions such as anger and depression.

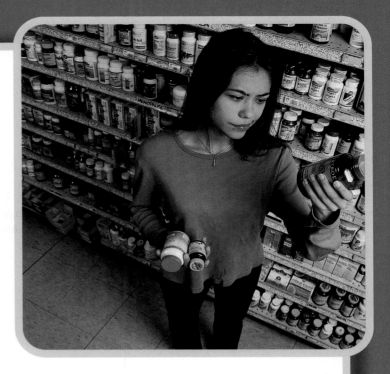

LIFE SKILL **Being a Wise Consumer** A consumer is a person who buys products or services, such as food, clothing, or CDs. A consumer also does things like get his or her car repaired. Being a wise consumer will allow you to buy health care products and services without paying too much money. It will help you decide what products are appropriate for you. It will also help you to determine if the claims an advertiser makes are true or false.

LIFE SKILL **Evaluating Media Messages** The media is all public forms of communication, such as TV, radio, movies, newspaper, and advertising.

Many times you are influenced by messages the media sends. This life skill will give you the tools to analyze media messages so you can make better judgments about the accuracy and validity of the message.

LIFE SKILL **Using Community Resources** A resource is something that can be used to take care of a need. Most communities offer a number of services that can help you maintain good health. This life skill will show you where to find these services and describe how they can keep you healthy.

LIFE SKILL **Making GREAT Decisions** Making decisions is something that you do every day. Making the right decisions can affect every aspect of your life. If you make the wrong decisions, the consequences can be tough. Use the Making GREAT Decisions model to help you make decisions and the STOP process to correct your mistakes.

LIFE SKILL **Using Refusal Skills** A refusal skill is a way you can decline to do something you don't want to do. Learning how to say no to others will help you make better decisions. Base your decisions on your values and on what is best for you— not necessarily what is more fun for you or for others.

LIFE SKILL **Setting Goals** A goal is something that you want to do or hope to achieve in the future. Setting goals helps you stay focused on the future. This life skill will show you how to set your long- and short-term goals.

For more information about the ten skills for a healthy life, see Chapter 2.

Making GREAT Decisions

Should I study for my exam or hang out with friends? Should I get a tattoo? Am I willing to smoke if it makes me look cool?

MAKING GREAT DECISIONS

Give thought to the problem.

Review your choices.

Evaluate the consequences of each choice.

Assess and choose the best choice.

Think it over afterward.

What's so GREAT about decision making?

Every day teens are faced with some very difficult choices. Some of the decisions you make can affect you for the rest of your life. The Making GREAT Decisions model is a tool that you can use to help make these difficult decisions a little easier. Taking the time to consider your goals and values can assist you in making the decisions that are right for you.

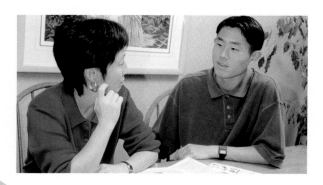

So how does using this model work in the real world?

Imagine you were trying to decide whether you should study for your exam or go to the movies. Look at the table below to see how the Making GREAT Decisions model can guide you through this decision-making process.

GIVE thought to the problem. Stop to think about the situation before making any hasty decisions.

REVIEW your choices. In this case, your choices are to stay home and study or go to the movies.

EVALUATE the consequences of each choice. Staying at home and studying will help you to get a good grade. If you go to the movies and then do poorly on the exam, you may not be allowed to participate in sports and other extracurricular activities.

ASSESS and choose the best choice. Staying home to study will help your grade and keep you out of trouble. If you do poorly on the exam, you'll probably lose privileges

THINK it over afterward. If you decided to study, think about how not only did you improve your chances for a good grade, you can go see the movie later. If you decided to go to the movie, think about how important your grades are and how your decision will affect you down the road.

If I use the Making GREAT Decisions model, will I always make the right decision?

Even if you use the model when you are trying to make a decision, it is still possible (and completely normal!) that you will make a wrong decision.

Sometimes the results of making the wrong decision can be embarrassment or humiliation. Don't worry! The feeling of embarrassment will pass, and friends won't hold your mistake against you or think less of you.

Sometimes, however, making the wrong decision can have serious consequences. When this happens, you can use the **STOP, THINK, GO** process. This process has three simple steps and can be very helpful in turning around the damage caused by a wrong decision. The steps of the process are as follows:

1. **STOP** and admit that you made a wrong decision. Take responsibility for what you've done. Stop whatever it was you were doing that was undesirable. This will help minimize the damage from the wrong decision and will allow you to start taking control of the situation again.

2. **THINK** about with whom you can talk about the problem. Usually a parent, guardian, or other responsible adult can help you. Tell this trusted adult about your decision and what its consequences are. Discuss with them ways to correct the situation, and what the possible outcomes are.

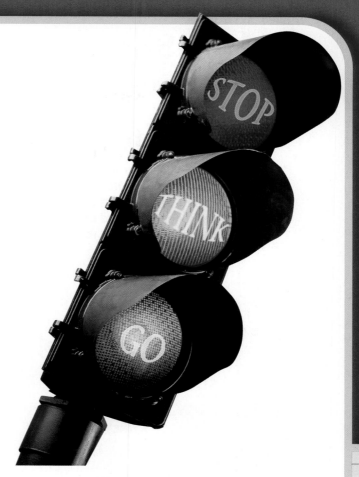

3. **GO** and do your best to correct the situation. Sometimes just walking away is the best way to deal with a situation. It may prevent the problem from getting worse.

Sometimes the only way to correct a situation is to "tell on" someone. Many times the decisions that we make are influenced by the actions of other people. Other times, it may be that you need to apologize to someone that you have hurt. This can be difficult, but both you and the other person will feel better afterward.

 For more information about making GREAT decisions, see Chapter 2.

Using Refusal Skills

Have you ever heard any of the pressure lines below? Every now and then, you may feel pressured to do something that you don't want to do or that goes against your beliefs and values. When you need to stand up to someone, it helps if you already know what you're going to say.

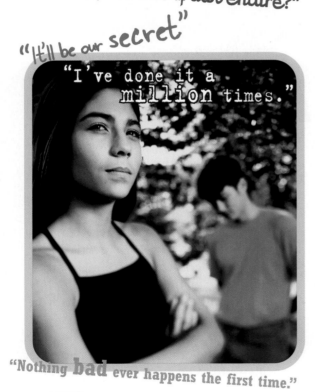

"*Don't be such a baby.*"

"*Where's your sense of adventure?*"

"*It'll be our secret*"

"I've done it a million times."

"Nothing **bad** ever happens the first time."

"**Everyone** is doing it."

How do I stand up to someone who is pressuring me?

Refusal skills are strategies a person can use to avoid doing something they do not want to do. Sometimes, certain strategies are more appropriate for certain situations. Sometimes, you might have to refuse in a couple of different ways for people to accept your answer.

Why do I need to practice using refusal skills?

Most people are a little uncomfortable saying no to their friends. Practicing refusal skills can help you know what to do if you are ever in a "real life" refusal situation. Practicing these skills in low-pressure situations increases the odds that you'll have the confidence to hold your ground when it really matters to you.

How can I resist pressure?

▶ Say no, and mean it. Keep saying no.

▶ Make up an excuse to leave the situation.

▶ Arrange a code beforehand with a parent or someone you trust that indicates that you need to be picked up to get out of a bad situation.

▶ Make a joke out of the situation, and change the subject.

▶ Practice responses like those in the table.

Some things crack under pressure. Will you?

If you hear this . . .	You can say this . . .
Do you always do what your parents tell you to?	Do you HAVE to do everything that everyone else does?
Come on, please? For me?	No! I'm thinking about ME because obviously YOU'RE not!
No one has to know.	I'll know, and that's one too many people for me.
You're just chicken.	It takes a lot more guts to hold out than to give in.
Don't you want to know what it's like?	Sorry guys, but I need to get going.
If you loved me, you'd let me.	If you loved me, you wouldn't ask.

What do I do if someone is pressuring me and won't stop?

The first thing you should do is seek help and advice from a trusted adult. See if the two of you can figure out why someone is so concerned with pressuring you. If the person pressuring you has been a friend in the past, you may need to stop hanging out with him or her. If the person is not a friend, you may need to take steps to try and avoid seeing this person.

How do I say no and still sound cool?

Here are 10 ways to insist that you do things your way:

1. **Blame someone else.** My parents would ground me for life. Besides, it's just not worth it.

2. **Give a reason.** No, my dad said he'll pay me if I stay home and help him.

3. **Ignore the request or the pressure.** Pretend you don't hear them and avoid talking about the issue.

4. **Leave the situation.** Sorry, guys, but I need to get going.

5. **Say no thanks.** No, thanks. I'm just not interested.

6. **Say no, and mean it.** No, I mean it! How many times do I have to say no?

7. **Keep saying no.** How many times do I have to tell you no? Forget it!

8. **Make a joke out of it.** Do you guys HAVE to do everything everyone else does?

9. **Make an excuse.** I can't tonight. I have football practice.

10. **Suggest something else to do.** Why don't we go get some pizza or something else instead?

11. **Change the subject.** So, anyway, what was Angela talking about today at lunch?

12. **Team up with someone.** Sarah and Marcia don't want to go either, so we're going to do something else. Do you want to come with us?

 TOPIC link For more information about practicing refusal skills, see Chapter 2.

10 Tips for Building Self-Esteem

How many times has there been something that you really wanted to do? Maybe you've wanted to try out for the track team or the band, but you just didn't feel like you had what it takes to make it. Feeling confident about yourself and your abilities is one important part of self-esteem.

What is self-esteem?

A very important part of your personality is your self-esteem. Self-esteem is a measure of how much you value, respect, and feel confident about yourself. The better you feel about yourself, the more self-confident you will feel and appear to others.

Where does self-esteem come from?

Self-esteem, as the name implies, comes from within a person. Others may help lift your self-esteem by giving compliments or by cheering you on, but you are the only one that will feel self-esteem's influence. You gain self-esteem by trying new things or by trying to improve the things that you already do.

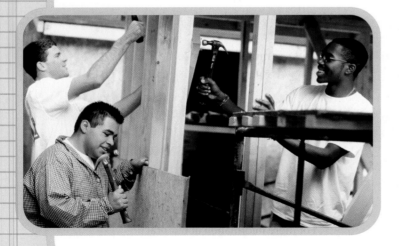

What are the benefits of high self-esteem?

People who have high self-esteem respect themselves and take better care of themselves. They are more likely to stick with their goals and try new things. People who have high self-esteem are also more likely to be valuable members of their family, school, and community.

How can I improve my self-esteem?

There are many ways that you can build your self-esteem.

1. **Make a list of your strengths and weaknesses.** Identify the things you are successful at and try to find time to do those things.

2. **Develop a support system of friends.** Choose friends who will support you and encourage you to do your best. Avoid people who put you down, even if they are joking.

3. **Practice positive self-talk.** Substitute positive thoughts like "I'll figure this out" for negative thoughts like "I'll never figure out how to do this."

4. **Practice good health habits.** A healthy diet, regular exercise, and good grooming habits will help you feel good about yourself. If you look bad, you'll probably feel bad.

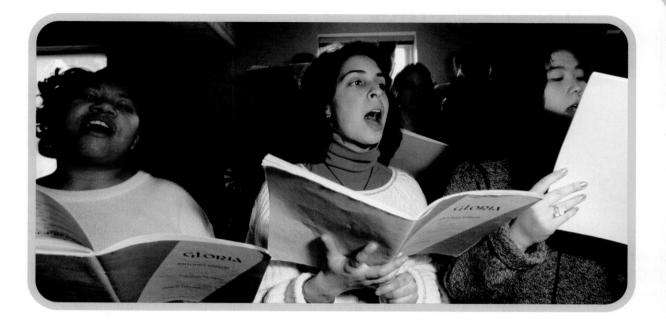

5. **Avoid doing things just to "go along with the crowd."** Sometimes people with low self-esteem do things they normally wouldn't do, just to fit in. In the short run, this may work, but in the long run, you'll feel better about yourself when you do the things that support your values.

6. **Give credit where credit is due.** Reward yourself for doing something well. Treat yourself to a movie, a meal at a restaurant, or a new CD. You worked hard and deserve a treat.

7. **Set short-term goals that will strengthen your weaknesses.** Map out a plan to help you reach your goals. Even small improvements are better than not trying at all.

8. **Don't be afraid to try something new.** Sign up for the class you have always wanted to take. Take a swimming or dance lesson. You'll never know if you're good at something until you try it.

9. **Nothing puts things in perspective better than volunteering for those in need does.** Spend time working at a soup kitchen, deliver meals to those who can't leave their homes, or spend time visiting people at a nursing home. Your problems will probably seem less significant than those of the people you help. Helping others can also give you a sense of purpose.

10. **If you experience defeat, don't dwell on it.** Try to learn something positive from the experience and move on. Don't make the mistake of running it over and over again in your mind. Remember, "If at first you don't succeed, try, try again!"

 For more information about self-esteem, see Chapter 3.

REFERENCE Guide

Calorie and Nutrient Content in Selected Foods

This table is organized into 14 categories: beverages; breads and grains; cereals; condiments; crackers; dairy and eggs; desserts; fast foods; fruits; meat, fish, poultry, and eggs; mixed dishes; nuts and seeds; snack foods; and vegetables.

Food and serving size	Calories (kcal)	Calories from fat (kcal)	% Calories from fat (%)	Total fat (g)	Saturated fat (g)	Cholesterol (mg)	Total carbohydrate (g)	Dietary fiber (g)	Protein (g)	Calcium (mg)	Iron (mg)	Vitamin C (mg)	Vitamin A (μg RE)
BEVERAGES													
Carbonated beverage (soda)													
12 fl oz	184	0	0	0.0	0.0	0	38	0.0	0.0	13	0.0	0	0
24 fl oz with ice (approximate values)	221	0	0	0.0	0.0	0	57	0.0	0.0	16	0.5	0	0
32 fl oz with ice (approximate values)	295	0	0	0.0	0.0	0	76	0.0	0.0	25	0.6	0	0
diet, 12 fl oz	0	0	0	0.0	0.0	0	0	0.0	0.0	0	0.0	0	0
Fruit punch, 1 cup	117	0	0	0.0	0.0	0	30	0.3	0.0	20	0.5	4	0
Milk													
chocolate, 2%, 1 cup	179	45	25	5.0	3.1	17	26	1.2	8.0	285	0.6	2	143
lowfat, 1%, 1 cup	102	27	26	3.0	1.6	10	12	0.0	8.0	300	0.1	2	144
reduced fat, 2%, 1 cup	122	45	37	5.0	2.9	18	12	0.0	8.1	298	0.1	2	139
skim (fat free), 1 cup	91	0	0	0.0	0.0	4	12	0.0	8.0	301	0.1	2	149
whole, 1 cup	149	72	48	8.0	5.1	33	11	0.0	8.0	290	0.1	2	76
Milkshake, 12 fl oz	414	90	22	10.0	6.0	25	60	1.5	10.6	459	0.4	0	72
Orange Juice, 1 cup	105	0	0	0.0	0.0	0	25	0.5	2.0	20	1.1	147	43
Sports drink, 24 fl oz	150	0	0	0.0	0.0	0	42	0.0	0.0	0	0.0	0	0
Tea, unsweetened, 1 cup	2	0	0	0.0	0.0	0	1	0.0	0.0	8	0.0	0	0
Water, bottled, 12 fl oz	0	0	0	0.0	0.0	0	0	0.0	0.0	5	0.0	0	0
BREADS AND GRAINS													
Bagel, plain, 4 in. diameter	314	16	5	1.8	0.3	0	51	0.1	10.0	50	2.4	0	0
Biscuit, 1 medium	101	45	45	5.0	1.2	1	13	0.4	2.0	67	0.8	7	0
Bread													
white, 1 slice	76	9	12	1.0	0.4	1	14	0.6	2.0	24	0.8	0	0
whole wheat, 1 slice	86	9	10	1.0	0.3	0	16	2.4	3.0	25	1.2	0	0
Doughnut													
cake type, with chocolate frosting	211	117	55	13.0	3.5	26	21	0.9	2.0	22	0.7	0	10
cake type, plain	204	99	49	11.0	1.8	18	25	0.8	2.0	15	0.6	0	16
yeast, with glaze	242	126	52	14.0	3.5	12	27	0.7	4.0	20	1.6	0	16
French Toast, plain, 1 slice	149	63	42	7.0	1.8	75	16	0.1	5.0	65	1.1	0	86
Fried rice, no meat, ½ cup	132	54	41	6.0	0.9	21	17	0.7	3.0	15	0.9	2	10
Muffin, blueberry	155	36	23	4.0	0.8	17	27	1.5	3.1	32	0.9	1	5
Pancake, 4 in. diameter	86	0	0	0.0	0.0	4	19	0.7	2.4	26	0.7	0	4
Pasta, noodles, ½ cup	99	0	0	0.0	0.1	0	20	1.2	3.0	5	1.0	0	0
Pita bread, wheat, 1 medium	165	9	5	1.0	0.1	0	33	1.3	5.0	52	1.6	0	0
Rice													
brown, ½ cup	110	9	8	1.0	0.2	0	23	1.8	2.0	11	0.7	0	0
white, enriched, ½ cup	133	0	0	0.0	0.1	0	29	0.3	2.0	3	1.5	0	0

Food and serving size	Calories (kcal)	Calories from fat (kcal)	% Calories from fat (%)	Total fat (g)	Saturated fat (g)	Cholesterol (mg)	Total carbohydrate (g)	Dietary fiber (g)	Protein (g)	Calcium (mg)	Iron (mg)	Vitamin C (mg)	Vitamin A (µg RE)
Roll													
dinner	141	31	22	3.4	0.8	0	24	1.0	3.0	1	1.0	0	0
hamburger/hot dog	123	20	16	2.2	0.5	0	22	1.3	3.0	56	1.3	0	0
Tortilla													
corn, plain, *6 in. diameter*	58	6	10	0.7	0.1	0	12	0.0	2.0	52	0.4	0	0
flour, *8 in. diameter*	104	20	20	2.3	0.6	0	18	1.7	3.0	71	1.9	0	0
Waffle, from frozen, plain	88	25	28	2.7	0.5	11	14	1.2	2.0	38	0.0	0	150

CEREALS

Food and serving size	Calories (kcal)	Calories from fat (kcal)	% Calories from fat (%)	Total fat (g)	Saturated fat (g)	Cholesterol (mg)	Total carbohydrate (g)	Dietary fiber (g)	Protein (g)	Calcium (mg)	Iron (mg)	Vitamin C (mg)	Vitamin A (µg RE)
Cereal													
corn flakes, not sweetened, *1cup*	91	0	0	0.0	0.0	0	22	0.7	2.0	1	7.8	12	188
cornflakes, presweetened, *1 cup*	146	0	0	0.0	0.1	0	34	0.8	1.0	1	5.5	18	274
Oatmeal													
flavored instant, *½ cup*	125	9	7	1.0	0.3	0	26	2.5	3.0	104	3.9	0	305
plain, *½ cup*	72	9	13	1.0	0.2	0	13	2.0	3.0	0	0.8	0	2

CONDIMENTS

Food and serving size	Calories (kcal)	Calories from fat (kcal)	% Calories from fat (%)	Total fat (g)	Saturated fat (g)	Cholesterol (mg)	Total carbohydrate (g)	Dietary fiber (g)	Protein (g)	Calcium (mg)	Iron (mg)	Vitamin C (mg)	Vitamin A (µg RE)
Butter, *1 tsp*	36	33	93	3.7	2.4	10	0	0.0	0.0	1	0.0	0	33
Honey, *1 Tbsp*	64	0	0	0.0	0.0	0	18	0.0	0.0	1	0.1	0	0
Ketchup, *1 Tbsp*	16	0	3	0.1	0.0	0	4	0.2	0.2	3	0.1	2	15
Margarine, stick or tub, *1 tsp*	34	34	101	3.8	0.7	0	0	0.0	0.0	1	0.0	0	50
Mayonnaise, regular, *1 Tbsp*	57	44	77	4.9	0.7	4	4	0.0	0.1	2	0.0	0	32
Salad dressing, Italian, *1 Tbsp*	69	64	93	7.1	1.0	10	1	0.0	0.1	1	0.0	0	11
Salsa, *1 Tbsp*	4	0	8	0.0	0.0	0	1	0.3	0.2	5	0.2	2	22
Spaghetti sauce, *½ cup*	136	36	26	4.0	1.5	0	21	4.0	2.2	35	1.4	13	96
Sugar, white, *1 tsp*	16	0	0	0.0	0.0	0	4	0.0	0.0	0	0.0	0	0
Syrup													
chocolate, *2 Tbsp*	50	1	3	0.1	0.1	0	12	0.7	0.6	4	0.0	0	0
pancake, *1 Tbsp*	25	0	0	0.0	0.0	0	7	0.0	0.0	0	0.0	0	0

CRACKERS

Food and serving size	Calories (kcal)	Calories from fat (kcal)	% Calories from fat (%)	Total fat (g)	Saturated fat (g)	Cholesterol (mg)	Total carbohydrate (g)	Dietary fiber (g)	Protein (g)	Calcium (mg)	Iron (mg)	Vitamin C (mg)	Vitamin A (µg RE)
Crackers													
cheese with peanut butter, *6*	210	90	43	10.0	2.5	0	23	1.0	5.0	80	0.9	0	0
graham, *4 crackers*	59	2	3	0.2	0.0	1	11	0.5	1.0	11	0.6	0	0
soda crackers, *5 squares*	70	18	26	2.0	0.0	0	12	0.6	1.0	18	0.7	0	4
Matzo, *1 matzo cracker*	111	1	1	0.2	0.0	0	22	0.8	3.5	11	0.8	0	0

DAIRY AND EGGS

Food and serving size	Calories (kcal)	Calories from fat (kcal)	% Calories from fat (%)	Total fat (g)	Saturated fat (g)	Cholesterol (mg)	Total carbohydrate (g)	Dietary fiber (g)	Protein (g)	Calcium (mg)	Iron (mg)	Vitamin C (mg)	Vitamin A (µg RE)
Cheese													
American, prepackaged, *1 slice*	70	45	64	5.0	2.0	15	2	0.0	4.0	100	0.0	0	46
cheddar, *1 oz*	114	81	71	9.0	6.0	30	0	0.0	7.1	204	0.2	0	78
cottage, lowfat, *½ cup*	102	12	12	1.4	0.9	2	4	0.0	7.0	78	0.2	0	82
cream, *1 Tbsp*	51	45	89	5.0	3.2	32	0	0.0	1.1	12	0.2	0	55
cream, fat free, *1 Tbsp*	13	1	8	0.1	0.0	0	1	0.0	2.0	26	0.0	0	130
string, *1 stick*	72	45	63	5.0	2.9	16	1	0.0	7.0	183	0.1	0	50
Egg, boiled, *1 large*	78	48	61	5.3	1.0	212	0	0.0	6.0	25	0.6	0	84
Egg, scrambled, plain, *¼ cup*	74	45	61	5.0	1.0	212	0	0.0	6.0	25	0.6	0	84
Frozen yogurt													
cone, chocolate, *1 single*	157	63	40	7.0	3.9	1	22	1.1	4.0	115	0.6	1	42
nonfat, chocolate, *½ cup*	104	9	9	1.0	0.5	1	21	1.5	5.0	163	0.9	1	2
Whipped cream, *2 Tbsp*	15	14	90	1.5	1.0	4	1	0.0	0.0	0	0.0	0	0
Yogurt, lowfat, fruit flavored, *1 cup*	231	27	12	3.0	2.0	12	47	0.0	12.0	372	0.2	1	27

Calorie and Nutrient Content in Selected Foods (continued)

Food and serving size	Calories (kcal)	Calories from fat (kcal)	% Calories from fat (%)	Total fat (g)	Saturated fat (g)	Cholesterol (mg)	Total carbohydrate (g)	Dietary fiber (g)	Protein (g)	Calcium (mg)	Iron (mg)	Vitamin C (mg)	Vitamin A (µg RE)
DESSERTS													
Brownie, 1 square	227	90	40	10.0	2.0	14	30	1.4	1.5	11	0.9	0	6
Cake, chocolate with chocolate frosting, 1 piece	411	153	37	17.0	5.0	45	61	3.1	4.6	48	2.5	0	25
Candy, candy-coated chocolate, 10 pieces	34	9	26	1.0	0.9	0	5	0.2	0.0	1	0.1	0	4
with peanuts, 10 pieces	103	45	44	5.0	2.1	1	12	0.7	2.0	20	0.2	0	5
Candy, chocolate bar, 1.3 oz	226	126	56	14.0	8.1	10	26	1.5	3.0	84	0.6	0	24
Cheesecake, 1 piece	660	414	63	46.0	28.0	220	52	0.2	11.0	106	2.0	1	520
Cinnamon roll with nuts and raisins, 2 oz	217	63	29	7.0	1.4	8	34	1.1	3.2	36	1.6	0	60
Cookies													
chocolate chip, 1 cookie	59	23	38	2.5	0.8	3	8	0.2	0.6	3	0.3	0	7
oatmeal, 1 cookie	113	27	24	3.0	0.8	9	20	0.3	1.0	10	1.3	0	1
sugar, 1 cookie	72	27	38	3.0	0.8	7	10	0.1	0.8	3	0.3	0	4
Fruit juice bar, 1 bar	63	0	0	0.0	0.0	0	16	0.0	0.9	4	0.1	7	22
Gelatin dessert, flavored, ½ cup	80	0	0	0.0	0.0	0	19	0.0	2.0	0	0.0	0	0
Ice cream bar, vanilla with chocolate coating, 1 bar	171	99	58	11.0	6.4	1	17	0.3	2.0	136	0.4	25	0
Ice cream cone one scoop regular ice cream, 1 single	178	72	40	8.0	4.9	32	22	0.1	3.0	102	0.2	0	84
Ice cream, chocolate, ½ cup	143	40	28	4.5	22.4	7	19	0.8	2.5	72	0.6	0	275
Ice slushy, 1 cup	151	0	0	0.0	0.0	0	63	0.0	1.0	4	0.3	2	0
Pie, apple, double crust, 1 piece	411	162	39	18.0	4.0	19	58	0.0	3.7	11	1.7	3	9
Pudding, chocolate, ½ cup	160	27	17	3.0	1.8	5	27	1.2	3.2	153	0.6	2	43
FAST FOODS													
Burrito, beef and bean	520	207	40	23.0	10.0	150	55	11.0	24.0	150	2.7	5	600
Cheeseburger ¼ lb, on bun, with lettuce, tomato, mustard, ketchup, and pickles	520	261	50	29.0	12.6	97	37	1.7	28.0	127	4.3	2	33
regular size mustard, ketchup, onions, pickles	319	117	37	13.0	5.6	42	36	1.9	15.0	144	2.7	2	64
Chicken nuggets, 4	198	108	55	12.0	2.5	42	10	0.0	12.0	9	0.6	1	0
Chicken sandwich													
breaded chicken breast on bun, with lettuce, tomato, and mayonnaise	492	261	53	29.0	5.5	52	42	1.7	17.0	129	2.5	1	29
grilled chicken breast, on bun, with lettuce, tomato, and mayonnaise	361	63	17	7.0	2.0	54	44	2.6	27.0	132	2.5	4	19
French Fries													
1 small order	199	90	45	10.0	2.0	0	26	2.0	2.0	10	0.4	10	1
1 large order	430	198	46	22.0	5.0	0	56	5.0	5.0	23	0.9	20	2
1 supersize order	545	234	43	26.0	6.0	0	67	6.0	6.0	27	1.0	25	2
Hamburger, regular size, on bun, with mustard, ketchup, and pickles	266	81	30	9.0	3.2	28	36	1.9	12.0	126	2.7	2	23
double meat, double bun, cheese, sauce, lettuce, and tomatoes	510	234	46	26.0	9.3	76	46	3.3	25.0	202	4.3	3	66

Food and serving size	Calories (kcal)	Calories from fat (kcal)	% Calories from fat (%)	Total fat (g)	Saturated fat (g)	Cholesterol (mg)	Total carbohydrate (g)	Dietary fiber (g)	Protein (g)	Calcium (mg)	Iron (mg)	Vitamin C (mg)	Vitamin A (μg RE)
Sub sandwich													
Italian, *6 in. long*	467	216	46	24.0	9.0	57	38	3.0	20.0	40	4.0	15	169
vegetarian, *6 in. long*	222	27	12	3.0	0.0	0	38	3.0	9.0	25	3.0	15	120
Taco													
crispy, with ground beef, cheese, lettuce, and tomato	180	90	50	10.0	4.0	25	12	3.0	9.0	80	1.1	0	100
soft, with beans and rice and no cheese	218	27	12	3.0	0.0	0	19	3.0	7.0	60	0.8	1	60
soft, with chicken, cheese, lettuce, and tomato	212	63	30	7.0	2.6	37	22	2.1	15.0	85	0.8	1	64

FRUITS

Food and serving size	Calories (kcal)	Calories from fat (kcal)	% Calories from fat (%)	Total fat (g)	Saturated fat (g)	Cholesterol (mg)	Total carbohydrate (g)	Dietary fiber (g)	Protein (g)	Calcium (mg)	Iron (mg)	Vitamin C (mg)	Vitamin A (μg RE)
Apple, raw, with skin, *1 medium*	81	1	1	0.1	0.1	0	21	3.5	0.2	9	0.2	8	7
Applesauce, unsweetened, *½ cup*	52	0	1	0.0	0.0	0	14	1.5	0.2	5	0.4	2	14
Banana, fresh, *1 medium*	114	9	8	1.0	0.2	0	27	2.7	1.0	7	0.4	10	9
Blueberries, *½ cup*	41	0	1	0.0	0.0	0	10	2.0	0.5	4	0.1	10	7
Cantaloupe, *¼ medium*	44	1	2	0.1	0.0	0	10	1.0	1.1	14	0.3	53	403
Cherries, sweet, fresh, *1 cup*	84	2	3	0.3	0.0	1	19	2.7	1.4	18	0.5	8	25
Grapes, *½ cup*	62	1	2	0.1	0.0	0	16	0.9	0.6	13	0.3	4	9
Mango, *½ medium*	68	1	1	0.1	0.0	0	18	1.9	0.5	1	0.0	23	321
Olive, ripe, *1 large*	5	9	178	1.0	0.1	0	1	0.2	0.0	4	0.1	0	1
Orange, fresh, *1 large*	85	0	0	0.0	0.0	0	21	4.3	1.7	52	0.1	70	28
Peach, fresh, *1 medium*	37	0	0	0.0	0.0	0	9	1.7	1.0	4	0.1	6	42
Pineapple chunks, canned in juice, *½ cup*	84	0	0	0.0	0.0	0	22	1.1	0.6	20	0.4	13	18
Plum, fresh, *1*	36	0	1	0.0	0.0	0	9	1.0	0.5	3	0.1	6	21
Raisins, seedless, dry, *1 cup*	495	2	0	0.2	0.0	1	131	6.6	5.3	81	3.4	6	1
Strawberries, fresh, *1 cup*	46	0	1	0.0	0.0	1	11	3.5	0.9	21	0.6	86	41
Watermelon, *½ cup*	26	0	0	0.0	0.0	0	6	0.4	0.0	6	0.1	8	30

MEAT, FISH, POULTRY, AND EGGS

Food and serving size	Calories (kcal)	Calories from fat (kcal)	% Calories from fat (%)	Total fat (g)	Saturated fat (g)	Cholesterol (mg)	Total carbohydrate (g)	Dietary fiber (g)	Protein (g)	Calcium (mg)	Iron (mg)	Vitamin C (mg)	Vitamin A (μg RE)
Bacon, *3 slices*	109	81	74	9.0	3.3	16	0	0.0	6.0	2	0.3	0	0
Beef jerky, *1 piece*	81	46	56	5.1	2.1	10	2	0.4	6.6	4	1.1	0	0
Bologna, beef and pork, *1 slice*	73	58	80	6.5	2.5	13	1	0.0	2.7	3	0.3	0	0
Chicken breast													
fried with skin, *1 split breast*	364	166	46	18.5	4.9	119	13	0.4	34.8	28	1.8	0	17
grilled and skinless, *1 split breast*	142	27	19	3.0	0.9	44	73	0.0	27.0	13	0.9	0	5
Chicken drumstick, fried, *meat and skin of 1 drumstick*	193	102	53	11.3	3.0	62	6	0.2	15.8	12	1.0	0	19
Chicken strips, breaded white meat, no skin, *2 strips, 3 in. × 1 in.*	218	54	25	6.0	1.7	102	0	0.0	37.0	18	1.3	0	33
Chicken wing, fried, *meat and skin of 1 wing*	159	96	61	10.7	2.9	39	5	0.1	9.7	10	0.6	0	12
Chorizo, *1 link*	273	207	76	23.0	8.6	53	1	0.0	14.5	5	1.0	0	0
Corndog, chicken	272	117	43	13.0	3.0	65	26	0.0	13.0	90	2.0	0	30
Ham, lunchmeat, *2 ounces*	70	27	39	3.0	1.0	30	1	0.0	10.0	0	0.7	0	0
Hot dog													
regular, *no bun*	220	153	70	17.0	6.0	50	5	0.0	6.0	0	0.7	0	0
low fat, *no bun*	70	23	32	2.5	1.0	2	7	0.0	6.0	0	0.7	2	0

REFERENCE Guide

Health Agencies and Organizations

The list of health agencies and organizations below can provide you sources for answering your health-related questions and finding information on a variety of health-related topics.

Agriculture Research Service USDA
3700 East West Highway
Hyattsville, MD 20782

Al-Anon, Alateen Family Group Hotline
1600 Corporate Landing Parkway
Virginia Beach, VA 23454-5617
(888) 4-AL-ANON (425-2666)

Alliance for Children and Families
11700 West Lake Park Drive
Milwaukee, WI 53224
(800) 221-2681

American Academy of Pediatrics
141 Northwest Point Boulevard
Elk Grove Village, IL 60007-1098
(847) 434-4000

American Anorexia/Bulimia Association, Inc.
165 W. 46th Street Suite 1108
New York, NY 10036
(212) 575-6200

American Association for Active Lifestyles and Fitness
1900 Association Drive
Reston, VA 20191
(800) 213-7193

American Alliance for Health, Physical Education, Recreation & Dance
1900 Association Dr.
Reston, VA 20191-1598

American Association for Health Education
1900 Association Drive
Reston, VA 22091
(703) 476-3437

American Association for Retired Persons
601 East Street NW
Washington, DC 20049
(202) 434-2277

American Cancer Society
1599 Clifton Road NE
Atlanta, GA 30329
(800) ACS-2345 (227-2345)

American College of Sports Medicine
P.O. Box 1440
Indianapolis, IN 46206
(317) 637-9200

American Council for Drug Education
164 West 74th Street
New York, NY 10023
(800) 488-3784

American Dental Association
211 East Chicago Avenue
Chicago, IL 60611
(800) 621-8099

American Diabetes Association
1701 N. Beauregard Street
Alexandria, VA 22311
(800) 342-2383

American Dietetic Association
216 West Jackson Boulevard
Chicago, IL 60606-6995
(800) 366-1655

American Foundation for the Blind
11 Penn Plaza
New York, NY 10001
(800) AFB-LINE (232-5463)

American Heart Association
7272 Greenville Avenue
Dallas, TX 75231-4596
(800) 242-8721

American Institute for Preventive Medicine
30445 Northwestern Highway
Suite 350
Farmington Hills, MI 48334
(800) 345-AIPM (345-2476)

American Institute of Stress
124 Park Avenue
Yonkers, NY 10703
(800) 24-RELAX (247-3529)

American Liver Foundation
75 Maiden Lane
Suite 603
New York, NY 10038
(800) GO LIVER (465-4837)

American Lung Association
1740 Broadway
New York, NY 10019-4274
(800) 586-4872

American Medical Association
515 N. State Street
Chicago, IL 60610
(312) 464-5000

**American Public Health
Association**
800 I Street NW
Washington, DC 20001-3710
(202) 777-APHA (777-2742)

**American Red Cross,
National Headquarters**
8111 Gatehouse Road
Falls Church, VA 22042-1203
(800) 375-2040

**American Running and Fitness
Association**
4405 East-West Highway
Suite 405
Bethesda, MD 20814
(800) 776-2732

**American School Health
Association**
7263 State Route 43
P.O. Box 708
Kent, OH 44240
(303) 678-1601

**American Society
for Deaf Children**
P.O. Box 3355
Gettysburg, PA 17325
(800) 942-ASDC (942-2732)

Arthritis Foundation
1330 West Peachtree Street
Atlanta, GA 30309
(800) 283-7800

**Asthma and Allergy Foundation
of America**
1233 20th Street NW
Washington, DC 20036
(800) 7-ASTHMA (727-8462)

**Centers for Disease Control
and Prevention**
1600 Clifton Rd.
Atlanta, GA 30333
(800) 311-3435

Eat Right Hotline
1675 University Boulevard
UAB Station
Birmingham, AL 35294
(800) 231-DIET (231-3438)

**Environmental Protection
Agency**
Ariel Rios Bldg.
1200 Pennsylvania Avenue NW
Washington, DC 20460

**Family Resource Center
on Disabilities**
Douglas Building
20 East Jackson Boulevard
Suite 900
Chicago, IL 60604-208
(800) 952-4199

Federal Trade Commission (FTC)
Consumer Response Center
Washington, DC
(202) 326-2222

Food Allergy Network
104000 Eaton Place
Suite 107
Fairfax, VA 22030-2208
(800) 929-4040

Food and Drug Administration
5600 Fishers Lane
Rockville, MD 20857-0001
(888) INFO-FDA (463-6332)

**Food and Nutrition
Information Center**
National Agriculture Library
Room 304
10301 Baltimore Blvd.
Beltsville, MD 20705

**Food Safety and Inspection
Administration**
USDA
Washington, DC 20250

**Juvenile Diabetes Foundation
International**
120 Wall Street
19th Floor
New York, NY 10005
(800) 533-2873

Lupus Foundation of America
1300 Piccard Drive
Rockville, MD 20850
(800) 558-0121

Lyme Disease Foundation
1 Financial Plaza
Hartford, CT 06103-2611
(800) 886-5963

Medic Alert International
2323 Colorado Ave
Turlock, CA 95382-2018
(800) ID-ALERT (432-5378)

Mothers Against Drunk Driving
511 E. John Carpenter Freeway
Suite 700
Irving, TX 75062
(800) GET-MADD (438-6233)

**National Association for
Family Child Care**
525 SW 5th Street, Suite A
Des Moines, IA 50309-4501
(800) 359-3817

**National Cancer Information
Center of the American
Cancer Society**
P.O. Box 142302
Austin, TX 78714-2302
(800) 225-2345

Medical and Dental Careers

Medical workers provide different types of care to improve a person's health. Many medical workers diagnose illnesses and injuries and provide specialized treatment. Others operate highly specialized medical equipment or work in laboratories.

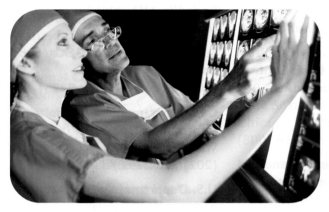

Physician

What Physicians Do

Physicians perform medical examinations, diagnose, and treat patients who have illnesses and injuries. They help people understand how to prevent disease. Physicians are also known as medical doctors (MDs) and they are licensed to perform surgery and prescribe medications. General practitioners or family doctors treat patients for a variety of illnesses. Other doctors choose an area of specialization, such as obstetrics and gynecology, dermatology, and neurological surgery.

Where Physicians Work

Some physicians have their own private practice. Others are employed at hospitals, research facilities, and different specialty clinics.

What Is Required to Become a Physician

▶ a bachelor's degree
▶ 4 years of medical school
▶ 3- to 5-year residency to specialize and be certified

Registered Nurse

What Registered Nurses Do

Registered nurses (RNs) interpret and respond to a patient's symptoms, reactions, and progress. They teach patients and families about proper healthcare, assist in patient rehabilitation, and provide emotional support to promote recovery. RNs use a broad knowledge base to administer treatments and make decisions about patient care. RNs may be responsible for supervising aides, assistants, and LPNs. Often nurses choose to work in specialized areas such as obstetrics (childbirth) or public health.

Where Registered Nurses Work

Registered nurses are employed in places such as hospitals, public health departments, nursing homes, and public schools.

What Is Required to Become a Registered Nurse

▶ associate's degree or bachelor's degree
▶ individual state licensing

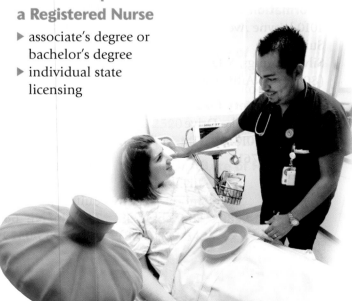

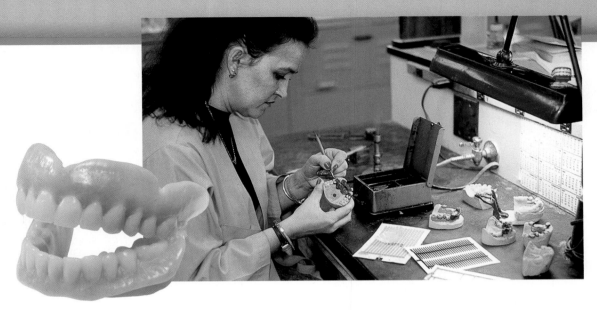

Emergency Medical Technician (EMT)

What Emergency Medical Technicians Do

Emergency medical technician (EMT) is a broad term used to address emergency medical staff. These technicians respond to healthcare crises. They drive ambulances, give emergency medical care, and, if necessary, transport patients to hospitals. EMTs respond to emergencies such as heart attacks, unexpected childbirth, car accidents, and fires. They explain the situation to local hospital staff. Under the direction of a physician, EMTs are told how to proceed with medical care. They perform CPR (cardiopulmonary resuscitation), control bleeding, place splints on broken bones, and check pulse and respiration. Paramedics receive additional training and therefore may be given more responsibilities.

Where Emergency Medical Technicians Work

Emergency medical technicians work in hospitals, for fire departments, or in an ambulance if they have more advanced training.

What Is Required to Become an Emergency Medical Technician

- ▶ training appropriate to duties
- ▶ basic classes for certification
- ▶ numerous college courses, depending upon career goal

Dental Laboratory Technician

What Dental Laboratory Technicians Do

Dental laboratory technicians construct and repair dentures, crowns, and other dental appliances for missing, damaged, or poorly positioned teeth. They follow a dentist's prescription to make plaster models of the patients' jaws and teeth. The technicians then use acrylic, molding equipment, and porcelain to create an exact copy of the teeth.

Where Dental Laboratory Technicians Work

Some dental laboratory technicians work in dentists' offices. Other technicians work for hospitals, including U.S. Department of Veterans Affairs' hospitals. Still other technicians work in laboratories or within their own homes.

What Is Required to Become a Dental Laboratory Technician

- ▶ a high school diploma
- ▶ 3 to 4 years as an apprentice or 2 years of college in an associate's degree or certification program

REFERENCE Guide

Healthcare Administration

Hospitals and other healthcare facilities must employ administrators to coordinate the activities of all employees—both medical and nonmedical—so that patients receive the best possible care. Healthcare administrators range from housekeepers and computer specialists to hospital directors.

Medical Transcriptionist

What Medical Transcriptionists Do

A medical transcriptionist listens to an audio-recorded summary of a patient's condition and treatment. The transcriptionist types the information and then places the information in the patient's permanent record. This typed information provides a clear, concise, written record, which must contain correct spelling, grammar, and punctuation. Transcriptionists use computers and word processors to complete many medical documents, which include medical histories, physicals, consultations, and operative reports. They record procedures and treatments for the medical record and for the medical staff's reference.

Where Medical Transcriptionists Work

Medical transcriptionists are employed by clinics, hospitals, insurance companies, physicians' offices, and private transcription companies, or they may be self-employed.

What Is Required to Become a Medical Transcriptionist

- ▶ high school diploma or equivalent
- ▶ classroom and clinical experience (from 9 months for a certificate to 2 years for an associate's degree)
- ▶ pass certification exam of the American Association of Medical Transcriptionists to become a certified medical transcriptionist (CMT)

Medical Coder

What Medical Coders Do

A medical coding professional uses a classification system to assign code numbers and letters to each symptom, diagnosis, disease, procedure, and operation that appears in a patient's chart. These codes are used for insurance reimbursement, for research, for health planning analysis, and to make clinical decisions. A high degree of accuracy and a working knowledge of medical terminology, anatomy, and physiology are important skills for these professionals to have.

Where Medical Coders Work

Medical coders are employed by hospitals, insurance companies, doctors' offices, and health maintenance organizations (HMOs).

What Is Required to Become a Medical Coder

- ▶ high school diploma or equivalent
- ▶ associate's degree or a 24- to 36-month home study course through the American Health Information Management Association
- ▶ certification by the American Health Information Management Association to work in certain states

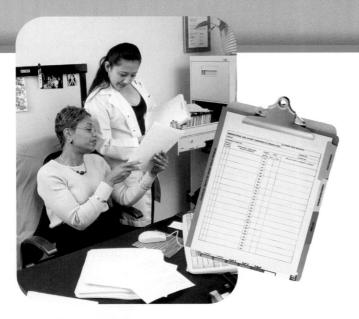

Medical Claims Examiner

What Medical Claims Examiners Do

Medical claims examiners review charges on health-related claims to see if the costs are reasonable based on the diagnosis. If a medical claims examiner feels that an error has been made on an insurance claim, he or she will try to work out the problem before the insurance company will pay the claim. Examiners will then either authorize the appropriate payment or refer the claim to an investigator for a more thorough review.

Where Medical Claims Examiners Work

Medical claims examiners work for insurance companies.

What Is Required to Become a Medical Claims Examiner

▶ a bachelor's degree (no specific course of study is required, but business or accounting courses may be useful)
▶ a general understanding of medical terminology and procedures

Systems Analyst

What Systems Analysts Do

Systems analysts solve computer problems and enable computer technology to meet the individual needs of an organization, including health care agencies. They help an organization realize the maximum benefit from its investment in equipment and personnel. Systems analysts also work on making the computer systems within an organization compatible so that information can be shared. This process may include planning and developing new computer systems or devising ways to apply existing systems' resources to additional operations. Systems analysts may design new systems, including both hardware and software, or add a new software application to harness more of the computer's power.

Where Systems Analysts Work

Most systems analysts work with a specific type of system such as business, accounting, financial, scientific, or engineering systems that varies with the type of organization they work for. Systems analysts who have a general knowledge of healthcare facilities and the functions the facilities perform usually find jobs in hospitals, insurance agencies, and health maintenance organizations.

What Is Required to Become a Systems Analyst

▶ a bachelor's degree in computer science, information science, or management information systems (MIS)
▶ other qualifications that vary with area of service

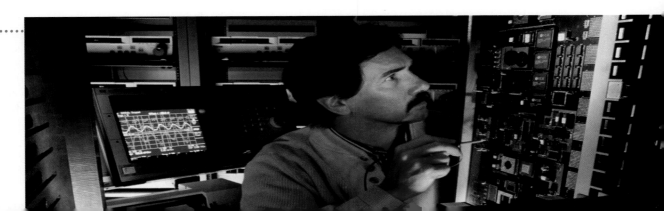

Health Education

There are many types of healthcare professionals who specialize in educating people about how to improve their overall physical and mental health. Education is part of almost any healthcare worker's job.

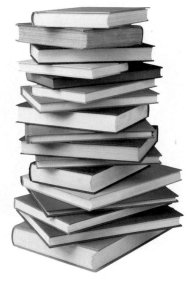

Community Health Educator

What Community Health Educators Do

Community health educators try to improve the general health of the community by informing people about important topics such as pollution, disease, drug abuse, nutrition, safety, and stress management. Community health educators try to teach people how to avoid contracting diseases and how to manage the disease when it is contracted. These educators lead presentations and write educational brochures and reports to teach people about health and disease and ways to meet specific health needs.

Where Community Health Educators Work

Community health educators usually work for local or state governments or for private organizations.

What Is Required to Become a Community Health Educator

- ▶ training appropriate to duties
- ▶ usually a bachelor's degree or a master's degree focusing on public health or education

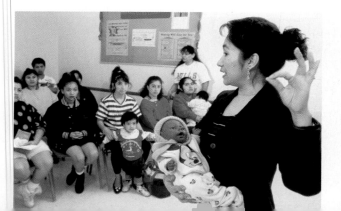

Mental Health Counselor

What Mental Health Counselors Do

Mental health counselors help people and their families cope with emotional and mental trauma. In individual or group counseling sessions, these counselors help patients learn how to manage problems with family, depression, stress, addiction, substance abuse and more. The counselors work closely with other health professionals to recommend treatments and assistance programs to patients. Mental health counselors are often referred to as therapists, psychologists, and analysts. Many mental health counselors specialize in areas of counseling such as family and parent-child relationships, domestic violence, or chemical dependency.

Where Mental Health Counselors Work

Some places where mental health counselors may work are private practices, clinics, and mental hospitals.

What Is Required to Become a Mental Health Counselor

- ▶ a bachelor's degree
- ▶ at least 2 years postgraduate study to achieve a master's degree or 3 to 5 years to achieve a doctoral degree (Ph.D)

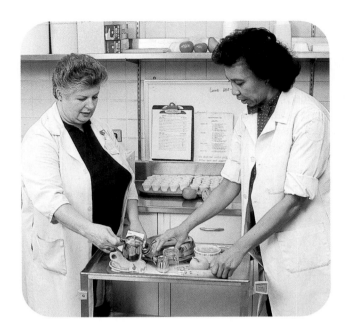

Dietitian

What Dietitians Do

Dietitians help people learn about and follow healthy eating habits. These professionals often create personalized diets for patients according to the person's health status and nutritional needs. Dietitians may also oversee a hospital or health clinic's food preparation service. Dietitians help to prepare and inspect food and help clients improve or create a personalized healthy eating plan. For example, a dietitian may work in a clinic or hospital teaching patients who have diabetes or high blood pressure about which types of food they should eat or try to avoid.

Where Dietitians Work

Dietitians work at places such as hospitals, health clinics, schools, public health agencies, or businesses, such as a food service management company.

What Is Required to Become a Dietitian

▶ a bachelor's degree in dietetics or nutrition (the program must be approved by the American Dietetic Association)
▶ a master's degree or doctoral degree, depending on career goals

Health Writer and Editor

What Health Writers and Editors Do

Health writers and editors research, write, and communicate health information. They contribute articles and other forms of writing to health-related publications such as hospital newsletters and medical journals. Health editors and writers also work writing and editing for health sites on the Internet. They may write about a specific health topic such as cancer or health insurance issues, or they may write about many different topics. They will often write for a specific audience (such as medical doctors). Therefore, they know how to use the same medical terminology and language used by doctors.

Where Health Writers and Editors Work

Health writers or editors work for publishing companies, radio or television stations, professional medical journals, Internet companies, universities, health foundations, or government agencies.

What Is Required to Become a Health Writer and Editor

▶ a bachelor's degree and coursework in science and health-related classes

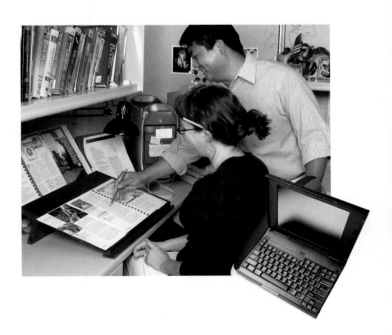

REFERENCE Guide

Community Service

Many people working in community service provide services and products to medical personnel, patients, and the general public. Some of these professions require extensive training, while others only require a few courses after high school.

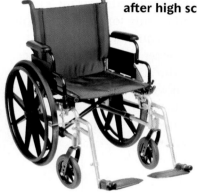

Home Health Aide

What Home Health Aides Do

Home health aides provide personal care in the home to people who are elderly, handicapped, or recovering from an illness or injury. The responsibilities of home health aides include getting the patient out of bed, as well as helping the patient bathe and groom, dress, and exercise. The aide also helps the patient remember to take his or her medication, helps with housecleaning and meal preparation, and provides emotional support.

Where Home Health Aides Work

Home health aides are usually employed by an agency but work in their patient's homes.

What Is Required to Become a Home Health Aide

▶ certification and training, which vary by state (federal law requires a person to have at least 81 hours of classroom and practical training under the supervision of a registered nurse for the person to be eligible to take the national certification exam)

Medical Social Worker

What Medical Social Workers Do

Medical social workers assist patients and their families with health-related problems and concerns. These social workers lead support group discussions, help patients locate appropriate healthcare and other health services, and provide support to patients who have serious or chronic illnesses. These professionals help patients and the patient's families find resources to overcome unhealthy conditions, such as child abuse, homelessness, and drug abuse. Social workers also help patients find legal resources and financial aid to pay for health services.

Where Medical Social Workers Work

Medical social workers usually work for hospitals, nursing homes, health clinics, or community health agencies.

What Is Required to Become a Medical Social Worker

▶ a bachelor's degree or a master's degree

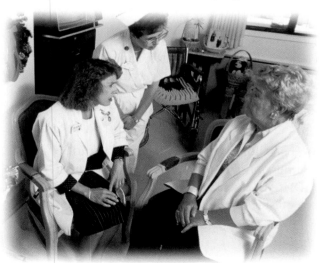

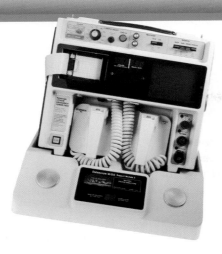

Biomedical Equipment Technician

What Biomedical Equipment Technicians Do

Biomedical equipment technicians specialize in electronic and mechanical equipment used to diagnose and treat diseases. These technicians work with equipment ranging from electronic switches to sophisticated diagnostic equipment. Biomedical equipment technicians adjust and test equipment for proper operation. They periodically inspect and repair machines. They also install new equipment, such as electrocardiographs (EKGs) and artificial kidney machines. These technicians also perform safety inspections on electrical and radiation equipment, demonstrate the use of equipment for other medical personnel, and propose new equipment purchases or modifications.

Where Biomedical Equipment Technicians Work

Biomedical equipment technicians work in places such as hospitals, clinics, and medical equipment manufacturing plants.

What Is Required to Become a Biomedical Equipment Technician

▶ 1 to 3 years in a technical program or a bachelor's degree

Health Insurance Agent

What Health Insurance Agents Do

Health insurance agents sell health insurance to the public. Health insurance is used to help pay for medical expenses if a person needs to go to the doctor or hospital or to receive some other type of medical treatment. A health insurance agent helps people determine what the proper insurance policy for them would be. They consider factors such as how many people are to be covered, what the ages of the people to be covered are, and what level of coverage is needed. Health insurance agents also help their customers by answering questions and acting as a liaison between the insurance company and a customer who needs to file a claim.

Where do Health Insurance Agents Work?

Health insurance agents are located throughout the country and usually work in a private office or in the office of an insurance agency.

What Is Required to Become a Health Insurance Agent

▶ a bachelor's degree or education needed per company of employment
▶ specified amount of continuing education (required per state)

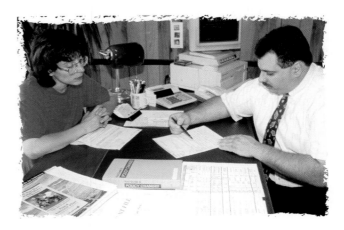

Sports and Recreation

Helping people maintain life-long health through sports and recreation is a rapidly growing area in health careers. The ability of exercise to reduce stress has also created an important new field of jobs. Occupations in this area range from trainers to therapists.

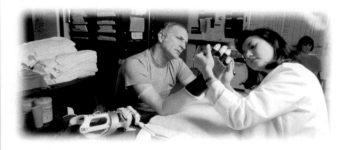

Occupational Therapist

What Occupational Therapists Do

Occupational therapists help patients adjust to and recover from physical illnesses and injuries, such as spinal cord injuries or partial paralysis. Occupational therapists lead patients through rehabilitative exercises and show the patients new ways to perform simple tasks such as getting dressed, cooking, and eating. These professionals also help people who have been injured at work find care and resources and to learn new work duties if necessary. Depending upon the patient's needs, the therapists provide each patient with a personalized rehabilitation plan and may teach him or her how to use equipment such as wheelchairs, walkers, and other aids.

Where Occupational Therapists Work

Occupational therapists work in hospitals, in clinics, or in private business.

What Is Required to Become an Occupational Therapist

▶ a bachelor's degree or a certification program in occupational therapy followed by passing a national certification exam

Certified Athletic Trainer

What Certified Athletic Trainers Do

Athletic trainers are health professionals who work with athletes from sports teams and organizations to prevent, recognize, treat, and rehabilitate sports-related injuries. They provide first aid and nonemergency medical services at sporting events and practices, and they help team members get long-term medical help, if needed.

Where Certified Athletic Trainers Work

Certified athletic trainers usually work for college or professional sport teams, or train amateur athletes.

What Is Required to Become a Certified Athletic Trainer

▶ a bachelor's degree from a National Athletic Trainer's Association (NATA) program or attendance at an NATA internship (Either path requires training in CPR and NATA certification.)

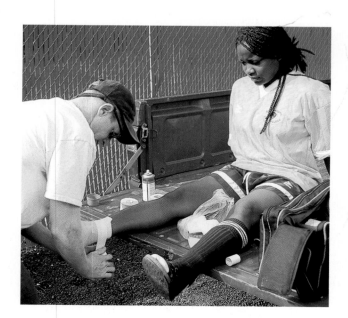

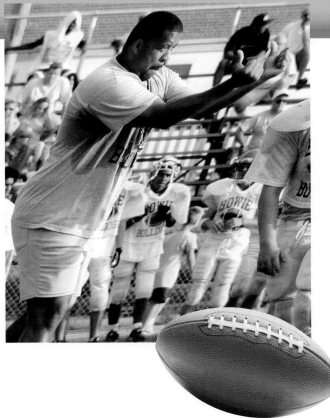

High School Coach

What High School Coaches Do

High school coaches are responsible for training young athletes to play sports well and safely. Coaches usually coach one or more sports, and they may have other duties, such as teaching or working in school administration. Coaches also teach sportsmanship, leadership, and how to work together as a team. High school coaches are responsible for the safety and well-being of their players both on the field and in transit to and from games or competitions.

Where High School Coaches Work

High school coaches work at public and private high schools.

What Is Required to Become a High School Coach

▶ a bachelor's degree
▶ sometimes a master's degree or a Ph.D.

Recreational Therapist

What Recreational Therapists Do

Recreational therapists plan and carry out treatment programs for people who have physical, mental, or social disabilities or for individuals recovering from substance, sexual, and physical abuse. Therapists use art, music, recreation, and dance to help patients relieve stress, express themselves, and build self-confidence. Motivational and creative programs are used to encourage behavior change, improve coordination, and increase social skills.

Where Recreational Therapists Work

Some places where recreational therapists work include hospitals, adult and child day care centers, and nursing homes.

What Is Required to Become a Recreational Therapist

▶ a bachelor's degree
▶ at least 6 months of clinical training

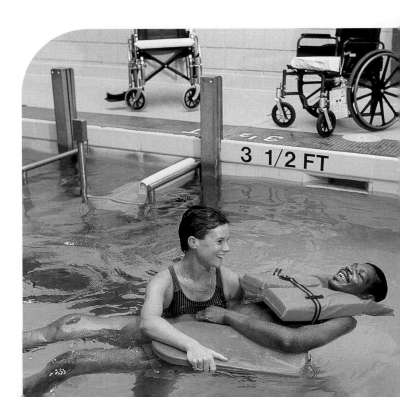

CHAPTER 1
Leading a Healthy Life

1. true
2. false, there are many behavioral risk factors for heart disease. You can follow healthy behaviors to help reduce your chances of developing heart disease
3. true
4. true
5. true
6. false, physical health is just one aspect of overall health

Knowledge—What's Your Health IQ? Scoring

Calculate the percentage of questions you answered correctly by dividing the number of questions you answered correctly by the total number of questions. Then, multiply that number by 100. Check your percentage correct below:

80–100 percent correct Excellent! Your high score shows you have a strong knowledge with the health topics in the chapter. Use this knowledge to make good health choices and you'll be on your way to leading a healthy life!

60–79 percent correct Good You are aware of some of the health topics in the chapter. Learning more about these issues can help you to make better decisions about your health.

0–59 percent correct Needs Improvement It is important to understand the health issues that affect you. Having a high health knowledge can influence you to choose healthy behaviors so you can enjoy a healthy life. Read the chapter carefully, and then retake the What's Your Health IQ? to see if your score improves.

CHAPTER 2
Skills for a Healthy Life

If you scored:

20–28 points You are doing an excellent job of evaluating and learning from the decisions you make that relate to your overall health.

11–19 points You are doing well overall. However, you have a number of areas in which you can improve decisions about your health.

0–10 points You may need to make some major changes in the way you make decisions. You can learn to make changes in your decision-making by reading Chapter 2.

CHAPTER 3
Building Self-Esteem and Mental Health

If you scored:

19–24 points You show respect for yourself and others and probably have high self-esteem.

10–18 points You probably have a healthy self-esteem but could improve the way you treat yourself and others.

0–9 points You should make some major changes in the way you treat yourself and others. You can learn about factors that affect your self-esteem and how to improve it by reading Chapter 3.

CHAPTER 4
Managing Stress and Coping with Loss

If you scored:

19–24 points You are doing an excellent job of managing stress.

10–18 points You are doing very well overall but have areas in which you can improve how you manage stress.

0–9 points You should be making some major changes in the way you deal with stress or you may develop a stress-related illness. You can learn more about how to manage stress by reading Chapter 4.

CHAPTER 5
Preventing Violence and Abuse

If you scored:

19–24 points You are doing an excellent job of avoiding conflict and violence.

10–18 points You are doing very well overall but have areas in which you could improve your interactions with other people.

0–9 points You should be making some major changes in the way in which you interact with other people. You can learn more about how to better avoid conflict and violence by reading Chapter 5.

CHAPTER 6
Physical Fitness for Life

1. false, benefits can be obtained from exercising less often (5 days a week)
2. true
3. false, girls will increase their muscle mass but will not develop bulky muscles typical of males
4. false, lifting weights is anaerobic exercise
5. false, the body needs rest from exercise or injury will occur
6. false, anabolic steroids are used to treat medical problems, but their use to improve athletic performance is illegal
7. true

To check your score, refer to Knowledge—What's Your Health IQ? Scoring on p. 642 under Chapter 1.

CHAPTER 7
Nutrition for Life

1. true
2. false, plant foods do not contain cholesterol
3. false, fiber is important because it enables food to move through the intestines efficiently
4. false, you need to consume vitamins and minerals in your diet because your body can't produce them and many of them cannot be stored very long in the body
5. true
6. true
7. false, choosing the right kind of snacks can provide energy and nutrients needed for active, growing people

To check your score, refer to Knowledge—What's Your Health IQ? Scoring on p. 642 under Chapter 1.

CHAPTER 8
Weight Management and Eating Behavior

1. true
2. true
3. true
4. false, a weight management program includes healthy eating and exercise habits that maintain a healthy weight

5. true
6. true
7. false, most food-borne illnesses are caused by foods that are prepared or eaten at home

To check your score, refer to Knowledge—What's Your Health IQ? Scoring on p. 642 under Chapter 1.

CHAPTER 9
Understanding Drugs and Medicines

1. false, minor side effects of OTC medicines are common
2. true
3. true
4. true
5. true
6. false, all drugs, despite their source, are made from chemicals
7. false, people can become addicted to prescription drugs such as painkillers

To check your score, refer to Knowledge—What's Your Health IQ? Scoring on p. 642 under Chapter 1.

CHAPTER 10
Alcohol

1. true
2. true
3. true
4. true
5. true
6. false, alcoholism affects all people who know the alcoholic
7. false, motor vehicle accidents is the No. 1 cause of death among teens; the majority of these accidents are alcohol related.

To check your score, refer to Knowledge—What's Your Health IQ? Scoring on p. 642 under Chapter 1.

CHAPTER 11
Tobacco

1. true
2. false, chewing tobacco causes serious problems to mouth, throat, and stomach
3. false, herbal cigarettes do contain tobacco

4. false, smoking can harm your lungs after smoking for only a short time
5. true
6. false, chemicals in tobacco smoke readily pass through the placenta
7. true

To check your score, refer to Knowledge—What's Your Health IQ? Scoring on p. 642 under Chapter 1.

CHAPTER 12
Illegal Drugs

1. false, most people try drugs for various reasons, such as peer pressure
2. false, marijuana is an addictive drug
3. false, stimulants can give you increased energy and alertness yet can be extremely harmful to the body
4. false, anabolic steroids can actually cause males to develop breasts, have a lower sperm count, and have shrunken testes
5. false, medicinal barbituates are given under physician supervision; however, they are still dangerous and addictive
6. true
7. false, damage to the brain due to drug use is usually permanent

To check your score, refer to Knowledge—What's Your Health IQ? Scoring on p. 642 under Chapter 1.

CHAPTER 13
Preventing Infectious Diseases

If you scored:

22–32 points You are doing an excellent job of preventing the spread of infectious diseases and of protecting yourself from infectious diseases.
11–21 points You are doing well overall. However, there are a number of areas in which you could improve your behavior to prevent the spread of infectious diseases.
0–10 points You should make some major changes in your behavior to protect yourself from infectious diseases and prevent the spread of infectious diseases. You can learn to protect yourself from infectious diseases by reading Chapter 13.

CHAPTER 14
Lifestyle Diseases

If you scored:

20–28 points You are doing an excellent job of protecting yourself from lifestyle diseases.
11–19 points You are doing well overall but have areas in which you could improve your health-related behaviors and protect yourself from lifestyle diseases.
0–10 points You have a number of areas in which you could make improvements in your health-related behaviors. You can learn how to protect yourself from lifestyle diseases by reading Chapter 14.

CHAPTER 15
Other Diseases and Disabilities

1. false, the development of some hereditary diseases is influenced by behavioral factors
2. false, scientists hope to develop such treatments but have not done so yet
3. false, autoimmune diseases are caused primarily by defective genes
4. false, allergies and asthma are types of immune disorders while rheumatoid arthritis is an autoimmune disease
5. true

To check your score, refer to Knowledge—What's Your Health IQ? Scoring on p. 642 under Chapter 1.

CHAPTER 16
Adolescence and Adulthood

1. true
2. false, girls naturally have more body fat than boys
3. true
4. false, the leading cause of death in young adults is unintentional injuries; in middle adulthood, the leading cause is cancer
5. false, most older adults do not experience Alzheimer's disease
6. true

To check your score, refer to Knowledge—What's Your Health IQ? Scoring on p. 642 under Chapter 1.

CHAPTER 17
Marriage, Parenthood, and Families

1. false, it's not realistic to expect one's spouse to meet all of his or her partner's needs
2. false, the consequences can also be felt by the couples children, family, and friends
3. false, a mature person initiates resolution to marital conflicts
4. true
5. true

To check your score, refer to Knowledge—What's Your Health IQ? Scoring on p. 642 under Chapter 1.

CHAPTER 18
Reproduction, Pregnancy, and Development

1. false, sperm are made in the testes
2. true
3. false, most cases of testicular cancer occur among men aged 15 to 35
4. false, testosterone is the primary hormone in males
5. true
6. true
7. false, women typically produce and release only one mature egg each month
8. true
9. false, the baby's major body structures are formed by the end of the first trimester

To check your score, refer to Knowledge—What's Your Health IQ? Scoring on p. 642 under Chapter 1.

CHAPTER 19
Building Responsible Relationships

1 . false, differences in values and personality are a significant thing to consider when dating someone
2. false, as in any situation in life, each individual has choices, and there are many ways to avoid the pressures of becoming sexually active

3. true
4. true
5. true

To check your score, refer to Knowledge—What's Your Health IQ? Scoring on p. 642 under Chapter 1.

CHAPTER 20
Risks of Adolescent Sexual Activity

1. true
2. false, only about 20 percent of teen mothers eventually marry the father of the child
3. true
4. true
5. false, abstinence eliminates all of the risks of teen sexual activity

To check your score, refer to Knowledge—What's Your Health IQ? Scoring on p. 642 under Chapter 1.

CHAPTER 21
HIV and AIDS

1. true
2. true
3. false, HIV is not transmitted through casual contact, such as shaking hands
4. false, HIV is not transmitted through casual contact, such as drinking from a water fountain after a person infected with HIV has
5. true
6. true
7. false, sterile, single-use needles are used during blood donations in the U.S., so blood donors are not at risk of HIV infection
8. false, many HIV-infected people are unaware of their infection and therefore cannot warn anyone else of their infection

To check your score, refer to Knowledge—What's Your Health IQ? Scoring on p. 642 under Chapter 1.

A

abdominal thrusts (Heimlich maneuver) the act of applying pressure to a choking person's stomach to force an object out of the throat

abstinence the conscious decision not to participate in sexual activity and the skills to support that decision

abuse physical or emotional harm to someone

acid rain any precipitation that has a below-normal pH (acidic)

acne an inflammation of the skin that occurs when the openings in the skin become clogged with dirt and oil

acquired immune deficiency syndrome (AIDS) the disease that is caused by HIV infection, which weakens the immune system

action plan a set of directions that will help you reach your goal

active ingredient the chemical component that gives a medicine its action

addiction a condition in which a person can no longer control his or her drug use

adolescence the period of time between the start of puberty and full maturation

advocate to speak or argue in favor of something

aggressive hostile and unfriendly in the way one expresses oneself

alcohol the drug in wine, beer, and liquor that causes intoxication

alcohol abuse drinking too much alcohol, drinking it too often, or drinking it at inappropriate times

alcoholism a disease that causes a person to lose control of his or her drinking behavior; a physical and emotional addiction to alcohol

allergy a reaction by the body's immune system to a harmless substance

alveolus a thin-walled air sac that is found in clusters in the lungs and that is the site of gas exchange

Alzheimer's disease a disease in which a person gradually loses mental capacities and the ability to carry out daily activities

amebic dysentery (uh MEE bik DIS uhn TER ee) an inflammation of the intestine that is caused by an ameba

Americans with Disabilities Act (ADA) wide-ranging legislation intended to make American society more accessible to people who have disabilities

anabolic steroid a synthetic version of the male hormone testosterone that is used to promote muscle development

anorexia nervosa an eating disorder that involves self-starvation, a distorted body image, and low body weight

antibiotic resistance a condition in which bacteria can no longer be killed by a particular antibiotic

antibody a protein that is made by the immune system in response to a specific antigen

antigen an identifying protein on the coating of every cell and virus

appetite the desire, rather than the need, to eat certain foods

artery a blood vessel that carries blood away from the heart to other parts of the body

arthritis inflammation of the joints

assertive direct and respectful in the way one expresses oneself

asset a skill or resource that can help a person reach a goal

asthma a disorder that causes the airways that carry air into the lungs to become narrow and to become clogged with mucus

asymptomatic showing no signs of a disease or disorder even though an infection or disease is present

asymptomatic stage a stage of an infection in which the infectious agent, such as HIV, is present but there are few or no symptoms of the infection

atherosclerosis (ATH uhr OH skluh ROH sis) a disease characterized by the buildup of fatty materials on the inside walls of the arteries

atrium a chamber of the heart that receives blood that is returning to the heart

autoimmune disease a disease in which the immune system attacks the cells of the body that the immune system normally protects

GLOSSARY

B

bacteria tiny, single-celled organisms, some of which can cause disease

basal metabolic rate (BMR) the minimum amount of energy required to keep the body alive when in a rested and fasting state

B cell a type of lymphocyte that is made in bone marrow and that makes antibodies

benign tumor (bi NIEN TOO muhr) an abnormal, but usually harmless cell mass

binge drinking the act of drinking five or more drinks in one sitting

binge eating/bingeing eating a large amount of food in one sitting; usually accompanied by a feeling of being out of control

blood a tissue that is made up of cells and fluid and that carries oxygen, carbon dioxide, and nutrients in the body

blood alcohol concentration (BAC) the amount of alcohol in a person's blood, expressed as a percentage

blood pressure the force that blood exerts against the inside walls of a blood vessel

blood vessels the tubes, including arteries, veins, and capillaries, through which the blood moves through the body

body composition the proportion of body weight that is made up of fat tissue compared to lean tissue

body image a measure of how you see and feel about your appearance and how comfortable you are with your body

body mass index (BMI) an index of weight in relation to height that is used to assess healthy body weight

bone marrow a layer of soft tissue at the center of many bones

brain the main control center of the nervous system that is located inside the skull

brain stem the part of the brain that filters and guides signals coming from the spinal cord to other parts of the brain

bronchiole the smallest of the tubes that branch from the bronchus in a lung

bronchus one of the two tubes that branch from the trachea and send air into each lung

bulimia nervosa an eating disorder in which the individual repeatedly eats large amounts of food and then uses behaviors such as vomiting or using laxatives to rid the body of the food

bullying scaring or controlling another person by using threats or physical force

burn an injury to the skin and other tissues that is caused by heat, chemicals, electricity, or radiation

C

cancer a disease caused by uncontrolled cell growth

capillary a tiny blood vessel that carries blood between arteries and veins and through which nutrients and waste pass into and out of the blood

carbohydrate a class of energy-giving nutrients that includes sugars, starches, and fiber

carbon monoxide a gas that blocks oxygen from getting into the bloodstream

carcinogen (kahr SIN uh juhn) any chemical or agent that causes cancer

cardiac pacemaker a group of cells that are at the top of the right atrium and that control the heartbeat

cardiopulmonary resuscitation (CPR) a life-saving technique that combines rescue breathing and chest compressions

cardiovascular disease (CVD) a disease or disorder that results from progressive damage to the heart and blood vessels

carotid pulse the pulse that is felt at the carotid arteries, the major arteries of the neck

cavity a hole in the tooth produced by tooth decay

central nervous system (CNS) the part of the nervous system made up of the brain and spinal cord

cerebellum the part of the brain that controls balance and posture

cerebrum the largest, most complex part of the brain that receives sensations and controls movement

cervix the narrow base of the uterus that leads to the vagina

chemotherapy (KEE moh THER uh pee) the use of drugs to destroy cancer cells

chlamydia (kluh MID ee uh) a bacterial STD that infects the reproductive organs and that causes a mucous discharge

chlorofluorocarbons (CFCs) pollutants released by certain coolants and aerosol sprays

choking the condition in which the trachea (windpipe) is partly or completely blocked

chronic disease a disease that develops gradually and continues over a long period of time

circadian rhythm the body's internal system for regulating sleeping and waking patterns

cirrhosis (suh ROH sis) a deadly disease that replaces healthy liver tissue with scar tissue; most often caused by long-term alcohol abuse

club (designer) drug a drug made to closely resemble a common illegal drug in chemical structure and effect

cochlea a coiled, fluid-filled tube that is found in the inner ear and that is involved in hearing

codependency a condition in which a family member or friend sacrifices his or her own needs to meet the needs of an addict

collaborate to work together with one or more people

collagen protein fibers that make skin flexible

colon the major part of the large intestine

consequence a result of one's actions and decisions

conservation the wise use and protection of natural resources

consumer a person who buys products or services

coping dealing with problems and troubles in an effective way

cross-contamination the transfer of contaminants from one food to another

daily value (DV) the recommended daily amount of a nutrient; used on food labels to help people see how a food fits into their diet

dandruff flaky clumps of dead skin cells from the scalp

date rape sexual intercourse that is forced on a victim by someone the victim knows

decibels (DES uh BUHLZ) the units used to measure sound

deductible the amount that the subscriber must pay before an insurance company begins paying for medical services

defense mechanism an unconscious behavior that is used to avoid experiencing unpleasant emotions

deforestation the clearing of trees from natural forests to make space for crops or development

dehydration a state in which the body has lost more water than has been taken in

depressant a drug that causes relaxation and sleepiness

depression sadness and hopelessness that keeps a person from carrying out everyday activities

dermis the functional layer of skin beneath the epidermis

designated driver a person who chooses not to drink alcohol in a social setting so that he or she can safely drive himself or herself and others

diabetes a disorder in which cells are unable to obtain glucose from the blood such that high blood-glucose levels result

diabetic coma a loss of consciousness that happens when there is too much blood sugar and a buildup of toxic substances in the blood

diaphragm the sheet of muscle that separates the chest cavity from the abdominal cavity and that functions in respiration

Dietary Guidelines for Americans a set of diet and lifestyle recommendations developed to improve health and reduce nutrition-related disease risk in the U.S. population

dietary supplement any product that is taken by mouth, that can contain a dietary ingredient, and that is labeled as a dietary supplement

digestive tract the series of organs through which food passes

direct pressure the pressure that results from someone who tries to convince you to do something you normally wouldn't do

disability a physical or mental impairment or deficiency that interferes with a person's normal activity

discipline the act of teaching a child through correction, direction, rules, and reinforcement

dislocation an injury in which a bone has been forced out of its normal position in a joint

distress a negative stress that can make a person sick or can keep a person from reaching a goal

divorce the legal end to a marriage

domestic violence the use of force to control and maintain power over a spouse in the home

drug any substance that causes a change in a person's physical or psychological state

drug abuse the intentional improper or unsafe use of a drug

drug combination therapy an AIDS treatment program in which patients regularly take more than one drug

drug interaction a condition in which a drug reacts with another drug, food, or dietary supplement such that the effect of one of the substances is greater or smaller

drug tolerance a condition in which a user needs more of a drug to get the same effect

ear the sense organ that functions in hearing and balance

eardrum a membrane that transmits sound waves from the outer ear to the middle ear

ecosystem a community of living things and the nonliving parts of the community's environment

egg (ovum) the sex cell that is made by the ovaries and that can be fertilized by sperm

electrocution a fatal injury caused by electricity entering the body and destroying vital tissues

embryo a developing human, from fertilization through the first 8 weeks of development

emotion the feeling that is produced in response to life experiences

emotional intimacy the state of being emotionally connected to another person

emotional maturity the ability to assess a relationship or situation and to act according to what is best for oneself and for the other person in the relationship

empathy the ability to understand another person's feelings, behaviors, and attitudes

emphysema a respiratory disease in which air cannot move in and out of alveoli because they become blocked or lose their elasticity

enabling helping an addict avoid the negative consequences of his or her behavior

endocrine gland an organ that releases hormones into the bloodstream or into the fluid around cells

endometrium the lining of the uterus

environment the living and nonliving things that surround an organism

environmental tobacco smoke (secondhand smoke) a combination of exhaled mainstream smoke and sidestream smoke

enzyme a protein or other type of molecule that helps chemical processes happen in living things

epidemic the occurrence of more cases of a disease than expected

epidermis the outermost layer of the skin, made of one to several layers of dead cells

epinephrine (EP uh NEF rin) one of the hormones released by the body in times of stress; also called adrenaline

esophagus a long, straight tube that connects the pharynx (throat) to the stomach and through which food moves to get into the stomach

estrogen a hormone that regulates the sexual development and reproductive function of females

eustachian tube the tube that connects the middle ear to the throat

eustress a positive stress that energizes a person and helps a person reach a goal

extended family the people who are outside the nuclear family but are related to the nuclear family, such as aunts, uncles, grandparents, and cousins

external bleeding bleeding at the surface of the body

external pressure pressure that a person feels from another person or group to engage in a behavior

eye the sense organ that gathers and focuses light, generates signals that are sent to the brain, and allows one to see

GLOSSARY

F

fad diet a diet that requires a major change in eating habits and promises quick weight loss

fallopian tube the female reproductive organ that connects an ovary to the uterus and that transports an egg from the ovary to the uterus

family counseling counseling discussions that are led by a third party to resolve conflict among family members

fat a class of energy-giving nutrients; *also* the main form of energy storage in the body

fee-for-service insurance plan a traditional insurance plan in which the patient must pay a premium and a deductible

fertilization the process by which a sperm and an egg and their genetic material join to create a new human life

fetal alcohol syndrome (FAS) a set of physical and mental defects that affect a fetus that has been exposed to alcohol because of the mother's consumption of alcohol during pregnancy

fetus a developing human, from the start of the ninth week of pregnancy until delivery

first degree burn a burn that affects only the outer layer of the skin and looks pink

FITT a formula made up of the four parts of fitness training: frequency, intensity, time, and type

follicle a tiny pit in the skin that holds the root of a hair

food allergy an abnormal response to a food that is triggered by the immune system

food-borne illness an illness caused by eating or drinking a food that contains a toxin or disease-causing microorganism

Food Guide Pyramid a tool for choosing a healthy diet by selecting a recommended number of servings from each of six food groups

fracture a crack or break in a bone

fraud the marketing and selling of products or services by making false claims

frostbite a condition in which body tissues become frozen

funeral a ceremony in which a deceased person is buried or cremated

fungus an organism that absorbs and uses nutrients of living or dead organisms

G

gene a segment of DNA located on a chromosome that codes for a specific hereditary trait and that is passed from parent to offspring

generic medicine a medicine made by a company other than the company that developed the original medicine

gene therapy a technique that places a healthy copy of a gene into the cells of a person whose copy of the gene is defective

genetic counseling the process of informing a person or couple about their genetic makeup

gingivitis a condition in which the gums become red and infected and begin to pull away from the teeth

goal something that you work toward and hope to achieve

gonorrhea (GAHN uh REE uh) an STD that is caused by a bacterium that infects mucous membranes, including the genital mucous membranes

grieve to express deep sadness because of a loss

H

hallucinogen a drug that distorts perceptions, causing the user to see or hear things that are not real

hand signals signals used by cyclists that show pedestrians, automobile drivers, and others on the road when they intend to make a turn or stop

hazardous weather dangerous weather that causes concern for safety

hazing harassing newcomers to a group in an abusive and humiliating way

head lice tiny parasites that feed on blood vessels in the scalp

health the state of well-being in which all of the components of health—physical, emotional, social, mental, spiritual, and environmental—are in balance

health literacy knowledge of health information needed to make good choices about your health

health maintenance organization (HMO) a managed-care plan in which patients must use a doctor who contracts with the insurance company

Health on the Net (HON) Foundation an organization of Web sites that agree to follow a code of ethics regarding health information

health-related fitness fitness qualities that are necessary to maintain and promote a healthy body

Healthy People 2010 a set of health objectives established by the U.S. Department of Health and Human Services for improving the nation's health by 2010

heart the organ that acts as a pump that pushes the blood through the body

heart attack the damage and loss of function of an area of the heart muscle

heartburn the pain that is felt behind the breastbone and that is caused by GERD (gastric esophageal reflux disorder)

heat exhaustion a condition in which the body becomes heated to a higher temperature than normal

heatstroke a condition in which body loses its ability to cool itself by sweating

helper T cell (CD4+ cell) white blood cell that activates the immune response and that is the primary target cell of HIV infection

hemoglobin the oxygen-carrying pigment in red blood cells

hepatitis an inflammation of the liver

hereditary disease a disease caused by abnormal chromosomes or by defective genes inherited by a child from one or both parents

heredity (huh RED i tee) the passing down of traits from parents to their biological child

high-risk population any group of people who have an increased chance of getting a disease

HIV-antibody test a test that detects HIV antibodies to determine if a person has been infected with HIV

HIV positive describes a person who tests positive in two different HIV tests

home healthcare services medical services, treatment, or equipment provided for the patient in his or her home

hormone a chemical substance that is made and released in one part of the body and that causes a change in another part of the body

Human Genome Project a research effort to determine the locations of all human genes on the chromosomes and to read the coded instructions in the genes

human immunodeficiency virus (HIV) the virus that primarily infects cells of the immune system and that causes AIDS

human papilloma virus (HPV) a group of viruses that can cause genital warts in males and females and can cause cervical cancer in females

hunger the body's physical response to the need for food

hypothermia a condition in which the internal body temperature becomes dangerously low

incest sexual activity between family members who are not husband and wife

incontinence loss of voluntary control of urination

indirect pressure the pressure that results from being swayed to do something because people you look up to are doing it

infectious disease (in FEK shuhs di ZEEZ) any disease that is caused by an agent that has invaded the body

inflammation a reaction to injury or infection that is characterized by pain, redness, and swelling

inhalant a drug that is inhaled as a vapor

inpatient care medical care that requires a person to stay in a hospital for more than a day

insomnia an inability to sleep even if one is physically exhausted

insulin a hormone that causes cells to remove glucose from the bloodstream

integrity the characteristic of doing what one knows is right

internal bleeding bleeding within the body

internal pressure an impulse a person feels to engage in a behavior

intervention confronting a drug user about his or her drug abuse problem to stop him or her from using drugs

intoxication the physical and mental changes produced by drinking alcohol

joint a place where two or more bones meet in the body

keratin a strong, flexible protein found in skin, hair, and nails

kidney organ that filters water and wastes from the blood, excretes products as urine, and regulates the concentration of certain substances in the blood

lactose intolerance the inability to completely digest the milk sugar lactose

leukemia cancer of the tissues that make white blood cells

life expectancy the average length of time an individual is expected to live

life skill a tool for building a healthy life

lifestyle disease a disease that is caused partly by unhealthy behaviors and partly by other factors

ligament a type of tissue that holds the ends of bones together at joints

lung the main organ of the respiratory system in which oxygen from the air is exchanged with carbon dioxide from the blood

lymph the clear, yellowish fluid that leaks from capillaries, fills the spaces around the body's cells, and is collected by the lymphatic vessels and nodes

lymphatic system a network of vessels that carry a clear fluid called *lymph* throughout the body

lymph node a small, bean-shaped organ that contains small fibers that remove particles from the lymph

lymphocytes white blood cells that destroy bacteria, viruses, and dead or damaged cells

mainstream smoke smoke that is inhaled through a cigarette and then exhaled by a cigarette smoker

malignant tumor (muh LIG nuhnt TOO muhr) a mass of cells that invades and destroys healthy tissue

managed-care plan a plan in which an insurance company makes a contract with a group of doctors

marijuana the dried flowers and leaves of the plant *Cannabis sativa* that are smoked or mixed in food and eaten for intoxicating effects

marriage a lifelong union between a husband and a wife, who develop an intimate relationship

media all public forms of communication, such as TV, radio, newspaper, the Internet, and advertisements

Medicaid a healthcare program available to people who are on welfare, have dependent children, or are elderly, blind, or disabled

Medicare a healthcare program available to people who are 65 years old or older and for younger individuals who are disabled

medicine any drug used to cure, prevent, or treat illness or discomfort

melanin a pigment that gives skin its color and shields skin from ultraviolet radiation

memorial service a ceremony to remember the deceased person

meningitis an inflammation of the membranes covering the brain and spinal cord

menopause the time of life when a woman stops ovulating and menstruating

menstrual cycle a monthly series of hormone-controlled changes that prepare the uterine lining for a pregnancy

menstruation the monthly breakdown and shedding of the lining of the uterus, during which blood and tissue leave the woman's body through the vagina

mental disorder an illness that affects a person's thoughts, emotions, and behaviors

mental health the state of mental well-being in which one can cope with the demands of daily life

midlife crisis the sense of uncertainty about one's identity and values that some people experience in the middle of their lives

mineral a class of nutrients that are chemical elements that are needed for certain body processes, such as enzyme activity and bone formation

motor nerve a nerve that carries signals from the brain or spinal cord to the muscles and glands

mucus a thick, slimy fluid that is secreted by the lining of organs and glands

multiple sclerosis an autoimmune disease in which the body mistakenly attacks myelin, the fatty insulation on nerves in the brain and spinal cord

natural disaster a natural event that causes widespread injury, death, and property damage

neglect the failure of a caretaker to provide for basic needs, such as food, clothing, or love

negotiation a bargain or compromise for a peaceful solution to a conflict

neonatal abstinence syndrome drug withdrawal that occurs in newborn infants whose mothers were frequent drug users while pregnant

nephron a tiny, blood-filtering unit in the kidney

nerve a bundle of nerve cells (neurons) that carry electrical signals from one part of the body to another

neuron a specialized cell that receives and sends electrical signals

neurotransmitter a chemical released at the end of a neuron's axon

nicotine the highly addictive drug that is found in all tobacco products

nicotine substitutes medicines that deliver small amounts of nicotine to the body to help a person quit using tobacco

nonrenewable resource a natural resource that can be used up faster than it can be replenished naturally

nuclear family a family in which a mother, a father, and one or more biological or adopted children live together

nutrient a substance in food that provides energy or helps form body tissues and that is necessary for life and growth

nutrient deficiency the state of not having enough of a nutrient to maintain good health

nutrient density a measure of the nutrients in a food compared with the energy that the food provides

nutrition the science or study of food and the ways in which the body uses food

obesity (oh BEE suh tee) the state of having excess body fat for one's weight; the state of weighing more than 20 percent above one's recommended body weight

Occupational Safety and Health Administration (OSHA) a government agency created to prevent work-related injuries, illnesses, and death

opiates a group of highly addictive drugs derived from the poppy plant that are used as pain relievers, anesthetics, and sedatives

opportunistic infection (OI) an illness that is due to an organism that causes disease in people with weakened immune systems; commonly found in AIDS patients

outbreak an unexpected increase in illness

outpatient care medical care that requires that a person stay in the hospital only during his or her treatment

ovary the female reproductive organ that produces eggs and the hormones estrogen and progesterone

overcrowding condition in which there are too many inhabitants in an area to live healthily

overdose the taking of too much of a drug, which causes sickness, loss of consciousness, permanent damage, or even death

over-the-counter (OTC) medicine any medicine that can be bought without a prescription

overpopulation the point at which a population is too large to be supported by the available resources

overtraining a condition that occurs as a result of exceeding the recommendations of the FITT formula

overweight heavy for one's height

ovulation (AHV yoo LAY shuhn) the process in which the ovaries release a mature egg every month

GLOSSARY

P

pandemic a disease that spreads quickly through human populations all over the world

parental responsibility the duty of a parent to provide for the physical, financial, mental, and emotional needs of a child

passive not offering opposition when challenged or pressured

pathogen any agent that causes disease

peer mediation a technique in which a trained outsider who is your age helps people in a conflict come to a peaceful resolution

peer pressure a feeling that you should do something because that is what your friends want

pelvic inflammatory disease (PID) an inflammation of the upper female reproductive tract that is caused by the migration of a bacterial infection from the vagina

penis the male reproductive organ that removes urine from the body and that can deliver sperm to the female reproductive system

peripheral nervous system (PNS) the part of the nervous system made up of the nerves that connect the brain and spinal cord to other parts of the body

physical dependence a condition in which the body relies on a given drug in order to function

physical fitness the ability of the body to perform daily physical activities without becoming short of breath, sore, or overly tired

placenta a blood vessel–rich organ that forms in a mother's uterus and that provides nutrients and oxygen to and removes waste from a developing baby

plaque a mixture of food particles, saliva, and bacteria on the tooth

platelet a cell fragment that is needed to form blood clots

poison a substance that can cause illness or death when taken into the body

preferred provider organization (PPO) a managed-care plan that offers the patient an option to see a doctor who does not contract with the insurance company; the patient pays a higher fee to use this option

premium the monthly fee for insurance

prenatal care the healthcare provided for a woman during her pregnancy

prescription (pree SKRIP shuhn) a written order from a doctor for a specific medicine

primary care physician (PCP) family doctor who handles general medical care

prioritize to arrange items in order of importance

prostate gland a gland in males that adds fluids that nourish and protect sperm as the sperm move through the female body

protective factor anything that keeps a person from engaging in a harmful behavior

protein a class of nutrients that are made up of amino acids, which are needed to build and repair body structures and to regulate processes in the body

psychoactive describes a drug or medicine that affects the brain and changes how a person perceives, thinks, or feels

puberty the period of human development during which people become able to produce children

public health the study and practice of protecting and improving the health of people in a community

public service announcement (PSA) a message created to educate people about an issue

purging engaging in behaviors such as vomiting or misusing laxatives to rid the body of food

Q

quackery a type of fraud; the promotion of healthcare services or products that are worthless or not proven effective

R

Recommended Dietary Allowances (RDAs) recommended nutrient intakes that will meet the needs of almost all healthy people

recovering the process of learning to live without drugs

rectum the last part of the large intestine in which undigested wastes are stored

recycling reusing materials from used products to make new products

red blood cell blood cell that carries oxygen to the body cells and that returns carbon dioxide to the lungs

reflex an involuntary and almost immediate movement in response to a stimulus

refusal skill a strategy to avoid doing something you don't want to do

relapse a return to using drugs while trying to recover from drug addiction

renewable resource a natural resource that can be replaced over a short period of time

repetitions the number of times that an exercise is performed

rescue breathing an emergency technique in which a rescuer gives air to someone who is not breathing

resiliency the ability to recover from illness, hardship, and other stressors

resource something that you can use to help achieve a goal

resting heart rate (RHR) the number of times that the heart beats per minute while the body is at rest

retina the light-sensitive inner layer of the eye, which receives images formed by the lens and transmits nerve signals through the optic nerve to the brain

risk factor anything that increases the likelihood of injury, disease, or other health problems

root canal a procedure in which a dentist drills into the pulp of a tooth to remove the infection from a cavity

salmonellosis a bacterial infection of the digestive system that is usually spread by eating contaminated food

sanitation the practice of providing sewage disposal and treatment, solid waste disposal, clean drinking water, and clean living and working conditions

scrotum a skin-covered sac that holds the testes and that hangs from the male body

sebaceous gland gland in the skin that adds oil to the skin and hair shaft to keep skin and hair looking smooth and healthy

second-degree burn a burn that extends into the inner skin layer and is red, swollen, and blistered

sedentary not taking part in physical activity on a regular basis

self-actualization the achievement of the best that a person can be

self-concept a measure of how one views oneself

self-esteem a measure of how much one values, respects, and feels confident about oneself

semen a fluid made up of sperm and other secretions from the male reproductive organs

sensory nerve a nerve that carries signals from a sense organ to the central nervous system, where the signals are processed or relayed

set a fixed number of repetitions followed by a rest period

sexual abuse any sexual act that happens without consent

sexual activity any activity that includes intentional sexual contact for the purpose of sexual arousal

sexual assault any sexual activity in which force or the threat of force is used

sexual harassment any unwanted remark, behavior, or touch that has sexual content

sexual intercourse the reproductive process in which the penis is inserted into the vagina and through which a new human life may begin

sexually transmitted disease (STD) an infectious disease that is spread by sexual contact

shock a condition in which some body organs do not get enough oxygenated blood

sibling a brother or sister related to another brother or sister by blood, the marriage of the individuals' parents, or adoption

side effect any effect that is caused by a drug and that is different from the drug's intended effect

sidestream smoke smoke that escapes from the tip of a cigarette, cigar, or pipe

skeleton a framework of bones that support the muscles and organs and protect the inner organs

sleep apnea a sleeping disorder characterized by interruptions of normal breathing patterns during sleep

sleep deprivation a lack of sleep

sperm the sex cell that is made by the testes and that is needed to fertilize an egg from a female

spinal cord the column of nerve tissue that runs through the backbone from the base of the brain

spinal nerves nerves that branch from the spinal cord and that go to the brain and to the tissues of the body

splint a device used to stabilize (hold secure) a body part

sprain an injury in which the ligaments in a joint are stretched too far or are torn

stimulant a drug that temporarily increases a person's energy and alertness

strain an injury in which a muscle or tendon has been stretched too far or has torn

stress the body's and mind's response to a demand

stressor any situation that is a demand on the body or mind

stroke a sudden attack of weakness or paralysis that occurs when blood flow to an area of the brain is interrupted

suffocation a fatal injury caused by an inability to breathe when the nose and mouth are blocked or when the body becomes oxygen-deficient

suicide the act of intentionally taking one's own life

symptom a change that a person notices in his or her body or mind and that is caused by a disease or disorder

synapse a tiny space across which nerve impulses pass from one neuron to the next

syphilis (SIF uh lis) a bacterial STD that causes ulcers or chancres; if untreated, it can lead to mental and physical disabilities and premature death

tar a sticky, black substance in tobacco smoke that coats the inside of the airways and that contains many carcinogens

target heart rate zone a heart rate range that should be reached during exercise to gain cardiorespiratory health benefits

T cell a white blood cell that is made in the thymus and that attacks cells that have been infected by viruses

tendon a strong connective tissue that attaches muscles to bones

testis (testicle) the male reproductive organ that makes sperm and testosterone

testosterone the male hormone that is made by the testes and that regulates male secondary sex characteristics and the production of sperm

third-degree burn a burn that penetrates all layers of skin as well as the tissue beneath the skin and appears pearly white, tan colored, or charred

tinnitus (ti NIET es) a buzzing, ringing, or whistling sound in one or both ears that occurs even when no sound is present

tolerance the ability to overlook differences and to accept people for who they are; *also* a condition in which a user needs more of a drug to get the same effect

tonsils small, rounded masses of lymph tissues found in the throat

tooth decay the process in which acid from plaque and tartar slowly dissolve the hard surfaces of the teeth

trachea the long tube that carries air from the larynx to the lungs; also called the windpipe

trigger lock a device that helps prevent a gun from being fired

ultraviolet (UV) radiation radiation in sunlight that is responsible for tanning and burning skin

universal precautions the set of procedures used to avoid contact with body fluids and to reduce the risk of spreading HIV and other diseases

urinary bladder the hollow, muscular sac that stores urine

urine waste liquid excreted by the kidneys, stored in the bladder, and passed through the urethra to the outside of the body

uterus the female reproductive organ that provides a place to support a developing human

vaccine a substance that is usually prepared from killed or weakened pathogens or from genetic material and that is introduced into a body to produce immunity

vagina the female reproductive organ that connects the outside of the body to the uterus and that receives sperm during reproduction

value a strong belief or ideal

vegetarian dietary pattern that includes few or no animal products

vein a blood vessel that carries blood toward the heart

ventricle one of the two large, muscular chambers that pump blood out of the heart

violence physical force that is used to harm people or damage property

virus a tiny disease-causing particle that consists of genetic material and a protein coat

vitamin a class of nutrients that contain carbon and that are needed in small amounts to maintain health and allow growth

wake a ceremony to view or watch over the deceased person before the funeral

weight management a program of sensible eating and exercise habits that keep weight at a healthy level

wellness the achievement of a person's best in all six components of health

white blood cell a blood cell whose primary job is to defend the body against disease

withdrawal uncomfortable physical and psychological symptoms produced when a physically dependent drug user stops using drugs

wound a break or tear in the soft tissues of the body

carcinogen/carcinógeno toda sustancia química o agente que causa cáncer

cardiac pacemaker/marcapasos cardíaco grupo de células que se encuentran en la parte superior de la aurícula derecha y controlan los latidos del corazón

cardiopulmonary resuscitation (CPR)/resucitación cardiopulmonar (CPR, por su nombre en inglés) técnica para salvar la vida que combina la recuperación de la respiración y compresiones en el pecho

cardiovascular disease (CVD)/enfermedad cardiovascular trastorno del sistema circulatorio causado por daño al corazón y vaso sanguíneo

carotid pulse/pulso carotideo pulso que se siente en las arterias de las carótidas, arterias principales del cuello

cavity/caries cavidad en la dentadura de una persona producida por la degeneración dental

central nervous system (CNS)/sistema nervioso central (SNC) el cerebro y la médula espinal

cerebellum/cerebelo parte del cerebro que controla el equilibrio y la postura

cerebrum/córtex parte más grande y compleja del cerebro que recibe sensaciones y controla el movimiento

cervix/cuello de la matriz base angosta de la matriz que conduce a la vagina

chemotherapy/quimioterapia uso de drogas con la finalidad de destruir células cancerosas

chlamydia /clamidia ETS causada por una bacteria que infecta los órganos reproductores y provoca la secreción de una sustancia mucosa

chlorofluorocarbons (CFCs)/clorofluorocarbonos (CFC) contaminantes que despiden ciertos pulverizadores en aerosol y líquidos refrigerantes

choking/atragantamiento trastorno en el que el tubo digestivo se obstruye de manera parcial o total

chronic disease/enfermedad crónica enfermedad que se desarrolla poco a poco y continúa durante un período prolongado de tiempo

circadian rhythm/ritmo circadiano sistema interno del cuerpo encargado de regular los patrones de sueño y actividad

cirrhosis/cirrosis enfermedad mortal que reemplaza los tejidos sanos del hígado por tejidos cicatrizados inservibles; en la mayoría de los casos es causada por el abuso de alcohol durante un largo período de tiempo

club (designer) drug/droga de club (de diseño) droga elaborada de modo que su estructura química y efectos son similares a los de una droga ilegal común

cochlea/cóclea tubo en forma de espiral, lleno de líquido, que se encuentra en el oído interno y participa en la audición

codependency/codependencia condición en la que un integrante de la familia o un amigo sacrifica sus necesidades para satisfacer las necesidades de un adicto

collaborate/colaborar trabajar juntos con una o más personas

collagen/colágeno fibras de proteínas que hacen que la piel sea flexible

colon/colon porción principal del intestino grueso

consequence/consecuencia resultado de las acciones y las decisiones de una persona

conservation/conservación uso correcto y la protección de los recursos naturales

consumer/consumidor persona que compra productos o servicios

coping/sobrellevar manejar los problemas y los inconvenientes de manera eficaz

cross contamination/contaminación cruzada traspaso de contaminantes de un alimento a otro

daily value (DV)/valor diario (VD) cantidad diaria recomendada de un nutriente; se utiliza en las etiquetas de los alimentos y permite a las personas saber qué aporta un alimento a su dieta

dandruff/caspa trocitos escamosos de células de piel muertas en el cuero cabelludo

date rape/violación en una cita relación sexual forzada por alguien que la víctima conoce

decibels (dB)/decibeles (dB) unidades utilizadas para medir el sonido

deductible/deducible monto que el abonado debe pagar antes de que una compañía de seguro comience a pagar los servicios médicos

defense mechanism/mecanismo de defensa pensamiento o conducta inconsciente que se utiliza para no experimentar emociones desagradables

deforestation/deforestación eliminación de árboles de los bosques naturales con la finalidad de hacer lugar para cosechas o construcciones

dehydration/deshidratación condición en la que el cuerpo no contiene suficiente agua

depressant/depresivo droga que produce relajación y somnolencia

depression/depresión trastorno del ánimo en el que una persona se siente muy triste y desesperanzada durante un período largo de tiempo

dermis/dermis capa funcional de la piel debajo de la epidermis

designated driver/conductor asignado persona que decide no beber alcohol en un evento social para poder manejar de manera segura, ya sea que viaje solo o acompañado

diabetes/diabetes trastorno en el que las células no pueden obtener glucosa de la sangre y que resulta en niveles altos de glucosa en la sangre

diabetic coma/coma diabético pérdida del conocimiento que ocurre cuando el nivel de azúcar en la sangre es muy alto y se forma una acumulación de sustancias tóxicas en la sangre

diaphragm/diafragma lámina de músculo que separa la cavidad torácica de la cavidad abdominal y que participa de la respiración

Dietary Guidelines for Americans/Guía Alimenticia para los Estadounidenses conjunto de recomendaciones alimenticias y sobre el estilo de vida desarrollado para mejorar la salud y reducir el riesgo de enfermedades relacionadas con la nutrición en la población estadounidense

dietary supplement/suplemento alimenticio todo producto que se tome vía oral y contenga un ingrediente dietario y lleve una etiqueta que lo identifique como un suplemento dietario

digestive tract/tracto digestivo serie de órganos por los que pasan los alimentos

direct pressure/presión directa presión ejercida por una persona para de convencer a otra de que haga algo que normalmente no haría

disability/discapacidad incapacidad o deficiencia mental o física que afecta la actividad normal

discipline/disciplina acción de enseñar a un niño a través de la corrección, indicaciones, reglas y refuerzo

dislocation/dislocación lesión en la que un hueso sale de su posición normal en una articulación

distress/alteración estrés negativo que puede hacer que una persona se enferme o no logre alcanzar una meta

divorce/divorcio terminación legal de un matrimonio

domestic violence/violencia doméstica uso de la fuerza para controlar y mantener poder sobre el conyuge en el hogar

drug/droga toda sustancia química que provoca un cambio en el estado físico o emocional de una persona

drug abuse/abuso de drogas uso indebido e intencional de una droga legal o uso de una droga ilegal

drug combination therapy/terapia de combinación de drogas programa de tratamiento para el SIDA en el que los pacientes toman más de una droga regularmente

drug interaction/interacción de drogas condición en la que una droga reacciona al ser combinada con otra droga, un alimento o un suplemento alimenticio; por ejemplo, el efecto de una de las drogas puede ser mayor o menor

drug tolereance/tolerancia a la droga condición en la que una persona necesita aumentar la dosis de droga para obtener el mismo efecto

ear/oído órgano sensorial que participa en la audición y el equilibrio

eardrum/tímpano membrana que transmite ondas de sonido del oído externo al oído medio

ecosystem/ecosistema comunidad de seres vivos y los elementos no vivientes de su entorno

egg (ovum)/óvulo célula sexual producida por los ovarios que puede ser fecundada por un espermatozoide

health-related fitness/estado físico relacionado a la salud cualidades de estado físico necesarias para mantener y promover un cuerpo sano

Healthy People 2010/Gente sana 2010 conjunto de objetivos para la salud establecidos por el Departamento de Salud y Servicios Humanos de Estados Unidos con el propósito de mejorar la salud de la nación para el año 2010

heart/corazón órgano que funciona como una bomba que hace fluir la sangre a través del cuerpo

heart attack/ataque al corazón condición en la que el corazón no recibe suficiente sangre y el tejido del corazón se daña o se destruye

heartburn/acidez estomacal dolor que se siente detrás del esternón provocado por el TREG (trastorno de reflujo esofagogástrico)

heat exhaustion/agotamiento por calor trastorno de salud en el que el cuerpo adquiere una temperatura superior a la temperatura normal

heat stroke/insolación trastorno de salud en el que el sistema que controla la capacidad del cuerpo para enfriarse mediante la transpiración deja de funcionar

helper T cell (CD4+ cell)/célula T colaboradora (célula CD4+) glóbulo blanco que activa la respuesta inmunológica y que es la célula objetivo principal de la infección por VIH

hemoglobin/hemoglobina pigmento presente en los glóbulos rojos encargado de transportar oxígeno

hepatitis/hepatitis inflamación del hígado

hereditary disease/enfermedad hereditaria enfermedad causada por cromosomas anormales o por genes defectuosos que un niño hereda de uno o ambos padres

heredity/herencia transmisión de rasgos de los padres a sus hijos biológicos

high-risk population/población de alto riesgo todo grupo de personas que tienen mayores probabilidades de contraer una enfermedad

HIV-antibody test/prueba de anticuerpo del VIH prueba que detecra los anticuerpos del VIH, lo que permite determinar si una persona está infectada por el VIH

HIV positive/VIH positivo describe a una persona que tiene dos pruebas diferentes de VIH con resultado positivo

home healthcare services/servicios de salud en el hogar servicios médicos, tratamientos o equipo que se le proporcionan al paciente en su casa

hormone/hormona sustancia química que se elabora y se libera en una parte del cuerpo y produce un cambio en otra parte del cuerpo

Human Genome Project/Proyecto del genoma humano trabajo de investigación con el objetivo de determinar las ubicaciones de todos los genes humanos en los cromosomas e interpretar las instrucciones codificadas en los genes

human immunodeficiency virus (HIV)/virus de inmunodeficiencia humana virus que infecta principalmente las celulas del sistema inmunológico y causa el SIDA

human papilloma virus (HPV)/virus de papiloma humano (VPH) grupo de virus que puede causar verrugas genitales en hombres y mujeres y cáncer de cuello de la matriz en las mujeres

hunger/hambre respuesta física del cuerpo a la necesidad de alimentos

hypothermia/hipotermia temperatura corporal inferior al valor normal

immunity/inmunidad enfermedad causada por un agente patógeno que se puede transmitir de una persona a otra

incest/incesto relación sexual entre los integrantes de una familia que no son marido y mujer

incontinence/incontinencia pérdida del control voluntario de la orina

indirect pressure/presión indirecta presión para hacer algo porque las personas que admiras lo hacen

infectious disease/enfermedad infecciosa toda enfermedad causada por un agente o un patógeno que invade el cuerpo

inflammation/inflamación reacción a una lesión o infección caracterizada por dolor, enrojecimiento e hinchazón

inhalant/inhalante una droga que se inhala en forma de vapor

inpatient care/hospitalización atención médica que requiere que una persona permanezca en el hospital durante más de un día

insomnia/insomnio incapacidad para dormir aun si la persona está físicamente agotada

insulin/insulina hormona que permite que la glucosa pase del torrente sanguíneo a las células

integrity/integridad característica de hacer lo que uno sabe que es correcto

internal bleeding/sangrado interno sangrado dentro del cuerpo

internal pressure /presión interna impulso que siente una persona de actuar de una manera determinada

intervention/intervención acción de enfrentar a un consumidor de drogas con su problema para que deje de consumirlas

intoxication/intoxicación cambios físicos y mentales producidos por beber alcohol

joint/articulación parte del cuerpo en la que dos o más huesos se encuentran

keratin/queratina proteína fuerte y flexible que se encuentra en la piel, el pelo y las uñas

kidney/riñón uno de los órganos que filtra el agua y los desechos de la sangre, elimina productos en forma de orina y regula la concentración de ciertas sustancias en la sangre

lactose intolerance/intolerancia a la lactosa incapacidad de digerir completamente la lactosa, el azúcar de la leche

leukemia/leucemia cáncer de los tejidos del cuerpo que producen glóbulos blancos

life expectancy/esperanza de vida tiempo de vida promedio que se espera viva una persona

life skill/destreza para la vida herramienta para construir una vida sana

lifestyle disease/enfermedad causada por el estilo de vida enfermedad causada en parte por conductas no saludables y en parte por otros factores

ligament/ligamento tipo de tejido que mantiene unidos los extremos de los huesos en las articulaciones

lung/pulmón órgano principal del aparato respiratorio en el que el oxígeno del aire se intercambia con el dióxido de carbono de la sangre

lymph/linfa líquido transparente y amarillento que sale de los capilares, llena los espacios alrededor de las células del cuerpo y es absorbido por los vasos y ganglios linfáticos

lymphatic system/sistema linfático red de vasos que transportan la linfa por todo el cuerpo

lymph node/ganglio linfático órgano pequeño en forma de frijol que contiene fibras pequeñas que eliminan partículas de la linfa

lymphocytes/linfocitos glóbulos blancos que destruyen bacterias, virus y células muertas o dañadas

mainstream smoke/humo emanado por fumador humo que un fumador inhala a través de un cigarrillo y luego exhala

malignant tumor/tumor maligno masa de células que invade y destruye el tejido sano

managed-care plan/plan de atención de salud administrada plan en el que una compañía de seguros firma un contrato con un grupo de médicos

marijuana/marihuana flores y hojas secas de la planta *Cannabis sativa*

marriage/matrimonio unión para toda la vida entre marido y mujer, quienes mantienen una relación íntima

media/medios de comunicación todas las formas públicas de comunicación; por ejemplo, televisión, radio, periódicos, Internet y avisos publicitarios

Medicaid/Medicaid programa del cuidado de la salud disponible para personas que tienen un plan de asistencia, tienen hijos dependientes, o son ancianos, ciegos o discapacitados

Medicare/Medicare programa de salud para personas de 65 años de edad o mayores y para personas más jóvenes con discapacidades

placenta/placenta organo rico en vasos sanguíneos que se forma en la matriz de la madre, proporciona nutrientes y oxígeno al bebé en desarrollo y elimina sus desechos

plaque/placa mezcla de bacterias, saliva y partículas de alimentos que se deposita en los dientes

platelet/plaqueta fragmento de célula necesario para formar coágulos de sangre

poison/veneno sustancia que puede ocasionar enfermedad o muerte si ingresa al cuerpo

preferred provider organization (PPO)/organización de proveedor seleccionado (PPO, por su nombre en inglés) plan de salud administrado en el que el paciente tiene la opción de consultar a un médico que no tiene contrato con la compañía de seguro; el paciente paga una tarifa más elevada por uilizar esta opción

premium/prima tarifa mensual de un seguro

prenatal care /atención prenatal cuidado de la salud que se proporciona a una mujer durante el embarazo

prescription/receta orden escrita de un médico para un medicamento específico

primary care physician (PCP)/médico de cabecera (PCP, por su nombre en inglés) médico personal o de la familia que se encarga de los cuidados médicos generales

prioritize/dar prioridad disponer elementos por orden de importancia

prostate gland/próstata glándula masculina que aporta líquidos que nutren y protegen a los espermatozoides a medida que se desplazan por el cuerpo de la mujer

protective factor/factor protector cualquier cosa que impide a una persona adoptar una conducta ofensiva

protein/proteína clase de nutrientes formados por aminoácidos, sustancias necesarias para construir y reparar estructuras del cuerpo y regular procesos del cuerpo

psychoactive/psicoactivo describe a una droga o un medicamento que afecta al cerebro, que cambia cómo percibimos, pensamos o sentimos

puberty/pubertad período del desarrollo humano durante el que las personas adquieren la capacidad de tener hijos

public health/salud pública práctica de proteger y mejorar la salud de personas en una comunidad

public service announcement (PSA)/anuncio de servicio público (PSA, por su nombre en inglés) mensaje creado para educar a las personas sobre un tema

purging/purgar llevar a cabo acciones tales como vomitar o consumir laxantes de forma indebida para eliminar la comida del cuerpo

quackery/curanderismo un tipo de fraude; promoción de servicios o productos de salud sin valor o comprobación

Recommended Dietary Allowances (RDAs)/cuotas dietarias recomendadas (CDR) consumo de nutrientes recomendados que satisfacen las necesidades de casi todas las personas sanas

recovering/recuperando proceso de aprender a vivir sin drogas

rectum/recto porción final del intestino grueso donde se almacenan los desechos no digeridos

recycling/reciclaje reutilización de materiales a partir de productos usados para elaborar productos nuevos

red blood cell/glóbulo rojo célula de la sangre que transporta oxígeno a las células del cuerpo y que transporta dióxido de carbono de regreso a los pulmones

reflex/reflejo movimiento involuntario y casi inmediato en respuesta a un estímulo

refusal skill/habilidad de negación estrategia para evitar hacer algo que no quieres hacer

relapse/recaída regresar a utilizar drogas mientras se recupera de una adicción

renewable resource/recurso renovable recurso natural que se puede reemplazar en un período corto de tiempo

repetitions/repeticiones número de veces que se realiza un ejercicio

rescue breathing/respiración de rescate técnica de emergencia mediante la cual una persona le proporciona aire a la que no respira

resiliency/resilencia capacidad para recuperarse de una enfermedad, una dificultad u otro factor estresante

resource/recurso algo que puedes utilizar para alcanzar una meta

resting heart rate (RHR)/índice de pulsaciones en reposo (IPR) número de veces que el corazón late por minuto mientras el cuerpo está en reposo

retina/retina capa interna del ojo que es sensible a la luz, recibe imágenes formadas por el cristalino y transmite señales nerviosas a través del nervio óptico al cerebro

risk factor /factor de riesgo todo aquello capaz de aumentar la probabilidad de lesión, enfermedad u otros problemas de salud

root canal/endodoncia procedimiento mediante el cual un dentista perfora la pulpa dental para eliminar la infeccíon producida por una caries

salmonellosis/salmonelosis infección del aparato digestivo causada por una bacteria que suele contraerse al comer alimentos contaminados

sanitation/saneamiento práctica de proporcionar drenaje y tratamiento de aguas residuales, el desecho de residuos sólidos, agua potable limpia y condiciones de trabajo y vivienda limpias

scrotum/escroto bolsa de piel que contiene los testículos

sebaceous gland/glándula sebáceas glándula que aporta grasa a la piel y al cuero cabelludo para mantenerlos suaves y saludables

second-degree burn/quemadura de segundo grado quemadura que atraviesa la primera capa de la piel y produce enrojecimiento, inflamación y ampollas

sedentary/sedentario persona que no practica ninguna actividad física regularmente

self-actualization/autorealización máximo potencial de una persona

self-concept/autoconcepto medición de cómo una persona se ve a sí misma

self-esteem/autoestima medición de cuánto se valora, respeta y cuánta confianza en sí misma se tiene una persona

semen/semen líquido formado por espermatozoides y otras secreciones de los órganos reproductores masculinos

sensory nerve/nervio sensorial nervio que transmite señales desde un órgano sensorial al sistema nervioso central, donde se procesan y se organizan

set/serie número fijo de repeticiones seguidas por un período de descanso

sexual abuse/abuso sexual acto sexual que se produce sin el consentimiento de una persona

sexual activity/actividad sexual toda actividad que incluye contacto sexual intencional con la finalidad de excitación sexual

sexual assault/agresión sexual toda actividad sexual en la que se utiliza la fuerza o se amenaza con hacerlo

sexual harassment/acoso sexual todo comentario, comportamiento o contacto no deseado que tenga contenido sexual

sexual intercourse/relación sexual proceso de reproducción en el que el pene se introduce en la vagina, y mediante el cual se puede dar comienzo a una vida humana

sexually transmitted disease (STD)/enfermedad de transmisión sexual (ETS) enfermedad infecciosa que se transmite por contacto sexual

shock/choque respuesta del cuerpo a un flujo de sangre reducido

sibling/hermano hermano o hermana relacionado con otro hermano u otra hermana de sangre, el casamiento de sus padres o la adopción

side effect/efecto secundario todo efecto producido por una droga que es diferente al efecto intencional de la droga

sidestream smoke/humo del cigarrillo humo que emana la punta de un cigarrillo

skeleton/esqueleto estructura de huesos que sostiene los músculos y órganos y protegen los órganos internos

sleep apnea/apnea del sueño trastorno del sueño caracterizado por interrupciones de los patrones de respiración normales durante el sueño

sleep deprivation/ausencia de sueño falta de sueño

sperm/espermatozoide célula sexual producida por los testículos necesaria para fecundar el óvulo de una mujer

INDEX

internal pressure, to be sexually active, 464
Internet, medical information on, 46–47, 564–565
intervention, 306
intestinal gas, 208
intestine, effect of tobacco on, 269f, 270
intoxication, 242
intravenous drug use, 503
iodine, 163t
iron, 163t, **165**, 179, 180–181, 182
iron-deficiency anemia, 165
iron supplements, 165
iron toxicity, 165
irradiated foods, 170f

jealousy, **65**, 458
jock itch, 333, 433t, 434
Johnson, Ervin "Magic," 510, 510f
joint injuries, 592–593
joints, **528–529**, 529f, 530
junk food, 155, **175–176**

Kaposi's sarcoma, 502
keloids, 569
keratin, 566, 570
Ketamine, 288t, 293
kidney, 540, 540f
kissing disease, 318
knee, 531, 531f
knuckles, cracking of, 528
kreteks, 265

lactic acid, 531
lacto-ovo vegetarian diet, 181
lactose, 156f, 170
lactose intolerance, 209
large intestine, 538, 538f, 539
larynx, 536, 536f
laughing gas, 291
LDL (low-density lipoprotein), 159
leukemia, 351t, 543
leukocytes, 535
LH (luteinizing hormone), 438, 525
lice, 317f
life change stressors, 79, 79t
life expectancy, 402
life skills, **26–28**, 27f, 614–615, 614f
lifestyle diseases, 66, **340–342**, 553
causes of, 340
risk factors for, 340, 341–342, 341f
life-threatening injuries, 576
ligaments, 129, 531f, 593
ligament sprain, 143t
lightening, 608
lipids, 158

liquid formula diet, 200t
listening skills, 59, 59f
liver, 538f
effects of alcohol on, 243, 245f, 246
loneliness, 65
look-alike drugs, 293
loss (emotional), 89–92
love
between family members, 421
in marriage, 411
low-density lipoprotein (LDL), 159
low sodium foods, 168
LSD, 300
lung cancer, 268, 271, 350, 351t
lungs, 536, 536f, 540f
effect of tobacco on, 268, 269f
luteinizing hormone (LH), 438, 525
Lyme disease, 319
lymph, 542
lymphatic system, 324, 542, 542f
lymphatic vessels, 542, 542f
lymph nodes, 324, 542, 542f
lymphocytes, 542, 543, 543t
lymphoma, 351t

macrophages, 543, 543t
macular degeneration, 377
MADD (Mothers Against Drunk Driving), 258
magnesium, 163t
magnetic resonance imaging (MRI), 352
ma huang, 144t
mainstream smoke, 270–271
major depression, 71t
Making GREAT Decisions model, **30–31**, 30f, 615, **616–617**
malaria, 317f, 318, 319, 333
male reproductive system, **430–435**, 522–523
anatomy of, 431–432, 431f, 432f
functions of, 430
preventing problems with, 434
problems of, 433, 433t
malignant tumor, 349
malnutrition, 164
maltose, 170
mammogram, 352, 442f
managed-care plans, 561
marijuana, 219, 231, 288t, **289–290**, 289f
marriage, 396, **410–414**, 461
teen, 412
Maslow's hierarchy of needs, 62–63, 62f
matrix of nails, 571
maximum heart rate (MHR), 134
MD (Doctor of Medicine), 556, **632**
MDMA (Ecstasy), 288t, 292
measles, 318, 332t
media messages, 28
about alcohol use, 257
about body image, 203
about drug abuse, 284

evaluation of, 27f, 28, 615
fast-food ads, 186–187
prescription drug ads, 238–239
pressure from, 34t
about tobacco use, 272
violence in, 102
Medicaid, 561
medical advances, 17, 17f, 18f
medical alert bracelet, 356f
medical emergencies, 576–579
medical history, 369
medical licensing, 555
medical research, 18
medical social worker, 638
Medicare, 561
medicines, 218–219, **222–229**. See also drugs
allergies to, 226–227, 226f
drug interactions, 227
over-the-counter, 220–221, 220t, 224–225
prescription, 220–221, 220t, 223, 228
types of, 220–221, 220t
wise use of, 228–229, 229f
melanin, 566, 568
melanoma, 568
memorial services, 91
menarche, 389
meningitis, 331
menopause, 397
menstrual cramps, 440t, 441
menstrual cycle, **438–439**, 439f, 525
hormones, 438, 439, 453f
menstruation, 389, 438, 439f, 525
mental benefits, of exercise, 127f, 128
mental changes
in adolescence, 390–392, 390f
in adulthood, 395, 397–398, 399–400
mental disorders, 12, **68–72**, 71t
mental health, 12, 12f, 26, **61**
metabolic rate, 127
metabolism, 155
metastasis, 350, 350f
methadone, 306
methamphetamine, 296t, 297
meth labs, 297
methylphenidate (Ritalin), 220t, 295, 297
MHR (maximum heart rate), 134
middle adulthood, 397–399, 399t
middle-age spread, 179
middle ear, 521, 521f
midlife crisis, 398
milk sugar, 156f
minerals, 154, **163**, 163t
food label information, 169
in vegetarian diet, 182
mineral supplements, 164
mini-bike safety, 600–601
minor in possession (MIP), 255
miscarriage, 271, 446, 447t
mistakes, Stop, Think, and Go process to correct, 32
mononucleosis, 318, 332t

Acknowledgments

ACADEMIC REVIEWERS

(continued from p. iv)

Richard Storey, Ph.D.
Professor of Biology
Colorado College
Colorado Springs, Colorado

Marianne Suarez, Ph.D.
Postdoctoral Psychology Fellow
Center on Child Abuse and
    Neglect
University of Oklahoma Health
    Sciences Center
Oklahoma City, Oklahoma

Nathan R. Sullivan, M.S.W.
Associate Professor
College of Social Work
The University of Kentucky
Lexington, Kentucky

Josey Templeton, Ed.D.
Associate Professor
Department of Health, Exercise,
    and Sports Medicine
The Citadel, Military College
    of South Carolina
Charleston, South Carolina

Marianne Turow, R.D., L.D.
Associate Professor
The Culinary Institute of America
Hyde Park, New York

Martin Van Dyke, Ph.D.
Professor of Chemistry Emeritus
Front Range Community College
Westminster, Colorado

Graham Watts, Ph.D.
*Assistant Professor of Health
    and Safety*
The University of Indiana
Bloomington, Indiana

MEDICAL REVIEWERS

David Ho, M.D.
Professor and Scientific Director
Aaron Diamond AIDS Research
    Center
The Rockefeller University
New York, New York

Ichiro Kawachi, Ph.D., M.D.
*Associate Professor of Health
    and Social Behavior*
School of Public Health
Harvard University
Boston, Massachusetts

Leland Lim, M.D., Ph.D.
Year II Resident
Department of Neurology and
    Neurological Sciences
Stanford University School
    of Medicine
Stanford University
Palo Alto, California

Iris F. Litt, M.D.
Professor
Department of Pediatrics and
    Adolescent Medicine
School of Biomedical and
    Biological Sciences
Stanford University
Palo Alto, California

**Ronald G. Munson, M.D.,
F.A.A.F.P.**
*Assistant Clinical Professor,
    Family Practice*
Health Sciences Center
The University of Texas
San Antonio, Texas

**Alexander V. Prokhorov, M.D.,
Ph.D.**
*Associate Professor of Behavioral
    Science*
M.D. Anderson Cancer Center
The University of Texas
Houston, Texas

Gregory A. Schmale, M.D.
Assistant Professor
Pediatrics and Adolescent Sports
    Medicine
University of Washington
Seattle, Washington

Hans Steiner, M.D.
*Professor of Psychiatry and Director
    of Training*
Division of Child Psychiatry
    and Child Development
Department of Psychiatry and
    Behavioral Sciences
Stanford University School
    of Medicine
Stanford, California

PROFESSIONAL REVIEWERS

Toni Alvarez, L.P.C.
Counselor
Children's Solutions
Round Rock, Texas

Nancy Daley, Ph.D., L.P.C., C.P.M.
Psychologist
Austin, Texas

Sharon Deutschlander
Executive Director
Alcohol and Drug Abuse Services
Port Allegany, Pennsylvania

Terry Erwin
*Hunter Educational Coordinator
    for the State of Texas*
Texas Hunter Education Program
Texas Parks and Wildlife
    Department
Austin, Texas

Linda K. Gaul, Ph.D.
Epidemiologist
Texas Department of Health
Austin, Texas

Georgia Girvan
Research Specialist
Idaho Radar Network Center
Boise State University
Boise, Idaho

Linda Jones, M.S.P.H.
*Manager of Systems Development
    Unit*
Children with Special Healthcare
    Needs Division
Texas Department of Health
Austin, Texas

William Joy
President
The Joy Group
Wheaton, Illinois

Edie Leonard, R.D., L.D.
Nutrition Educator
Portland, Oregon

JoAnn Cope Powell, Ph.D.
*Learning Specialist and Licensed
    Psychologist*
Counseling, Learning and Career
    Services
University of Texas Learning
    Center
The University of Texas
Austin, Texas

Hal Resides
Safety Manager
Corpus Christi, Texas

Eric Tiemann, E.M.T.
Emergency Medical Services
Hazardous Waste Division
Travis County Emergency
    Medical Services
Austin, Texas

Lynne E. Whitt
Executive Vice President
National Center for Health
    Education
New York, New York

TEACHER REVIEWERS

Dan Aude
Magnet Programs Coordinator
Montgomery Public Schools
Montgomery, Alabama

Andrew Banks
Sexuality Educator
LifeGuard Character and Sexuality
    Education
Austin, Texas

Robert Baronak
Biological Sciences Teacher
Donegal High School
Mount Joy, Pennsylvania

Judy Blanchard
District Health Coordinator
Newtown Public Schools
Newtown, Connecticut

David Blinn
Secondary Sciences Teacher
Wrenshall High School
Wrenshall, Minnesota

Johanna Chase
School Health Educator
Los Angeles County Office
    of Education
Downey, California

Michelle Deery
*Health and Physical Education
    Teacher*
Donegal High School
Mount Joy, Pennsylvania

Donna DeFriese
Communications Teacher
Soddy Daisy High School
Soddy Daisy, Tennessee

Stacy Feinberg, L.M.H.C.
Family Counselor for Autism
Broward County School System
Coral Gables, Florida

Arthur Goldsmith
Secondary Sciences Teacher
Hallendale High School
Hallendale, Florida

Calvin Gross
Sports Coach and Health Teacher
Rochester High School
Rochester Hills, Michigan

Jacqueline Horowitz-Olstfeld
Exceptional Student Educator
Broward County School District
Fort Lauderdale, Florida

Jay Jones
Sports Coach and Health Teacher
Olathe North High School
Olathe, Kansas

Lincoln LaRoe
*Coach, United States Olympic
    Rowing Team*
Milwaukee, Oregon

Steward Lipsky
Secondary Sciences Teacher
Seward High School
New York, New York

Alyson Mike
Science and Health Teacher
East Helena Public School System
East Helena, Montana

Donna Norwood
Secondary Sciences Teacher
Monroe High School
Monroe, North Carolina

Jenna Robles
Health Teacher
Escondido High School
Escondido, California

Denice Lee Sandefur
*Secondary Sciences and Health
    Teacher*
Nucla High School
Nucla, Colorado

Bert Sherwood
Science and Health Specialist
Socorro Independent School
    District
El Paso, Texas

Carla Thompson
Health Teacher
Antioch Community High School
Antioch, Illinois

Dan Utley
Sports Coach and Health Teacher
Hilton Head High School
Hilton Head Island, South
    Carolina

Alexis Wright
Principal
Rye Country Day School
Rye, New York

Joe Zelmanski
Curriculum Coordinator
Rochester Adams High School
Rochester Hills, Michigan

CREDITS

Illustration Credits

Frontmatter: Page xii, Morgan-Cain & Associates; xvii, Ortelius Design. **Chapter 1:** Page 9, Leslie Kell; 10, Gary Locke/Suzanne Craig Represents Inc.;13, Fian Arroyo; 23, Leslie Kell. **Chapter 2:** Page 26, Fian Arroyo; 27, Leslie Kell; 38, Marty Roper/Planet Rep. **Chapter 4:** Page 87, Gary Locke/Suzanne Craig Represents Inc.; 99, Leslie Kell. **Chapter 5:** Page 121, Leslie Kell. **Chapter 6:** Page 139, Dan Vasconcellos; 151, Leslie Kell. **Chapter 7:** Page 158, Leslie Kell;165, Leslie Kell;167, Marty Roper/Planet Rep; 185, Leslie Kell. **Chapter 8:** Page 193-194, Leslie Kell; 213, Leslie Kell. **Chapter 9:** Page 221, Articulate Graphics/Deborah Wolfe Ltd.; 231, Articulate Graphics/ Deborah Wolfe Ltd.; 224, Marty Roper/Planet Rep; 237, Leslie Kell. **Chapter 11:** Page 265, Leslie Kell; 275, Gary Locke/Suzanne Craig Represents Inc.; 280, Rick Herman. **Chapter 12:** Page 291, Articulate Graphics/Deborah Wolfe Ltd.; 290, Leslie Kell; 311, Leslie Kell. **Chapter 13:** Page 322, Dan Vasconcellos; 337, Leslie Kell. **Chapter 14:** Page 345, Articulate Graphics/Deborah Wolfe Ltd.; 346, Leslie Kell; 361, Leslie Kell. **Chapter 15:** Page 373(tr), Leslie Kell; 373(tl), Articulate Graphics/Deborah Wolfe Ltd.; 383, Leslie Kell. **Chapter 16:** Page 405, Leslie Kell. **Chapter 17:** Page 425, Leslie Kell. **Chapter 18:** Page 431-432,Christy Krames; 437-439,Christy Krames; 439, Leslie Kell; 448-449, Christy Krames; 453, Leslie Kell. **Chapter 19:** Page 457, Dan Vasconcellos; 462, Dan Vasconcellos; 471, Leslie Kell. **Chapter 20:** Page 481,Leslie Kell; 493, Leslie Kell. **Chapter 21:** Page 497, Argosy; 498, Leslie Kell; 501, Leslie Kell; 513, Leslie Kell. **HOW YOUR BODY WORKS:** Page 516, John Karapelou; 517, Morgan-Cain & Associates; 518, Christy Krames; 519(tr), Articulate Graphics/Deborah Wolfe Ltd.; 519(tl), John Karapelou; 520-521, Keith Kasnot; 522, Christy Krames; 524, Christy Krames; 525, Christy Krames; 527, John Karapelou; 528, Network Graphics; 529-531, John Karapelou; 532, Morgan-Cain & Associates; 534, Christy Krames & Morgan-Cain & Associates; 536-538, John Karapelou; 540, John Karapelou; 541, Christy Krames; 544, Articulate Graphics/ Deborah Wolfe Ltd.; 545, John Karapelou; **FIRST AID AND SAFETY:** All illustrations in the chapter done by Marcia Hartsock/The Medical Art Company. **WHAT YOU NEED TO KNOW ABOUT:** Page 566, Morgan-Cain & Associates; 572, Articulate Graphics/ Deborah Wolfe Ltd. **YOUR HEALTH YOUR WORLD:** Gary Locke/Suzanne Craig Represents Inc.

Photography Credits

Abbreviations used: (t) top, (b) bottom, (c) center, (l) left, (r) right, (bkgd) background

Border design on Contents in Brief page, Table of Contents pages, Analyzing Data features, Real Life Activity features, and Life Skills features, Digital Image ©2004 EyeWire

i (c), Scott Van Osdol/HRW; ii (tr), ©Chad Slattery/Getty Images/Stone; v (all), Peter Van Steen/HRW; v (bl), Peter Van Steen/HRW

TABLE OF CONTENTS: vi (tl), Corbis Images; vi (bl), David Young-Wolff/PhotoEdit; vii (br), John Langford/ HRW; viii (tl), ©Clay Patrick McBride/Photonica; viii (cl), Digital Image ©2004 Artville; ix (cr), Digital Image ©2004 EyeWire; ix (bl), ©Ariel Skelley/CORBIS; x (tl), John Langford/HRW; xi (tl), ©Don Smetzer/Getty Images/ Stone; xi (cr), Catrina Genovese/Index Stock Imagery/ PictureQuest; xi (br), Digital Image ©2004 PhotoDisc; xii (bl), K. Beebe/Custom Medical Stock Photo; xiii (tr), ©Ariel Skelley/CORBIS; xiv (tl), Mary Kate Denny/ PhotoEdit; xiv (bl,bc), ©2004 Luciano A. Leon c/o MIRA; xiv (br), Michael Newman/PhotoEdit; xv (cr), ©Bob Daemmrich/The Image Works; xvi (c), Digital Image ©2004 PhotoDisc

UNIT 1: 2-3 (all), ©Werran/Ochsner/Photonica **Chapter 1:** 4-5 (all), Digital Image ©2004 PhotoDisc; 6 (bl), Grantpix/Index Stock Imagery, Inc.; 8 (t), John Langford/ HRW; 11 (cr), Digital Image ©2004 Artville; 12 (tc), ©David Young-Wolff/Getty Images/Stone; 14 (bc), Corbis Images; 16 (tl), Victoria Smith/HRW; 17 (cr), ©Richard Radstone/Getty Images/Taxi; 18 (tcr), ©Martin H. Simon/ Corbis SABA; 18 (tr), ©Rob Gage/Getty Images/Taxi; 18 (tcl), ©Saturn Stills/ SPL/Photo Researchers, Inc.; 18 (tl), ©V.C.L./Getty Images/ Taxi; 19 (br), David Young-Wolff/ PhotoEdit; 20 (tl), David Weintraub/Stock Boston **Chapter 2:** 24-25 (all), ©Nancy Richmond/The Image Works; 29 (br), Robert Wood/HRW; 31 (br), Jonathan Nourok/PhotoEdit; 32 (cl), Corbis Images/HRW; 33 (cr), Spencer Grant/PhotoEdit; 34 (tr, cr), Digital Image ©2004 PhotoDisc; 34 (cl), John Langford/ HRW; 35 (tr), Myrleen Ferguson Cate/Photo Edit; 36 (bl), Mary Kate Denny/PhotoEdit; 39 (tr), Peter Van Steen/HRW; 40 (b), ©Bob Daemmrich/The Image Works; 41 (br), ©Bob Daemmrich/The Image Works; 42 (tl), Peter Van Steen/ HRW; 43 (tr), Robert Wood/HRW; 43 (cl), Corbis Images/ HRW; 47 (tr), Sam Dudgeon/HRW **Chapter 3:** 48-49 (all), David Young-Wolff/PhotoEdit; 50 (cl), ©Dick Clintsman/ Getty Images/Stone; 51 (all), ©Stockbyte; 52 (tr), Michael Newman/PhotoEdit; 53 (br), Victoria Smith/HRW; 55 (cr), Spencer Grant/PhotoEdit; 56 (cl), John Langford/HRW; 58 (bl), John Langford/HRW; 59 (tr), ©Reed Kaestner/CORBIS; 60 (tl), ©Bruce Ayres/Getty Images/Stone; 61 (cr), Digital Image ©2004 EyeWire; 64 (bl), Digital Image ©2004 PhotoDisc; 65 (tr), Jim Cooper/AP/Wide World Photos; 67 (tr), Ralf-Finn Hestoft/Index Stock Imagery, Inc.; 68 (cl), ©Lisette Le Bon/SuperStock; 69 (tl), ©Arthur Tilley/Getty Images/ Taxi; 70 (bl), ©Charles Nes/Getty Images/Stone; 72 (tl), ©Jon Bradley/Getty Images/Stone; 73 (tr), ©Lisette Le Bon/SuperStock; 73 (cl), ©Dick Clintsman/Getty Images/ Stone; 73 (bl), ©Arthur Tilley/Getty Images/Taxi **Chapter 4:** 76-77 (all), Digital Image ©2004 PhotoDisc; 78 (cl), ©Benelux Press/Getty Images/Taxi; 80 (tl), ©Chris Shinn/ Getty Images/Stone; 81 (all), John Langford/HRW; 83 (br), ©Lori Adamski Peek/Getty Images/Stone; 84 (cl), ©Jack Hollingsworth/CORBIS; 86 (bl), ©David Rosenberg/Getty Images/Stone; 88 (tl), ©Color Day Production/Getty Images/ The Image Bank; 89 (cr), age fotostock/Jonnie Miles; 90 (b), ©Ewa Grochowiak/Corbis Sygma; 91 (br), ©Annie Griffiths Belt/CORBIS; 93 (cr), ©Richard Lord/The Image Works; 94 (b), ©Laurence Monneret/Getty Images/Stone; 96 (tl), ©Christian Lantry/Getty Images/Stone; 97 (tr), ©Benelux Press/Getty Images/Taxi; 97 (cl), ©Ewa Grochowiak/Corbis Sygma; 97 (bl), ©Richard Lord/The Image Works **Chapter 5:** 100-101 (all), ©Lucidio Studio Inc./CORBIS; 102 (tl), ©Seth Kushner/Getty Images/Stone; 103 (bl), George Emmons/ Index Stock Imagery, Inc.; 104 (tl), ©Spencer Rowell/ Getty Images/Taxi; 105 (tr), Robert F. Bukaty/AP/Wide World Photos; 106 (b), John Langford/HRW; 108 (cl), ©Robert Essel/Corbis Stock Market; 109 (bc), ©Lawrence Manning/ CORBIS; 110 (tl), ©Karine Dilthey/Getty Images/Taxi; 111 (bl), Digital Image ©2004 PhotoDisc; 112 (br), John Langford/HRW; 113 (tr), ©Bruce Ayres/ Getty Images/Stone; 114 (cl), ©Denis Felix/Getty Images/ Taxi; 117 (br), Grantpix/ Index Stock Imagery, Inc.; 118 (tl), SW Production/Index Stock Imagery, Inc.; 119 (tr), ©Lawrence Manning/CORBIS; 119 (cl), Digital Image ©2004 PhotoDisc; 119 (bl), ©Denis Felix/Getty Images/ Taxi

UNIT 2: 122-123 (all), ©Dick Clintsman/Getty Images/ Stone **Chapter 6:** 124-125 (all), ©Lori Adamski Peek/ Getty Images/Stone; 126 (cl), Scott Vallance/HRW; 127 (bc), John Langford/HRW; 127 (cl), ©V.C.L./Getty Images/Taxi; 127 (cr), ©SPL/Photo Researchers, Inc.; 127 (br), ©Photo Researchers, Inc.; 128 (bl), ©Lawrence Migdale/Getty Images/Stone; 129 (tr), ©Michael Darter/ Photonica; 130 (bl), ©Syracuse Newspapers/The Image Works; 131 (tl), David Young-Wolff/PhotoEdit; 132 (tl), Mary Steinbacher/ PhotoEdit; 132 (cl), Bob Daemmrich/ Stock Boston, Inc./PictureQuest; 133 (cr), ©James Muldowney/Getty Images/Stone; 134 (bl), Michael Newman/PictureQuest; 136 (cr), Mark Gibson Photography; 136 (cl), David Schmidt/ Masterfile; 136 (br), Steve Fitzpatrick/Masterfile; 136 (bl), Andrew Olney/ Masterfile; 140 (b), Mark Gibson Photography; 141 (tr), ©Terje Rakke/Getty Images/The Image Bank; 142 (bl), ©Bob Daemmrich/The Image Works; 144 (cl), Custom Medical Stock Photo; 146 (cl), ©David Lassman/ Syracuse Newspapers/The Image Works; 147 (tr), Digital Image ©2004 PhotoDisc; 147 (br), ©Malcolm Piers/Getty Images/The Image Bank; 149 (tr), Bob Daemmrich/Stock Boston, Inc./PictureQuest; 149 (cl), ©James Muldowney/ Getty Images/Stone; 149 (bl), ©Bob Daemmrich/The Image Works **Chapter 7:** 152-153 (all), Carl A. Stimac/ The Image Finders; 154 (cl), Scott Lanza/FoodPix; 155 (tl, br, bl), Sam Dudgeon/HRW; 155 (tr, bc), Digital Image ©2004 PhotoDisc; 156 (cl), Peter Van Steen/HRW; 157 (tr), Digital Image ©2004 PhotoDisc; 157 (tc), Sam Dudgeon/HRW; 158 (tc), Digital Image ©2004 PhotoDisc; 159 (cr), Digital Image ©2004 PhotoDisc; 160 (all), Sam Dudgeon/HRW; 161 (cr), Sam Dudgeon/ HRW; 162 (tr), Sam Dudgeon/HRW; 162 (c), Corbis Images; 162 (br, bc), Digital Image ©2004 PhotoDisc; 163 (tr), ©Stockbyte; 163 (cr, bc), Digital Image ©2004 PhotoDisc; 164 (cl), Peter Griffith/Masterfile; 164 (tr, br), ©Dr. M. Klein/Peter Arnold, Inc.; 165 (tr, br), Sam Dudgeon/ HRW; 165 (tl), John Langford/HRW; 166 (tl), ©Robert Daly/Getty Images/Stone; 168 (tl), Victoria Smith/HRW; 171 (oil), Digital Image ©2004 PhotoDisc; 171 (yogurt), Sam Dudgeon/HRW; 171 (milk), Corbis Images; 171 (cheese), ©Stockbyte; 171 (fish), ©Stockbyte; 171 (chicken), David Bishop/FoodPix; 171 (eggs), Corbis Images; 171 (broccoli), Corbis Images; 171 (potato), Christina Peters/FoodPix; 171 (carrot), ©Burke/Triolo Productions/Getty Images/FoodPix; 171 (grapes), ©Stockbyte; 171 (tomato), ©Stockbyte; 171 (strawberries), Corbis Images; 171 (orange), ©Stockbyte; 171 (oatmeal), Sam Dudgeon/HRW; 171 (pretzel), Digital Image ©2004 PhotoDisc; 171 (bread), Victoria Smith/ HRW; 171 (candy), Digital Image ©2004 PhotoDisc; 171 (pasta), ©Stockbyte; 172 (tl), Sam Dudgeon/HRW; 172 (tc, bc), Peter Van Steen/HRW; 173 (tc, c), Peter Van Steen/HRW; 173 (cl, br), Sam Dudgeon/HRW; 175 (br), John Langford/HRW; 177 (b), ©Jon Riley/Getty Images/ Stone; 178 (br), Digital Image ©2004 PhotoDisc; 179 (cr), ©Tom Hauck/Allsport/ Getty Images; 180 (tr), ©Peter Cade/Getty Images/Stone; 181 (tr), Sam Dudgeon/HRW; 182 (tl), Peter Van Steen/HRW; 183 (tr), Digital Image ©2004 PhotoDisc; 183 (tl), Peter Van Steen/HRW; 183 (bl), ©Tom Hauck/Allsport/Getty Images; 186 (bl), Victoria Smith/HRW; 187 (tr), Digital Image ©2004 PhotoDisc **Chapter 8:** 188-189 (all), Rubberball Productions®; 191 (t), Ed Lallo/HRW; 193 (tl, cl), Digital Image ©2004 PhotoDisc; 193 (c, cr), ©Scott Markewitz/Getty Images/Taxi; 193 (br), Jonathan Nourok/ PhotoEdit/Picture-Quest; 194 (tl), Victoria Smith/HRW; 195 (tr), Merritt Vincent/PhotoEdit/PictureQuest; 196 (cl), ©Layne Kennedy/ CORBIS; 197 (br), ©V.C.L./Getty Images/Taxi; 200 (br), Peter Van Steen/HRW; 202 (cl), Digital Image ©2004 PhotoDisc; 203 (br), Ed Lallo/ HRW; 204 (b), ©Charles Thatcher/Getty Images/Stone; 205 (tr), Nina Berman/SIPA Press; 207 (cr), Victoria Smith/HRW; 208 (cl), ©Zigy Kaluzny/Getty Images/ Stone; 209 (bc, br), John Langford/HRW; 211 (tr), ©Scott Markewitz/Getty Images/Taxi; 211 (cl), Digital Image ©2004 PhotoDisc

UNIT 3: 214-215 (all), ©David Job/Getty Images/Stone **Chapter 9:** 216-217 (all), ©Romilly Lockyer/Getty Images/ The Image Bank; 218 (cl), Bob Daemmrich/Stock Boston; 219 (tc), Digital Image ©2004 Artville; 219 (tl), ©Richard Hamilton Smith/CORBIS; 219 (tr), ©R. Laurence/Photo Researchers, Inc.; 222 (cl), Sam Dudgeon/HRW; 223 (tr), ©CC Studio/SPL/Photo Researchers, Inc.; 225 (t), Victoria Smith/HRW; 226 (bl), ©Dr. P. Marazzi/Photo Researchers, Inc.; 227 (tr), ©Color Day Production/Getty Images/The Image Bank; 229 (cr), Digital Image ©2004 Artville; 230 (cl), Digital Image ©2004 PhotoDisc; 232 (br), ©Clay Patrick McBride/ Photonica; 235 (tr), Bob Daemmrich/Stock Boston; 235 (cl), Digital Image ©2004 Artville; 235 (bl), ©Clay Patrick McBride/Photonica; 238 (bl), Victoria Smith/ HRW; 239 (tl), Victoria Smith/HRW **Chapter 10:** 240-241 (all), Mike Derer/AP/Wide World Photos; 242 (cl), Sam Dudgeon/ HRW; 243 (tr), ©Chad Slattery/Getty Images/ Stone; 244 (bl), ©Simon Battensby/Getty Images/Stone; 247 (bl), Digital Image ©2004 PhotoDisc; 249 (tr), ©Nick White/Getty Images/Taxi; 250 (cl), Peter Byron/ PhotoEdit; 252 (tl), Mary Kate Denny/PhotoEdit; 253 (br), Paul Conklin/PhotoEdit; 255 (b), Digital Image ©2004 PhotoDisc; 256 (cl), Steven Skjold/Painet; 257 (br), ©Syracuse Newspapers/Kevin Jacobus/The Image Works; 258 (tr, tc), ©2004 Luciano A. Leon c/o MIRA; 258 (tl), Michael Newman/PhotoEdit; 259 (tr), ©Syracuse Newspapers/Kevin Jacobus/The Image Works; 259 (cl), Peter Byron/PhotoEdit; 259 (bl), Digital Image ©2004 PhotoDisc **Chapter 11:** 262-263 (all), ©SuperStock; 264 (cl), ©Terry Williams/Getty Images/The Image Bank; 265 (tr), Photo courtesy of Oral Health America/Romano & Associates; 266 (tr), Louie Balukoff/AP/Wide World Photos; 268 (tl), Victor R. Caivano/ AP/Wide World Photos; 269 (tr), Gladden Willis/Visuals Unlimited; 269 (bc), ©Martin M. Rotker/Photo Researchers, Inc.; 269 (tc), Carolina Biological/Visuals Unlimited; 269 (bl), Visuals Unlimited; 269 (tl), Custom Medical Stock Photo; 269 (c), Victoria Smith/HRW; 270 (br), Custom Medical Stock Photo; 271 (tr), ©Collection CNRI/ Phototake; 272 (cl), ©Peter Poulides/Getty Images/Stone; 273 (bl), Bruce Coleman, Inc.; 276 (bl), ©Image 100/ CORBIS; 277 (br), Don Couch/HRW; 278 (tl), Bill Haber/AP/Wide World Photos **Chapter 12:** 282-283 (all), ©Spencer Rowell/Getty Images/Taxi; 284 (tr), ©Ted Horowitz/Corbis Stock Market; 284 (cl, cr), ©2002 PhotoAlto; 284 (bl), ©Ariel Skelley/ Corbis Stock Market; 284 (br), Corbis Images; 285 (tl), Digital Image ©2004 PhotoDisc; 286 (tl), Digital Image ©2004 PhotoDisc; 287 (br), Darrin Jenkins/Pictor/Image State; 289 (b), ©Phil Schermeister/CORBIS; 292 (tl), Eric Mason/AP/Wide World Photos; 293 (cr), Patriot-News, Joe Hermitt/ AP/Wide World Photos; 294 (tl), Corbis Images/ HRW; 295 (br), William F. Campbell/TimePix; 297 (tr), ©Clay Patrick McBride/Photonica; 298 (b), Victoria Smith/

CREDITS

HRW; 299 (tr), Gari Wyn Williams/Pictor/Image State; 300 (tl), Chuck Nacke/Woodfin Camp/PictureQuest; 301 (cr), Robert F. Bukaty/AP/Wide World Photos; 302 (bl), Don Couch/HRW; 303 (tr), ©Annie Griffiths Belt/ CORBIS; 304 (br), Akos Szilvasi/Stock, Boston Inc./ PictureQuest; 305 (tr), Paul Conklin/ PhotoEdit/PictureQuest; 305 (tl), ©Moritz Steiger/Getty Images/The Image Bank; 306 (b), Mary Kate Denny/PhotoEdit; 307 (br), Digital Image ©2004 PhotoDisc; 308 (tl), ©Lori Adamski Peek/Getty Images/Stone; 309 (tr), ©2002 PhotoAlto; 309 (cl), Eric Mason/AP/Wide World Photos

UNIT 4: 312-313 (all), ©R.W. Jones/CORBIS **Chapter 13:** 314-315 (all), ©Jim Sulley/The Image Works; 316 (bl), ©Dr. P. Marazzi/SPL/Photo Researchers, Inc.; 316 (br), ©Lowell Georgia/Photo Researchers, Inc.; 316 (bc), ©Oliver Meckes/ Photo Researchers, Inc.; 316 (c), ©Oliver Meckes/ Gelderblom/Photo Researchers, Inc.; 317 (cl), ©John Watney/Photo Researchers, Inc.; 317 (cr), NMSB/Custom Medical Stock Photo; 317 (br), ©Oliver Meckes/Photo Researchers, Inc.; 317 (bl), ©David Scharf/Peter Arnold, Inc.; 317 (c), ©Meckes/Ottawa/ Photo Researchers, Inc.; 317 (bc), ©Mark Clarke/SPL/ Photo Researchers, Inc.; 319 (cl), ©Matt Meadows/Peter Arnold, Inc.; 319 (bc), Michael Newman/ PhotoEdit; 319 (cr), John Langford/HRW; 319 (br), ©Jack K. Clark/The Image Works; 323 (tc), ©Don Smetzer/Getty Images/ Stone; 323 (tl), Custom Medical Stock Photo; 323 (tc, tr), Sam Dudgeon/HRW; 324 (cl), ©Bill O'Conner/Peter Arnold, Inc.; 325 (tr), Michelle Bridwell/PhotoEdit; 326 (b), Kenneth Jarecke/Contact Press Images; 327 (br), Peter Van Steen/HRW; 328 (tl), Digital Image ©2004 PhotoDisc; 329 (bl), Davis Barber/PhotoEdit; 330 (bkgd), Sam Dudgeon/ HRW; 330 (bl), Bob Daemmrich/ Stock Boston; 332 (tl), Mary Kate Denny/PhotoEdit; 333 (br), ©Andrew Syred/ SPL/Photo Researchers, Inc.; 334 (tl), ©S. Nagendra/Photo Researchers, Inc.; 335 (tr), NMSB/Custom Medical Stock Photo; 335 (cl), Sam Dudgeon/HRW; 335 (bl), ©S. Nagendra/ Photo Researchers, Inc. **Chapter 14:** 338-339 (all), ©Peter Cade/Getty Images/The Image Bank; 341 (bl), Digital Image ©2004 EyeWire; 342 (tl), Digital Image ©2004 PhotoDisc; 343 (cr), Peter Van Steen/HRW; 344 (c), Victoria Smith/HRW; 344 (tc), Art & Science/Custom Medical Stock Photo; 344 (bc), ©Adamsmith/SuperStock; 345 (tr), Digital Image ©2004 PhotoDisc; 347 (tr), ©Geoff Tompkinson/SPL/ Photo Researchers, INC.; 348 (tl), Mark Gallup/Pictor/Image State; 349 (br), AP Photo/Midland Daily News/Jan-Michael Stump; 351 (bc), ©Triller-Berretti/Barts Medical Library/ Phototake; 351 (tr), ©Photo Researchers, Inc.; 353 (br), Sam Dudgeon/HRW; 355 (br), ©Yoav Levy/Phototake; 356 (cl), Michael Newman/PhotoEdit; 357 (tl), Jan Sonnenmair/ Aurora; 358 (tl), ©Tim Bieber/Getty Images/ The Image Bank; 359 (tr), ©Photo Researchers, Inc.; 359 (cl), Peter Van Steen/HRW; 359 (bl), Michael Newman/ PhotoEdit; 362 (bl), Laurie Bayer/Image State; 362 (cl), ©David Parker/SPL/ Photo Researchers, Inc.; 362-363 (b), ©Dept. Of Clinical Cytogenetics, Addenbrookes Hospital/SPL/Photo Researchers, Inc. **Chapter 15:** 364-365 (all), ©Ariel Skelley/CORBIS; 366 (cl), ©Arthur Tilley/Getty Images/Taxi; 367 (tr), ©Meckes/Ottawa/Photo Researchers, Inc.; 368 (bl), ©James King-Holmes/ Photo Researchers, Inc.; 368 (bc), ©Dept. of Clinical Cytogenetics, Addenbrookes Hospital/ SPL/Photo Researchers, Inc.; 370 (tl), ©Ken Eward/BioGrafx/ Photo Researchers, Inc.; 371 (cr), ©Jennie Woodcock/Reflections Photolibrary/CORBIS; 372 (tl), Sam Dudgeon/HRW; 372 (cl), ©Ralph C. Eagle, Jr./Photo Researchers, Inc.; 374 (tl), ©Ed Kashi/CORBIS; 374 (tr), ©Salisbury District Hospital/Photo Researchers, Inc.; 375 (tr), David Zalubowski/AP/Wide World Photos; 376 (bl), Chuck Close, Self-Portrait, 1993, oil on canvas, 72 x 60", Portrait of the artist with work in progress, Photograph by Ellen Page Wilson, Courtesy of PaceWildenstein ©Chuck Close; 377 (br), Peter Van Steen/HRW; 378 (bl), Steph/VISUAL/ZUMA Press; 379 (b), ©Tim Wright/ CORBIS; 380 (cl), ©Jack Kurtz/The Image Works; 381 (tr), ©Meckes/Ottawa/Photo Researchers, Inc.; 381 (cl), David Zalubowski/AP/Wide World Photos; 381 (bl), ©Tim Wright/CORBIS

UNIT 5: 384-385 (all), ©Rob Lewine/CORBIS **Chapter 16:** 386-387 (all), John Langford/HRW; 388 (cl), Digital Image ©2004 PhotoDisc; 389 (br, bl), Digital Image ©2004 PhotoDisc; 390 (cl), Digital Image ©2004 PhotoDisc; 395 (cr), John Langford/HRW; 396 (bl), Digital Image ©2004 PhotoDisc; 397 (br), ©Steven Peters/Getty Images/Stone; 398 (tl), ©Laurence Fleury/ Explorer/Photo Researchers, Inc.; 399 (br), ©Nick Sinclair/Photonica; 400 (tl), Digital Image ©2004 PhotoDisc; 401 (br), ©Mark Scott/Getty Images/Taxi; 402 (tl), ©vq production/Iconotec; 403 (tr), ©Mark Scott/ Getty Images/Taxi; 403 (cl), Digital Image ©2004 PhotoDisc; 403 (bl), ©Laurence Fleury/Explorer/Photo Researchers, Inc.; 406 (bl), Victoria Smith/HRW; 406 (cl), Digital Image ©2004 PhotoDisc; 407 (tr), Paul Perez-www.latinfocus.com **Chapter 17:** 408-409 (all), ©Kaluzny-Thatcher/Getty Images/ Stone; 410 (bl), Peter Van Steen/HRW; 410 (bc), ©Bruce Ayres/Getty Images/ Stone; 410 (br), Diana Goetting/HRW; 411 (tr), ©Steve Chenn/CORBIS; 412 (cl), Ed Lallo/HRW; 413 (cr), Michael Newman/PhotoEdit; 415 (cr), ©Ron Chapple/ Getty Images/Taxi; 417 (tr), ©Stephanie Rausser/Getty Images/Taxi; 418 (bl), AP/Wide World Photos; 419 (bl), Bill Bachmann/PhotoEdit; 420 (bl), Robert Wood/HRW; 422 (tl), ©Tom Stewart/Corbis Stock Market; 423 (tr), ©Stephanie Rausser/Getty Images/Taxi; 423 (cr), ©Ron Chapple/Getty Images/Taxi; 423 (bl), Bill Bachmann/ PhotoEdit

UNIT 6: 426-427 (all), ©Saul Bromberger & Sandra Hoover/Raw Talent Photo **Chapter 18:** 428-429 (all), Jim McGuire/Index Stock Imagery, Inc.; 430 (bl), ©AFP/CORBIS; 432 (tl), ©Jason Burns/Dr. Ryder/ Phototake; 433 (bl), ©Quest/SPL/Photo Researchers, Inc.; 434 (tl), ©Jake Martin/ Allsport/Stone; 435 (tr), Sam Dudgeon/HRW; 436 (cl), AP Photo/Stuart Ramson; 438 (tl), ©Professors P.M. Motta & J. Van Blerkom/SPL/Photo Researchers, Inc.; 440 (br), ©SPL/ Photo Researchers, Inc.; 441 (cr), ©Neo Vision/ Photonica; 442 (tl), K. Beebe/ Custom Medical Stock Photo; 443 (cr), ©Dennis Kunkel/ Phototake; 445 (tl, tc, tr), Lennart Nilsson/Albert Bonniers Publishing Co.; 446 (bl), ©Leland Bobbe/Getty Images/Stone; 447 (tr), ©David H. Wells/ CORBIS; 449 (cr), ©Dianne Fiumara/Getty Images/Stone; 450 (tl, cl), Gene Whitworth/HRW; 450 (bl), Susan Feldkamp/HRW; 451 (tr), ©Dennis Kunkel/Phototake; 451 (cl), ©AFP/ CORBIS; 451 (bl), ©Dianne Fiumara/Getty Images/Stone **Chapter 19:** 454-455 (all), ©Chad Slattery/ Getty Images/Stone; 456 (tl), Catrina Genovese/ Index Stock Imagery/PictureQuest; 458 (tl), Digital Image ©2004 PhotoDisc; 460 (cl), Digital Image ©2004 PhotoDisc; 461 (tl), ©Richard Shock/Getty Images/Stone; 463 (tr), George Emmons/Index Stock Imagery, Inc.; 464 (br), Digital Image ©2004 PhotoDisc; 464 (cl), ©Stockbyte; 465 (bl), Digital Image ©2004 PhotoDisc; 467 (br), ©Bob Daemmrich/The Image Works; 468 (tl), ©Tom McCarthy/ PhotoEdit; 469 (tr), Catrina Genovese/Index Stock Imagery/PictureQuest; 469 (cl, bl), Digital Image ©2004 PhotoDisc; 472 (bl), Nostalgia Cards ©SuperStock; 473 (tl), Ewing Galloway/Index Stock Imagery, Inc.; 473 (tr), ©Image 100/CORBIS **Chapter 20:** 474-475 (all), ©Charles Gupton/CORBIS; 476 (all), Peter Van Steen/HRW; 477 (all), Digital Image ©2004 PhotoDisc; 478 (all), Peter Van Steen/HRW; 480 (cl), John Langford/ HRW; 481 (tr), John Langford/HRW; 483 (tl), ©Don Smetzer/ Getty Images/Stone; 484 (cl), Digital Image ©2004 PhotoDisc; 485 (cr), Digital Image ©2004 PhotoDisc; 486 (br), Siebert/Custom Medical Stock Photo; 487 (c), ©SIU/ Peter Arnold, Inc.; 487 (br), Science VU/Visuals Unlimited; 488 (br), DR. P. Marazzi/SPL/Custom Medical Stock Photo; 490 (tl), Victoria Smith/HRW; 491 (tr, cr), Peter Van Steen/ HRW; 491 (cl), ©Don Smetzer/ Getty Images/Stone; 491 (bl), Digital Image ©2004 PhotoDisc **Chapter 21:** 494-495 (all), Aaron Haupt/Stock Boston; 496 (bl), Digital Image ©2004 PhotoDisc; 499 (t), Digital Image ©2004 PhotoDisc; 500 (cl), ©Nibsc/ Photo Researchers, Inc.; 502 (tl), ©Bruce Ayres/Getty Images/Stone; 503 (cr), ©Conor Caffrey/SPL/ Photo Researchers, Inc.; 504 (tl), Ed Zurga/AP/Wide World Photos; 505 (cr), Digital Image ©2004 Artville; 507 (tr), ©Tony Craddock/SPL/Photo Researchers, Inc.; 508 (b), Jakub Mosur/AP/Wide World Photos; 509 (br), ©David Lassman/ The Image Works; 509 (c), Digital Image ©2004 PhotoDisc; 510 (tl), Ed Bailey/AP/Wide World Photos; 511 (tr), Digital Image ©2004 PhotoDisc; 511 (cr), ©Bruce Ayres/Getty Images/Stone; 511 (bl), Jakub Mosur/AP/ Wide World Photos

INTRODUCTION TO HEALTH HANDBOOK: 514-515 (all), Sam Dudgeon/HRW

EXPRESS LESSON/HOW YOUR BODY WORKS: 516 (br), David Young-Wolff/PhotoEdit; 523 (tr), Michael Newman/ PhotoEdit; 525 (tc), ©Dennis Kunkel/ Phototake; 526 (bl, bc), Digital Image ©2004 EyeWire; 529 (all), Sergio Purtell/ Foca/HRW; 531 (tr), ©Nathan Bilow/Allsport/Getty Images; 534 (cr), ©Ed Reschke/Peter Arnold, Inc.; 535 (tl), Robert Caughey/Visuals Unlimited; 535 (cl, bl), David M. Phillips/ Visuals Unlimited; 535 (tr), ©Spencer Rowell/Getty Images/ Taxi; 539 (tr), ©Roy Morsch/CORBIS; 541 (tr), SW Production/ Index Stock Imagery, Inc.; 542 (bl), Carol Guenzi Agents/ Index Stock Imagery, Inc.; 543 (tl), ©Juergen Berger, Max-Planck Institute/SPL/Photo Researchers, Inc.; 544 (tl), ©Richard Price/Getty Images/Taxi; 547 (tr), ©Spencer Rowell/Getty Images/Taxi

EXPRESS LESSON/WHAT YOU NEED TO KNOW ABOUT: 548 (b), ©Jamsen/Premium/Panoramic Images, Chicago 2004; 550 (bl), ©Kelly-Mooney Photography/ CORBIS; 552 (bl), Custom Medical Stock Photo; 554 (tl), Mark Richards/ PhotoEdit; 554 (cl), Laurent Rebours/AP/Wide World Photos; 554 (cr), Custom Medical Stock Photo; 554 (tr), ©Howard Davies/CORBIS; 555 (tr), ©Digital Vision; 556 (br), Digital Image ©2004 PhotoDisc; 557 (tl), ©Chronis Jons/Getty Images/Stone; 558 (bl), ©COMSTOCK, Inc.; 560 (tr), Digital Image ©2004 Artville; 563 (tc), Sam Dudgeon/ HRW; 567 (tr), Digital Image ©2004 PhotoDisc; 568 (tl), David Young-Wolff/PhotoEdit; 569 (tr), Digital Image ©2004 EyeWire; 570 (bl), ©Donna Day/Getty Images/Stone; 571 (tr), Randy Taylor/Index Stock Imagery, Inc.; 573 (tc), K. Beebe/Custom Medical Stock Photo; 573 (tr), ©Jennie Woodcock/Reflections Photolibrary/CORBIS; 574 (bl, cl, bc), Peter Van Steen/HRW; 574 (br), Corbis Images/ HRW; 574 (cr), ©Peter Gridley/Getty Images/Taxi

EXPRESS LESSON/FIRST AID & SAFETY: 578 (bl), ©Ariel Skelley/CORBIS; 586 (t), Custom Medical Stock Photo; 586 (br), A. Bartel/Custom Medical Stock Photo; 587 (tr), ©Ken Lax/Photo Researchers, Inc.; 588 (bc), Bob Winsett/Index Stock Imagery, Inc.; 590 (br), Bob Daemmrich Photo, Inc.; 591 (tr), Lisa Davis/HRW; 593 (tr), ©SPL/Photo Researchers, Inc.; 594 (tc), ©Sinclair Stammers/SPL/Photo Researchers, Inc.; 594 (c), ©Dr P. Marazzi/SPL/Photo Researchers, Inc.; 594 (bc), ©John Radcliffe Hospital/SPL/Photo Researchers, Inc.; 596 (t), ©Garry Watson/SPL/Photo Researchers, Inc.; 596 (tc), ©Michael & Patricia Fogden/CORBIS; 596 (bc), Digital Image ©2004 EyeWire; 596 (b), Mr. Yuk is a registered trademark of Children's Hospital of Pittsburgh.; 597 (cr), ©Larry West/Getty Images/Taxi; 598 (bl), ©Tim Wright/ CORBIS; 599 (br), Digital Image ©2004 PhotoDisc; 599 (tr), ©Marc Romanelli/Getty Images/The Image Bank; 600 (tr), ©Marc Romanelli/Getty Images/The Image Bank; 602 (tc), Sam Dudgeon/HRW; 602 (bl), ©Ariel Skelley/CORBIS; 603 (all), Victoria Smith/HRW; 604 (tr), John Langford/HRW; 604 (cr), Peter Van Steen/ HRW; 604 (br), Corbis Images/ HRW; 605 (tr), Susan Van Etten/PhotoEdit; 606 (bl), Spencer Grant/PhotoEdit; 607 (tr), Digital Image ©2004 PhotoDisc; 608 (br), Victoria Smith/HRW; 608 (bc), Digital Image ©2004 Artville; 609 (tc), Digital Image ©2004 PhotoDisc; 609 (c), Sam Dudgeon/HRW; 609 (br), Victoria Smith/HRW; 609 (tr), Digital Image ©2004 EyeWire; 610 (tr), ©Getty Images; 612 (br), Digital Image ©2004 PhotoDisc; 613 (tr), ©Richard Hutchings/CORBIS

LIFE SKILLS QUICK REVIEW: 615 (tr), Peter Van Steen/HRW; 616 (bl), David Young Wolff/PhotoEdit; 617 (tr), Corbis Images/HRW; 618 (cl), ©Brad Wilson/ Photonica; 620 (bl), ©Areil Skelley/CORBIS; 621 (t), ©David H. Wells/CORBIS

REFERENCE GUIDE/HEALTH CAREERS: 632 (br), Spencer Grant/PhotoEdit; 632 (bc), Digital Image ©2004 PhotoDisc; 632 (tl), Digital Image ©2004 EyeWire; 633 (tr), Jeff Greenberg/Visuals Unlimited; 633 (tl), Digital Image ©2004 Artville; 634 (tr), Digital Image ©2004 PhotoDisc; 635 (tl), Michael Newman/PhotoEdit; 635 (b), ©John Madere/Corbis Stock Market; 635 (tc), Digital Image ©2004 Artville; 636 (bl), A. Ramey/PhotoEdit; 636 (tr), Digital Image ©2004 PhotoDisc; 637 (tl), Jeff Dunn/Stock Boston; 637 (br), Sam Dudgeon/HRW; 637 (inset), Digital Image ©2004 PhotoDisc; 638 (br), A. Ramey/PhotoEdit; 638 (tl), Digital Image ©2004 PhotoDisc; 639 (br), Jeff Greenberg/PhotoEdit; 639 (tl), Digital Image ©2004 Artville; 640 (tl), Mark Richard/PhotoEdit; 640 (br), Mark Gibson Photography; 641 (tl), Tom Carter/PhotoEdit; 641 (br), Charles Gupton/ Stock Boston; 641 (c), Digital Image ©2004 Artville

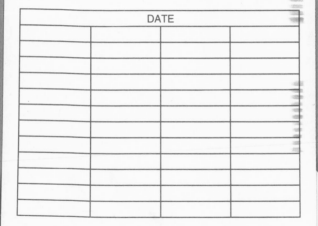

SIGNS

OF

LIFE

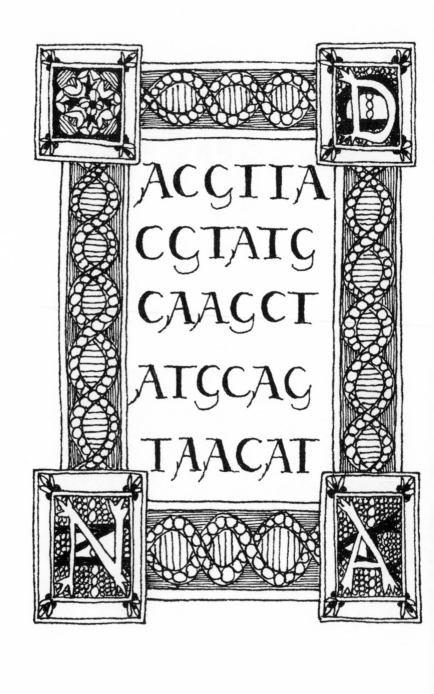

SIGNS
OF
LIFE

THE
LANGUAGE
AND
MEANINGS
OF
DNA

ROBERT POLLACK

HOUGHTON MIFFLIN COMPANY

Boston   New York

1994

Copyright © 1994 by Robert Pollack

For information about permission to reproduce selections from
this book, write to Permissions, Houghton Mifflin Company,
215 Park Avenue South, New York, New York 10003.

Library of Congress Cataloging-in-Publication Data
Pollack, Robert, date.
Signs of life : the language and meanings
of DNA / Robert Pollack.
p. cm.
Includes bibliographical references and index.
ISBN 0-395-64498-4
1. Genetics — Popular works.   2. DNA — Popular works.
I. Title.
QH437.P65 1994
575.1 — dc20   93-32474
CIP

Printed in the United States of America

BP 10 9 8 7 6 5 4 3 2 1

Frontispiece by Amy Pollack

Book design by Anne Chalmers

CONTENTS

ACKNOWLEDGMENTS

At the heart of this book is a gift from my wife, Amy, and our daughter, Marya: the time, space, and freedom to write, and the encouragement to begin again.

It was an immense privilege to work with John Sterling at Houghton Mifflin, whose insight and talents have surely made this a better book. I am indebted as well to my agents, Anne Engel and Jean Naggar, and to our mutual friends, Penny and Horace Judson, without whose kind and thoughtful help little would have been possible.

I thank the Alfred Sloan Foundation, the Howard Hughes Medical Institute, the Abe Wouk Foundation, the John Simon Guggenheim Foundation, and the Dartmouth College Department of Anthropology for their support, and Columbia Science Librarian Kathleen Kehoe for engaging the metaphor of this book so congenially by eagerly getting me every book and paper I ever needed.

David Albert, Akeel Bilgrami, Suzie Chen, Eric Holtzman, Nancy Hopkins, Ken Korey, Joshua Lederberg, Madeline Lee, Michelle Mattson, Alan McGowan, Don Melnick, Hugh Nissenson, Bruce Pipes, Michael Rosenthal, Charles Sheer, Ted Tayler, Jim Watson, Amy, Marya, and my brother Barry were all kind enough to make many useful suggestions; all the oversights, wrong guesses, and misunderstandings that slipped past me are my own responsibility.

SIGNS
OF
LIFE

INTRODUCTION

THIS BOOK BEGAN in the late 1970s, when my family and I first learned that my father was afflicted with Alzheimer's disease. He has since died, after a long period during which he hadn't enough of a mind to recognize us, a source of much despair for my family and me as we pondered the mystery of this slow, sad end to his life. When he was diagnosed with the disease, I did what any sensible molecular biologist would do. Trained to read the literature of science and medicine for clues on how to attack such a problem, I spent much time in the library of Columbia's College of Physicians and Surgeons. Not realizing how unhappy this was making me, I persisted in the notion that I could help my father if only I could find the pattern that I knew had to be hidden in the published research literature. I was wrong; there was no discernible path to reversing the course of this disease ten years ago, and while there have been some recent tantalizing flashes in the fog, there is no path I can see today. This was hard for me to believe then, and it still is. But believing it, and accepting it, was necessary to having any sort of a life for myself. The life I have had since his disease was diagnosed is quite similar to the one I had before, with one clear difference: I still believe we can figure out how the natural world works through science, but its limits have become as interesting to me as its powers, as I realize that scientific discoveries cannot protect me from the pain of loss.

I have always loved books: I have been a scientist since high school; before then I read omnivorously and wanted to be a writer. My grandparents had been driven from Eastern Europe at the turn of the century, arriving at Ellis Island with little besides hope for an auspicious future in America for their children if not for themselves. Like so many other children of immigrants who fell short of their parents' dreams by leaving school to work, my parents held tightly to the nineteenth-century notion of science as the motor of progress and the leveler of hierarchies. The authors they read and passed on to me — H. G. Wells, Paul de Kruif, J. B. S. Haldane — led me to believe for a short while that scientific laws had been found to govern all history and all behavior and these laws were as predictable and general as those that governed energy and matter. My adolescent rebellions had a peculiar twist: as my friends broke the dietary rules of their parents, tremulously eating their first pork in a Chinese restaurant, I staked out my independence by insisting that scientific laws did not extend to human affairs and that history was not predictable. From this mutiny I formed the idea of becoming a scientist myself, a radical notion for a boy whose pleasure came from reading and whose parents had not finished high school.

I was just preparing for high school myself in the spring of 1953 when James Watson and Francis Crick published a nine-hundred-word prose poem in the British journal *Nature* that established the symmetrical, twisted structure of the chemical deoxyribonucleic acid — DNA — and showed that the way it was made explained how it could serve as the chemical of the gene. Of course, this purest and most beautiful example of the inextricable intertwining of form and function in biology made no quick headway in the educational establishment responsible for my schooling, so biology remained for me a confused subject full of lists and mysteries. At Columbia College I chose physics as my science, because it seemed to me to be of the greatest generality and therefore most likely to yield the underlying laws of nature I had decided to pursue. But by the time I graduated, the explosion of new ideas and results in molecular biology and genetics had reached even me. I turned to biology as a graduate student early enough to learn about genes and their chemistry from research papers and seminars given by their authors, not from textbooks. From physics I brought two contradictory lessons: to guard against unnecessary complexity and to be constantly aware that what was easily observable was no guide to what was invisibly small.

I began my career as a biologist studying the genetics of bacteria and the viruses that live within them. But as soon as I finished the project in bacterial genetics that earned me a Ph.D. from Brandeis University, I found myself drawn ineluctably to the border where science touches directly on matters of human concern. I joined the Pathology Department at New York University School of Medicine to begin what would be a thirty-year project: to unravel the molecular events that led to the appearance of a cancer in an otherwise healthy tissue.

In the late 1960s, after two years of work, I made my first personal contribution to the problem in a paper showing that within a tumor there would always be more normal cells, and that these spontaneous revertant cells had regained the growth controls that kept a normal tissue from overgrowing its boundaries. This paper caught the eye of James Watson. After one seminar and two beers, he invited me to join a small group of young scientists at Cold Spring Harbor Laboratory, a private research institute on the North Shore of Long Island that had, as I remember, two Nobel laureates on its permanent staff of twelve when I arrived.

In this way I enlisted in President Nixon's War on Cancer, a baroque moment in the history of American science that provided hundreds of young scientists with jump starts to our careers. When I ran a lab at Cold Spring Harbor in the early 1970s, my family and I lived in a set of converted stables. There were weeks when I would walk from our apartment down the laboratory's main road to my dishes of normal and cancer cells, then back up the road at night to our vegetable garden, not knowing which day of the week it was, not carrying any money or keys (let alone any ID or credit cards), just drunk on science all the time.

I would sometimes meet Barbara McClintock — perhaps the most original geneticist since Mendel and certainly the most self-disciplined person I have ever known — on my walk to the lab if I were up early enough, and she would show me her flowers. She was interested in the genetics underlying the appearance of the little red flowerlets at the center of a bunch of Queen Anne's lace. She would offhandedly teach me about those flowers along the road in ways that quietly conveyed to me that she knew each of them, personally and by name, and that she also knew every other plant within sight and its family history as well.

At home in this scientist's Arcadia, I continued my work on simple versions of cancer, imitations of the disease in a dish. I grew cells from mice and people, from normal tissue and tumors, seeing to it that each cell preserved the characteristics reminiscent of its status in the body. I took DNA from various sources — a cell, a virus, a bacterium — put it into another cell, and followed the inherited changes. Over the years, this premeditated genetic transformation brought on by moving DNA from one cell to another permitted my colleagues and me to describe in daunting detail the genes that change when a normal cell of the body turns into a cancer cell.

In the 1970s and later, as my father was dying his slow death, scientists in my field added to DNA transformation a second skill of comprehensive importance when they learned how to change a gene as they desired. Since then, the direct manipulation of inheritance — an impossibility when I was a graduate student — has become the stuff of high school laboratories. Molecular biologists, including younger colleagues who were not even born when I was in high school, now hold great power over inheritance. Some have begun to transliterate the entire sequence of human DNA — the human genome — into a string of English letters; others have succeeded in recasting the DNA of other species of plants and animals, including many of the ones we eat.

I'd bet that if we survive long enough to be able to look back, the second half of this century will be known, not as the Age of Atoms, but as the Age of DNA. Just forty years ago Watson and Crick were making tin and paper models of DNA and uncovering the set of laws that govern all inheritance, the base-pairing rules that make DNA the perfect self-copying text. Watson's life has encompassed the Age of DNA: a few years ago, he brought together the people and the money necessary to launch the comprehensive transliteration of human DNA, the Human Genome Project. Already, the new tools of molecular biology are capable of making profound changes in the human genome, of changing us and giving us the capacity to change our children for better or worse. This new capacity has come upon us very quickly: it is as if we had just deciphered a few words in a new language and begun rewriting ancient texts before understanding their full meaning. The task that lies beyond the Human Genome Project is not merely to transliterate, nor simply to comprehend a cell's way of reading its DNA, but also to translate, and then to read, the DNA within ourselves with the full analytical power we might bring to any of our own texts.

My science — molecular biology — has become to a large extent a project to understand fully how our bodies read the unique and uniquely interesting chemical texts within each of our cells. The meanings we have begun to draw from human DNA and the changes we have begun to make in it are important and should be understandable to everyone, which is one reason I have organized this book around the notion of human DNA as a work of literature, a great historical text. But the metaphor of a chemical text is more than a vision: DNA is a long, skinny assembly of atoms similar in function, if not form, to the letters of a book, strung out in one long line. The cells of our bodies do extract a multiplicity of meanings from the DNA text inside them, and we have indeed begun to read a cell's DNA in ways even more subtle than a cell can do.

The reality of "deep time" — that is, that the history of the planet goes back tens of thousands of millions of years and that life has been on the planet for thousands of millions of years — is at first difficult to comprehend. Looking at life in all its variety and complexity, the alternative is to believe in magic. The notion of DNA as a text makes it possible to imagine natural selection as an author in deep time, writing at the rate of perhaps a letter every few centuries to produce the instruction books for all the living things we are among today. Just as an analysis of the fossils in rocks that now show themselves on the surfaces of the planet gives us the actual historical record of mountains and oceans as they formed and reformed over the last couple of billion years, so an analysis of DNA texts will provide direct information about events in biological evolution that shared the same deep times. Before long, museums of natural history will be in practice what they have always been in theory: libraries of DNA, with holdings that range from current editions to the ancient and unexpected DNAs of fossils.

Our own species is young only in comparison with life itself; we are all the children of ancestral peoples who walked the earth hundreds of thousands — perhaps even millions — of years ago. Each living person's DNA is rich in specific passages derived from a particular genealogy. Yet at the same time we can be sure that the texts we find will all refer to the same past, a past of branching descent. We must begin to see the texts of an individual and the texts common to members of a species as a form of literature, to approach them as one would approach a library of precious, deep, important books. A proper appreciation of molecular biology as one of the arts — a branch of history — as well as one of the sciences may provide the burgeoning field of molecular medicine with the manifold vision of the world that both science and medicine need if they are to honor the great Hippocratic constraint, to do no harm.

∾

When a colleague in Columbia's Philosophy Department asked me what this book was about, I said that it was an attempt to explore the implications of the fact that we are on the verge of grasping at least some of the multiple meanings of our DNA. He responded, "Must I find out?" We both laughed, but afterward I could not shake off the troubling sense that he was casually conveying a deeply felt but usually silent doubt that many sophisticated people have about the utility and necessity of understanding even the science most likely to affect their lives. In a 1993 national Louis Harris poll sponsored by the March of Dimes, 86 percent said that they know "almost nothing" or "relatively little" about gene therapy. Scientists too have often remained silent, by and large failing to make clear to a larger audience what it is they do, why they do it, what they expect to accomplish, and what they fear. Why has it been so hard for scientists and nonscientists to communicate productively? There is no simple answer, but in writing about the meanings of our genes I have found it necessary to push against three barriers to mutual comprehension, even with the metaphor of DNA as text to ease the problem of translating the jargon of my field.

First, many nonscientists are wary of scientific language, often recoiling from its authority and sometimes fearing that complicated notions are being used to legitimize unspoken political agendas. Without an understanding of the underlying science, wariness turns to an unfocused distrust. In the same Harris poll, 73 percent agreed "strongly" or "somewhat" with the statement that "the potential danger from genetically altered cells is so great that strict regulations are necessary"; the poll did not ask about the internal inconsistency of the majority's response, which coupled an admission of ignorance about genetics with a certainty of its riskiness. But wariness has been called for in the past, and if science is to be kept honest, there is no harm in approaching it with a well-informed skepticism.

Consider, for example, the damage done by geneticists in the period leading to the U.S. immigration laws of the 1920s. These laws were "scientific" since they drew their rationale from the sworn congressional testimony of many highly regarded biologists and physicians. Committees of Congress heard "scientific" proof that similarities of language, religion, or ethnicity were inherited expressions of a small number of underlying "genes," that such undesirable traits as laziness, drunkenness, avariciousness, and poverty were simple genetic traits. In this way, scientists gave intellectual cover to the decision to exclude immigrants on the basis of their skin color, religion, nationality, and language: it was Italians who were genetically more likely to be poor, Jews from Eastern Europe who were genetically greedy, and so forth. The inaccuracy, intellectual sloppiness, and prejudices of these scientists and like-minded members of Congress converged in the Immigration Law of 1926, which codified the most crudely racist and biologically foolish distinctions since the Constitution's definition of a slave as 60 percent of a human being. By the

1940s, this eugenically correct law had blocked the escape to the United States of many people who subsequently died in actions carried out according to the more activist laws of the German Third Reich.

This impulse to misuse the language of genetics for political purposes has not disappeared: the "ethnic cleansing" of Bosnia is built on the same misguided dream of biological purity. Nor has the United States freed itself of the problem. In 1992, federally sponsored meetings were called to discuss the likelihood of discovering "genes for violent behavior" and the ways in which such genetic information — not that it is likely to exist — might be used to finger "susceptible" people and their families even before any crime had been committed. The resulting publicity led the granting agency — the National Institutes of Health — to cancel one of these meetings, but we have no assurance that it was the last of its kind.

Practicing science is an analytical act and also a creative one. The second barrier to understanding is that scientists' endless rounds of "on the other hand" are often mistaken for an inability to be certain about the meaning of an experiment. It is as though every professor of English were at once a writer of novels and an interpreter-theorist of those very novels. Such people are rare in the humanities and social sciences, but all productive scientists are quite resigned to oscillating between creation and criticism, knowing that public recognition without continued carping from one's peers is useless and empty praise.

The basic problem is that most nonscientists do not have a very clear understanding of the paradox underlying all scientific advances: namely, that scientists love to do experiments that show their colleagues to be wrong. By this adversarial process, science gradually reveals the way nature works. The notion that published science must be free of error, and that error itself indicates sloppy thinking or fraudulent intent, is misguided. Bystanders often misunderstand the place of error in science and imagine that scientists who override one another's findings are in some way not entirely serious about their work or that no scientific statement can be true if any one is false.

The willful disregard by society at large of what has been

discovered by science is the third barrier to serious discourse. When political representatives ignore the facts they pay scientists to discover, those scientists who wish to help society benefit from their discoveries feel duped. Take the matter of prenatal care: bad or nonexistent prenatal care can cause a lifetime of misery, often accompanied by a huge societal bill. Scientists have explained this perfectly well at the cellular level: the final organization and function of the cells of the body are at greatest risk when tissues are being formed, and such cellular organization continues into the period immediately after birth. Prenatal care begins before a woman becomes pregnant: to assure that her newborn child will have the full use of its endowment of intelligence and good health, a woman must eat proper food and abstain from drugs and alcohol. Yet our country still refuses to acknowledge a nonjudgmental duty to educate every woman about her body and to nurture every pregnant woman and every newborn child.

Or take the issue of biological diversity. The 1973 Endangered Species Act is based on the notion — endorsed by most members of the scientific community and buttressed by new information at the level of DNA — that the loss of a species may affect all other living things, including people, because species evolve and survive through mutual interactions and competition. During George Bush's term as president, Manuel Lujan, Jr., the secretary of the interior, was in charge of enforcing the act. In May of 1992 the *New York Times* reported that "Secretary Lujan in fact does not believe in Darwin's theory of evolution, with the rise and extinction of species." We can only wonder whether the secretary — and through him the Department of the Interior — saw the Endangered Species Act as sensible or whether to him it was fatally flawed by virtue of its grounding in the fact of evolution. In the face of such official attitudes, one can easily understand why many of my colleagues have little incentive to try to explain their work to the world at large.

∿

In the early 1970s, when every transformation of a cell by an altered DNA was a novel event, I found myself in a situation that altogether changed my way of seeing science as a calling and as a profession. One of the first genomes to be spliced into a recombinant DNA molecule belonged to the tumor-causing virus SV40, which was joined to the genome of a plasmid of the bacterium *E. coli* in Paul Berg's laboratory at Stanford in 1971. This new genome combined genetic information from a bacterium with genetic information from a virus that normally lives in the kidneys of African monkeys. Such information had never been found in one genome before; the closest version of it in nature had not existed since the age when the only living things were neither bacteria nor animal cells nor their viruses, but some precursor of them all.

News of this accomplishment reached me at Cold Spring Harbor, where I was teaching Janet Mertz, then a graduate student of Paul Berg's, now a professor at the University of Wisconsin. I was also studying SV40 and thought it possibly a dangerous virus; closely related viruses, called JC and BK, had been found at autopsy in the brains of many people. It seemed to me that to put SV40 genes inside a laboratory culture of one of the bacterial species that colonize our intestines risked accidentally transforming someone's colon cells by SV40 DNA. This would be a new route for these genes, one our bodies were not prepared to defend against. Concerned, I called Professor Berg and asked him whether he had thought about the possibility of these risks. His first reaction was one of controlled astonishment at my sheer effrontery, but he did listen. After a few more phone conversations, he agreed to suspend further experiments, and to recommend that others do the same, until the recombinant plasmid could be tested for safety.

Berg's statesmanlike willingness to pull back voluntarily from an exciting line of work on the basis of a totally hypothetical and certainly low risk was unprecedented and significant. It led to a program of tests carried out for the NIH in military facilities like Fort Detrick in Maryland, where workers were protected by vents and shields that had been developed to insulate technicians engaged in producing germ warfare agents. The very air leaving these facilities was passed through a flame to prevent the escape of any microorganisms. After more than a year the results were clear: the many recombinant plasmids, viruses, and bacteria tested were each no more — and sometimes were less — infectious than the most infectious of their original sequences. More to the point of my initial concern, the intestines of volunteers who ingested laboratory strains of recombinant *E. coli* did not, in fact, become overgrown with these bacteria; the normal bacteria of the gut prevailed. Once the test results were in, the NIH decided to allow recombinant DNA research to go forward, but it established a Recombinant DNA Advisory Committee to serve as a watchdog and clearinghouse for new developments. In the past fifteen years the group has not had much to do, and its purview has been slowly but steadily reduced; whether this is wise remains to be seen.

Professor Berg was able to continue his work unimpeded by further phone calls until 1980, when Stockholm called to say he had won the Nobel Prize in Chemistry for his discoveries in recombinant DNA. But from the time I called him to the present day, I have never been able to feel entirely comfortable with one of the basic premises of science as it is currently practiced. The concept of peer review is built on the notion that scientists alone should judge one another's work, but that phone call to Professor Berg was just too hard for me to make. And though I am sure I had every right to query him as I did, I have often wondered whether I would have called if I had been competing directly with him at the time. I think not; after all, it was Berg, not I, who agreed even temporarily to stop a most interesting line of work.

❧

Back to the philosophy professor's question: Why poke around inside myself to get at a biological text, magically small though it might be? Are we so driven by hubris? Why not leave the text alone, unread? Curiosity is one reason, but humility is a better one, and awe is better still. Evolution has taken about four billion years to write the set of texts we can find in the DNA of creatures alive today. We are about to be able to read them in much the same manner we read any book of our own creating. This is a daunting prospect, but I cannot imagine any people so devoid of curiosity about their own bodies that they are not interested in what the text says. Nor is there really any choice in the matter: once we begin to read the book that describes how we ourselves are made, it is unlikely we will stop in the middle. The real question is not whether, but how, to read the human genome.

In *Signs of Life* I have tried to show how biology and medicine have come together in the project to understand how our bodies read DNA and how this new biology may be superseded by yet another perspective, as boundaries to the meanings we have begun to draw from DNA and the editorial changes we have begun to make in it become apparent. I have also considered the implications of one unexpected consequence of the new biology: its intersection with another, completely separate intellectual movement that has grown and flourished in the last few decades. With the discovery that a set of symbols has been used by nature to encode the information for the construction and maintenance of all living things, semiotics — the analysis of languages and texts as sets of signs and symbols — has become relevant to molecular biology. Semiotics has given students of the DNA text a new eye for reading, allowing us to argue for the validity of a multiplicity of meanings, or even for the absence of any meaning, in a stretch of the human genome.

Although semiotics and molecular biology both have been remarkably fertile in recent years, few scientists or literary critics have been prepared to move out of their own familiar territories to learn from the other. As a result, each kind of text has usually been analyzed by someone trapped in one or the other set of unnecessary intellectual constraints: the critic does not know that nature too has invented ways to read meanings into a text, and the scientist does not fully take the point that the transliteration of a DNA sequence into a string of four letters is no more likely to reveal the multiplicity of meanings in a gene than the transliteration of a poem by Pushkin from Cyrillic to English letters would enable an English-speaking person to see the layers of meaning in the poem. Yet if each strongly believes one type of text is worth reading, it is because both types of text — literary and genetic — may touch on the same matters of consciousness and mortality.

Despite my often-recollected helplessness in the face of my

father's illness and death, I have tried to keep molecular biology in perspective. I have never seen science as a religion or merely as a business or a game. Nor have I ever been tempted to join my colleagues from the other side of campus who dismiss science as "nothing important — life is not an experiment." Now past fifty, I am as certain as I was thirty years ago that this branch of science will continue to yield answers to ever more important questions. Once DNAs are read like books, whole new worlds of discourse will open up as we borrow from various disciplines involving textual analysis to interpret nature's text. How does a cell read its DNA? Certainly with great precision and with greater fastidiousness than we can read and agree on the meaning of our books. Are cells reading, exactly, or are they merely decoding? If DNA encodes our ability to read, how can we read that information itself? Will there be, for instance, a "canon" of DNA texts? Will DNA texts allow themselves to be analyzed for their meaning, or will meaning be evanescent and in the mind of the reader, as audience theorists today would predict? When we can read DNA the way we read a book, we will have to address these questions.

Though the metaphor of DNA as text opens many doors, the walls of ignorance and indifference between science and the rest of our culture make it hard for anyone to feel comfortable with the complex task at hand. Humanists shirk a text constructed by natural selection and written in an invisible chemical medium. Scientists avoid projects that cannot be framed as questions to be answered by controlled experiments. Still, the effort will have to be made. We and other living things are, after all, united by a common past and a common chemistry: we are related enough to a duck and an orange that we can eat them both. Now that we can make an original text by hooking together DNA from ducks, DNA from oranges, and, if we wish, DNA from people, it is time for everyone to learn about the language these DNAs share, the dialects they have evolved, and the arguments they articulate.

As the chance to determine our origins and our history becomes a necessity, we will all have to change the way we understand the essential nature of our bodies and our minds.

In my own effort to do so, I have taken inspiration from the English poet Robert Graves, who once wrote to me:

> Poets and physicians are closely allied in thought. Diagnostics and cure (truth and love, in essence) belong to both professions. In fact I find real doctors far closer to me in spirit than musicians or painters or sculptors. By "doctor," of course, I include all scientists who are not routineers of science, but have hearts and minds and are finding out the relations between mind and its physical concomitants.

1

~

INVISIBLE CITIES AND

CRYSTALLINE BOOKS

MANHATTAN IS A ROCKY ISLAND at the mouth of the Hudson River. Since 1810, when it was cut up into convenient rectangular blocks for future sale, it has accumulated large buildings. The two largest — not the most beautiful, but the largest — are located on the Hudson shore at the southern tip of the island. There, on their own windblown, rather desolate plaza, stand the twin towers of the World Trade Center. They are huge. Close up, they loom over a visitor and seem to be toppling from their own vast bulk. Inside, they are like most other office buildings of the late twentieth century: anonymous, filled with endless offices, each in turn brightly lit, well vented, but depressingly the same from floor to floor for more than a hundred stories. Each floor of each building covers almost an acre, which is cut up into a three-dimensional rectilinear grid pierced by dozens of elevator shafts. The outer wrapping of each building is made of metal and glass and is permanently sealed against the elements except at the base, where pipes bring in and take out the necessary fluids, energy, and heat, and at the top, where the buildings vent their excess heat. Prodigious numbers of people and vast amounts of information and money move in and out of these buildings every day, but at the end of each day they remain, quite unperturbed, much as they were on the day they opened.

Now imagine for a moment that we have slipped into a

slightly altered version of reality: we visit the World Trade Center plaza and find only one tower before us. Confused, because we recall there ought to be two towers, we go inside. We find the expected warrens, corridors, elevators, and such, but no sign of another tower. In our wandering, we come upon an unexpected set of barriers. We have entered the central core of the building, which is set off from the rest of the floors by an elaborate array of restraints. Authorized personnel scurry back and forth through sets of double doors, carrying sheaves of computer printouts. It is not at all clear what work they are performing.

Sneaking past the barriers, we find ourselves in an odd sort of library. We wander around the stacks, noticing that there are almost no books. In fact, the stacks themselves hold only duplicate sets of a series of books, two copies of each volume of what looks very much like the 1969 edition of the *Encyclopaedia Britannica*. Officious staff are carefully taking down one or another volume, photocopying an article, and replacing the volume. These clerks come and go, carrying out photocopies of pages of the library's twenty-three-volume encyclopedia and coming back with instructions for more copies, perhaps of the same article, perhaps of another. It all looks very orderly but also peculiar. It seems odd that the library should be sealed off, and odd also that so many copies of so few articles are being made.

Exploring further, we come to a separate sector of the library, where volumes of the encyclopedia are being painstakingly reproduced, bindings and all. This work is nearly complete: as we watch, the final volume in this duplicate set of volumes is finished, and all forty-six books are bundled off to a far corner of the library. We try to follow, but a sealed door stops us. Behind us, the library staff is suddenly excited; some people are scurrying out of the library, and we slip out in their wake.

We walk toward the elevators, puzzled by a certain soft vibration underfoot. The elevators are all temporarily out of order, so we enter an office to look out the window. We are just beginning to count ferries in the harbor when, quite smoothly and silently, the entire tower splits down the middle from top to bottom. There, just out the window and neatly aligned with ours, is a second tower on its own place on the plaza. No one in the building but us seems to find anything unusual about this quiet, massive, precise doubling of a sky-scraper. The elevators start up again; we return home to take a troubled nap, dreaming of the moment when the two towers will each divide again, cramming four onto the plaza overlooking New York Harbor.

~

Living objects all share four attributes: they can produce off-spring, they have a history of common descent from shared ancestors, they are made of invisible soft building blocks called cells, and each cell carries within itself a singular chemical called deoxyribose nucleic acid, or DNA, a large molecule assembled from the atoms of just five elements — carbon, phosphorus, nitrogen, hydrogen, and oxygen. The eye has its limits: without help it cannot see the parts — the atoms linked to one another as molecules, the molecules gathered into cells — of which it and all other living tissue is built. As a result, it has taken us a long time to see that the first three attributes are consequences of the fourth: of all the molecules in every cell, DNA alone unites all life in a common history, because every cell of every living thing has for about the past four billion years contained a version of DNA.

In human beings, as in every other living thing, DNA tells each cell exactly how to produce the thousands of other molecules that maintain the cell's shape and its place in the body. It is DNA that tells a liver cell to stock the blood with fresh proteins and to store sugar, a nerve cell to stretch itself out into long threads whose tips communicate with the others they touch. And as the metaphor of the replicating towers suggests, the DNA of a cell contains the instructions for making precise copies of itself and of the cell it is in. Each of us has always had, in each of our cells, a DNA text that guided our development from fertilized egg cell to embryo, fetus, and person; it is a precise copy of our sole and complete inheritance, one that is far more ancient than any human artifact. Because of its remarkable ability to command its own precise replication, DNA has sustained and linked all people since our beginnings as a single species at some time over the past million years.

DNA governs the operation of every cell in our bodies. A cell is a busy place, a city of large and small molecules all constructed according to information encoded in DNA. The metaphor of a city may seem even more farfetched than that of a skyscraper for an invisibly small cell until you consider that a cell has room for more than a hundred million million atoms; that is plenty of space for millions of different molecules, since even the largest molecules in a cell are made of only a few hundred million atoms. DNA ensures that a cell is not just a chemical soup but a molecular city with a center from which critical information flows, a molecular version of King David's Jerusalem. That walled city, with its supply of food and water entering through special portals and channels, had a great temple at the center and a book at the very center of the temple. A cell's version of the temple is the nucleus, a membrane-wrapped receptacle enclosing the cell's DNA. The nucleus is also the hub from which portions of the text are delivered to the cell, just as the sacred scripts were read to the people of Jerusalem from the entrances of the temple.

Observed through a powerful microscope a cell looks very complicated, and it is. It is wrapped in a fatty outer membrane pocked and studded with molecules — gates, channels, receptors and probes — that enable cells to be in contact with one another and with their immediate surroundings. The territory between the nucleus and the cell's outer membrane is called the cytoplasm — a maze of rods, balls, and sheets studded and filled with enzymes and various other proteins, all suspended in a salty gel.

Early analysts of the body's chemical composition did not place much importance on DNA, since it makes up such a small fraction of the material of the cell compared to its salts, proteins, carbohydrates, and fats. If a cell were as big as the Old City of Jerusalem, each chemical "letter" in the cell's DNA text — consisting of a few hundred atoms — would be about as big as a letter in a word of any familiar book. Yet every part of the cell, no matter how complex its form or function, is made according to information contained in the DNA folded into its nucleus. To appreciate this triumph of molecular origami, consider that the DNA in one human cell, if unwound and straightened out, would be a pair of molecules each about one yard long. A yard of DNA is a hundred million times longer than it is wide, and this exquisite thinness is the key to its ability to fit inside the nucleus. The pair of yard-long DNAs in a human cell are so slender that about ten billion copies, laid side by side like the wires of a telephone cable, would fit inside a waist-length human hair. That is about as many pairs of human DNA as there are people on the planet today; a genetic archive of our entire species could therefore be tightly packed into one long human hair if we had the means (and the desire) to do it.*

The DNA in every cell of a person — called the person's genome — is close to an encyclopedia in design and content. Like any proper encyclopedia, a human genome is divided and subdivided into volumes, articles, sentences, and words. And as in an encyclopedia written in English or Hebrew — but not a logographic language such as Chinese — words are further divided into letters. Biologists call the volumes in a genome chromosomes, a word derived from the Greek for "colored bodies," because they were large enough to be seen as dark dots by the first people to look at cells under a microscope. The articles in a genomic DNA text are the sets of genes that interact to give a cell or a tissue its specific character, and the sentences are the genes themselves. The words are called do-

---

* We are very big compared to a cell, and cells are very big compared to the atoms of which they, and we, are composed. We are made of about 100 million million, or 10^{14} cells, and each cell is made up of about 10^{14} atoms. Put another way, the complexity of a cell in molecular terms is about as great as the complexity of a person — brain and all — in cellular terms. This is as hopelessly unintuitive as the fact that the universe is hundreds of millions of times older — and life on earth is tens of millions of times older — than the oldest living person. The universe is about 3×10^{10} years old. The planet Earth has spun around the sun for about 4.5×10^9 years; life has left remnants of its existence that are at least 3.8×10^9 years old, telling us that Earth spent relatively little time as a lifeless planet. The billions of years that have gone by since Earth first held life make up the "deep time" of joint geological change and biological evolution, against which all human time, measured in millennia, is as leaves of grass.

mains, and the letters, base pairs. The concatenation of letters into words, words into grammatical sentences, and sentences into articles occurs in DNA, but in order to see how, we will have to first know how the letters themselves are formed and how they can make good copies of themselves.

～

The 1969 edition of the *Encyclopaedia Britannica*, which played the role of the human genome in the story of the replicating towers, has twenty-three alphabetically ordered volumes of articles that altogether contain about two hundred million letters. Most of our cells have pairs of each chromosome; the twenty-three pairs contain about six billion base pairs, so a single human genome is a text about three billion letters long. In each volume of an encyclopedia the string of letters is organized into thousands of separate articles about discrete subjects. In the long string of DNA letters in a chromosome, there are thousands of stretches of letters — genes — that each address a particular topic: how to make a particular protein perhaps, or how to find another stretch of DNA. The index of the *Britannica* has about two hundred thousand entries. Altogether, the chromosomes of a person contain at least a hundred thousand genes; we do not yet know exactly how many there are.

The topics in an encyclopedia are ordered by their spelling, rather than their meaning, so that a reader can quickly find the right place without knowing much about any given topic. Sometimes, especially when the topic words themselves have a common origin, adjacent topics may be related by meaning. Similarly, the genes in each chromosome are present in a precise order that seems usually — but not always — to be arbitrary; when genes that do similar things are next to each other, they are likely to be related by common descent from a single gene. The orderliness of genes in each chromosome shows up during the division of one cell into two, when the DNA of each chromosome coils up on itself, giving each one a characteristic set of crosswise bands. Each band marks the presence of a few hundred genes; the pattern of bands on each chromosome is very regular from person to person.

The constancy of chromosome banding from one to another individual within a species establishes that the genes are in a specific order, but it also masks a great deal of individuality in each person's DNA. Because the genes themselves are too small to see with a regular microscope, their textual differences from person to person are not normally visible within the bands, just as the differences among people on the ground are not visible from the top of a tall building. Rarely, a person is born with one or more chromosome bands out of place, snipped from one chromosome and attached to another, or duplicated as an extra copy within the genome. Such errors are like blocks of articles accidentally bound out of alphabetical order in an encyclopedia volume. Perhaps because misplaced genes cannot be found by the body in much the same way users cannot easily find an article if it is not in its proper — though arbitrary — alphabetical place, such anomalies are almost always accompanied by abnormalities at birth.

The notion of DNA as a text is far more than a metaphor. The letters of a human genome do encode more information than the *Britannica,* and both genome and encyclopedia carry their information in a single string of letters. We don't think of the book's letters as a single string because they are separated into words, sentences, lines, and pages. While the paper, the size and font of the type, the length and number of lines, the amount of white space between the letters and lines of type, and the binding all contribute to the pleasure of holding and reading a book, they serve first and foremost to preserve the correct sequence of letters and spaces from beginning to end.

DNA and the letters of a book are alike in function though not in form: the meaning in a DNA molecule emerges only when its genes are read in a useful — not necessarily alphabetical — order. The linear order of genes in a chromosome band need not be the order in which they are read out in any cell; genes, like sentences, are separate and separable passages, each critical to the way different cells derive different meanings from the same long, complicated text. In each chromosome, line and page breaks do not occur; the letters form one continuous line. But along that line, the genes are separated by other sequences that serve as molecular punctuation marks. Sets of genes form arguments the way sentences form paragraphs and articles.

Magnified a million times, the letters in DNA would be about the same size as the letters in this sentence, but the text would not look the same at all. The linear sequence of letters on a page is two-dimensional. We read with our eyes, seeing and understanding sets of letters and spaces as words. Then we use a mental lexicon and the syntax of our language to understand: first we grasp the words and the grammatical sentences they form, then the paragraphs and chapters, and then, finally, the arguments of the entire book. DNA too has words, syntax, and meanings, but as a text it is a molecular LEGO set, a sculpture whose information — encoded in its very shape — cannot be read at a distance. It has to be "felt" by other molecules in the cell in order to be read. DNA's letters are three-dimensional; they are read and understood by touch, the way a blind person reads a Braille text.

Now imagine DNA enlarged a hundred times more — a hundred million times altogether — so that its letters are as big as pizza pans. At this magnification, the human genome would have about the same circumference as a person's waist: it would be about fifty thousand miles long, and its atoms would be the size of marbles or golf balls. Its surface would be knobby, not at all smooth, and you would immediately notice two twisted ridges running the length of the DNA, like two vines wrapped around a tree trunk. Looking closer, you would see that the twisted ridges — each as thick as your arms — were a repeating chain of carbon, hydrogen, oxygen, and phosphorus atoms. When you felt along the two lengthwise grooves between the ridges, you would discover stacks of molecular disks called bases between the twisted vines, looking like thick, stiff leaves. These leaves would appear much alike, but on close examination you would see four different kinds: two bigger bases named adenine (abbreviated A) and guanine (G) and two smaller ones named thymine (T) and cytosine (C). Each base is made of nitrogen, hydrogen, oxygen, and carbon atoms and is flat, but because their atoms are arranged in slightly different ways, the bases have distinctly different outer edges. The bases are attached to the two twisted ridges by very short, stubby stems made of carbon, hydrogen, and oxygen atoms.*

A careful look at the bases themselves would reveal a considerable regularity in the pairs they form across the vines. Wherever an A comes from one stem, it is met by a T coming from the other strand; and if a G is coming from one strand, it always meets a C attached to the other strand. Anywhere you look along the double vine, you may find any sequence of leaves along one strand, but only two kinds of leaf pairs — G:C and A:T — would link the two strands. All in all, DNA would present itself to you as a pair of twisted vines, with G:C, C:G, T:A, and A:T pairs of inward-facing leaves coming off each vine to touch one another, making one complete turn of the double helix for every ten pairs of leaves. If you looked at the leaves on edge you could see through them, like venetian blinds.

If this is a text, where is the information? Information cannot be found in sameness. All the parts that are exactly the same from region to region on the DNA cannot hold information any more than a book of identical blank pages or a book filled with nothing but the same letter over and over. Where, then, is this double vine different?

Grab one of the two vines and climb on it; as you do, feel again the contours of the grooves that run between the vines. The flexible vines themselves are a simple repeat of oxygen, phosphorus, carbon, and hydrogen, the same everywhere along their length. But the grooves do not feel the same; they are wavy in a complicated way, like the grooves of a phonograph record. Looking inside the grooves, you see that the complex ripple is the surface of the outer edges of the four kinds of inward-pointing leaves, the four base pairs. Moving along the DNA, you feel the edges of the base pairs as a contour, and each is different, the way the milled edge of a quarter is differ-

---

* Names carry an evolved history of meanings. Adenine is a chemical that was first isolated from various glands: the Latin prefix for "gland" is *adeno*. Purified thymine too first came from a gland, the thymus. Cytosine was thought at first to come specifically from the cytoplasm, not the nucleus of a cell; guanine comes from guano (bird dung), which is rich in it.

ent from the smooth edge of a nickel. The sequence of ripples or contours you feel as you run your hand along the edges of a stretch of base pairs is the three-dimensional medium in which DNA stores its information. With a little bit of practice, you can recognize each of the four base pairs by feel, then transliterate this three-dimensional text by writing down the sequence in which the bases appear on one of the two vines as a string of English letters: AGCTA, and so forth.

The double helix of vines is a completely repetitive, stable structure, but the sequence of base pairs linking the vines needs not follow any pattern or order at all. Just the opposite: the sequence of base pairs in a DNA molecule is free to change without any effect on the structure of the outer double helix. Therefore, though at first the stack of leaves may appear to be an endless repetition of the four bases, you will discover as you write down the order of the base pairs that DNA is different from region to region. Sometimes you will feel a quite regular pattern of bumps in the groove as the base pairs run through a simple sequence over and over. Such a repeat is similar to a pitch pipe sounding a single note so that the instruments of an orchestra can tune up — it is necessary for the musicians, perhaps, but not the music. Sometimes, though, you will come upon a run of thousands of bases in which each of the four bases appears in approximately equal frequency but in no predictable order. Such a sequence of bases is precisely like the sequence of notes in a concerto or the letters in a book: no matter whether we look at a stretch of ten, one hundred, or one thousand notes or letters, the remainder of the sequence is not predictable from any of its parts. The absence of a repeating and therefore predictable pattern to the sequence of its bases is the sign that a particular stretch of DNA carries unique information. These are the genes.

If one strand can carry information in the sequence of its bases, why does DNA have two vines and a groove in which to feel the contour of a run of base pairs instead of just one vine with a sequence of bases appended, to be felt like beads on a rosary? The answer lies in DNA's double role as a text and as an inheritance: it has to have its own way of making copies of itself, to be delivered by parents to the first cell that will be their child, then copied thereafter by each cell so that it is present in all the cells of the body at all times in the life of the offspring. DNA's double-strandedness is its machinery for copying itself. In his firsthand account of the discovery of DNA's structure, *The Double Helix*, James Watson explained DNA's two strands with a wink: "Important biological objects come in pairs." By this glancing reference to the ubiquity of sex, he also meant to convey that each of DNA's two strands can be the source of an identical, new DNA molecule, so that the genetic information in one DNA molecule can be passed from one generation of cells — and individuals — to the next.

The clue to how this copying machine works lies in the special way DNA has of resolving what would seem to be an unnecessary ambiguity in the information it carries. A sequence of bases in a stretch of DNA can be read forward or backward; how does a cell know in which direction the DNA is correct? If you climbed along one of the DNA vines and came across a sequence like GGGAA, you could go backward and read it as AAGGG or you could jump to the other vine and feel the base-paired sequences CCCTT or TTCCC, depending which way you went. The base-pairing rules may predict a lot, but alone they leave the information in DNA ill defined. The ambiguity is resolved — and the copying mechanism revealed — by a closer examination of the vines. A real vine grows from the ground up and so has a natural top and bottom, but a molecule of DNA has no preferred direction. This is so for an unexpected reason: each strand of DNA does have an intrinsic direction, but the two strands always run counter to each other. Consequently, like the king of hearts in a deck of cards, a batonlike molecule of DNA can be twirled halfway around and still look the same.

Objects like DNA that retain their shape after a half rotation are said to have dyad symmetry. Imagine two trains on adjacent tracks leaving a station but traveling in opposite directions. At the windows of each train are passengers waving good-bye to the other train. If the trains were to stop and the passengers were to clasp hands across the platform, then the trains and their passengers, like the helical vines of DNA and their base pairs, would be in a state of dyad symmetry. A photograph taken from the air would show the trains linked by pairs of arms, and if there were no other landmark, one would not be able to tell which train was heading in which direction.

Look more carefully at those passengers reaching toward the hands of the passengers heading in the opposite direction. Their hands — palms facing in opposite directions — barely meet. As the tips of their fingers touch, each pair of hands forms an extended flat surface with fingers in contact running down the middle. To allow these flat surfaces to form, every person's elbow and shoulder must jut forward at a sharp angle from a window of one of the trains. Indeed, one could tell which end of the train held the locomotive, and which direction the train was about to go, simply by observing the angle made by each person's arm as it stretched to meet another's palm. Similarly, DNA's four bases all jut from their pair of vines at the same angle, meeting in between as a succession of flat base pairs. The base pairs have to be flat and stack perfectly, for if they puckered or met at an angle, DNA as a whole would not have dyad symmetry; rather, the direction of the bend or the angle of the base pairs would give DNA a built-in directionality, just as we could tell which train was which in our aerial photograph if the passengers on both trains were all pointing in the same direction instead of shaking hands across the platform. But the bases come off both vines at the same angle, so molecules that read the sequence of base pairs of DNA can first point themselves in the proper direction on either strand by recognizing this angle.

The base-pairing rules assure that the sequence on one strand will predict the sequence on the other. But because the molecules that read DNA in our cells always proceed from front to back, as seen from either DNA strand, and because dyad symmetry assures that front to back on one strand is the opposite direction from front to back on the other, special DNA sequences must first align these molecules so that they can only read the DNA of a gene in one of two possible directions, the so-called sense direction. By convention, the sequence of base pairs read in the sense direction is written from left to right. For instance, consider a DNA that has the sequence of base pairs G:C, C:G, A:T, T:A. The bases along one strand could be transliterated left to right as GCAT or right to left as TACG; the other strand could be transliterated as CGTA or ATGC. Let us say that the proper direction on one strand gives the sequence GCAT and indicate this by an arrowhead: GCAT>. Then the base-pairing rules tell us that the other strand would be properly transliterated as <CGTA. In order to follow a convention familiar to readers of the Romance, Slavic, and Germanic languages, transliterated DNA sequences are written from left to right, so the base-paired complement of GCAT> would be written as ATGC> rather than as <CGTA. This convention is awkward, but the arrowheads assure that the complementarity of two base-paired DNA strands is not forgotten.

Just as one set of molecules can use the fixed and constant elements of DNA's structure to align themselves for transliteration of the variable, informationally rich sequence of base pairs, other molecules see any double-stranded DNA molecule as the parent of two identical daughter molecules and carry out this doubling, called replication. The molecules of replication unzip the two strands of a DNA so that each can become the template for the construction of a new double-stranded DNA, whose sequence of base pairs will be identical to that of the original. Before a cell is fully prepared to duplicate its genes this way, it must stock up on a fresh supply of the four subunits of a new DNA strand. These subunits, called nucleotides, are made of a base already linked through a sugar to a phosphate group. Then, at the moment that one DNA is about to become two, the two strands separate.

Imagine a typesetter who places letters in a rack that will not take just any letters but will only accept a single, specific sequence of letters. The base-pairing rules leave no choice to the sequence of nucleotides that assemble as second strands on each of the two parental strands of a replicating DNA molecule. Each strand is the rack on which the nucleotides with proper bases line up to form a run of base pairs; each base on the original strand serves as a template for the addition of the proper nucleotide to the growing second strand. As new bases are appended to each strand to form a brand-new second strand, the base-pairing rules assure that each new double-stranded DNA molecule will be an exact replica of its parent.

All DNA, whether or not it encodes a gene, replicates this way. For most stretches of DNA, biologically useful information is held on only one strand, but the ubiquitous second strand, the way the two strands run in opposite directions, the law that G must pair with C and A with T — these three constraints mean that the information along an old strand of DNA is kept with fidelity by the new strand so that the informational strand — whichever it may be — is always assured of faithful replication as one molecule of DNA becomes two. The second strand is the minimum imaginable amount of extra molecular baggage necessary to make either strand's information self-replicating.

In 1944 the Austrian physicist Erwin Schrödinger predicted that the material of the gene would both be very stable and contain much information, despite the contradictory quality of these two attributes. Schrödinger captured the genetic material's exquisite requirement for both stability and meaning in an oxymoron, describing genes as being made of an "aperiodic crystal." By aperiodic, Schrödinger meant that the gene's material had to carry information. In this sense, any text in any alphabet must be aperiodic if it conveys information. A typical sentence, this one for instance, has information in proportion to its total length, because for every letter in the sentence, any of the other twenty-five letters might have been used to make any one of a very large number of alternative sentences, some of them with quite different meanings, others with no meaning at all. By calling the gene a crystal, Schrödinger meant that a gene needed the regularity and stability of crystals, the only other large things in nature that have lasted as long as life. The paradox was this: the gene had to have crystalline stability but it could not take the form of a crystal's purely periodic, informationally barren repeat. DNA — the base-paired double helix — completely removes the sting of paradox from Schrödinger's prediction. DNA is, precisely, an aperiodic crystal.

DNA's elegant architecture was worked out in the early 1950s. The first sign that it provided the solution to the problem of gene replication — albeit one that made the daring assumption that a gene's information resided entirely in its DNA — appeared as a brief poetical note to the April 25, 1953, issue of the scientific journal *Nature* by James Watson and Francis Crick. With this singular understatement, Watson and Crick opened the age of modern biology:

> The novel feature of the structure [of DNA] is the manner in which the two chains are held together by the . . . bases. . . . The sequence of bases on a single chain does not appear to be restricted in any way. However, if only specific pairs of bases can be formed, it follows that if the sequence of bases on one chain is given, then the sequence on the other chain is automatically determined. . . . It has not escaped our notice that the specific pairing we have postulated immediately suggests a copying mechanism for the genetic material.

$\sim$

Some kinds of bacteria — small, single-celled creatures with a single molecule of DNA for a chromosome — have survived for billions of years. No one bacterium lives very long, but through DNA replication and cell division, the population persists. One bacterial cell becomes two by duplicating its chromosome, moving each new copy to opposite ends of the cell and splitting down the middle; each daughter bacterium then carries away one of the two new chromosomes. At every generation, the molecules of DNA replication use an old strand of DNA as a template for a new one. Consider what this means for these bacteria: among the ones alive today may be a rare bacterium that carries one of the two DNA strands from one of its ancient ancestors. In the extreme case, somewhere on Earth might be a bacterium with DNA made up of two strands of absurdly different ages: one made twenty minutes ago and the other almost as old as the planet itself.

Even if such a rarity exists, we have no way of discovering it; the base-pair sequence in the ancient DNA strand would not be chemically distinguishable from that of any other bacterium of the same species. The planet's surface has changed many times over, but DNA and the cellular machinery for its replication have remained constant. Schrödinger's "aperiodic crystal" understated DNA's stability: no stone, no mountain, no ocean, not even the sky above us, have been stable and constant for this long; nothing inanimate, no matter how complicated, has survived unchanged for a fraction of the time that DNA and its machinery of replication have coexisted.

But nothing alive is ever perfect. Though the backbones of DNA strands may last for a very long time, the information within DNA can change by accident at any time. The rigid base-pairing rules, which enable information to be copied from one DNA double helix to two, can also fix in place any error that occurs. Sometimes such an error can be calamitous. The word "mutation" was coined in 1901 by the Dutch botanist Hugo De Vries to describe the sudden appearance of a new variant form or behavior that did not go away but rather bred true in successive generations. The best-known single mutation is the one first seen by one of the founders of modern genetics, Thomas Hunt Morgan. In 1910 Morgan reported that he had found a single white-eyed fruit fly among the tens of thousands of little red-eyed fruit flies that his laboratory maintained. In short order he showed that this fly was genetically different from normal; that is, its descendants would sometimes — but not always — have white eyes as well, and, like color blindness in humans, this mutation affected males much more frequently than females. Descendants of the first white-eyed fruit fly are still giving their cells, chromosomes, and DNA to scientists in hundreds of laboratories throughout the world today.

Mutations are changes in the sequence of bases in the DNA of a gene. Even a single base pair, if copied or repaired wrong just once, can completely change the meaning of a stretch of DNA and preserve that changed meaning in all subsequent generations of that DNA. These changes are often harmful, and our cells have many ways of preventing them. For example, consider the possible consequences of a summer spent enjoying long, lazy days of sunshine at the beach. Your skin responds by darkening to protect the DNA in the dividing cells beneath the skin from the errors an invisible fraction of sunlight called ultraviolet can introduce. Everyone's skin is made of many kinds of cells. The cells whose clumps we shed as dandruff are cross-linked to form the waterproof layer that keeps us from melting in the rain. Beneath these dead cells lies a single layer of living, dividing cells, whose daughter cells push up to replace the dead and dying skin cells as they are shed. The layer of live cells also contains a number of pigmented cells called melanocytes, from the Greek for "black cells."

As each melanocyte fills with tiny sacs of black pigment, it hands these off to brand-new skin cells. The skin cells of populations raised far from equatorial sunlight receive relatively few sacs of black pigment from their melanocytes, so their skin looks beige or pinkish from the blood vessels beneath; the skin cells of populations close to the equator receive many packets of pigment, so their skins range from brown to black. In all people, melanocytes respond to sunlight by dividing and by increasing the number of pigment granules they place in skin cells, further darkening the skin to shield the DNA of the dividing skin cells.

When the melanocyte shield fails, the ultraviolet portion of sunlight can lead to changes in the DNA of a cell that has yet to divide, introducing an error in one or more of its genes. In a sequence that contains two A:T base pairs in a row, the two thymines lie so closely on top of each other that the energy of ultraviolet sunlight can form a bond directly between them, called a thymine dimer. The molecules that carry out DNA replication cannot get past this unexpected compound, so usually replication ends at that point, and a skin cell dies. Sometimes a cell can suffer a self-inflicted wound: it can inadvertently change its DNA sequence as it tries to repair the damage done by ultraviolet light.

Repair enzymes are always on the job, snipping into DNA's backbone and removing mismatched or damaged bases, replacing them with new, proper bases, and then sealing up the loose ends on the damaged strand. If the repair of a thymine dimer is successful, then the skin cell and its descendants will be normal. But if the repair enzymes responsible for fixing a thymine dimer snip it out and reseal the strand without first inserting two good thymines, the "fixed" strand suffers the loss of two Ts, a change as consequential to the DNA's meaning as to the meaning of a sentence in which "tattle" becomes "tale." If the deletion is faithfully copied into a full double-stranded DNA during DNA replication, it will then be propagated in one of the two daughter DNAs and its descendant cells. The change in base sequence would no longer be seen by the repair systems of daughter cells as an error to be fixed, so it would be propagated thereafter as long as the cells in which it resided were viable. In this way, a change in base sequences, or a mutation, can be locked in DNA for many generations.

One rare but dangerous consequence of such a sunlight-induced error is a cluster of rapidly growing variant cells, which we call skin cancer; when the cancer grows from a mutated melanocyte, it is called a melanoma. Often, the cells of tumors — including tumors of the skin — show a rearrangement of chromosomes. Not surprisingly, then, agents we know as causes of cancer, such as the tars in cigarette smoke, are capable of damaging and rearranging our chromosomes. Sunlight, chemicals, and other forms of radiation can also cause complete breaks in DNA. The faulty repair of such breaks can also massively rearrange the sequence of DNA in a genome. Large enough rearrangements can actually change the gross appearance of chromosomes, as pieces of DNA millions of base pairs long break away from one chromosome and attach to another. When such rearrangements, called chromosome translocations, occur in the cells that will merge to begin a developing embryo, they are often fatal; where they are not, they will often result in serious illness from birth on.

Mutations are rare if we measure their rate of appearance relative to the lifetime of an organism. But life is old, and in the course of its existence some new sequences of base pairs have survived for a long time; others have been lost quickly and forever. While some, perhaps most, mismatches of base pairs during DNA replication generate neutral or lethal mutations, beneficial mutation is the underlying cause of life's diversity. If DNA replication were perfect, without error, life would have died out long ago from its failure to adapt to the fluctuations in temperature, atmosphere, and water level the earth has seen over the ages. With slight but continuous mutation, however, the descendants of some organisms have been able to survive myriad environmental perturbations to become the millions of species of flora and fauna we recognize today.

DNA's wasteful but so far successful strategy for surviving environmental stress and competition through less than perfect replication is the fuel that powers Darwinian natural selection. For example, where stereotypical altruistic behavior has been examined carefully, it has been found to enhance the survival of close relatives of the altruistic individual. Kin selection, as it is called, takes place at the cost of one individual's life but raises the probability that some of that individual's unique DNA sequences will survive, passed on by relatives. Since the sequences of DNA in the chromosomes of any organism are the sole vehicle for transmitting viability through time, we must grapple with a depressing, reductionist summary of natural selection: all life is DNA's way of making more DNA. To those of us who choose to make it so, life is more than that; but we cannot call on biological justifications for our choice.

Without exception, members of all living species carry shared DNA sequences, a fact that is consistent with the bracing notion that a single DNA-based life form was the ancestor of all living things — the Big Birth theory, as it were. Just as paleontologists sometimes can accurately date the fossilized remains of an ancient species using geological markers, molecular paleontologists can determine the rates at which DNA sequences for the same gene have diverged over time. They have found that many groups of ancient genes have diverged very slowly, changing about one to ten base pairs per million years. From such rates, called molecular clocks, they can propose how long it has been — usually in millions to hundreds of millions of years — since the last common ancestor between two living species was itself alive. Given the difficulties of getting exact dates and clear identifications for ancient remains and the risks of idiosyncrasy in the choice of genes to analyze, it is remarkable how often molecular and field paleontologists can roughly agree on the age of a long-vanished species.

Darwin assumed that natural selection would generate a slow but smooth appearance of new species, but in some cases the fossil record suggests that species may be stable for very long periods of time, only to be supplanted in short bursts of species proliferation. These often follow hard upon cataclysmic extinctions of many species. Niles Eldredge and Stephen Jay Gould have a name for this staircase variant of Darwin's smooth ramp of speciation: punctuated equilibrium. Certainly the lifetime of some living species can be very long: the fairy shrimp has been around for more than two hundred million years, or about one twentieth of the entire time life has been present on Earth. The oldest fairy shrimp fossils look slightly smaller than living samples but are otherwise indistinguishable from them. Perhaps the stability of their environment over unusually long periods has contributed to the longevity of the species by forcing the loss of what must have been, over all those years, a number of individuals bearing a very large collection of different spontaneous mutations.

∿

Rich in variations on the theme of life as DNA has become, most DNA sequences never existed and never will. In order to appreciate the abundance of untapped possibilities in the DNA of our chromosomes, consider a very short sequence of bases that runs 17 base pairs long. A small calculation reveals that there are 4^{17}, or approximately 17 billion, different sequences of seventeen base pairs. Since there are only about three billion base pairs in any one set of twenty-three human chromosomes, any particular stretch of seventeen base pairs should appear at random no more than once in any human genome. There are about six billion people alive today; each one can be identified by a single unique string of seventeen base pairs, with more than that number of unused sequences left over.

With so many sequences possible, the discovery that our chromosomes carry many long stretches of DNA with almost identical sequences comes as a bit of a surprise. Names help to explain multiple mentions, or families, of DNA sequences. The six billion people on the planet can get by with rather short names. In no more than seventeen letters we can usually get both a first and second name and a middle initial. Since the purpose of names is to distinguish us from one another while retaining information about our family origins, the uniqueness of names is consistent with the improbability of repeating two long stretches by accident. Only rarely do two unrelated people have identical full names, and when the situation arises, we can be pretty sure it is not entirely a random occurrence but the result of one or both of two possibilities: either the two people are related or the name is quite common, or both. Similarly, when human gene sequences are deciphered, some that are a few dozen to a few hundred bases long are present throughout the human genome, in thousands or even hundreds of thousands of copies. Other sequences are found in sets of genes that have a common ancestry or a common function or both. In these cases, we assume that the multiple sequences arose by duplication and reduplication from a single sequence, not by the vanishingly small possibility of coincidence.

Looking at the richness of life on Earth today, it is hard at first to believe that natural selection — which permits the survival of some but not all randomly occurring sequence differences in DNA — is responsible for so many elegant designs. But every mutation may be a new design, and each mutation that survives must make sense in its own context before it can serve as the new baseline for the next mutation. In this way, a series of changes will accumulate over time in remarkable mimicry of intelligent design. We can get the same effect by selecting from a set of slightly variant words, all of which make sense. Consider the following statement, which ought to be clear to every reader at this point: "A base in DNA encodes the data of a gene, storing information in the text of life." We can also get from the word "base" to the word "life," passing through the words "data," "gene," and "text," in a series of single-letter mutations, all of which generate new words that make sense. One of several ways is: *base>* bale> dale> date> *data>* date> Dane> cane> cant> cent> gent> *gene>* gent> tent> *text>* tent> cent> cant> cane> lane> line> *life*. My sentence using the five words is reasonable and logical. In comparison, the sequence of words in the selective sequence makes no sense, although each word has meaning. Both reach the same words in the same order. In the same way — locally smooth while globally random — the natural selection of a meaningful minority of changes in DNA generates spectacularly complex structures, which seem in retrospect — but only in retrospect — to be the result of an intelligent plan.

⁓

Earth spins in a void as cold as any the Universe allows, which presents a time paradox. No matter how hot Earth once was, it should have cooled, skin first, rather rapidly once it formed, like a potato removed from the stove. Darwin was unable to explain how the Earth's surface could have remained temperate for long enough to allow life to evolve. The answer to this puzzle was provided about a century ago from a wholly unexpected source, one full of resonance in our atomic age: the discovery of radioactive elements and of their capacity to release vast amounts of energy from the disintegration of their atomic nuclei. The core of our planet is full of radioactive materials, and the heat they slowly release has warmed its surface over the billions of years since it formed. More recently natural selection, building on the mutation of DNA, broadened the spectrum of living DNA sequences until they arrived at those encoding us.

We — in the briefest instant as measured on this scale of time — have now learned how to transmute both atoms and DNA for our own purposes. While natural selection continues, and will continue while life on Earth remains, it will never again be entirely constrained by random mutation nor entirely protected from self-induced catastrophe. If all other species can be born, live a certain amount of time, have offspring, and one day die, then we must consider the likelihood that this will be the fate of our own species. The big brains that have brought us to consciousness, memory, and the dream of immortality have given each of us a deep sense of individuality, a sense that makes it difficult for us to grasp the notion that our species — not any one of us, nor any one family, race, religion, or nation — is the smallest unit of survival through natural selection and that its survival is anything but assured.

2

~

CHROMOSOMES

AND CANONS

HUMAN GENOMES ARE PLENTIFUL but fleeting. At the conception of every child, a distinctly different human genome is bound and issued for the first and only time. There are as many human genomes as there are persons: six billion drafts of the human DNA text are clustered over every part of the planet not covered by water. Each human genome differs from all the others because — while each is made of the same set of about a hundred thousand genes — a gene need not be restricted to a single version of its precise text. Indeed, many genes denote themselves in different versions, called alleles (pronounced ah-*leels*; from the Greek for "of one another").

To see how different versions of a gene coexist, we can compare the text of the human genome to another ancient (or at least very old) text, the New Testament. First set down in Greek, the New Testament has been translated and retranslated into English for the past five centuries. Each translation, from the Tyndale Bible of 1525 to the 1960 Revised Standard Version, has held great meaning for millions of faithful Christians. But though they are all the New Testament, each version is different. For example, here are the six versions — alleles — of a single sentence from the Book of James, Chapter 4, verse 5:

TYNDALE, 1525 *(the first English Bible):* "Either do ye think that the scripture sayeth in vayne. The sprite that dwelleth in you, lusteth even contrary to envye."

GENEVA, 1562 *(Shakespeare's Bible):* "Do yee think that the scripture saith in vaine, the spirit that dwelleth in us, lusteth after envie?"

DOUAY, 1582 *(the first Catholic translation):* "Or do you thinke that the Scripture saith in vaine: To envie doth the spirit covet which dwelleth in you?"

KING JAMES, 1611: "Do ye think that the Scripture saith in vain, the spirit that dwelleth in us lusteth to envy?"

AMERICAN STANDARD VERSION, 1901: "Or think ye that the scripture speaketh in vain? Doth the spirit which he made to dwell in us long to envying?"

REVISED STANDARD VERSION, 1960: "Or do you suppose it is in vain that the scripture says, 'He yearns jealously over the spirit which he has made to dwell in us?'"

With the help of a good concordance we find that within each allelic version of James 4:5 is a reference to an earlier work: the phrase "the spirit he planted within us" comes from "the breath of life," the divine spark in each human being first mentioned in verse 2, line 7, of Genesis, one of the five books of the Torah at Jerusalem's center. Genes, too, carry earlier sequences from other, earlier genes; deriving the full historical meaning of a gene can begin only when a full concordance of the genome is available.

A comparison of these six biblical sentences shows us that this single line from James has no single, perfect translation. Since the Greek is ambiguous about whether "the spirit" is the subject or object of the verb "to yearn," the sentence was given two quite different meanings by its last two translators. Does this mean that the Bible read by Shakespeare was "incorrect"? Not at all. And what is true for sentences in any important book — but especially for a book that has been important for a long time and has gone through many editions, reprintings, and translations — is also true for genes: meanings will multiply with time, and no single allele is ever going to be the sole "correct" version.

The process of natural selection confirms this point. If two or more alleles work equally well in terms of fecundity and the survival of offspring, no single allele is "normal" or "bad." It is therefore not surprising that any two healthy people are likely to carry different, distinctive alleles for many genes. Blood type, for instance, is largely determined by which of three normal alleles — A, B, or O — a person carries. Until the discovery of blood groups A, B, and O at the turn of the century led to safe blood transfusion, these alleles were a set of distinctions without a difference.

The existence of several alleles for a single gene is the basis of human individuality: a person can inherit two alleles for any gene but can only pass along one of these to a descendant. The inheritance of one or the other allele is a matter of chance at the moment of conception; as a result, no child is the exact genetic copy of either parent. Multiple alleles have been found for almost half the human genes studied so far; just as a vast number of hands can be dealt from only fifty-two cards, the number of possible assortments of alleles is large enough to assure that no two people will ever be born by coincidence with exactly the same genomes.*

Any change in a DNA text that generates a new allele — even a change as simple as the addition, removal, or substitution of a single base pair — is a mutation. Some mutational misprints of DNA's less than perfect copying machine leave a gene's meaning intact, but others can make its message dangerous or even lethal to the organism. Single base-pair mutations in the genes that encode hemoglobin — the oxygen-binding pigment inside red blood cells that gives them their color and us the oxygen we need to convert our food to energy — can have quite dramatic effects. One such typo produces the sickle-cell mutant allele of a hemoglobin gene, which makes abnormal hemoglobin molecules that lock into stacks, distorting the normal bagel shape of a red blood cell into a pointy-

---

* If no more than three hundred of the hundred thousand human genes — instead of the tens of thousands we expect — were found to be multi-allelic, then there would be at least 2^{300}, or 10^{100}, different human genomes possible. Compared to this absurdly large number of possibilities, the fraction of possible genomes that have actually existed is vanishingly small: only 10^{80} atomic particles are said to make up the entire known universe.

ended croissant. The bent blood cells pile up in the tiniest blood vessels, shoving as ineffectually as a crowd of tourists trying to get through a revolving door. A person who inherits two sickle-cell alleles for the hemoglobin gene — and therefore no normal alleles — will have sickled red blood cells and will suffer from crippling bouts of anemia, tiredness, and internal organ damage. But if a person's genome includes one normal allele and one sickle-cell allele for the hemoglobin gene, enough normal hemoglobin will be made to allow for a nearly normal life.*

Whether normal or damaging, alleles are gifts we receive from our parents and give to our children. Both parents inherit twenty-three pairs of chromosomes, but because sperm and egg cells are haploid — meaning they carry only one copy of each gene — each parent can give only one half of each chromosome pair to a child. To a parent, this means that as much genetic information will be cast off as passed on each time a child is conceived. To a grandparent the message is even more severe: because a baby's cells can have only one of each parent's two alleles, the alleles from two of its four grandparents cannot be included in the genome of a child. Worse yet, the choice of which allele is sent on to a child — mother's mother's, mother's father's, father's mother's, or father's father's — is entirely random, and the choice usually differs from gene to gene and child to child.

Parental chromosomes are not delivered unchanged from the bodies of a mother and father into the sperm and egg that fuse to make a child. Instead, as sperm and egg cells are made — the process is called meiosis — pairs of chromosomes carrying the same genes lie next to each other and exchange DNA. Alleles of genes that lie next to each other are then switched

---

* Why has the sickle-cell allele not been lost? While a double dose of the sickle-cell allele usually results in early death, a single allele confers some protection against malaria. The tiny, single-celled animal that causes malaria lives for a time in red blood cells and finds sickle-cell hemoglobin inhospitable. People with one sickle-cell allele therefore suffer fewer and less severe bouts of malaria than those with two alleles for normal hemoglobin. Not surprisingly, carriers of one sickle-cell allele — as well as children born with sickle-cell anemia — are both common in the parts of Africa, the Middle East, and South Asia where malaria is endemic.

about. Once the new sperm or egg cell is created, a gene on one of its chromosomes may be represented by an allele that came from the parent's mother, whereas the next gene may be an allele that originally belonged to the parent's father.

All alleles come from a grandparent; this is the genetic basis for the closeness of a family's resemblance. Traits that involve the expression of great numbers of genes are the clearest indicators of the role of inheritance in the choice of alleles. Facial appearance is the most obvious one: overall, children do resemble their parents and grandparents more than their other relatives. Nevertheless, every baby is an assemblage of choices from the chromosomes of its parents. The process of shuffling the alleles from each parent's two parents — called recombination — assures that every chromosome that goes into egg or sperm will carry an assortment of alleles that never existed in the chromosomes of any of the new child's four grandparents.

At the level of individual genes, a baby is no more related to its parents than it is to anyone else who carries the same pair of alleles for a particular gene. This counterintuitive notion kills all hope that studying the sequences and mechanisms of action of a small number of human genes will allow us to understand the wellsprings of human individuality. While it is becoming possible sooner and sooner after conception to determine which alleles of a gene a fetus has inherited, recombination during meiosis randomizes the allotment of grandparental alleles to each child in a way that cannot be controlled by any technology we can envision. Recombinant DNA — produced at every meiosis — is not so much a human creation as an ancient and necessary step in the development of a unique genome for every person.

For any gene, the particular pair of alleles in a person's genome is called the genotype. When two people differ in form because they carry different genotypes, their genotypes are said to result in different phenotypes. (The word "phenotype" contains the notion of appearances as distinct from their underlying realities; it comes from the same Greek root as "phantom.") Phenotypes like eye color show themselves in the outward appearance of a person; others, like blood type, are hidden beneath the skin. The distinction between inherited alleles and their visible consequences — between genotype and phenotype — raises a deep question about DNA as a text: why do we need the word, and the notion, of a phenotype at all? In principle, if all forms are encoded in DNA, should not every outward phenotype imply a single, distinct genotype? Why not, then, simply speak of genotypes and drop the redundancy of the phenotype, the phantom of appearances?

The answer is simple but surprising: a crucial ambiguity allows different genotypes to generate the same phenotype. This ambiguity arises whenever either one or two copies of an active allele produce the same phenotype: a person with the phenotype of type A blood may be carrying either one A and one O allele or two A alleles. Usually, an allele that has no effect on the phenotype unless it is present in both copies is inactive. For example, while the A and B alleles are responsible for two slightly different chemicals on the surface of a red blood cell, the O allele is silent and inactive, neither adding nor subtracting anything. In its silence it offers no barrier to the function of a second allele of either the A or the B type, so genotypes of AO and BO generate phenotypes indistinguishable from AA and BB, respectively. An active allele producing the same phenotype, whether present on one chromosome or both — like the one for blood type A — is called dominant. The phenotype resulting from the presence of two inactive alleles — type O blood — is called recessive, and the inactive allele itself — like the one for blood type O — is often called a recessive gene.*

Though we cannot tell by looking at a person with a dominant phenotype whether the gene for that phenotype is present on both chromosomes or only one, the distinction may have consequences in future generations. Take eye color. The same pigment cells that give the skin a tint of beige or brown or black also sit at the back of the iris. When the appropriate allele commands them to hand off pigment sacs to the cells of

---

* If a person inherits a matched pair of alleles for a particular gene, he or she is said to be homozygous for that gene (from the Greek for "identical" and "joined together"); a person inheriting a dominant allele from one parent and a recessive allele from the other is said to be heterozygous for the gene (from the Greek for "different" and "joined together").

the iris, we see a brown- or black-eyed person. When an inactive allele cannot give this command, we see a blue- or green-eyed person, because by itself the unpigmented iris, like a swimming pool, reflects the bluish colors of light and absorbs the red. Although more than one gene contributes to the phenotype of eye color, the dominant allele of the major gene puts pigment into the iris, while the recessive allele of this gene does not. Blue-eyed people are therefore certain to have inherited two recessive alleles, while brown-eyed people may have inherited one or two active copies of this gene; they cannot tell which by looking each other in the eye.

Two blue-eyed people can be fairly certain that all their children will share their eye color, since all four possible alleles of the eye pigment gene in all of their sperm and eggs are going to be silent. But two brown-eyed people who hope all their children will inherit their brown eyes cannot predict that this will always happen. If both parents have genomes containing one dominant and one recessive allele of the eye pigment gene, they stand a good chance of having a blue-eyed baby. After meiosis puts the silent, recessive allele for eye color in half of the father's sperm and in half of the mother's eggs, a quarter of their children are likely to have blue eyes.

Something esoteric is going on here: the silence of the recessive allele need not be permanent. Recessive and dominant alleles are just slightly different sequences of DNA, and both are equally stable through any number of generations. A recessive allele may be passed from parent to child again and again, silent but persistent. Then, when two random parental throws of the allelic dice bring one parent's recessive blue-eye allele together with the other's recessive allele, blue eyes surface, as blue as any other, even though the child's genealogy may show nothing but brown-eyed ancestors. If such parents are surprised by the eye color of their baby, it is because they did not know that each of them was carrying a silent allele in addition to the dominant one that gave them their brown eyes.

The persistence of recessive alleles also belies the common notion that our form — the shapes and colors and traits that make us who we are — is inherited by some sort of blending of ancestral fluids. The womb is not a genetic mold into which a child's future constitution is poured; there is no mixing of two inheritable liquids, no "blood," no "blue bloods," no "bloodlines." Children are assembled as a collection of discrete, randomly assorted, stable, dominant and recessive ancestral alleles. The difference in these two notions of form is important. One can imagine an undesirable trait encoded in the genetic fluid of an ancestor eventually being diluted out simply by the passage of generations. But the stability of recessive alleles means that the silent texts in a person will not necessarily be diluted away in the children and grandchildren arising from the marriage of that person to someone of the "right blood." Well bred as some of us may wish to think we are, the genomes of each of us and each of our children remain mosaics containing some large number of inescapable, undilutable recessive alleles. Single copies of recessive alleles, silent in the presence of their dominant alternatives, keep us from being able to judge all genotypic books by their phenotypic covers.

We have had evidence of the difference between genotype and phenotype since 1863, when Gregor Mendel described the hidden inheritance of recessive alleles and elevated genetics from an accumulation of farmers' habits to a quantitative science. Mendel carefully recorded the phenotypes of many generations of experimentally mated pea plants. In all, he followed seven pairs of alleles and found that in each case one allele — smooth peas, say — was dominant and the other — wrinkled peas — recessive. A cross between parents carrying one of each allele always produced a mixture of offspring, with about one in four showing the recessive phenotype. Since genes that are on the same chromosome travel together from generation to generation unless recombination separates them, it is quite remarkable that he obtained such clear statistical data for each pair. Apparently, although he could not have known it — chromosomes had not yet been described when he did his work — the species of pea he used had seven chromosome pairs, and each gene he studied happened to be on a different chromosome pair.

The wrinkled pea allele itself has an interesting story. The strain arose when a foreign piece of DNA inserted itself into

the middle of a gene that makes starch, rendering it inopera-
tive. Starch is one of the foods a pea seed stores for later use
by the growing seedling, and storing starch is a major job for
the pea: many genes encode the molecules that link sugar
molecules into the great chains and webs we see as starch
granules. If both alleles of one of these genes are disabled, a
pea's capacity to make starch is ruined. Starch will hold water
and swell — think of tapioca pudding. Simple sugars, though
sweet, will not hold water as starch does. Failing to convert
sugar into starch, doubly recessive peas show not one but two
phenotypic differences from dominant, smooth peas: they do
not stay plump as they grow in the pod, and they taste much
sweeter than smooth, starchy peas. The sweetness of wrinkled peas no doubt made them desirable to cultivate, which is
probably why Mendel had true-breeding recessive strains of
wrinkled peas for his work.

Mendel was a farmer, priest, and schoolteacher in Brno, a
city then in the Moravian portion of the Austro-Hungarian
Empire and now in the Czech Republic. He must have been a
person of great observational skill, almost unimaginable pa-
tience, and great good fortune. A student at the University of
Vienna for two years, he knew the work of other European
botanists. How pleasantly unexpected that this celibate scientist, and not any of his more worldly peers, had the wit and
perseverance to discover the mechanism that governs inheritance from pea plant to pea plant — and from parent to child.
And how fitting that a priest should have found that this
mechanism is built on a text that can remain silent for any
length of time but then speak out again with full force.

∾

The most dramatic phenotypic difference determined by the
presence of a single allele is sex: boys are male like their
fathers and grandfathers; girls are female like their mothers
and grandmothers. This pattern of inheritance suggests that
the choice between male and female in a developing embryo,
like the choice of wrinkled or smooth in a developing pea seed,
is underwritten by a choice from a single pair of alleles. This
is true, but the gene that determines the sex of a child differs

from other pairs of alleles in one important way: it has its own chromosome. While women have twenty-three pairs of matched chromosomes, including one pair called X and X, men have twenty-two pairs plus one mismatched set, called X and Y.

The normal allele for male sex on the Y chromosome is dominant: in its presence an early embryo grows into a male; embryos that lack it grow into females. The biblical story of Eve's creation from a part of Adam's body is thus backward; all human embryos begin by looking female. The action of the sex-determining gene on a male embryo's Y chromosome transforms an initially female body into one that will belong to a little boy. This gene — called SRY — acts by turning on a cascade of other genes, beginning with the ones that form the testes, in a precisely timed fashion throughout the developing male embryo. The human genome must contain two interleaved texts, one to be read only in male cells and the other only in female cells; both are present in interdigitated form in the DNA of all cells of both men and women. How much of what we assume is a common genome is in fact held in reserve for one sex? It speaks to the subtlety of our genomes that all of us have DNA sequences our bodies will never read — sequences that can be read only by cells in a person of the other sex.

The cells of girls as well as boys use the information on only one X chromosome. Early in the development of a female embryo, one X chromosome in every cell is rendered permanently silent by a chemical coating called methylation. Since the inactive X chromosome is chosen at random in each of its cells, the female embryo grows up to be a mosaic of cell patches expressing different X-associated alleles: a tabby coat, for example, is seen only on female cats. Short regions of many other chromosomes are methylated even earlier, during the formation of sperm and egg. This localized methylation — called imprinting — can make two identical alleles behave differently in the developing human embryo, and the embryo's normal development requires both the maternally and the paternally imprinted versions of each gene.

The inheritance of a Y chromosome is almost always

sufficient for the inheritance of a male body, and exceptions confirm the dominance of the Y gene. Rarely, a human egg is successfully fertilized by a mismade sperm bearing an X chromosome but also — stuck onto another chromosome — the critical piece of DNA from a Y chromosome. A person who develops from such a fertilized egg will be physically male even with two X chromosomes in each of his cells. Conversely, a person born from an egg fertilized by a sperm carrying neither the X nor the Y chromosome will have only a single maternal X chromosome in each cell but will be physically female. Normally, though, the choice between the conception of a girl or a boy is simply a matter of whether an egg is fertilized by a sperm carrying an X or a Y chromosome.

About half of the sperm in a normal man carry his X chromosome and half his Y. If X sperm and Y sperm each fertilized eggs with the same efficiency, half of the children born should be of each sex. In fact, about 5 to 10 percent more boys than girls are born, suggesting that the Y sperm may have a slight competitive advantage or that a male embryo does slightly better in the womb. However, once born, males are at greater risk of dying. By the time people are old enough to have children, the ratio of mothers to fathers has settled back to about even numbers, then keeps dropping with increasing age. As anyone who has visited southern Florida knows, there are many more retired grandmothers than grandfathers. Perhaps this is partly the consequence of culture or of the hormonal balances of men and women, but recessive alleles on any man's X chromosome certainly take their toll as well. While a boy and his sister may both inherit the same recessive allele with their mother's X chromosome, the girl can — but the boy cannot — look to a second X chromosome from their father to provide a functional allele of the gene. Boys will therefore have a higher probability than girls of displaying the consequences of such X-linked alleles as red-green color blindness and hemophilia.

Soon after Mendel's discovery of recessive alleles was absorbed by the scientific community — it took more than thirty years — alleles that were neither recessive nor fully dominant began to turn up. The inheritance of one recessive allele and one of these incompletely dominant alleles produces a third phenotype, different from those generated by two normal or two mutant alleles. For example, a cross of red and white snapdragons produces pink flowers. The white-flowered snapdragons have two copies of a silent allele for a gene that normally produces red pigment, and red-flowered plants have two copies of an active, pigment-producing allele. But as it happens, one active allele for the red pigment is not sufficient to fully saturate the petals with color, so we can see at a glance that pink flowers have one allele that produces the pigment and red flowers have two. The "pink snapdragon" phenotype, with one allele functional but unable to serve for two and the other silent or missing, can sometimes be less than completely healthy. For example, even in the presence of normal hemoglobin encoded by a single functional allele, the sickle-cell allele produces enough abnormal hemoglobin to cause difficulties at high altitudes, where oxygen is in shorter supply.

Even when a functional allele is fully dominant, the inheritance of only one copy instead of two can lead to problems, especially when that remaining copy must function throughout the body in order to maintain an essential aspect of normal form. For example, the family of genes that works together to keep cells in our body from dividing out of turn also keeps tumors from arising in our bodies. One member of this gene family, p53, has been studied with particular care. When mutations — like the ones caused by the ultraviolet component of sunlight — damage both alleles of p53 in the chromosomes of any cell of the body, that cell and its descendants can begin to divide in an uncontrolled way until they grow into a malignant tumor. Biologists know that p53 plays a major role in keeping tumors from sprouting, since both copies of the gene are damaged or lost in a majority of human tumors.

Normally, when a person inherits two functional alleles of the p53 gene, the second allele of p53 provides the body with a valuable redundancy. Mutations in a tissue cell may inactivate one of its p53 alleles, but the cell will not become a tumor because the remaining allele will still produce enough p53 to keep it in check. A person born with only one functional allele of p53 will appear healthy at first, because one p53 allele can hold all the body's cells together. But any time a cell anywhere in the body loses its sole active p53 allele through mutation, a tumor is likely to grow. The phenotype of people with only one functional p53 gene is therefore abnormal in an insidious way: at all times they are highly susceptible to developing a tumor. Some families with this propensity share the Li-Fraumeni syndrome: its victims develop multiple tumors early in childhood. The phenotype of increased susceptibility to cancer reappears in Li-Fraumeni children as frequently as if it were a dominant allele: a man or woman with one damaged p53 allele will inevitably put that allele into half his sperm or half her eggs, so about half of his or her children will inherit a tendency to develop cancer even if their other parent has two functional p53 alleles. P53 is not the only gene linked to the dominant inheritance of cancer susceptibility in this way. Another, RB, is even nastier: when active from conception in only a single allele, it gives children tumors in their eyes before their first birthday.

~

No one wants to inherit a disease, and no one wants to pass on the susceptibility to one to their children. It would be handy to be able to take the sperm or eggs from a person and select only "desirable" sperm to fertilize a "desirable" egg, so that every baby was healthy. But recombination and recessiveness together mean that we cannot prepare a cell to become the sperm or egg we wish. Alleles are tucked away in the chromosomes of sperm and egg cells; like an electron resisting any effort to pin down its position and direction of movement, any allele in an egg or sperm would escape from our grasp as we opened up and killed the cell that carried it. Along with the recombination of alleles and the random assortment of chromosomes during meiosis, this makes it hard to imagine how prospective parents will ever be able to choose an egg and sperm free of any particular pair of recessive alleles that might make for an unhealthy baby.

While the selection of alleles before conception seems unlikely, DNA analysis of blood or biopsy cells can reveal which alleles a person received at conception. The equipment for doing this requires a very small amount of tissue, in some cases no more than a single cell. With this capacity in the hands of a wide range of professional people, from molecular biologists to physicians to lawyers to the FBI and the army, two distinctly different terrains lie ahead. Both involve interpreting DNA from people at risk, and both are likely to be full of legal, ethical, and political potholes. Since it has never been a habit of scientists to sit with an idling engine at a turn in the road, for better or worse both are likely to be well traveled.

Down one road, the tools of DNA analysis are being used to detect and recover defective alleles from the tissues of persons already afflicted with genetic diseases. The goal is to learn how a specific allele differs from normal, then to create drugs that might block or reverse the effects of the abnormal alleles in people — or embryos — who would otherwise be vexed with one or another inherited disease. This calls for some tough choices: every time the DNA sequence of a defective allele for an incurable disease is found, potential carriers may be obliged to learn of their gloomy inheritance before research has given them any way to ameliorate it.

Scans of disease-related alleles, especially when they run ahead of treatments for the disease, often have serious and unintended consequences, damaging the lives of those they were designed to help. In a classic example from the early 1970s, the U.S. government mandated that certain arbitrarily chosen and poorly defined groups of healthy citizens — prisoners, African Americans, Hispanic Americans — would have to be tested for the presence of a sickle-cell allele. Although the stated aim was to help reduce the number of children born with sickle-cell anemia, no counseling or any medical care was tendered. After a few years of considerable outcry, the government ended the mandatory program.

The road to early detection started out a few decades ago as a set of assays of phenotype that could be carried out on children just after birth. For instance, a drop of blood must be taken at birth from every child born in some states — California comes to mind — and tested for the presence of chemicals that signal the inability to properly digest foods containing the common ingredient phenylalanine. This inherited disease, called phenylketonuria or PKU, profoundly retards children who eat foods containing phenylalanine in their first ten years, while the brain is still growing. Magically enough, PKU children can have a normal life if they are spotted immediately and given foods with little or no phenylalanine until they are about ten years old. Spared by proper diet in childhood, many women carrying two PKU alleles have reached childbearing age. Providing they drop their dietary intake of phenylalanine around the period of pregnancy and make sure that their children are tested for PKU at birth, both mothers and children can be protected from the consequences of their mutant alleles.

Tay-Sachs disease is another syndrome that ends in retardation and death, but we have no cure for it. It is the lethal consequence of an unlucky union of two silent alleles for a gene that helps complete the outer surfaces of growing nerve cells. The nervous system of a person who inherits either one or two functional alleles for this gene is normal, but a child born with two defective alleles lives only a few years before fading into profound retardation and death. From a small blood sample it is easy to tell whether a potential parent has one or two normal alleles for this protein: like the pink and red snapdragons, one or two functional alleles have different levels of activity, both compatible with normal nerve cell development. While a carrier with one normal allele married to a person with two normal alleles can be sure that all of his or her children will be free of the disease, two carriers run a one-in-four risk of creating a doomed and tragic little life. For the past thirty years, potential parents from families at risk have been encouraged to take a test before conceiving a child. Couples who find they are both carriers of a defective Tay-Sachs allele may choose to have the cells of a fetus tested as well, and if it lacks the critical enzyme, to have it aborted.

Tay-Sachs disease can occur in anyone, but it appears with a very high frequency among the children of Europeans of Jewish ancestry.* Parental testing and counseling, and prenatal

---

* Like African Americans whose ancestors were made somewhat resistant to endemic malaria by one sickle-cell allele, many American Jews of European descent inherit the Tay-Sachs gene today because it gave some advantage to their ancestors. According to the anthropologist Jared Diamond, one Tay-Sachs allele — but not two — conferred some resistance to tuberculosis, a plague endemic to the ghettos of Europe.

testing and abortion, have together dropped the incidence of children born with Tay-Sachs in the American Jewish community by more than tenfold. In one famous example of sensitive genetic counseling, eligible young members of an Orthodox Jewish community were at great risk of having Tay-Sachs children but were opposed to abortion and in any case would not subject themselves to testing for fear that it would ruin their chances of marriage. Their predicament was solved by their creative rabbi. Himself a carrier of a mutant allele for the Tay-Sachs gene, the rabbi arranged a matchmaking service that would test its subscribers under conditions of total confidentiality, revealing the results only to him. Then, once a match was arranged, he would tell the bride and groom to consult a genetic counselor only if both carried a defective allele. Otherwise, he said nothing. In this way, two people learned about a potentially disastrous situation in private, when it could do no harm and only when it was necessary for them to know. If they then chose not to marry, only the rabbi would know the reason. From 1983 to 1987, more than four thousand young people were secretly tested in this way; six couples discreetly backed out of marriages that would have put them at risk of having a Tay-Sachs child, and not one child with Tay-Sachs was born to the community. This sort of sensitivity to the needs and fears of potential parents will be hard to match as the technology for detection of carriers of various inherited diseases improves, and genetic counseling will become more difficult to accomplish without imposing unexpected choices.

The alleles that cause PKU and Tay-Sachs need not be sought after as DNA sequences in chromosomes, because they signal themselves reliably in the bodies of their carriers. Most diseases, though, are not so flashy. We suspect they are inherited because they run in families, but in the absence of a chemical marker like the missing enzymes of PKU and Tay-Sachs, the complex phenotypes of such diseases do not shed light on the genomic problem. Cystic fibrosis is the most common inherited disease among Americans of European descent. About fifteen million Americans carry one allele for cystic fibrosis; among European Americans, the disease occurs in about one in sixteen hundred births. The symptoms are complex, including difficulty in breathing because of a thick mucus that fills the lungs. Current treatments prolong life and ease the pain, but they do not cure this disease. One ancient diagnostic sign prevails in all victims of cystic fibrosis, even infants: their sweat is excessively salty, suggesting that the disease may be the consequence of damage in some part of the cellular machinery responsible for moving salts in and out of cells.

The DNA difference responsible for the most common cystic fibrosis allele was recently discovered through the direct analysis of the genomes of carriers and victims. A team of Canadian and American physicians and geneticists succeeded in isolating a large, new gene from a chromosome band that had been associated with cystic fibrosis. Once it was recovered from the DNA of a healthy person, the sequence of bases in its DNA was deciphered, and from that, its encoded protein was predicted. Then the sequence of DNA in the same gene from patients with cystic fibrosis was deciphered. The DNA of more than 70 percent of these patients differed from normal in exactly the same way, showing a loss of three base pairs in the same place along the gene. With the normal and mutant alleles of this gene in hand, scientists have been quick to find, name, and study the normal and mutant versions of the protein it encodes. The protein normally sits in the membranes of the cells that line the airways and intestinal tract, regulating the amount of salt — or, more precisely, chloride ions — that can leave the cells. The cystic fibrosis mutant fails to regulate this flow properly, and the symptoms of cystic fibrosis ensue from this defect. This protein, called cystic fibrosis transmembrane conductance regulator or CFTR, had not been known to exist until this work.

Despite these discoveries, the treatment for cystic fibrosis still cannot go beyond the temporary amelioration of symptoms. In the near future we should see a new class of drugs that treat the cause, not the consequence, of this mutation; for example, drugs capable of restoring CFTR activity, if not CFTR itself, in the cells of cystic fibrosis victims. Also, in short order, tests for mutant CFTR activity carried out on cells and fetuses from potential carriers should become straightforward.

Such tests would give the much larger number of Americans who carry the cystic fibrosis mutant allele the same early warning available to carriers of the Tay-Sachs mutant allele.

The CFTR story is an early example of what has been called reverse genetics: the discovery first of the DNA difference associated with an inherited disease; then, by the comparative analysis of normal and mutant DNA, discovering the gene responsible for the disease and elucidating its normal role in healthy people. The allelic error of a disease turns out to be a good hook with which to fish out hitherto unknown human genes, and we can expect to see many more genes isolated, sequenced, and understood through reverse genetics.

~

The second road from the analysis of the human genome to medical practice also presents difficult choices. The road begins with the technique of fertilization *in vitro* (from the Latin for "in glass"), or IVF. Until about twenty years ago, there were only two ways for an infertile couple to raise a child: adoption or — if the man's sperm cells were not viable — insemination with another man's semen. In either case, the child was still conceived and carried in the uterus. Then a burst of implausible but basically straightforward technology enabled physicians to stimulate a woman's ovary to produce egg cells that could be harvested from her body and mixed with a man's sperm in a glass dish. As soon as the first sperm deposited its nucleus inside an egg cell in one of these dishes, *in vitro* fertilization was complete; a new human genome had been launched into the world from the oddest of harbors. To ensure that this embryo had a chance to develop, it was then kept under the microscope for a few hours or days before being placed in the sort of environment every embryo its age takes for granted, a woman's uterus.

IVF is not a molecular technique, but the full panoply of analytical machinery based on DNA can be brought to bear on the naked, glass-enclosed, microscopically observed embryo as it goes through its first divisions. The same scans for aberrant alleles that work on one cell taken from the million billion cells of an adult will also work on one of the eight cells of an embryo whose entire existence began a few hours earlier in a glass dish. Although this point has an obvious logic, it may be harder to comprehend that an embryo can surrender one eighth of its substance without ill effect. But a very young embryo can afford to sacrifice one cell with no effect on its later development. Identical twins, for example, each grow up from one of the first two cells of a fertilized egg without any of the material, genetic or otherwise, in the other cell.

The technology for safely removing one cell from an eight-cell embryo is now well established: after several years of testing and use in animal husbandry, the technique was adapted for human embryos and successfully applied in 1991. If a test of the embryonic DNA finds at least one functional allele for the gene at risk, the remaining cells are watched for a while and then implanted to become a baby. If the DNA test shows that the alleles in the seven remaining cells lack, for example, even one normal allele for the CFTR or Tay-Sachs gene, they are forfeited — not aborted so much as never allowed to get fully under way.

Early detection and IVF are both becoming more common, but neither is becoming any simpler in its consequences. Will IVF technology move beyond its accepted role in countering infertility to become widely used by couples who are, or think they are, at some genetic risk? Each time a new gene is discovered, prenatal genetic testing looms larger as an issue; more choices open up for everyone, but they are not necessarily choices anyone would want. Who has the right to know the result of a prenatal DNA test: the mother, the father, the sperm donor, the egg donor, the bearer of the IVF fetus, the State, or — when they are all different — all of them? Who decides which alleles, and which embryos, escape abortion or qualify for reimplantation after IVF and DNA testing? As the technology for recovering mutant genes by reverse genetics improves, more and more women and men will face one or another Hobson's choice.

Also troubling is the high cost of these new tests and treatments. Many of these choices, difficult though they may be, are simply not available to Americans who lack medical insurance or even a job. In the United States today, more than forty million people are without any form of health insurance. Among them are likely to be perhaps a million carriers of a mutant cystic fibrosis allele. Without an agreement among the president, the Congress, and the nation's physicians to change the way medical care is provided, these citizens will never be able to afford a test for the mutant CFTR allele, let alone be given the guidance and facilities to act on the basis of its result. In the absence of insurance to pay for CFTR testing, IVF, or the eight-cell embryo test, they will become the parents of tens of thousands of carriers and thousands of children with cystic fibrosis each year, few of whom are likely to have access to any future gene-based tests or therapies to reverse their disease's fatal course.

~

These difficult issues seem benign when compared to those raised by a third road from the genetics laboratory to the world beyond, the one that goes through eugenics. Soon after Mendel's work was rediscovered a century ago, politicians as well as physicians saw uses for the knowledge of recessive alleles; inevitably, perhaps, patriots in several countries envisioned the possibilities inherent in a rational plan to improve the genetic quality of a nation. This third road has been little traveled lately, but in the first part of this century, the eugenics movement brought together some of the best geneticists and physicians and the worst chauvinists in the Western world. It was (and for some people still is) easy to endorse their early agenda: civilized people have an obligation to minimize the number of defective alleles in their chromosomes and in those of their descendants, replacing them with good, better, and best alleles.

Some eugenicists, however, were impatient with simple testing and counseling. Would it not be easier to cultivate the best selection of human alleles, they asked, if the wasteful, genetically risky business of having children were put under rational control, and easier still if the results of genetic analysis were fed into a state apparatus that would decide who could be born and who not? Germany was the most hospitable to the eugenics movement in the 1920s and 1930s. As they thought of ways to accomplish the "weeding and seeding" of human alleles, German eugenicists were first assisted, then taken over, by a political movement, a government, and a leader all driven by the crudest and most naive notions of national and racial purity. In that time and place it was only a short walk for many physicians, and for some professors of psychiatry, anthropology, zoology, and genetics, to go from theories of eugenics to the practice of mass murder.

Their downward spiral can be reconstructed from their writings and from the grim record they left behind in other ways. It went from an appreciation of the ability of recessive phenotypes to reappear unexpectedly after generations of silence to the clinical observation that certain mental diseases and physical deformities were inherited in this way; then to acquiescence in the nonsensical notion that some alleles observed national boundaries and religious distinctions; to the endorsement of the even more bizarre notion that within a country, a measurable set of alleles marked the national "type," so that persons whose phenotypes revealed their lack of these alleles could never be brought into the national fold; to the solemn decision that a life without such alleles was simply not worth living; to participation in the sterilization, and then the murder, of millions of people presumed — on the basis of such markers as the shape of their noses or the lilt to their voices — to lack these alleles in their chromosomes. When Adolf Hitler said "Politics is applied biology" in one of his most popular and successful slogans during Germany's fateful 1933 election campaign, he meant it.*

How could this happen? It is easy to see — standing on a mountain of ashes — where the scientists and doctors of Germany went off the deep end. But only twenty years before Hitler came to power, eugenics was a recognized, legitimate branch of genetics, and in Germany, the United States, and

---

* Benno Müller-Hill points out in his book *Murderous Science* that in March 1943 the internationally renowned human geneticist Professor Doctor Eugen Fischer, previously editor of the authoritative 1940 text *Human Heredity and Racial Hygiene*, wrote, "It is a rare and special good fortune for a theoretical science to flourish at a time when the prevailing ideology welcomes it, and its findings can immediately serve the policy of the state." A few months later the infamous Dr. Josef Mengele, then a young scientist at Fischer's Kaiser Wilhelm Institut in Berlin, was appointed the camp doctor in Auschwitz.

many Western countries it drew the attention of reasonable, educated people. Andrew Carnegie, for instance, was a generous and enthusiastic supporter of the international eugenics movement. He founded the Carnegie Station for Experimental Evolution at Cold Spring Harbor, Long Island, at the turn of the century. Charles Davenport, the director of the Cold Spring Harbor laboratory in the 1920s, contributed heavily to Congress's decisions in that decade to restrict immigration to the United States on "national" grounds. His testimony before Congress, and that of others, was full of eugenic contentions couched in the most scientific tone; for example, alcoholism, poverty, and avarice were argued to be "genes" inherited by people born of Irish, Italian, and Jewish parents, respectively.

The first wave of American eugenics was bad genetics, which caused a lot of suffering before it ran its course, but at least it stopped short of overriding our tradition that citizenship for immigrants and their children was a matter of law. The European eugenics movements of that period were not inhibited by such laws; in many countries they were given strength and legal standing by laws that inextricably linked full citizenship to notions of race and "blood." This coincidence of political and eugenic agendas helped eugenics in Germany to go off the tracks, derailed by an explosive combination of two mistakes. The first was the belief that an ideal human type exists. As a piece of science this makes little sense, flying as it does in the face of the first tenet of natural selection, that the survival of a species over the long term will depend above all on the existence of a maximum of variation from individual to individual. However, the notion took hold, and from it came the German eugenicists' notion of *Ballastexistenzen*, or "lives not worth living." In the years between Hitler's rise to power and the beginning of World War II, hundreds of thousands of Germans hospitalized with various genetic and mental ailments, others afflicted with alcoholism and the like, and still others with no particular problem except that they were attracted to people of the same sex were sterilized without their knowledge or acquiescence but with the agreement of their doctors. With the invasion of Poland in 1939, sterilization was succeeded by wartime euthanasia; these Germans died in hospitals and nursing homes by gas and lethal injection before the killing squads were vetted to new jobs in the concentration camps of the East.

The second error arose from the choice of phenotypes that would identify an individual whose appearance approached this ideal. In order for a program of controlled reproduction to be effective, all such ideal phenotypes had to breed true. The only phenotypes that are certain to breed true are those made by pairs of recessive alleles; dominant alleles cannot produce the surprise-free stability of phenotypes needed for a breeding agenda. Not surprisingly, then, German eugenicists planned to breed for the recessive phenotypes of tall height, blue eyes, straight blond hair, small ears, and a small nose. But choosing these as the desirable features of an ideal German also meant identifying the genetic, biological enemy. Each ideal phenotype could be overwhelmed at any time by a single unwanted but dominant allele that might come from a short, dark-eyed, curly-haired, large-eared, long-nosed wanderer. That was enough to ignite the interest of Hitler and anyone else short and dark who had notions of ethnically cleansing Germany of such people in order to build a "master race" of tall, blond, blue-eyed people.

Under Hitler the next step — marshaling the efforts of a nation behind a program of human breeding for recessive phenotypes — needed only one piece of scientifically meaningless, emotionally charged nonsense to throw the whole enterprise into malignant focus. This was the notion that despite all appearances to the contrary, every potential Jewish parent was inevitably the bearer of an undesirable, alien allele that would crush the ones Germany needed, the crazy idea that Jewishness was a single allele of a single gene. However inarticulately stated by Hitler's propagandists, this was the academically certified eugenic argument for the destruction by bullet, gas, and fire of German and then European Jewry, of Germans and others who had one Jewish grandparent, and especially of about a million Jewish children, some of them exactly my age.

∾

Eugenic programs need heading off early. Once established in the bureaucracy of a modern nation-state, any such agenda — especially one buttressed by the technological powers of modern biology — is likely to be able to survive war's defeat, dozens of elections, and decades of rejection by a multitude of governments. For example, almost sixty years after the Nürnberg Laws, the codification of "German-ness" as an inherited trait and the notion that the presence of "German" genes may be predicted from characteristics that are precisely only skin deep still inform contemporary German law. Passport laws automatically confer German citizenship on a class of people outside the national boundaries who are defined more or less as *eindeutschfähig*, "biologically eligible," to be German. All "non-Germans," on the other hand — including German-born, German-speaking people who do not fit this category — have a special set of questions to answer in applying for citizenship. Until 1991, one of these questions was, "What is the shape of your nose?"*

Nor did the egregious application of eugenics in the Third Reich vaccinate us against other pathological applications of biology to human affairs. Consider the common use of skin color as a marker of complicated, partly inherited, partly culturally modulated phenotypes, in particular the vastly complex and uniquely human traits of character and intelligence. This habit lives on even though there can be no impersonal, molecular shortcut to discovering a person's abilities. Indeed, many medical conditions — and most traits we dislike or qualities we admire — are not the products of single alleles, recessive or otherwise. To the extent that they are inherited at all, they are the consequence of the expression of large and unidentified assemblages of genes as well as of a lifetime of unpredictable interactions with other people. Even such a simple marker as an adult's height, for example, is determined in part by a set of about a hundred genes and in part by circumstance, upbringing, nutrition, and the like.

---

* In response to my request in 1992 for details on changes in German law regarding "non-Germans," the Ministry of the Interior in Berlin elaborated as follows: "Information on the shape of the face or nose may no longer be requested. However, unified forms for the new travel documents have not yet been introduced. Last year the federal government and the states agreed therefore, that until the design of the new travel documents had been decided upon, the old forms should be used. This decision was taken for reasons of thrift."

We can expect the genetic component of the human condition to become larger as we learn how to track alleles for numbers of genes at once. Aspects of sexual behavior, in particular, are likely to be mapped to the genome; after all, no part of behavior is likely to contribute more to the survival of a species than the will and the capacity to bear progeny. Dean Hamer of the NIH recently found, for instance, that some men displaying a common variant of sexual behavior in males — early-onset male homosexuality — inherit a specific small region of their mother's X chromosome. The search is on for the allele or alleles in this region of the X chromosome that contribute to male sexual behavior; the best bet is that these alleles will be different in heterosexual and homosexual men.

Every soldier surrenders his or her DNA to the military at recruitment, so that wartime casualties may be unambiguously identified. The policy of the U.S. armed forces toward homosexuals who wish to serve has recently become "Don't ask, don't tell, don't pursue." This policy, which now requires abstinence on the part of enlisted troops, will soon require abstinence of a different sort from the Pentagon: will the armed forces be able to avoid scanning millions of DNA samples for the appropriate sequences once a DNA associated with homosexual behavior becomes available? DNA differences as such cannot legitimately order humans in any hierarchy of present or future value, but it nevertheless seems likely that homosexual Americans will enjoy the same rights of privacy as do heterosexuals only if the president, the courts, and Congress agree in fairly short order that such DNA scans may not be carried out. Otherwise, homosexuals are likely to be the first Americans to become members of a new, DNA-based, genetic underclass.

Another lesson that must be drawn from this century's earlier, disastrous romance with applied eugenics is that we cannot possibly distill from the billions of evanescent drafts of the human genome a single, canonical text. "The human genome" does not exist except as an abstract notion, and while one or even a few alleles may one day be isolated and sequenced for every human gene, even this collection would be different in revealing and interesting ways from the particular human genome in you, or me, or anyone else who has ever lived or ever will live. Perhaps because they have to live with the shame of the Holocaust, postwar scientists and politicians in Germany have to this day shied away from concerted, large-scale work on the human genome, and German practices in genetic counseling are heavily tilted toward individual privacy. But in the United States — and surely eventually in Germany as well — future genetic counseling will inevitably provide the sort of information earlier eugenicists could only imagine.

About four hundred and fifty human diseases have already been linked to specific alleles of human genes, and there is every reason to suspect that mutations in many of the other hundred thousand or so human genes will also be associated with human disease in time. For instance, the special sort of mistake in DNA — extra repeats of a three-base sequence — that generates the Huntington's disease allele in one gene and the mental retardation of the Fragile X syndrome in another is also present in another hundred human genes, all of which wait to be analyzed and linked to their particular syndrome. The temptation to apply basic research on the human genome first to medicine, then to social policy, and then to traditionally private choices is sure to grow with time.

Neither great fame nor a track record of profound scientific insight is proof against this temptation. Consider this report of Sir Francis Crick's 1968 Godlee Lecture, taken from a news article in *Nature*, the same journal that fifteen years earlier had published his and Watson's discovery of DNA's structure and function:

> If new biological advances demand a continuous readjustment of ethical ideas, how are people to be persuaded to adapt to the situation? Clearly by education, and Dr Crick did not think it right that religious instruction should be given to young children. Instead they should be taught the modern scientific view of man's place in the universe, in the world and in society, and the nature of scientific truth. Not only traditional religious views must be re-examined, but also what might be called liberal views about society. It is obvious that not all men are born equal and it is by no means clear that all races are equally gifted. . . . So important is it to

understand the genetics of human endowment that parents should perhaps be permitted, Dr Crick said, to dedicate one of a pair of identical twins to society so that the two twins could be brought up in different environments and compared.

But do "new biological advances demand a continuous readjustment of ethical ideas"? The human genome is a text, but not a sacred one. As the six versions of one line from the Book of James show, even words held sacred by millions of people turn out to have many equally valid versions when examined closely; how much less likely is it that there will ever be a single, canonical human genome whose precise alleles we might hold up as perfect, sacred, or even special? Yet that assumption underlies a significant portion of current biomedical research and development. Each newly isolated and sequenced human gene invites the speculation that we have been brought closer to understanding what the ultimate, supremely "gifted" genome would be. Every time science gives us a new chance to dream this way, we are all obliged — as bearers of different but equally valid versions of the genomic book — to recognize the temptation, and to forswear it. Leaving the boundary between public and personal access to our genomes to the experts — biologists, physicians, lawyers, even Nobel laureates — will not do.

3

SENTENCES, SCULPTURES,

AND THE AMBIGUITIES

OF TRANSLATION

A COMPARISON OF DNA'S LANGUAGE with English helps put the genomic language and its meanings in their proper context. Like any other spoken language, English is a series of overlapping sounds issued in long streams carrying information, more like music than text; descriptions of the muscular movements giving rise to speech lie at the root of the English words "language" and "tongue." While we are born with the capacity to make about two hundred sounds, most languages use a duller spectrum of pops and whistles; spoken English, for instance, uses only about forty. Written English chops the flux of speech into separate sounds and captures them in a set of only twenty-six symbols. Using the sounds and twenty-six letters, we can speak and write all the hundreds of thousands of words in the English language and make up new ones at any time.*

Other languages follow the same pattern: whether spoken or written, they all assemble long strings of a rather small number of sounds or symbols; the various vowels and consonants of English, the consonant-vowel symbols of Korean, and the word symbols of Chinese are examples of how writing quan-

---

* Take the word "scientist," for instance. It did not exist until 1840, when the president of the Geological Society in London coined it to describe "a cultivator of science in general" and Charles Darwin in particular.

tizes spoken speech. Why are languages constructed this way? Why aren't they short agglomerations of ever larger numbers of different sounds or symbols? The rich informational content of a stretch of base pairs in a DNA molecule suggests the answer. The number of possible concatenations of a small number of symbols — or sounds — grows very rapidly with the length of the chain, whether it is a DNA sequence, a word, a sentence, or a song. For example, a speaker of English, using forty sounds, can assemble billions of "words" only six sounds in length.

Of course, almost all of these have never been said and never will be. Words are different from the vast excess of possible arbitrary strings of sounds or symbols in one critical way: each word has at least one meaning to the speaker. The concatenation of words affords great flexibility in the construction of different, unambiguous statements for different, unpredictable purposes. The principle of concatenation is so strong that human languages — and the genomic language — apply it twice. At the primary level, sounds or symbols are strung together to assemble a word, the minimal free form, the shortest natural figure of speech that can be spoken with meaning. Then words are strung together to make sentences; the possibilities for meaning in a sentence are greater than the sum of the meanings of its words. A language can be understood only by defining words by their functions in a sentence and studying the meanings of sentences.

The meanings of words can be classified according to any number of lexicons and dictionaries. Together, meanings define the conceptual system of a human language — the mental lexicon of that language — which resides in the minds of its speakers. Our mental lexicons seem constructed according to a basic rule that frees us from any limitation in how we choose to represent meaning. As the Swiss linguist Ferdinand de Saussure first pointed out in 1916, no sets of sounds or letters are restricted to a particular concept, nor is any concept naturally expressed only by one particular group of sounds or letters. Saussure gave the name "signifier" to the form of a word and "signified" to its concept. In his view, there can be no intrinsic link between the signified and the signifier, between the form of a word and its meaning. Despite the apparent arbitrariness of a language freed of any obligatory link between signifier and signified, languages do have a coherent structure, because both forms and meanings can be defined in terms of their relations with other forms and meanings, fusing signifier and signified in a set of "signs." Once these definitions are in place for a language, the mental lexicon stores them. The similarity of the lexicons in the minds of two people is what allows them to exchange meaningful conversation, and one person to comprehend what another has written.

The books people read and the words they speak may look and sound completely different as we go from one language to the next, but the attributes that define English as a language — letters concatenated into words and words into sentences; a syntax that defines meaningful sentences; a grammar for the parts of the sentence; a lexicon of meanings that carry over from one language to another; a later, archival, written version capturing the earlier spoken one — are shared by the other languages humans speak and write. Complex, complete meaning never resides at the level of sounds and symbols; it only begins at the secondary level of words.

The division between signifier and signified is deep and runs from philosophy to physiology. Fluency with signifiers can be measured by a capacity to spell words correctly; fluency with the signified concept is captured through a facility with analogies. Remarkably, lesions of the brain can affect one skill while leaving the other intact, suggesting that we keep signifier and signified separate even as we think. In philosophical terms, the lack of any direct, logical link between word and concept raises the stark obligation of the speaker and the hearer to confer agreed-upon meanings to the words they use. If audiences — you and I — cannot agree on a common set of signified meanings, our discourse must collapse into mere word play, a chaos from which words themselves cannot preserve us.

The deepest syntactical division in any language separates how words can be used in a sentence, distinguishing nouns from verbs. English syntax shares one universal rule with the syntax of all other spoken languages: every sentence has at least one noun part and one verb part. In English, a further syntactical rule puts the noun part before the verb part: the simplest grammatical English sentences take the form "noun verb," as in the laconic "He died." Beyond this, syntax provides hierarchical rules for the formation of more complex sentences; these rules — together with word endings that convey tense, number, and gender — make English highly complex and flexible. But all English sentences, like those in all other languages, are built from nested sets of one basic unit, a noun part with a verb part.*

Even though a sentence is more than the sum of its words, the concepts the words conventionally express must be part of the sentence's meaning. The semantics of a language define the meanings of its sentences in spite of the ambiguity and multiplicity of meanings carried by many words. For example, when the distinction between two meanings of "see" is intentionally blurred — "I see your point" — the power of the mixed use of the verb lies in its ability to convey the concrete meaning of seeing something with one's eyes along with the abstract notion of agreement. Context removes ambiguity from the meaning of a sentence, as it does for the words in a sentence.

Because words can have more than one meaning — this is called polysemy — sentences of great similarity may have completely different meanings. Polysemy is common in all languages, although more so in some (like Chinese) than others. My favorite example of the potential for confusion created by polysemy is a pair of sentences of the sort designed to stymie computers that try to read English by word comparison rather than meaning and syntax: "Time flies like an arrow" and "Fruit flies like bananas." In the first, "flies" is the verb; in the second it is a portion of the noun part. In the first, "like" is an element of the noun part, comparing the subject of the

---

* In English and other members of the Indo-European family of languages, gender is based on distinctions between the male and female sexes, so that nouns may be masculine, feminine, or neuter. But gender is a linguistic class of noun forms, not necessarily the same as sex. In Bantu, for instance, nouns fall into one of nineteen genders, including thin, human, female, animal, body part, and location.

sentence to another noun; in the second, it is a portion of the verb. The fact that languages permit polysemy is an independent confirmation of the distinction between signifier and signified and of the existence of signified meanings: in order for polysemy to be a problem, we must be storing polysemous words in our heads in more than one "place" according to their different signified meanings.

~

To understand the linguistic properties, syntax, grammar, and semantics of a human genome, we have to look at how a gene speaks to a cell and at the meanings of what it says. When we look inside the nucleus of one of our cells we see — after a moment to adjust for the necessary shift in scale — DNA in letters that connect to form words and words that connect to form sentences. We have already encountered these sentences: they are alleles, the specific versions of a gene. We know from genetics that alleles lie on a chromosome one after another in no particular order; they rarely form paragraphs or longer blocks of meaningful text when transliterated in the order we find them on a chromosome. The genome is not a book, composed to be read from beginning to end, but a lexicon, a collection of arbitrarily ordered sentences, similar to the arbitrary alphabetical order of entries in an encyclopedia.

The written lexicon of DNA that fills the nucleus of every cell in our bodies will remain silent until each cell uses it by excerpting its own set of transcribed and edited quotations called messenger RNAs. Messenger RNAs are signifiers as well, evanescent strings of gene domains. The cell shows its interpretation of their underlying meanings by converting them into proteins, which behave like portable, three-dimensional signified concepts. While every gene is a double helix no matter what its information, different proteins have different shapes, and each shape confers a capacity to carry out the actions described in its encoding gene. This leap from DNA to protein, from line to shape, from signifier to signified, makes a spectacular difference between linguistic and genomic texts: it is as if each sentence in an encyclopedia were folded into a unique origami sculpture that carried its meaning in its shape.

By translating enough texts into proteins with various shapes and consequent functions, a cell draws from its genome the capacity to carry out the multiplicity of interactive chemical changes that allow us to call it a living thing.

Bent, knotted, and folded, a cell's protein sculptures look like the animals in Alexander Calder's wire circus. They are made of thin molecular chains — thinner even than DNA's double helix — whose twenty links are different from one another and as bumpy as the wire that carries Christmas lights around a tree. These links are called amino acids. Like the four bases on a strand of DNA, the twenty amino acids can be hooked together in any order; they can appear at different places on the chain any number of times; and, like the four base pairs, each of the amino acids has a different molecular shape. But nothing prevents each sequence of amino acids from folding into three dimensions. In fact, the sequence of amino acids in a protein completely determines its final shape as it folds up on itself in its own specific way.

The specificity of protein folding is startling: billions of copies of a single protein can be purified from the cell and merged together in perfect alignment as a crystal. Such crystallization would be impossible if two copies of the same protein folded up even slightly differently. Each meaning of a sentence in the written language of DNA is thus manifested in a protein, because the sequence of DNA base pairs determines the sequence of amino acids in a protein, and the sequence of amino acids determines the three-dimensional shape into which the protein will fold.

Just as we can transliterate a sequence of base pairs in DNA from the full complexity of its three-dimensional, molecular shape into a sequence of four letters, we can convert the sequence of amino acids making up a protein into a string of twenty English letters. In this transliteration, A is the amino acid alanine instead of the base adenine, C is cysteine instead of cytosine, D is aspartic acid, and so forth, ending with Y for tyrosine. Though some of the letters are the same for both DNA and protein sequences, the twenty possible amino acids available for each position in a protein's chain mean that an amino acid sequence of any length can have many more possible meanings than a DNA sequence of the same length. For example, in DNA the sequence CGAT — cytosine-guanine-adenine-thymine — is one of 256 possible DNA sequences that can be constructed from four base pairs, whereas the same sequence in a protein — cysteine-glycine-alanine-threonine — is one of 160,000 possible stretches of four amino acids.

As with a DNA sequence, the letters of an encoded amino acid sequence are signifiers; only the three-dimensional shape of a protein carries the meaning of its encoding DNA. The freedom to fold and twist into three-dimensional structures gives a protein its capacity to express the meaning of the DNA that encoded it. Any two proteins can be very different in overall shape, and significant differences can occur with only very small differences in amino acid sequence. Hemoglobin, for example, is an amino acid chain with 141 links; a switch of only one amino acid in the chain distinguishes normal hemoglobin from its sickle-cell variant, yet the two proteins fold into shapes so different that a red blood cell containing the variant is distorted in shape.

What the folding chain of amino acids does so precisely, it does by rules we do not yet understand. Schrödinger's oxymoron about DNA was resolved when we understood how a double helix could be, in fact, an aperiodic crystal. The proteins encoded by the aperiodic crystal are also oxymoronic: their individual shapes are precisely unpredictable. So long as this is true, the genomic language, like our own languages, will not have a logical link between signifier and signified. This will not prevent its being read or understood; rather, it will assure that DNA remains a language expressing as full a range of meanings through arbitrary signifiers as any other language.

∽

The DNA language of the cell, and the way it is made manifest in protein, find parallels in the Greek, cursive Egyptian, and hieroglyphic Egyptian inscriptions found on the Rosetta Stone. Unearthed in 1799, the stone had been inscribed by the priests of Memphis about eight hundred years earlier, when Greek — the dominant language of coastal Egypt — was used even by priests of the ancient Egyptian religion. The stone had three texts in horizontal bands: fourteen lines of hieroglyphic bas-reliefs on the top, thirty-two lines of incised cursive, demotic Egyptian text in the middle, and fifty-four lines of the Greek of the day at the bottom. The Greek stated that the document set forth the same text concerning royal matters in three scripts. Nevertheless, its translation from Greek to the other two scripts was problematic. Hieroglyphs seemed too subtle and mysterious for simple translation. The demotic and Greek scripts were understood to encompass words by a similar use of symbols for sounds, but ever since Pythagoras, each hieroglyphic symbol was thought to be a complete, allegorical message, and the discoverers knew no way to translate between letters and allegorical symbols.

Fifteen years after it had been discovered and taken to Europe, the Rosetta Stone's translation was begun by Thomas Young, an English physician and physicist. Young saw that the hieroglyphs representing royalty were surrounded by a carved protective cord called a cartouche. He correctly guessed that at least within a cartouche, hieroglyphs had the values of sounds after all, in particular the consonant sounds of such royal names as Ptolemy and Cleopatra. Young was only partially successful in decoding these sounds, misattributing about as many sounds as he got right. The young French historian and linguist Jean-François Champollion — master of Latin, Greek, and six Oriental languages by the age of sixteen — broke the Rosetta Stone's code in 1821–22 by showing that hieroglyphic writing was a rebus. Some signs were alphabetic, as Young had inferred, but others were syllabic and still others were indeed symbolic, representing and summarizing a whole idea or object previously expressed alphabetically. In decoding the stone, Champollion also showed that it had been written first in Greek, then translated to hieroglyphics — that is, from alphabet to rebus, not the other way around. Although Greek was the prevailing language when the stone was carved, the full religious meaning of the text could only be found in its hieroglyphic representation, and the priests had taken care to preserve that meaning.

As with the Rosetta Stone, the last translation of a gene is the most complicated. DNA and the stone both carry a linear representation of a text into a sculptural one. In both, information is translated from an alphabetic sentence of many letters (base pairs or the Greek alphabet) to a second alphabetic language of letters (amino acids or the demotic Egyptian alphabet), then to a three-dimensional, sculptured figure (protein or hieroglyph). While we cannot yet unpack the meanings of a gene the way a protein does each time it folds into its native, active form, we have learned how a protein is put together from the information in a gene. This is called translation, but it is an inexact use of the word, since the process does not merely carry the meaning of a sentence from one alphabet to another — although it does do that — but also allows the string of letters in the second, protein alphabet to immediately fold itself up, thereby enacting each sentence's meaning.

If a protein is like a hieroglyph in the sense of being sculpted rather than written, the analogy ends there. A protein *is* the meaning of the DNA word, not just its translation into a pictographic language. Proteins can move about, and they are sent from the genome to a particular audience far from the chromosomes of the cell. Wherever it goes, a protein conveys the meaning of its gene, whether to other proteins, to DNA, or even to other cells, and it speaks in a language to which genes, cells, tissues, and organs all respond. The DNA genome of a cell is in constant conversation with itself through the translation of particular genes into DNA-binding proteins. Through other proteins, every genome is also in dialogue with other regions of its cell beyond the nucleus and with genomes of other cells of the body. The interplay between genes and their proteins in the genome can be as simple as the operation of a thermostat or as complex but orderly as the proceedings of a courtroom. Genes make proteins, proteins make genes; together they make a cell: a chemical dialectic makes us all, because a gene speaks only when it is spoken to.

The cell's language is grammatical, with a simple syntactical structure. Genes — the stretches of DNA that are capable of speaking through the proteins they encode — are divided into words, called domains, which are quite like verbs and nouns. Just as an English sentence must have a noun and a verb, so proteins must have at least two functional parts. Verb domains ("do this") convey the specific action a protein will take, while noun domains ("to that") convey the target of the protein's action. The minimal protein domains for "do this" and "to that" may be given greater specificity — or more subtle meanings — by other protein domains. A gene's domains are laid out in a row in its DNA as contiguous sequences of base pairs. But because a protein is capable of folding into three dimensions, its domains need not be formed out of one continuous run of amino acids. A protein can fold over itself, bringing together the front and back ends of the amino acid chain into a single, crisscrossed basket of meaning. Grammar is preserved despite the non-linear connection of genes to their protein domains. The part of a gene that is translated will yield at least one verb domain and one noun domain within the protein, and the positions of these domains, like the order of words in a Latin sentence, are less important than the precise form of each.

Proteins and their domains work by recognizing the three-dimensional shapes of other molecules. The proteins called enzymes change the molecules that fit into them. The outer surface of an enzyme is indented with pockets of various sizes that fit with remarkable exactitude around another molecule. What happens after the instant of recognition by touch depends on the rest of the enzyme's structure. Some enzymes break a bond between atoms in the molecule they bind to and then let the broken pieces go. These enzymes are the digestive apparatus of a cell, reducing large molecules to small ones. Other enzymes accomplish the reverse, finding two smaller molecules and linking them by abetting the formation of a specific chemical bond between them; the DNA polymerase that creates two molecules of DNA from the separated strands of one DNA is such an enzyme. But not all proteins are enzymes; indeed, the most common protein in our bodies is collagen, which is more commonly known as the primary material of Jell-O. Collagen accumulates in the spaces between cells. One thread of collagen recognizes another in such a way that a multiplicity of threads line up, coil around one another, and weave a thick mat around the cells, holding the entire body together.

Our immunity from infection depends entirely upon the

ability of proteins to recognize one another. All living things, ourselves included, are no more than fertilizer beds for other, smaller organisms. These invisible creatures — viruses, bacteria, protozoa, yeasts, and molds — can quickly and completely break down the cells of our bodies, using us as food just as we use dead plants and animals to feed ourselves. While we are alive, our blood wards off these invaders with a complicated set of cells and secreted proteins, the immune system. Cells in our blood can rapidly and efficiently engulf and kill any invading microorganism, providing we can tag the invader with another set of proteins called immunoglobulins or antibodies. We carry millions of immunoglobulins in our blood; there are very few foreign organisms whose surface molecules cannot be recognized by at least some immunoglobulins.*

Each of the immunoglobulins in our blood has one or more regions, called antigen-binding sites, which can recognize a single patch about twenty by twenty atoms in area on the surface of another molecule. Further, each immunoglobulin is always testing the blood for foreigners from its perch on the outer membrane of a few immune system cells. When a particular cellbound immunoglobulin recognizes an invading molecule, the cell producing that immunoglobulin is stimulated to divide, generating a clone of identical cells that make precisely the right immunoglobulin to bind to the offending molecule. We can feel this happening during a viral infection when we notice we have "swollen glands." These are nodes of immune system cells, growing and secreting antibodies.

In the immune system, as everywhere else in the body, the protein-encoding domains of a gene are silent until they are translated, like the unspoken words of a written sentence. Or think of an orchestra: when it performs — no matter how

---

* How do we manage to make millions of different immunoglobulins with a genome that has no more than about a hundred thousand different genes altogether? Think of the children's book that has a set of drawings of fanciful people and animals, with each page slit horizontally in thirds. By combining the top of one drawing with the middle of a second and the bottom of a third drawing, one can assemble a vast assortment of amusing recombinant portraits, many more than could be printed and bound in one book. Our bodies follow this strategy to distribute millions of reassembled immunoglobulin genes into cells of the immune system so that each new gene is in at least a few immune cells.

atonal the composition — most of the notes from most of the instruments are not played most of the time. If all the notes were played all the time, the result would be not music but noise. So it is with the genome: every cell of the body has the same full set of genes capable of ordering the construction of an entire body, but most of the time, most genes in most cells are silent.

Before a gene can be translated, a set of proteins must act on its regulatory region, a stretch of DNA next to the gene itself. Binding to this silent DNA, a paragraph's worth of regulatory proteins — which are themselves made from information in the DNA of the cell — together determine whether a gene's single sentence will be translated. Some of these proteins are tissue specific, others respond to environmental or hormonal signals: certain plant genes, for example, are sensitive to sunlight. Shaded endive is white rather than green because its pigment genes have been regulated to keep silent in the dark.

The regulatory region of a gene has a second syntactical structure of its own, one that is not limited by the requirements of communication at a distance through translation. While the spoken, translated portion of a gene is syntactically of the form "do this to that," the unspoken regulatory portion is a different sort of command: "Now, here, begin translation." The syntactical rule for the regulatory portion of a gene sentence is that the domain for "here" must follow the domain for "now" and immediately precede the first domain of the translated portion of the gene. Following a rule reminiscent of the way an English sentence must have the noun before the verb, the untranslated command of a gene sentence always precedes the translated portion, so that the complete written DNA sentence we call a gene will have the regular form "Now, here, begin translation: do this to that."

The domain for "here" is typically the same from gene to gene, and because it includes a string of alternating A-T and T-A base pairs, the domain is called the TATA box. But the "now" domain that begins a gene's sentence is notoriously complicated and different for every gene. In fact the "now" domain is often really a group of domains called response elements, and a gene with a large number of response elements that together mean "now" will be translated only in response to a set of regulatory proteins. Some genes that are active only in liver cells, for example, have at least five different "now" domains. While cells of many tissues make one or more of the regulatory proteins needed to activate a liver-specific gene, only liver cells contain all the proteins necessary to signal that translation should occur from these genes.

Some DNA sequences can be recognized only by a complex of two or more regulatory proteins, just as some locks may need two keys to be opened or some checks two signatures to be cashed. One way two regulatory proteins can join and together bind to a response element involves a protein domain called the leucine zipper, a long coil of amino acids with a particularly oily one, leucine, at every seventh place. When the coiled leucine zipper domains of two proteins meet, their leucines interdigitate like the teeth of a zipper, each supplying the other's leucines with a comfortably oily environment. Zipped together, two leucine zipper molecules can gain the ability to bind to a jointly recognized response element. Domains like the leucine zipper allow for combinations of regulatory proteins to address a large number of specific regulatory sequences.

Without a score, an orchestra must be silent or risk disharmony. But even with a completely annotated and fully rehearsed composition, no orchestra plays music unless all of the musicians are prepared to be silent much of the time, responding only when the score calls for their contribution. In the same way, the machinery of the cell is silent until the genome conducts an orderly dialogue between regulatory domains and DNA-binding proteins. That exchange determines which genes get translated at what moment in a given tissue; the resulting cascades of activation — especially of the genes coding for regulatory proteins themselves — can order the formation of a complex tissue. Symphony or embryo, the principle is the same: the more complex the pattern, the more important the silences.

∾

Once regulatory proteins bind to the appropriate region of a gene, it is ready for translation. Like the hands of a pianist playing one complicated chord again and again, the proteins play the "now and here" chord, thus permitting the gene to express itself. As that chord plays, a disposable copy of the information needed to complete the gene's sentence is sent from the gene's base sequence to the cytoplasm, where the machinery of translation sits. Making this disposable copy is called transcription, and the copy is assembled out of RNA, ribonucleic acid, an ancient cousin of DNA. RNA is usually found in the cell as a single strand rather than a double helix, although a strand of RNA with the proper sequence of complementary bases can fold back on itself to form a short hairpin of double helix.* RNA transcripts are copied from a DNA template by an enzyme called RNA polymerase. As it begins to travel along the gene, RNA polymerase twists the DNA so that its two strands are slightly unwound, separating a dozen or so bases on each strand from their paired bases on the other. The enzyme then brings complementary RNA bases to one of the two naked DNA strands and links them to create a new RNA, whose base sequence is complementary to one DNA strand. For instance, whenever the RNA polymerase detects a G on the DNA strand, it grabs a C from the soup of molecules swimming in the vicinity and pairs it to the G. Every T, likewise, gets an A. But when there is an A in the DNA sequence, the paired base is not T but a close analog called uridine (U). So, for example, if the template DNA strand had the sequence GCAT>, its transcript would have the sequence <CGUA rather than <CGTA. The RNA polymerase continues down the gene, stitching together this complementary RNA transcript, until it reaches a short sequence that signals it to stop. At this DNA domain the RNA polymerase lets go of both DNA and the transcript, and the DNA rewinds itself into a double helix.

The notion of a polymerase grabbing on to a DNA strand is more than a metaphor. Two relatives of RNA polymerase — DNA polymerase and the reverse transcriptase (RT) enzyme from the HIV virus — attach to DNA the way a sailor's hand catches a rope: the domains of these proteins both take the

---

* Some RNAs take on sculptural shapes by the interaction of hairpin loops. These folded RNAs can be recognized by specific proteins and assembled into complex RNA-protein structures.

precise form of a person's right hand. The structures of these two polymerases confirm that the order of domain words is not critical to a gene's meaning. The DNA polymerase gene encodes the domains in the order thumb-palm-fingers-palm, whereas the RT gene has its hand in the domain order: finger-palm-finger-palm-thumb. But because similar meanings are expressed by similar forms, these two proteins both fold into tiny, hand-shaped sculptures.

Before translation can begin in the cytoplasm, the RNA transcript of a gene must be edited and bound within the nucleus. The editing is accomplished by a set of RNA-protein complexes called sNRPs (pronounced *snurps*, short for small nuclear ribonucleo-proteins). These sNRPs bind to particular stretches of RNA in a transcript called introns, clip them out, and discard them. Once sNRPs reconnect the free ends of the remaining transcript, the edited strand of RNA no longer carries a base sequence identical to its gene, or to any other gene. Editing thus changes a transcript profoundly, deleting a portion of the text as a newspaper editor would to make a headline fit. And since introns can be spliced out in various ways from a single transcript, editing introns is a source of polysemy in DNA sentences as well, multiplying the final meanings of a gene before translation by unpacking two or more edited versions of a transcript from a single gene's DNA sequence. To protect edited transcripts from getting dog-eared, nuclear proteins add a chemical cap to one end of each and a tail — a stretch of As — to the other. Finally, the clipped, coiffed transcripts — now messenger RNAs — are ready to be sent to the cytoplasm to be translated.

Just as cells containing different mixes of regulatory proteins will open different genes, cells with different mixes of sNRPs may edit a transcript from the same gene differently, thereby making different proteins from the same opened gene. In just this way, for example, the gene for the muscle protein tropomyosin provides a panoply of proteins to different cells of the body. Tropomyosins regulate the speed and strength of muscle contraction. In some tissues, like the light meat of a chicken, the muscle must contract forcefully and quickly. In other tissues — the dark meat — the muscle contracts more slowly. In still other tissues, like the smooth muscle lining arteries, muscle cells are subject to hormonal regulation. Finally, fibroblasts, the cells that secrete collagen, must migrate to fill a wound. These cells too have a form of tropomyosin that is different from all the others.

The tropomyosin gene has a set of thirteen protein domains, each separated by an intron. The ability to make a particular set of splices in the transcripts of genes like tropomyosin allows us to make different kinds of muscle cells in different parts of the body. By alternative splicing in different tissues, any one of at least seven messenger RNAs is made in one or another tissue, generating different versions of tropomyosin, each conveying a slightly different meaning in its own cellular context. Imagine a conversation among various regulatory proteins and sNRPs concerned with muscle development as a chick is developing in its egg. Converting the tropomyosin gene's information into English, where "Now, here," is the gene's regulatory sequence, the gene would be read as "Now, here, begin translation: Make [intron] some [intron] light [intron] dark [intron] gizzard [intron] meat." When regulatory proteins bind to "Now, here," RNA polymerase begins transcription of that sentence. In breast muscle, editing the introns would generate a messenger with the intron-free instruction "Make some light meat," while leg muscle would edit the same transcript into "Make some dark meat." Both tissue-specific readings — and the other variants in gizzards and the like — would conserve the domains for "make," "some," and "meat."

∽

The common meanings of transcription and translation imply a certain rigidity in the former and the possibility of creative variation in the latter. Just the reverse is true for the molecular events we give these labels to. After an immensely complex series of interactions among many proteins, each carrying the meaning of its own gene, a cell decides when and where to transcribe a gene and how to splice the transcript, and different cells make different decisions. But once a cell does make and edit a transcript into a messenger RNA, translation into pro-

tein proceeds at once. A messenger RNA, like a grooved phonograph record, is the portable representation of the base-pair
bumps of its gene, and the translating machinery of the cell,
like a juke box, will play the music of any record the cell
brings to it. It will convert the messenger RNA's linear text,
its sequence of base bumps, into a chain of amino acids. These
will then become the meaning of the gene as they fold up into
a fully articulate, movable, active protein.

To put the messenger RNAs created by transcription and
editing to work, proteins shuttling between nucleus and cytoplasm carry them by cap and tail through doorlike pores out
of the nucleus into the cytoplasm. The cytoplasm lies between
the nucleus and the cell's outer membrane; to return to the
comparison between a cell and old Jerusalem, the cytoplasm is
the part of the Old City outside the Temple but inside the
walls. There messenger RNAs are fed into the machinery that
will convert their sequence of bases into a chain of amino
acids. Like everything else that is big and complicated in a cell,
this machinery is built from prefabricated modules, and the
translation modules are another large, complex collection of
RNAs and proteins, called ribosomes.

The cytoplasm's assembly line of ribosomes takes hold of
the front end of a messenger RNA and uses base pairing once
again, this time to bring amino acids together in the order
directed by the messenger. By themselves, amino acids cannot
enter this assembly line, because they are the wrong shape for
base pairing. To prepare for their concatenation into a protein,
each of the twenty amino acids is first attached to its own
special small RNA, called a transfer RNA. Each transfer RNA
has a run of three bases that can form base pairs with three
complementary bases on the messenger RNA. Accuracy in
translation is assured because only one amino acid can be
connected to a given transfer RNA; moreover, the correspond-
ing set of three complementary bases on the messenger RNA
encodes only that particular amino acid. The assembly line
uses this method of base pairing to align and link a string of
amino acids that matches the sequence of bases of a messenger
RNA.

Transfer RNAs embody the act of translation: each is bilin-
gual and unambiguous. They function a lot like a Chinese

chop block, a handy carved stone about the size and shape of a knife handle that combines the functions of seal, stamp, and signature. Like the name of a person incised in Chinese ideograms on the bottom of the chop block, an amino acid sits at one end of a transfer RNA. The set of RNA bases that form base pairs with the messenger RNA at the other end of a transfer RNA is like a label on the top of the block with the same name in English letters; a person who reads English but not Chinese could string together a row of these blocks to print a list that would be clear to a person who read Chinese.

The cytoplasm of every cell has many copies of each amino acid as well as many copies of sixty-one kinds of transfer RNAs. Though small, each transfer RNA is flexible enough to fold back on itself into three short base-paired stems and three RNA loops; the flattened, two-dimensional path of the bases in a transfer RNA looks like a cartoon drawing of Mickey Mouse's glove or a three-leaf clover. One end of each transfer RNA — the stem of the clover — is a site for the attachment of an amino acid. An enzyme recognizes each transfer RNA and attaches a specific amino acid to its stem. Each kind of transfer RNA has a different sequence of three RNA bases at the outer edge of one of its loops; the base sequence of this triplet predicts with certainty which amino acid will be attached to a given transfer RNA's stem.

The correspondence between the diagnostic triplet in a transfer RNA and the amino acid bound elsewhere permits the ribosomal machinery to translate accurately from base sequence to amino acid sequence. There are sixty-four possible ways to make messenger RNA triplets by connecting three RNA bases in a row, by choosing one of four (A, G, C, or U) for the first base, one of four for the second, and one of four for the third. All but three triplets are complementary to one or another transfer RNA's diagnostic triplet. In the ribosomal machine, each of the coding sixty-one triplets will base pair with a particular transfer RNA by its diagnostic triplet and thereby recognize a particular amino acid. The sixty-one messenger RNA triplets coding for amino acids in this fashion are called codons, and the table of correspondences between codons and amino acids is called the genetic code.

The translation of a gene sentence into protein according to this code — a pretty much universal, four-billion-year-old molecular Esperanto — begins as the transfer RNA–amino acid hybrids and the messenger RNA enter the ribosome assembly line. A ribosome brings two transfer RNAs, with their amino acids in place, into base-pairing contact with two successive triplets of messenger RNA bases. Gripped by the ribosome, the amino acids attached to the two transfer RNAs find themselves so close together that the chemical bond holding the first amino acid to its transfer RNA is broken, at which point it attaches instead to the second amino acid, which remains attached to its transfer RNA. With the transfer of a chemical bond, the first transfer RNA is no longer connected to an amino acid, and it no longer fits in the ribosome. It immediately falls out, displaced by the second transfer RNA, the tail of which now carries not one but two amino acids. The ribosome then ratchets the messenger RNA along by precisely three bases, the way the pawls of an escape mechanism advance a clock's gears.

As the ribosome travels in three-base jumps along the messenger RNA, it holds on to the transfer RNA attached to the growing protein's most recently added amino acid. Each transfer RNA that comes into the ribosomal machinery adds its amino acid to the growing end of the protein and in turn becomes the temporary link holding the growing protein to the machinery. Each time the assembly line adds a new amino acid to the growing chain in this way, it pulls the messenger RNA three bases farther along. These jumps enable the ribosome to base pair the proper transfer RNA — with its attached amino acid — to each successive triplet along the messenger RNA, at each step adding the proper amino acid to a growing protein. The assembly line is a zipper with a difference: the ribosome unzips a succession of transfer RNAs from the messenger RNA, growing a new protein as it goes.

The ribosome cannot know where to end the translation; such punctuations are encoded in the messenger RNA by UGA>, UAA>, or UAG>, the remaining three of the sixty-four possible codons. The three stop codons, as they are called, do not bind any transfer RNA. Instead, each binds a cytoplasmic protein that dislodges the new amino acid chain from its transfer RNA. This disassembles the entire machine, freeing messenger RNA and ribosomes for another round of translation. Stop codons usually restrict protein coding to one strand of a gene's DNA. Even though in principle both strands of a gene might carry coding information, once one strand uses certain triplets to code for amino acids, the base-pairing rules make it likely that stop codons will be present on the other strand. For example, the stop codon UGA> will be present on a strand of DNA each time the other strand uses UCA> to encode the amino acid serine.

With sixty-one transfer RNAs and their complementary messenger RNA codons but only twenty amino acids, all but two of the twenty amino acids are able to find and attach to more than one transfer RNA. Three amino acids (serine, leucine, and arginine) are encoded by six codons; five amino acids (valine, alanine, glycine, proline, and threonine) are encoded by four codons; one (isoleucine) is encoded by three codons; and nine (phenylalanine, tyrosine, cysteine, lysine, histidine, glutamine, glutamic acid, asparagine, and aspartic acid) are encoded by two codons. Only methionine and tryptophan are encoded by unique codons. Francis Crick first pointed out the special nature of a codon's first two bases in assigning amino acid specificity: the alignment of transfer RNA and messenger RNA on the ribosome depends critically on pairing to the first two bases of a messenger RNA's triplet, permitting a certain degree of "wobble" between transfer RNA and messenger RNA at each third base. The redundancy of the genetic code, coupled with wobble, allows more than one transfer RNA to place the right amino acid in the right place along a messenger RNA–ribosome assembly line, speeding up translation.

The polysemy interjected by editing adds to an ambiguity already brought on by redundancy in the genetic code: two or more DNA sequences may in fact encode the same protein by using redundant codons to order the assembly of the same amino acid sequence. This ambiguity is one way: looking at a protein's amino acid sequence, it is not possible to predict the DNA sequence that encoded it. In contrast, every messenger sequence is unambiguous: it leads to only one protein. A one-way ambiguity of this sort is called a degeneracy, and we say that the genetic code is degenerate. This degeneracy enables a stretch of DNA to encode two different proteins on its two strands by allowing each strand to avoid the use of the three complementary codons that would bring a stop to the translation of a messenger made from the other strand.* In certain small genomes whose reading space is cramped, in particular those of some viruses, genes are indeed transcribed from both strands, and small regions of transcriptional overlap may be generated by DNA double entendre. Besides viruses, each of us also carries many copies of an overlapped, bidirectionally coding genome in the cytoplasm of each of our cells, in hundreds of energy-producing machines called mitochondria.

Because all living things use the genetic code, it must have originated very early in the history of life on Earth. Presumably the twenty amino acids were each essential to the development of cells, and the proteins of living things have been made of all twenty ever since. But it is easy to imagine that, originally, life may have been based on a much simpler genetic code. If the earliest forms of life could have existed with only fifteen instead of twenty amino acids, a minimal genetic code may have had fifteen codons for the amino acids and one for a stop. Sixteen codons can be encoded by the sixteen possible doublets of bases (four possibilities for the first base times four for the second), so such a code could have been, not only simpler, but unambiguous and nondegenerate as well; each gene would be only two thirds the length of genes today, a considerable saving of molecular materials over time. But the genetic code, like much else in life, is historical rather than rational, and once twenty amino acids worked, natural selec-

---

* The codon UCA>, for example, codes for serine. DNA encoding it on one strand must insert the complementary stop codon <AGU (or UGA>) in a messenger made from the complementary strand. The degeneracy of the code, however, allows the serine to be coded for by five other codons: UCU>, UCC>, UCG>, AGU>, or AGC>; these choices would put the codons for arginine, glycine, arginine, threonine, or alanine in the complementary messenger RNA rather than the stop codon UGA>. Similarly, UUA> and CUA> both code for leucine but would insert the complementary stop codons UAA> or UAG>; therefore DNAs that use both strands to code for different proteins must use the other four codons for leucine: UUG>, CUU>, CUC>, or CUG>.

tion did not have occasion to discard any of them. The degeneracy of the genetic code tells us that natural selection is profoundly conservative. It does not abandon old mechanisms easily, even in the process of assembling a rational human being who might imagine a more efficient translation system.

~

Mutations provide natural opportunities for interpretation, and we can use them to tease out some of the subtleties of a cell's reading of its DNA. For instance, the fact that codons are three base pairs long means that while any gain or loss of base pairs will be a mutation, the gain or loss of one or two base pairs may have a far greater effect on the gene's encoded protein than the gain or loss of three, six, or any multiple of three base pairs. The translating assembly line can accommodate the addition of an extra amino acid, or the loss of a few, and still turn out a respectable if queer version of a protein. These changes, called missense mutations, may generate a phenotype that is indistinguishable from normal or one that is clearly wrong from the start; there is no way to predict the consequences to a protein of losing a single amino acid. If a missense mutation damages or deletes a protein's "do this" domains, the mutant protein will be inactive. If the "to that" domains are hit, an active but poorly focused protein, worse than none in some cases — such as sickle-cell anemia — will still be made. In the case of cystic fibrosis, missense opens the gates of the cell to a cascade of damaging phenotypes: in 70 percent of persons with cystic fibrosis, the mutation is a deletion of three bases, eliminating a single tryptophan from a critical domain.

Nonsense mutations — which generate silent, recessive phenotypes — jam up the translation machine with unwanted stop codons. To begin translation, the universal assembly line needs to come upon the codon AUG in the messenger RNA. This codon encodes methionine and also the beginning of translation, assuring that all proteins will have methionine as their first amino acid. As Sidney Brenner and Francis Crick — again — first pointed out, the first AUG in a messenger RNA determines how the subsequent sequence will be divided into codons, setting the reading frame of all subsequent codons. If one or two bases are added or subtracted from a messenger RNA, then the translation assembly line will simply roll over the point of deletion or insertion, and continue to put an amino acid in for every three bases. As a result, all the codons from the point of mutation will be out of phase. A deletion of the sixth base in the message that begins AUG GAG CAG CUG AAC, for example, changes the message entirely, to AUG GAC AGC UGA AC. This mutation encodes an abortive, tiny protein that ends when the messenger comes to UGA after only three amino acids. Stop codons that are not in phase with a messenger's first AUG — like the ". . . UG A . . ." of the normal message in this example — have no effect on translation and can therefore accumulate along a gene's sequence, hidden until a nonsense mutation reveals them to the machinery of translation.

Mutations also reveal that the meanings of a gene are not limited to its encoded proteins, complex as those meanings can be. Mutations in noncoding DNA — introns, regulatory regions, and the DNA between genes — may create abnormal forms or amounts of proteins, whose aberrant functions we see as diseases. Thalassemia, a hemoglobin disorder common to people of Mediterranean descent, results from an error in editing the introns of a hemoglobin transcript. In the earlier example involving the tropomyosin gene, a deletion in the regulatory region might produce the truncated, contradictory "No" in place of "Now, here"; a nonsense mutation in the coding region might abort the message at "Ma" so that no meat at all would be made; while a missense mutation might produce the weird "Make some dark mead." A mutation that damaged a splice junction might create the confusing request "Make some light dark meat" or the possibly lethal "Make some dark."

Knocking out the "here" domain of a gene's regulatory region usually just shuts off one gene, but if the regulatory region serves more than one gene in tandem, more than one protein can be eliminated by a single regulatory mutation. For example, our perception of color begins with a network of three sets of cells in the back of the eye. Each set is filled with a different pigment, sensitive either to red, green, or blue light. The genes encoding the red and green pigment genes are on the X chromosome; nonsense mutations in either the red or the green pigment gene generate one of the common color blindnesses, in which a person — usually a man — cannot fully distinguish among colors that differ by the presence or absence of red or green. Such men can still distinguish between blue and red or blue and green, so they see a reduced but still colorful world. In a rare and far more debilitating form of color blindness, a mutation in the regulatory region that simultaneously controls the synthesis of messenger RNA for both the red- and green-sensitive pigments leaves a person facing a blue-gray world, unable to see red, green, or any other color.

A mutation in one of the regulatory proteins that work on the "here" domains of other genes will disrupt the normal discussion among the sets of proteins that determine when and where a gene should be transcribed. This can generate a spectacular case of inadvertent polysemy: the same regulatory protein can have two effects in two parts of the body. For example, if a member of one family of genes encoding DNA-binding, regulatory proteins is mutated or absent, other genes that should be turned off or on are not, and as a result, entire blocks of tissue in the body may be assembled in the wrong place as an embryo develops.

Even completely silent DNA can be the source of new phenotypes. Scattered throughout the genome are short, silent sequences, islands of Cs and Gs that act as spacers between genes. Sequences of -CCG- repeated between thirty and fifty times, for example, are characteristically found between many genes. DNA polymerase must every once in a long while stutter a bit over these runs of CCG, because the lengths of CCG repeats are different from one person to another. These different lengths are inherited from parents as a silent allelic difference that is normally of no consequence. But should DNA polymerase stutter a bit too long, making a sequence of fifty or more CCGs in a row in one place on the X chromosome of an egg or sperm cell, that sequence becomes dangerous. A woman inheriting such a long CCG repeat may be healthy, but as her egg cells are made, the repeat will double and double again, becoming thousands of base pairs long. Her X chromosome cannot carry this pathologically long stretch of repeated DNA without difficulty; its last chromosome band dangles from the string of useless DNA, and genes nearby cannot be properly transcribed. If her child inherits this dangling chromosome, it will be born with the Fragile X syndrome, a common cause of mental retardation.*

These sorts of mutations tell us that our normal health depends on proper conversations among regulatory proteins and noncoding DNA sequences as much as or more than it does on the proteins — like collagen — that get exported by the cell. Noncoding sentences in the DNA language may never get read aloud as protein, but they are nonetheless essential for the maintenance of proper discourse in and among the cells of our bodies.

~

Translation — both the fact of it and the way it is carried out — makes the complete meaning of a DNA sequence impossible to predict and difficult to fully fathom. The redundancy of the genetic code in the protein-to-DNA direction means we can never be in a position to predict the exact DNA sequence of a gene from its protein. In particular, we may not draw the conclusion that two people with identical protein phenotypes carry identical DNA sequences; the redundancy of the code assures that there will be a vast number of alleles encoding the same normal protein. The exactness and nonredundancy of the genetic code in the DNA-to-protein direction may permit us to predict the amino acid sequence encoded in a transliterated stretch of DNA base pairs, but RNA splicing and editing make this, too, a less than certain thing.

The multiple alleles encoding specific proteins, the sculptural individuality of each protein's folding, the redundancies of codon degeneracy, and the ambiguities of splicing together

---

* The discovery of a runaway simple repeat in the fragile X chromosome opened a successful search for such sequences in the chromosomes of families with other inherited diseases. For instance, the gene that is mutated in Huntington's disease carries a pathological repeat, as does the gene for Kennedy's disease, a complex set of symptoms including progressive muscle weakness and, in men, feminized breasts and reduced fertility.

give the human genome its richness and depth as a text. They also assure that the transliteration of DNA sequences only begins the hugely complex job of reading a genome; indeed, looking at any new sequence of base pairs, no matter how long, is like discovering a written text inscribed in letters that form words whose meanings we cannot fully grasp. Even when the entire sequence of a human genome is transliterated into a string of English letters, that long list of As, Gs, Cs, and Ts will be a lexicon of genomic words and sentences, the meanings of which we cannot predict. The panoply of meanings in any DNA text — from a gene to the whole genome — will be clear to us only when we know, not just its complete sequence of base pairs, but also the full three-dimensional meanings of all its proteins.

4

THE MOLECULAR
WORD PROCESSOR

FOR BILLIONS OF YEARS, cells have transliterated a chosen set of genes into messenger RNAs, translated messages into strings of amino acids, and allowed each amino acid chain to manifest a gene's meanings by folding itself into an interactive protein. The meanings of a gene in a cell's DNA are for the most part hidden from us today, because no linear sequence, whether of DNA, RNA, or amino acids, can reveal the meaning of a protein any more than we might grasp from its letters the meaning of a new word in a foreign language. Proteins, like the meanings of words, can take on additional layers of meaning quite distinct from their primary intention: mutations that permit the transcription of a gene in the "wrong" cell or at the wrong time, followed by others that slightly change a protein's three-dimensional structure, can capture a protein for a completely new use. Even when different proteins are similar in shape, each will still take a unique set of specific actions on a unique set of target molecules. The only way to build a vocabulary of protein meanings has been to discover the three-dimensional structure and the final functions of individual proteins, one by one. This has been a slow, and for the most part unrewarding, enterprise, but we have to learn a new language, and there is unlikely to be a shortcut for the painstaking work of building a vocabulary.

When a stretch of DNA — even a very long DNA, even the

entire human genome — is converted into English letters, it has been transliterated, not translated. Though the translation of the human genome is still at best a distant target, transliteration is at hand. The U.S. government has been giving English letters to the base pairs of a human genome since 1988, when Congress and the president — undaunted by the inability of the National Cancer Act of 1971 to meet its goal of winning the war on cancer by directed research — established the Human Genome Project in a new division of the National Institutes of Health. The project began as one of James Watson's many ideas; to no one's surprise, Watson became its first director. The Human Genome Project is expected to cost several billion dollars — whether in addition to or instead of money that would have been spent for other NIH research remains a sore point for many scientists — but if Watson gets his dream, it will complete the transliteration of a human genome by 2003, in time for the fiftieth anniversary of his discovery of DNA's elegant, functional form.

How will the project avoid assigning false canonical status to one allele of each multi-allelic gene? The human genome would more easily be understood as a legacy of the entire species if the sequences assembled by the project were to come from the DNA of a single anonymous person. The project's goal is less ambitious but just as ponderous as the transliteration of any one person's genome: to place a correct letter — G, C, A, or T — in every position of a consensus three-billion-letter string. A consensus transliteration is not in any real sense a transliteration of *the* human genome. That would have to include the base-pair sequences, imprintings, and methylation patterns of a full, diploid set of twenty-two pairs of maternal and paternal chromosomes plus an X and a Y chromosome. Even then, about one base pair in a thousand is different from person to person, in genes and out. Realistically speaking, there are simply too many available versions of the genome — about ten billion, at least — to sequence them all.

The project has been expensive to set up; working toward a targeted cost of less than a dollar per base pair, it has so far recorded a million or so human base pairs at a cost of tens of millions of dollars. When it is complete, the resulting printout of three billion As, Ts, Gs, and Cs will be a triumph of trans-literation and a catalogue of at least one allele for all human genes. The letters of such a catalogue are each about a million times larger than a base pair; this presents immediate problems of storage and access. Like the National Security Agency, the Human Genome Project has turned to powerful computers to store and retrieve its rapidly growing skein of base-pair sequences.

As with any laborious deciphering job, surprises are inevitable: in 1992, three dozen research groups around the world laid out chromosome III of yeast as a string of 315,000 base pairs, less than one tenth the length of a bacterial chromosome and about one ten-thousandth the length of the human genome. When this relatively short genomic excerpt was put through a computer search for stretches that could be translated into protein, all thirty-seven known genes of chromosome III showed up, but so did many other long stretches without stop codons. Some of these are certain to be yeast genes that had never shown themselves by mutation and so were completely unexpected. If larger human chromosomes carry as many surprises, we can expect to find we are carrying, not the current estimate of one hundred thousand genes, but at least four hundred thousand genes, the majority of them unexpected and unknown.

On the way to complete transliteration, the organizers of the project have wisely set some important intermediate tasks. The first is to construct a sequence-based map of the human genome that would locate every known human gene to the left or right of all others in the genome. About a thousand human genes are already known through disease-related phenotypes generated by their mutant alleles. Most of them have been localized to one chromosome and quite a few to one chromosomal band, but our current encyclopedia of genes holds no more than 1 or 2 percent of the genes we all carry; the rest are somewhere in our chromosomes, and we don't know where. To speed the construction of a map that will locate new genes, the project aims to extract short DNA sequences — called sequence-tagged sites — spaced about a hundred thousand base pairs apart, order them in terms of their place in the genome, and link each to the nearest gene. Since each chromosome band has millions of base pairs, scientists seeking the DNA sequence of one of the mapped genes will be able to focus their attention on a stretch of DNA no bigger than a small fraction of a band. At the same time, the tagged sequences will provide an ordered set of landmarks for the localization of genes as yet undiscovered.

Many genes, and certainly all strings of DNA that contain more than one gene, are too large to be purified and studied easily. Instead, scientists store them as a set of DNAs inside bacteria or yeast cells. A collection of DNA fragments that includes all the sequences of a larger DNA is called a library. The term is optimistic; a fragment library is just that, a library of fragments. The DNA-based map will be the concordance that tells us the proper order of fragments in the human genome. The process of lining up contiguous DNA fragments is called walking the genome: each mapped fragment becomes a tool to find the next in line, much the way the aborigines in Bruce Chatwin's *Songlines* remember their way across the great outback of Australia by matching overlapping songs to pieces of terrain. Walking allows very dense, very long maps to be drawn up; the five-million-base-pair *E. coli* genome has been mapped in this way. Walking a library of the human genome allowed scientists to obtain the giant gene for cystic fibrosis and to assemble a map of the human Y chromosome. But even after being fully mapped, large genomes remain tough to transliterate; not even one bacterial genome has yet been transliterated and filed in a central computer bank.

No matter how fine the resolution of genomic maps, they will stay just that — maps of a territory we want to explore, not the territory itself. Furthermore, even the best map of genes will leave most of the human genome in the dark. We can safely bet that no more than 5 percent of the DNA in our chromosomes is transcribed anywhere in our bodies, while the remaining 95 percent is silent. Even if our chromosomes turn out to have four times as many genes as we now think they do, 80 percent of our chromosomes would be silent. Not all of this silent DNA is useless: in addition to the regulatory regions and introns of all our hundreds of thousands of genes, the human genome's silent sequences include the parts of each chromosome given over to proper movement and separation during mitosis and meiosis, as well as about fifty thousand other sequences that DNA polymerase molecules must find to start and stop replication, and the telomeres, a set of repeated short sequences at the ends of each chromosome.*

Despite their occasional capacity to surprise us, the vast stretches of silent sequences in the human genome are boring, and being chosen to transliterate them is no one's idea of a prize assignment. Predictably, most scientists involved in the project hope to work on sequences that speak to the body; especially interesting are those conversing with the brain. A large minority of all the genes we have are active only in our brains. The best way to find them is to treat a preparation of messenger RNAs from the brain with reverse transcriptase to produce a mixture of messenger-size DNAs, each carrying the edited text of one of the tens of thousands of messenger RNAs made only by the brain. Together these complementary DNAs — or cDNAs, as they are usually called — hold all the genomic information a grown brain uses to maintain itself. A few years ago, some members of the project working at the NIH decided to nibble while they sorted through this miscellany of cDNAs: they partially transliterated hundreds of short cDNA sequences made from brain-specific messenger RNAs, leaving the complete transliteration of each gene for some future time. Since each of these short sequences is different and each comes from a brain-specific gene, grazing in this way will eventually tag the full complement of genes expressed in the brain.

Tagging the DNA sequences of brain-specific cDNAs would seem to be a benign goal for the NIH, but it became a source of much controversy. Over Watson's objection, in 1992 the NIH applied for a patent on each of the short sequence tags. Within weeks of the announcement of the government's inten-

---

* The repeated DNA sequences of telomeres each fold into a knot that resists degradation. Telomeres are critical to the long-term integrity of a genome. As we age, our cells have a greater chance of finding themselves unable to divide, because their telomeres get tattered over time. It may even turn out that the loss of telomeres causes our cells to age; if so, drugs that would block telomere degradation might give us a way to slow the arrival of de Gaulle's "shipwreck," the decrepitude of aging bodies.

tions Watson stepped down, refusing to participate in what he saw as a land grab, an illegitimate block to the free exchange of data among scientists in different countries. For Watson — a blunt man of absolute integrity — the project should have been the culminating phase of his life's work, one that began for him forty years earlier with the discovery of the double helix. Instead, because he could not accommodate a political agenda that valued the rights of state ownership above open-ended scientific inquiry, the project lost one of this century's great visionaries.

Two years earlier Watson had written, "The nations of the world must see that the human genome belongs to the world's people, as opposed to its nations." For now, his own nation has failed to get the point. The NIH has stood firm despite initial reservations on the part of the U.S. Patent Office, and scientists engaged in similar genome research in the United Kingdom, Europe, and Japan have pressed it to reconsider. It remains to be seen whether the office will award any patents for incompletely sequenced genes; regardless, it is difficult to understand why even a complete sequence of a normal allele of any human gene should be claimed by any one person, laboratory, government, or nation, for it will always be present and available in the bodies of people all over the world.

In 1993 the Human Genome Project was taken over by Francis Collins, one of the discoverers of the CFTR gene that is mutated in patients with cystic fibrosis. As transliteration and mapping get cheaper and easier each year, it seems clear that the project will continue even without Watson's special blend of political naiveté and scientific vision, although — perhaps inevitably — both its budget and its hopes have been lowered a bit. While it is unlikely that all three billion base pairs of human genomic sequence will be in any one computer by 2003, by then scientists may well have mapped not only the human genome but also the genomes of many of their favorite experimental organisms: maps of the chromosomes of yeast, fruit fly, roundworm, and mouse are filling in rapidly, and maps of the genes of some plants are also under construction. Maps have always been freely available since their information cannot be patented. But because any gene on a map may yield a profitable product, we must hope that in using maps to obtain the expressed genes, scientists involved in the project will refuse to trade their own freedom of expression for a miscellany of patents.

~

Transliterations of human genes will be followed by attempts to understand what they say and do. The tools and techniques used to carry out this work amount collectively to a new machine, what I would call a molecular word processor. The machine — which is really not an artifact but an agglomeration of several technologies devised by microbiologists — is still rather crude; it will be a long time before anyone can transliterate and manipulate the text of the human genome with the ease and convenience of a word processor. But it is a powerful instrument: to use the molecular word processor is to write in the language of DNA, freed from the constraints that natural selection has placed on the possible meanings a cell can put into or draw from its genomic texts. With it, we can insert or read new meanings into existing genes, and construct new contexts in which gene sentences can take on new meanings. We can also create new meanings by rewriting old proteins. To enable us to do this, the machine recombines DNAs that encode the wordlike domains of a gene, writing a new sentence in DNA that yields a novel chain of amino acids. As our tiny vocabulary of protein meanings grows, we will inevitably be drawn to the idea of a molecular literature entirely of our own creation.

Borrowing current computer technology, the molecular word processor now available can be imagined as follows. It has a keyboard of only five letters: the four bases of DNA and the U that RNA takes in lieu of a T. With the letter keys we can synthesize a stretch of DNA or RNA that is dozens or even hundreds of bases long and carries any sequence of our choice. The apparatus that does this imitates DNA polymerase by hooking up a chain of bases, but it does so in the order we choose rather than by complementing the bases on an existing single strand. The result is a wholly synthetic single strand of DNA. To make an RNA, the machine is fed the four RNA subunits along with a desired order of bases. Just as "natural" vitamins are no different from synthetic ones, synthetic RNA or DNA strands have no difficulty being recognized by enzymes. For instance, DNA polymerase will easily convert a single synthetic strand of any DNA sequence into a regular, double-stranded DNA molecule.

The keyboard also has six function keys that carry out the commands to Cut, Paste, Search, Undo, Print, and Copy DNA sequences. Applying the function keys to the human genome and to DNA sequences created with the proper four letter keys, we can find stretches of DNA, remove them from the genome of a cell, splice them to sequences of either nature's making or our own, and transliterate the new genes into English letters as we go. For example, Cut and Paste applied to DNAs from a duck and an orange would give us a novel sequence containing genes from both, one that might be able to make an orange's protein in a duck's cell or vice versa.

The molecular word processor's software is wet: two of its function keys — Cut and Copy — come from microbial enzymes, proteins made by bacteria much like the ones that live in our own bodies, and Undo depends on an enzyme isolated from the kind of virus that causes AIDS. These tools are available to us because bacteria and other invisible life forms use the same genetic code and the same machinery of replication, transcription, and translation that our cells do.

Bacteria are extraordinarily prolific assemblers of genes and proteins: they can divide a few times in an hour. In each short period between divisions, the bacterium has to double everything within itself, including its chromosome. Genes are transcribed and proteins translated at a furious rate; even while the swollen, doubled bacterium pinches itself in two, it is busy making new proteins for the next division. Should life get hard — if the fluid it is in loses necessary nutrients or the temperature departs from a narrow range of comfort — a bacterium will shut down the transcription and translation of most genes, turn on a small set of other genes, and settle down inside a thick wall as a spore in hibernation.

A typical bacterium is a dirigible supported by a framework of proteins and sugars, with a rubbery sac just beneath the shell to regulate the flow of food and waste molecules. Bacteria have little experience of the world except through what is soluble and small enough to reach them in one or another watery environment. Food to them is a set of small molecules, sugars, salts, some vitamins perhaps, and oxygen in some cases to help burn the food. Stripped down to a single circular chromosome a few million base pairs around and an economy that tightly links self-expression to available resources, a bacterium might seem to lead a life of dull perfection. But bacteria are at risk from the same sort of biological extremism that we are: infection by viruses and parasites.

A bacterial virus carries an even smaller piece of DNA or RNA for a genome. As small as a few thousand bases, it encodes little more than the proteins necessary for its own outer coat and the enzymes necessary for its assembly. Inside its coat, its genome is dormant, but if a virus can place its genes inside a bacterium, the perfect if boring life of that bacterium is nearly over. Like a piece of luggage containing a bomb, invading viral genes are innocently handled by the unsuspecting bacterium's DNA-replicating and DNA-transcribing proteins. The result is the rapid proliferation of the virus's genes, messenger RNAs, and proteins, followed by a silent explosion as the bacterium, converted to a bag of viruses, bursts to release them.

The molecular word processor's Cut key is a plowshare beaten from the swords of an invisible war between bacteria and the viruses that infest them. The Cut key depends on a set of bacterial proteins called restriction enzymes, weapons that disarm viral DNA by chopping the genome of an invading virus to bits before it can damage the bacterial cell. Most restriction enzymes find and cut inside palindromes, DNA sequences that read the same on each strand. Acting as DNA scissors, these enzymes are actually pairs of identical proteins, each of which binds to one strand of the palindrome and cuts it.

For example, the common intestinal bacterium *E. coli* is the source of the restriction enzyme EcoRI (pronounced *ee*-koh-are-*one*). When EcoRI cuts inside the palindromic sequence

$$\ldots \text{GAATTC} \ldots >$$
$$< \ldots \text{CTTAAG} \ldots$$

a pair of EcoRI molecules first binds to the same GAATTC> sequence, then each breaks its strand between the G and the first A. This generates a staggered cut in the double-stranded DNA, with each strand carrying the sequence AATT hanging from a double-stranded stretch that ends with a C:G base pair.*

To protect its own DNA from being cut — all short sequences occur frequently in all genomes — every bacterial species that carries a restriction enzyme also carries another enzyme that camouflages the target sites on its own DNA, so that the hand of a restriction enzyme passes over the bacterial genome, remaining free to cut down invading, uncoated DNA. Bacteria that have EcoRI, for instance, cover every occurrence of GAATTC> on their own chromosomes. Restriction enzymes have been purified from hundreds of kinds of bacteria; each cuts DNA at a specific run of four to eight base pairs. Because every restriction enzyme will cut decisively at every occurrence of its target sequence, each enzyme will split a genome into small, precisely edged pieces.

Any two pieces of DNA that have been cut with a particular restriction enzyme have the same trailing, single-stranded palindromic ends, no matter which species they came from. The Paste key uses base pairing to bring together the fragments of DNA created by the same restriction enzyme: the single-stranded loose ends will spontaneously form base pairs, linking the two fragments. Two different fragments of DNA cut by EcoRI, for instance, will connect to each other as the single-stranded AATT> tail of one fragment forms base pairs with the <TTAA tail of the other fragment. Once held together by base pairing, the two pieces of DNA will look normal to the cell, except for a pair of breaks in the backbones of the two strands, displaced from each other by a few base pairs. These can be closed — pasted — by DNA repair enzymes, to create a clean, single piece of DNA. When a new DNA sequence is pasted together this way from the restriction fragments of different organisms' genomes, it is called a recombinant DNA.

---

* That is, the off-center cut
<pre>
      ...G|A A T T C...>
     <...C T T A A|G...
</pre>
generates two identical, single-stranded ends:
<pre>
      ...G>   AATTC...>
     <...CTTAA   <G...
</pre>

Recombinant DNAs become interesting when they are introduced into cells, where their novel combinations of regulatory regions and genes form sentences no cell would ever come across in nature.

Bacteria also harbor parasites, small loops of DNA called plasmids that coexist with bacterial DNA and get copied at each generation by the same enzymes. Plasmids do not kill the bacteria they infect but slow them down, like DNA worms in a bacterial puppy. A plasmid's infection of a bacterium may be dangerous for us, because some plasmids encode proteins that break down our antibiotics. Bacterial plasmids that encode resistance to an antibiotic are natural carriers of recombinant DNA. Once such a plasmid is slipped into a cell, it replicates and confers permanent resistance to the same antibiotic on all that cell's descendants, making its presence easy to track.

Making plasmids into carriers of recombinant DNA is another example of the recycling of microbial swords into molecular plowshares. Ordinarily, plasmids are a molecular burden on a bacterium, but in the topsy-turvy body of a patient treated with antibiotics, the circular genome of a plasmid can be a bacterium's lifesaver. An infected person receiving antibiotic treatment often becomes a culture vessel for the enrichment of bacteria that carry a drug-resistant plasmid: as other bacteria die from the antibiotic, resistant ones may thrive. But, using the Paste key, we can insert a DNA of our choosing into a drug-resistant plasmid, then feed it to a culture of bacteria. Only the bacterial cells that take in the plasmid and express its recombinant genes will be able to survive a dose of the antibiotic, thus turning an infectious bacterium's life preserver into a productive parasite of our own making. Bacteria, yeast, and even human cells — grown in dishes, tubes, and vats — have produced a multitude of novel, biologically active proteins from recombinant genes inserted into drug-resistant plasmids, opening a new era of molecular pharmacology.

The Search key also depends on the tendency of two bare but complementary strands of DNA to connect by their base pairs as a double-stranded DNA helix, a property called molecular hybridization. If the two strands of a DNA molecule are separated from each other by heat or by a strong solution of salts, they will each flop around aimlessly. When the temperature is lowered or the salts diminished, the two complementary strands will zip back up again, to form a regular double helix. This coming together can occur only if the two strands match exactly into G:C and A:T base pairs. A synthetic strand of DNA can be used to search for its complement anywhere in the genome: the letter keys of the molecular word processor allow us to make a short stretch of single-stranded DNA that carries a portion of the sequence of a gene we are after. If we chop up the whole genome with a restriction enzyme, separate the pieces into single strands using heat or salt, mix them with the synthetic DNA, and allow the mix to hybridize into double-stranded DNAs, the synthesized probe will hybridize only to its complementary sequence, forming a stable double-stranded DNA of the gene we are looking for.

The function key Undo is the enzyme reverse transcriptase. With it we can get back a DNA sequence from its messenger RNA so that the other keys will be able to work on it. The Undo key can be used to capture in DNA form — for later recombinant editing with the other keys — the set of messenger RNAs produced by any cell from any active gene. For example, we've already seen how the Undo key, followed by Cut and Paste, was used to produce a library of plasmids carrying cDNAs of the thousands of edited messenger RNA sequences produced by brain cells.

To print means to transliterate a DNA's sequence of base pairs into a string of Gs, Cs, As, and Ts. The Print key uses DNA polymerase to produce a nested set of partial-length copies of a restriction fragment. When these copies are separated and displayed in order of size, they reveal the sequence of bases in the original fragment. The trick to printing — as opposed to merely using the DNA polymerase to copy the fragment — is to give it a solution containing all four DNA bases as well as a calibrated dose of a mock version of one of the four, an unnatural caboose that connects to a growing DNA strand and then prevents further synthesis. Whenever the polymerase needs to insert that base — G, say — the new strand has a chance to get a mock G instead and be forced to end at that point. Four separate runs of DNA polymerase with the four mock bases produce four sets of nested partial sequences, each starting at the same place and ending at one or another occurrence of a particular base. When separated by size, the four sets of smaller fragments reveal by their locations the location of each of the four bases in the original fragment, and hence its sequence.

The machinery for printing DNA is quite accurate. But mistakes happen, and in practice the best sequencing laboratories report error rates in excess of one base in a thousand, which is worrisome, given that even simple genes can often run to thousands of base pairs. If even one base of a coding region is misread or skipped, the transliterated sequence will be as different from the real one as if the real one had suffered a frame shift or missense mutation. The most effective, if expensive, way to avoid such errors is to sequence both strands of a DNA fragment. If no errors have been made, Gs sequenced from one strand will always match up with Cs on the other, and As on one strand will match up with Ts on the other. Any deviation from the sequences predicted by the base-pairing rules signals the great likelihood of an error in one of the complementary transliterations, since such an error is far likelier than a mispaired DNA. And these errors matter: any hypothesis about a gene's function built on an erroneous transliteration — even one with just one skipped or added base pair in a thousand — may be wrong.

The sixth function key allows us to make many copies of any string of DNA letters: the Copy key also uses DNA polymerase but combines it with cycles of hybridization to produce huge numbers of copies of one stretch of DNA. When a cell is dividing and all its descendants are dividing in turn, the total number of cells will double and redouble each time a cycle of division is completed. This is a chain reaction: in only twenty doublings from one cell a million cells are born, and in thirty doublings a billion. The polymerase chain reaction, or PCR, forces the two strands of a fragment of DNA into a similar chain reaction of replication. In the presence of primers — short single-stranded DNAs that hybridize to the ends of the fragments — a single restriction fragment molecule will serve to start the chain reaction, which will create billions of copies in a few hours. The root of a single hair or the tiniest drop of blood has many copies of a person's entire genome and much more to tell — with the right PCR primers — than a fingerprint.

The Copy function of PCR depends on the molecular word processor's Print key to reveal the base sequences at the ends of a restriction fragment and its letter keys to chemically synthesize primers of single-stranded DNA that will base pair to these ends. Once primers have been made and tested on a restriction fragment, they can be applied directly to genomic DNA, where they will amplify whatever sequence sits between them. The case the NIH has made for patenting partial sequences of genes expressed in the brain depended on the latent power of PCR; patented sequences could be made into primers and probes that could be used to recover an entire gene's sequence from a preparation of human genomic DNA at any time.

Our molecular word processor is now complete. Let us say we want to make a vat of bacteria into a factory pumping out insulin, a human protein that people need, and one they are willing to pay for. Using Undo, then Cut and Paste on the messenger RNAs of a tissue means recovering a messenger RNA, turning it back into coding DNA, and inserting the coding DNA into a plasmid. Using Undo, we can make a collection of DNAs from the different messenger RNAs extracted from the insulin-producing cells of the pancreas. Since we know the amino acid sequence of insulin, we can use the genetic code as a guide to type in the right DNA sequence to synthesize a set of PCR primers. By applying the primers to our cDNA, we can use the Copy key of PCR to make many copies of the insulin gene's messenger RNA sequence in DNA format. Using Print we can transliterate this messenger RNA sequence, and using Search, we can then find the entire insulin gene in the human genome, complete with its regulatory regions. We can then use Cut and Paste to obtain the complete insulin gene and insert its coding region into a plasmid, next to regulatory sequences that the bacterium will recognize, being careful not to disrupt the plasmid's gene for antibiotic resistance. After recovering a bacterium that has taken in the plasmid by passing a culture through the antibiotic, we can transcribe the insulin gene from the plasmids that must be in surviving bacteria. Finally, we can provide these bacteria with a favorable culture fluid; as they rapidly reproduce, we have a microbial factory — built on a natural version of the Copy key — that pumps out human insulin. Human insulin made this way — Humulin is its trademarked name — has been on sale for some years.

Should we choose to change the amino acid sequence of the insulin our bacterial factory makes, hoping perhaps for a pseudo-insulin with interesting new properties — stability without refrigeration, perhaps — we need only go back to the plasmid, use our keyboard, make a variant DNA, and cycle it through the same bacterial machinery. We could also try for a more elegant solution to diabetes: delivery of the gene for insulin to cells in a patient's pancreas or liver. Keeping in mind the need for complete gene sentences ("Now, here, do this to that"), we could make a coding sequence for insulin follow its own regulatory sequence, or a regulatory sequence that activates transcription in a liver cell, or some third set of regulatory domains of our choosing. Each variant would be a different sentence, which may have a new meaning in a cell.

The first electronic word processors had keyboards and screens much like those of today's sleek, portable machines, but they had to be wired to boxes of electronic circuitry that filled a large room. Today's molecular word processor is like the lumbering, vacuum tube computers of the 1960s, but in place of wires and racks of diodes, ours have glass tubes that bring a DNA text to various chemical and enzymatic reactions. Cut, Paste, and Undo take place at body temperature in plastic and glass tubes that resemble nothing so much as crack vials. Copy and Search use benchtop instruments that flicker and hum as they work, much like the memory banks of the early computer. The fanciest parts of the molecular word processor are attached to the letter keys, which synthesize short runs of DNA to order, and to the Print key, which reads a DNA sequence from a set of nested fragments; both of these can actually have their own keyboards and video display screens.

Thirty years ago, few computer scientists foresaw cheap portable computers with random-access memories carrying whole books and the programs to write them with; with this history in mind, it is not very daring to predict that the Human Genome Project will bring down the size and cost of the molecular word processor fairly dramatically. Since all the function keys except Search are based on bacterial or viral enzymes, in principle the whole machine could become very small indeed.

≈

Beyond its evolving role in the Human Genome Project, today's molecular word processor is used in two other major developments at the boundary of science and public policy: identifying specific DNA sequences in samples of a person's genome, and creating new sequences to insert into the genomes of various kinds of cells. As an identifier, the word processor has been used to tell whether a person is the perpetrator of a crime, the parent or grandparent of a child, or the bearer of an allele of interest to physicians and insurance companies. As a gene recombiner, the word processor has inserted genes into bacteria to produce proteins for sale, into cells for possible injection into a person, and even into an embryo cell whose descendants can become a whole organism.

The molecular word processor can be used as an identifier because everyone's genome is different: about one base pair in a thousand on average is different between two unrelated people. Since even siblings inherit different sets of alleles from each parent, the DNA sequences of any two people — except, of course, for identical twins, who are the offspring of a single fertilized egg — will be unique. Because of its usefulness as an identifier, various models of the molecular word processor are in constant use in district attorneys' offices, personnel offices, hospitals, and insurance companies around the country; the FBI and the Pentagon sport particularly powerful ones.

Very small differences in sequence from person to person can be amplified by the Cut key. Each restriction enzyme cuts only at a specific, short sequence; even though these targets are as long as eight base pairs, a single base-pair difference anywhere in a site may either generate or remove the site from a stretch of DNA. As a result, single base-pair differences between two genomes will sometimes show up as large differences in the size of genomic DNA fragments produced by a restriction enzyme. Differences from person to person in the size of a particular fragment can be picked up by hybridization with a probe to sequences that surround the restriction enzyme's cutting site — in other words, by using the Cut and then the Search keys. Every combination of restriction enzyme and probe will reveal a new pattern of allelic differences — called restriction fragment length polymorphisms, or RFLPs (pronounced *riff*-lips) — between the DNAs of two people. RFLP analysis can be used to distinguish between the DNA of a rape victim and the DNA of sperm left by her attacker; it can also be used to match a tissue sample with its donor and thus identify — or exonerate — a man suspected of the rape.

RFLP analysis is also used to track down the gene responsible for a dominant inherited disease, and to determine — before symptoms appear — whether a child at risk of inheriting the disease received the damaged allele from the affected parent. When a family of many generations is available and members are willing to donate blood samples, their DNAs can be analyzed with a broad spectrum of RFLP probes that seek out allelic differences throughout the genome. If one set of probes picks out differences that are consistently correlated with the presence or absence of the disease through many generations, these probes are likely to base pair to sequences relatively close to the gene that causes the disease. At the request of a family carrying the alleles of an inherited disease, for instance, a doctor can easily and safely sample the amniotic fluid bathing a first-trimester fetus. From the DNA of cells shed by the fetus into the fluid, a lab can tell whether a child will develop Tay-Sachs disease, cystic fibrosis, or Huntington's disease.

In the late 1980s many young Argentineans, who had been kidnapped when their parents were killed during the "great disappearance" of the 1970s, were reunited with their grandparents by RFLP analysis. At first it seemed impossible that the real families of any of these children could be unambiguously identified, but when living grandparents insisted that they knew of their grandchildren's whereabouts, RFLP analysis with a twist provided an unambiguous test. The twist was to examine the small circular DNAs in the child's mitochondria. Because every woman puts hundreds of her mitochondria into each of her egg cells while a sperm donates only its nucleus to the fertilized egg, all of our mitochondria are inherited from our mothers, who in turn inherited them from their mothers. When the mitochondrial RFLP pattern of a child of "disappeared" parents matched the pattern of a grandmother's mitochondrial DNA, a family could be reunited.

To anyone wishing to know a person by his or her genome, RFLP analysis has two drawbacks: it is slow and expensive. Another method of identification using PCR — the Copy key — allows quick and cheap amplification of the short repeats of simple sequences that litter everyone's genome. These silent, stuttering runs have proved to be useful in rapid identification. With some pathological exceptions, like the growth of a CCG repeat in Fragile X families, differences in variable number tandem repeats (VNTRs) are inherited with the same stability as any other allele, so every length of a simple repeat can be treated as a different allele. Amplifying three or four VNTRs by PCR and separating them by size on a gel is a rapid and reliable way to get a record of bands unlikely to appear by chance a second time in anyone else. The result of the test, looking to the uninitiated like the Universal Product Code on a box of cereal, is the hottest ticket in forensic technology: the DNA fingerprint.

DNA fingerprinting is not absolutely unambiguous, but it comes close: only identical twins will have identical DNA fingerprints, and only people who come from very inbred groups are likely to share more than a few VNTR lengths. VNTR analysis is largely the invention of Alec Jeffreys of the University of Leicester in England, a scientist who instantly became an expert on forensics. Jeffreys is probably best known for identifying a disinterred South American skeleton as the remains of the much-sought-after Dr. Josef Mengele of Auschwitz. Jeffreys used VNTR analysis of DNA from the body's bones and from samples donated by his surviving wife and son. Only a fraction of a percent of the DNA from the remains was human; more than 99 percent was from the microorganisms of the grave. Nevertheless, the son's VNTR alleles could all be accounted for in the DNA of the mother and the DNA of the remains, which assured the identification of the body. It is fitting that traces of the genes of this terrible doctor, who killed so many in the name of genetic experimentation and then hid from responsibility for his actions, have been made to speak his name.

Since tracking a disease-related allele requires the cooperation — and the DNA — of many family members, some people have proposed that hospitals take a DNA sample of everyone at birth. But surrendering your genome, whether to a hospital, an insurance company, or an employer, may well mean surrendering your privacy. Once you provide your genome for analysis, your DNA can be tested for the presence of other alleles, now or in the future. Already the FBI and many large police departments have begun to assemble the molecular fingerprints of convicted criminals from DNA samples taken in prison, and the armed forces take and store a DNA sample from every person they recruit. Today, millions of Americans have their DNA on file in a public or private molecular word processor; with the federal government about to take new responsibility for controlling our country's trillion-dollar health care budget, setting the boundary between the voluntary submission and the compulsory surrender of one's genome is likely to become important in the near future.

Perhaps the most dangerous abuses of DNA identification using the molecular word processor will be those built on the correlation of sets of RFLP or VNTR bands in healthy people with differences in complex behavior, especially if the behavior can be shown to be, not only the result of experience, but also the consequence of any number of particular alleles. The human brain, which uses so much of the genome's information, is not likely to play out any of its sophisticated programs — intelligence, memory, humor, creativity — through a single gene, so it would be wise to look skeptically at any behavioral or intelligence tests designed to provide data for correlation to single DNA markers. But it takes only a little imagination to foresee a time when some organization will try to correlate a

RFLP or VNTR pattern with scores on a battery of tests designed to measure intelligence, or sexual preference, and then use this genetic marker to encourage or deny entrance to its ranks.

Assuring that a DNA sample is discarded after an RFLP or VNTR analysis ought to be the legal obligation of every insurance company, hospital, and prosecutor's office. But so far it is not, and because the probes that might be applied to it in later years cannot be predicted, the availability of DNA samples is likely to lead to many surprises, not all of them pleasant. The latent risk of loss of privacy is growing rapidly; keeping and analyzing people's DNA without specific, agreed-upon legal authority is like reading their mail or tapping their phones without a warrant. In France, by comparison, the right to privacy is so guarded by law that scientists and physicians have been prevented from notifying families at risk of inherited disease unless they ask for the information.

Even a single allele in the wrong hands can set unexpected limits on a person's future. If health and life insurance companies are ever permitted to demand a qualifying medical examination that includes family DNA analysis, they will be able to establish whether a prospective client is free of propensities to develop one or another disease, which then allows for the possibility that they would refuse insurance or raise the premium for a person who has no outward signs of disease. It is a bit ominous that the 1992 Persons with Disabilities Act, which provided so much in the way of equal rights and opportunities to people with manifest disabilities, offered no protection against the denial of access to health or life insurance.

Beyond its capacity to restrict access to insurance or health benefits, a test is a powerful instrument of control. Each test's results can be interpreted only by comparing an individual's outcome to the "normal" result, so whoever defines the limits of "normal" can easily stick permanent labels on young children. In *Dangerous Diagnostics*, Dorothy Nelkin offers a taste of the way economic incentives can distort the testing process. When the government introduced programs for children with learning disabilities in the 1970s and schools began to receive funds in proportion to the number of their affected students, the percentage of children called "learning disabled" by school tests increased threefold from 1976 to 1982.

In the absence of clear legal boundaries, we are at risk of developing a de facto national eugenics policy after all, not because we wish to identify and then eliminate people as undesirable members of "lesser races," but because some alleles will be considered undesirable by organizations in a position to limit their replication. We are now on the verge of developing cheap, comprehensive assays for hundreds of allelic differences, some of which will be associated with diseases and all of which will be inherited. The temptation to use this information irresponsibly will be great. It is ever more clear that our laws have lagged behind our technology; they do not recognize the power of the molecular word processor to force individuals and governments into making new kinds of decisions. Dean Hamer, who discovered DNA sequences that are inherited by a subgroup of homosexual men, saw this risk and said so in a blunt coda to his paper:

> We believe it would be fundamentally unethical to use such information to try to assess or alter a person's current or future sexual orientation, either heterosexual or homosexual, or other normal attributes of human behavior. Rather, scientists, educators, policy makers and the public should work together to ensure that such research is used to benefit all members of society.

~

Neither law nor custom stands in the way of using the molecular word processor to make money. Genes have been converted into cash, as pharmaceutical firms sell drugs and chemicals that can be produced only through recombinant DNA technology. Pharmaceutical hormones, for example, are always in short supply; they are difficult to isolate because of their potency in the body. To make a human hormone by recombining its gene into a plasmid costs less than to isolate it from the tissues of animals or recently dead people, and it is less dangerous. Gene-spliced hormones available to date include human growth hormone for dwarfism, erythropoietin for life-threatening anemia, and human insulin for diabetes. Not all have been profitable. Human growth hormone, called humatrope, cost the Lilly company about $100 million to produce; even with federal subsidies provided by the "Orphan Drug Act," it does not appear that the company will make back its investment before its patent runs out.

Several companies have used cells to produce human tissue plasminogen activator, or TPA, an enzyme that dissolves blood vessel clots on contact. TPA and an analogous enzyme from bacteria called streptokinase can both dissolve a new atherosclerotic clot and end a heart attack before great damage is done to the heart itself if they are injected at the earliest moment after a heart attack begins. But human TPA costs ten times more than streptokinase, and the pharmaceutical firms that spent large sums to develop and test recombinant TPA can legitimately recover their investment only if TPA proves to be considerably more successful at saving and prolonging lives than the less expensive bacterial enzyme, without showing any unexpected long-term side effects. Long-term survival rates will only be known after many more years, but recent large-scale, short-term studies in Europe revealed small improvements in survival when optimal doses of TPA were used instead of optimal doses of streptokinase. Since the annual market for the drug of choice to dissolve clots after a heart attack is likely to be in the billion-dollar range, and since so many millions of Americans already cannot cover the costs of their medical care, ongoing cost-benefit analyses of the optimal medical response to a heart attack are unlikely to generate a clear choice between TPA and streptokinase for many years.

Sometimes a recombinant DNA product can be useful to people and profitable to its manufacturers even if it is neither from a human gene nor intended for use as a drug; for example, recombinant genes that improve one or another property of a food crop have been put into many different plants. Though initial experiments of this sort have not caused big problems, they have given rise to periodic sentiment for molecular censorship to keep "unnatural" genes and gene products out of our food supply. Any actual problems to date have stemmed, not so much from the creation of "unnatural" foods, but from the ways in which this new technology has been made to serve the established order of agribusiness. For example, food plants — and tobacco — have been genetically modified to carry genes conferring resistance to various pesticides. These plants certainly do better than "natural" ones in fields heavily burdened with pesticide, but such a use of the molecular word processor does not speed the day when pesticide use can be reduced without loss of profitability.

In another case, companies producing animal feed and antibiotics for veterinary use have pioneered in the development of a gene-spliced, bacterially grown version of a hormone from cows called bovine somatotrophin, BST for short. Periodic injections of BST make cows eat a great deal and give much more milk. Studies done in the mid-1980s at the direction of the U.S. Food and Drug Administration found that milk from cows treated with BST was safe to drink. But the FDA recently acknowledged that BST causes some unexpected problems: the animals eat an extraordinary amount, their immune systems are stressed, udder infections are more common, and, as a result, their milk and milk products are more likely to be adulterated with residual antibiotics.

The FDA has been responding to these new issues raised by BST in a curiously halfhearted way. For more than a decade, four drug companies and their university subcontractors carried out tests on cows to accumulate information about BST and milk from BST-treated cows for the FDA. In 1986 the FDA allowed these companies and their contractors to recoup the costs of their tests by selling the milk and cheese from BST-treated cows without labeling the material as being from animals treated with an as yet unlicensed drug. It would be useful for all of us — and certainly BST's manufacturers — to know which children drank the BST cows' milk and ate their cheese, but FDA secrecy prevents this. If all goes well, we'll never notice, but if a statistical excess of some odd disease ever hits young adults in places like Wisconsin and Vermont, no one should be totally astonished to discover a connection with the milk sold during proprietarily secret early trials of BST.

The social consequences of BST are more immediate and more certain. Farmers in our country already produce so much milk that they can sell it only at a loss; government subsidies keep many dairy farms from bankruptcy. Estimates of the cost to a dairy farmer for BST range from ten cents to a dollar a shot, and the drug has to be administered every few days. This high cost threatens to put some small dairy farmers out of business, meaning that BST is less likely to raise total milk production than to maintain current production with a drop in the number of small dairy farms. BST is thus anything but a miracle drug for regions like rural New York and Vermont; for the rest of the country, the net effect may be higher milk prices. BST may turn out to be one of those advances that takes us in the wrong direction, a drug that costs everyone money but benefits only its manufacturers.

~

Genes modified in the molecular word processor have also been taken from their test tubes and their plasmids and returned to cellular genomes. I hesitate to call these new sequences genes, though they may be equivalent, because our technology and not nature has written them out in DNA for our own purposes. Although the technology for inserting sequences into a cell's genome is well understood, the eventual consequences of this genetic editing are not. Since we do not know in advance the full meaning of most sequences, we cannot fully predict how the new text will be understood by the cell that has been compelled to take it in.

Inserting recombinant DNA into cells may seem exotic, but it is in fact not very difficult. In 1944 Oswald Avery and his associates at the Rockefeller Institute (now the Rockefeller University) in New York showed that when bacteria took up very pure DNA, the bacterial phenotype changed in a predictable, permanent way. These experiments were the first to demonstrate that DNA — until then a molecule assumed to be as uninteresting as starch, hence given a name based on the deoxyribose sugars of its backbones — carried genetic information. We now know that bacteria and other cells — even human cells — require little convincing to incorporate foreign genes: in various salt solutions they take in all DNA with alacrity, not distinguishing "natural" genes from synthetic stretches or recombinant plasmids.

The name for the insertion of DNA into a cell — transformation — is Avery's, and with slight variations, Avery's chemical solutions perform on cells as well as they do on bacteria. Other techniques also work: if certain crippled viruses are loaded with a new gene, like a Trojan horse they will get it into a cell by infection. One tedious but absolutely certain way to get DNA into a single cell's nucleus — in particular, the nucleus of a fertilized egg cell — is simply to inject it through a very fine glass needle. The nucleus swells as if a mosquito had bitten it, and within hours the cell is expressing the injected gene. More techniques for getting DNA into cells appear every few months; among the more curious is an electric gun that shoots tiny glass beads covered with DNA into a plant cell and the successful injection of purified DNA by hypodermic syringe directly into the muscle of a mouse.

However the DNA gets into a cell, its promiscuous incorporation into the cell's genome assures that from then on a new DNA — whatever its provenance — will be replicated and passed on to all that cell's descendants. Human alleles returned to human cells can themselves be the source of medical treatment, without any bacterial interlocutors. Blood reaches every cell in the body, so it is not surprising that scientists have concentrated on getting the normal, functional alleles of a mutant gene into two kinds of cells from the blood system, white blood cells and the cells that line the insides of blood vessels. In 1989 researchers at the NIH carried out the first approved experiment in humans along these lines. They put a foreign gene that encoded a harmless, easily detected protein into human lymphocytes, then injected the DNA-transformed cells into patients already terminally ill with cancer. The experiment worked, since cells with the marker protein could be found in the patient's bloodstream for many days after the injection.

In 1990 the NIH authorized the same researchers to put new genes in the cells of a young girl sick with an inherited, incurable immunodeficiency syndrome. Due to a mutation, this child's blood cells could not produce the enzyme adenosine deaminase; as a result, the child had little to no ability to make and use antibodies. Her white blood cells were placed in a test tube and infected with a virus whose genome had been recombined with DNA coding for the missing enzyme and its adjacent regulatory sequences. The cultured cells and their descendants made the adenosine deaminase; they were then injected back into the child. She regained a partial immune response quickly, and according to a recent report, after two years "she is able to participate fully in school and social activities." A second child received the same therapy in early 1991 and is also doing well; in 1993 the NIH authorized immediate gene therapy for a small number of newborn victims of the disease. With the discovery of the gene for CFTR, scientists have begun to test DNA sequences that may provide a similar gene therapy for victims of cystic fibrosis. Because human adenovirus naturally infects the bronchial linings, its genome — recombined with a normal CFTR gene — is being tested in cultured cells from the lungs and bronchial tubes. Early reports suggest that this viral carrier can restore CFTR function to such cells, opening the way for clinical tests of gene therapy for cystic fibrosis.

Despite the promise of unique cures for intractable diseases through recombinant DNA therapy, we have to be careful not to step too quickly over the many boundaries we have set on human experimentation. For example, PCR has given us the capacity to diagnose whether an eight-cell embryo has at least one functional allele for the CFTR gene or whether the embryo would grow up to be a child with cystic fibrosis. Currently, embryos that lack a functional CFTR gene are simply not implanted *in utero*. While it may seem a reasonable extension of these studies to try instead to transform such an embryo cell with CFTR DNA and then to implant it with the rest of the embryo, such an attempt would amount to the sort of experiment on a person that most scientists and physicians now choose not to perform.

∾

In mathematics, one plus one equals two. In science and technology, one plus one can sometimes come to seven, or any other number, as synergistic interactions emerge from the combination of new tools and discoveries. We entered a magically fertile period of this sort as soon as the science of the Human Genome Project met the technology of the molecular word processor. The results have been considerably less scary than our worst fears but not at all as glorious as the promises made by those who foresaw an immediate revolution in medicine, agriculture, and the like. The science of recombinant DNA has been remarkably conservative in its infancy. It has made only the smallest emendations and changes so far — when measured against the vast unknown stretches of the genomes that fill the living world — but the pace is accelerating. Wheat that grows in herbicide-laced soil has been followed by more than forty species of DNA-modified food and fiber crops; by late 1992 there were more than six hundred tests of such crops under way in twenty countries.

We can expect new meanings to emerge from a new DNA text when commercially viable products have untoward and unexpected consequences in the marketplace. For example, one of the earliest products of genetically modified bacteria to reach the market was the amino acid tryptophan. Overproduced by genes inserted through recombinant DNA, the amino acid was sold as a treatment for insomnia. One batch turned out to contain an unexpected compound as well, two tryptophans hooked together. This new chemical caused serious brain damage to many people before tryptophan was taken off the shelf and destroyed; it seems that the recombinant bacterium made so much of the amino acid that the poison was produced as a completely novel by-product.

The story of bovine somatotrophin also illustrates the problem of unintended consequences. Because cows on BST get udder infections, they have to be treated with antibiotics. Unless farmers are very careful to withhold milk from the market for a day or so after antibiotic treatment, the drug will get into the milk, and children drinking large amounts of milk — or eating a lot of ice cream — will take in antibiotics. That, in turn, would make the consumers inadvertent breeders of antibiotic-resistant bacteria in their intestines; if they were to contract a bacterial infection, common antibiotics might not be effective. This scenario is all too reminiscent of the problem of hospital infections caused by antibiotic-resistant bacteria, and for the same reason: antibiotic-resistant plasmids won't go away just because we have figured out how to use them for our own purposes.

Transliterated human DNA has given us a set of powerful insights into our bodies even without giving up many of its meanings. Recombining genes and inserting them into bacteria will always depend on a very small number of profitable proteins, compared to the hundreds of thousands of different proteins that combine and interact to create each of us; the path to profitable products is never going to lead us to understand the meanings of the human genome. Identifying people by the sequences in their genomes will no doubt grow as an industry too, delicately balanced — if we are careful to maintain the balance — between individual privacy and communal needs. But the sequences used to identify a person, or even to identify a gene in a person, need not be understood at all in terms of their actions in the body. To read the human genome, though, we have no choice: we will have to make our DNA talk to us in words we can understand, words conveying the meanings our bodies have given to each of our genes. That conversation is taking place inside us every minute, but we have only just begun to understand it.

5

~

TEXTS, CONTEXTS, AND THE

TRANSGENIC STAGE

NATURE HAS BEEN a reclusive author, filling cells with magical effects and hidden intentions. A word processor makes it easy to put sentences together, but a machine cannot give meaning to a set of new words; only the author and the reader together can agree to do that. We will not learn the meaning of a gene by playing with it in our laboratories or computers; we have to put it back in a cell and allow it to show us what it means. This work has begun, as the protein-coding regions of genes assembled by the molecular word processor — in combination with various regulatory regions — have been let loose in one or another kind of cell. The first such gene transformations showed that context is as critical to the meaning of a gene as it is to a word: a gene may mean two completely different things in two different cells or even in the same cell at two different times. To translate the full, four-dimensional meaning of even one gene, we will need to see the pattern of cells in which it is expressed in various parts of the body at various times as well as the consequent interactions of its proteins with other molecules and cells.

When this motion picture of gene expression is played out in full color with a cast of every gene, we call it the life of an organism. Unless we somehow contrive to see that movie in its entirety, we will never accumulate a vocabulary sufficient for a complete reading of the human genome. So far, we have only prepared short, sketchy film clips, focusing on one gene at a time, running them at our own speed over and over until we get each part and subplot down pat, watching single genes play out their meanings in single cells or in whole animals. These short subjects — the lives of a single gene — have already taught us how a gene may kill one cell and force another to live when it should not; how we are built up, front to back and side to side, by a remarkably old set of genes; and how a brain may go bad from the overproduction or absence of a single gene's protein. When we transform cells or organisms with the genes we have first modified in our word processor, we may say that we are transliterating DNA into English letters, writing in the genomic language and, with the help of cells, learning to translate our own scripts a few words at a time.

I spent many years trying to understand a simple DNA sequence, the T-antigen gene of a virus called SV40, a small but subtle infectious agent first identified in the 1950s as a contaminant of cultured monkey kidney cells. Like any other parasite, a virus cannot live except by capturing and subverting a more complex form of life: viruses can make copies of themselves only after first getting into a cell and taking it over. The viruses that plague us take many paths into our bodies. The influenza virus likes the cells that line the nose, the throat, and the pipes that lead from neck to lungs. The polio virus likes the cells that line the intestine, but it will sometimes jump from there to the nerve cells that signal movement from the spinal cord to the limbs. HIV, the virus that causes AIDS, is today the most studied and most feared of human viruses and is among the most finicky. It grows in — and kills — only one of the hundreds of different kinds of cells in the blood. The body's immune system topples from this loss, which is followed quickly by the devastating and eventually lethal consequences of unchecked microbial opportunism.

Some viruses, like HIV, are little shapeless drops of fatty membrane wrapped around a protein coat containing a lethal genome; others, like SV40, are soccer balls of DNA and protein. Viruses like HIV milk their cell slowly, letting it shed millions of viral particles from its surface into the bloodstream. SV40 prefers the blitzkrieg, overthrowing a cell so quickly that in a few days it becomes a bag of viruses. These are not pretty life cycles, but from the viral point of view they are satisfactory examples of form following function, when function is no more than replication. Nothing about any virus is elegant or complex beyond the biochemistry of self-absorption and self-magnification; viruses are the purest product of evolutionary cynicism. Vaccines may lull us into temporary complacency, but we should respect viruses and expect them to be with us for the indefinite future. They, no less than we, have survived to this day; we have no reason to think we will last any longer than they will.

Viruses are the most efficient parasites: they occupy an entirely molecular niche and are free to completely ignore any other part of the body but the molecules they need in the cell they happen to invade. This molecular focus gives viruses their stunning specificity: the meaning of a viral protein can usually be understood only by a limited number of different cells. No amount of SV40 virus, for example, will make a bacterium or any cell of a bird take notice. A few human cells will grudgingly give in to SV40; most will ignore it. In fact, only certain cells of certain monkeys — the kidney cells of African Green monkeys are best — respond with dispatch to SV40's genes.*

To make visible a cell's response to SV40 T-antigen, let us scale up virus and cell, once again making atoms about as big as marbles and turning DNA back into a thick double vine. SV40 wraps and protects its DNA in a knobby spherical shell; enlarged one hundred million times, it would be a decorated balloon about eight feet in diameter, as big across as the thickness of the cell's outer membrane. The rigid viral shell, a mosaic of many copies of a viral protein jigsawed together by the bumps and hollows of their folded shapes, bears an uncanny resemblance to one of Buckminster Fuller's smaller ra-

---

* When two species share a recent common ancestor they are also likely to share susceptibility to more than one virus. It is not surprising, therefore, that African Green monkeys are also among the few higher primates — we are another — to be infected with an immunodeficiency virus; HIV and simian immunodeficiency virus (SIV) are very much alike.

dar domes. Hanging down into it like chandeliers are a few dozen copies of two other viral proteins. These scaffolds pin the virus's circular genome safely in place inside the shell.

Now imagine this virus coming up against a cell in a monkey's kidney. The cell's membrane, eight feet thick and many miles around, encloses a city of cytoplasm, itself surrounding a walled library within, the nucleus. The proteins of the virus's coat stick to the proteins protruding from the cell's membrane, like weather balloons caught in clumps of trees. The cell's response to the presence of an SV40 virus particle is fatally ambivalent. Neither fully welcoming nor sufficiently hostile, the cell draws in the membrane where the virus is stuck to it, bringing the virus into the cytoplasm wrapped in a coat of inside-out membrane. To dispose of this package of litter, the cell begins to chew it up with protein-destroying enzymes. This is just what the virus wants. As its hard shell is shredded, it releases the SV40 genome into the cytoplasm of the cell.

Now seen by the kidney cell not as litter but as a set of genes that has lost its way, the viral genome is carted through the cytoplasm into the cell's nucleus. There, the monkey's chromosomes are a barn-size accumulation of linked bales of carefully folded DNA. The DNA of each chromosome would be anywhere from five hundred to five thousand miles in length; uncoiled and laid end to end, the DNA in the chromosomes of the magnified monkey cell would have a total length of fifty thousand miles. At about five thousand base pairs, the SV40 genome — a zeppelin's necklace — is eventually picked up by molecules of RNA polymerase transcribing their way through the barns of chromosomal DNA. Helped by other DNA-binding proteins that recognize a proper starting point for transcription, RNA polymerase loosens the two strands of viral DNA, then transcribes down the viral DNA until a signaling sequence in the DNA stops it about halfway around the circle. So, in all innocence, the kidney cell opens a gene that will — as soon as its message is properly spliced to be translated by the cell's own cytoplasm into protein — seal its fate.

The viral transcript contains one splice start site and two splice end sites. In the nucleus the cell's sNRPs — artlessly compounding the folly of RNA polymerase — remove one of the two possible introns, turning the transcript into one or another messenger RNA. Carried to the cytoplasm, one messenger RNA is translated into the SV40-coded protein we are interested in, T-antigen. Soon enough, the kidney cell will read this protein as a molecular terrorist's note that says, "Make my proteins, copy my DNA, and when you're done, you're dead." The other messenger RNA encodes a smaller viral protein, unimaginatively called small-t-antigen. Not much is known about small-t-antigen except that it is small, shares a protein domain with T-antigen, and may assist it in some particularly subtle way.

Newly made T-antigen is a DNA-binding protein. The cell, recognizing this, must truck it back into its nucleus. There T-antigen finds its own small circle of a genome among the bales of chromosomal DNA and binds to it at two small response elements — the very regulatory domains that RNA polymerase used to begin T-antigen's own transcription. They are multiple runs of the five-base-pair phrase GAGGC, short passages inside a larger regulatory region of the viral genome called the Origin. By binding inside the Origin, T-antigen starts the process that will reduce the cell from an absentminded host to a zombie.

T-antigen's mere presence at the Origin stops RNA polymerase from beginning any more T-antigen transcripts and shuts down the synthesis of new T-antigen protein. Then, by forcing the cell's blocked, Origin-bound RNA polymerase to flip over, turn around, and transcribe viral DNA along the other half of the SV40 circle, T-antigen generates a new viral transcript. Copies of this RNA are also capable of a variety of different splices, each of which converts a molecule of transcript into a different messenger RNA. Once in the cytoplasm, these different messengers are translated into three new viral proteins. As they are made, they fold up and link to one another to form the hollow shells of new SV40 viruses, empty mine casings waiting only to be charged up with genomes of SV40 DNA.

Back at the SV40 Origin, T-antigen next tricks another set of the cell's own proteins, including its DNA polymerase, into copying the viral genome. From the Origin around to the far side of the genome's circle, DNA polymerase molecules begin to work in both directions until they meet, making two circles from the original SV40 DNA. As soon as T-antigen tricks it into replicating the first SV40 genome, the cell is doomed. In a natural version of PCR, one DNA genome becomes two, two become four, until — in only a few days — the nucleus is packed with millions of circles of SV40 DNA, all spinning off their own copies of RNA to be translated into yet more coat proteins to be assembled into millions of hollow casings. Finally, the new viral genomes start to wrap themselves into tight knots and slip into the waiting coats. The cell is reeling but still alive; T-antigen has one more meaning, and that will finish it off.

Cells are usually at rest in the monkey's kidney; division is a rare event for them. They impose this rest on themselves by making regulatory proteins — p53 is one we have already met, RB is another — to block the transcription of genes needed for cell division. Animals and people depend on these proteins and others like them to keep cancers from springing up; not surprisingly, many cancers contain mutations in one or both proteins. As it happens, T-antigen opens both RB and p53 locks, avidly binding to both of them and distracting them from their cellular tasks. As soon as p53 and RB are taken from their posts by T-antigen, the kidney cell, though eaten from within by the SV40 virus, nevertheless must begin to divide.

This last selfish grab by T-antigen is remarkable for its specificity: p53 was first discovered as a protein tenaciously stuck to T-antigen. Forcing the dying cell to attempt division pumps up its level of DNA polymerase; more DNA polymerase means more viral DNA replication and more viruses, and that speeds the moment of the cell's death. The burden is overwhelming. The kidney cell, deranged by the ever-increasing demand on its resources, breaks open and dies. The library that is the nucleus has been forced to make and deliver millions of DNA circles into the giant balloons that fill the few square miles of cell surrounding it; library and city both are dying of the unending outpouring of new SV40 viruses even as the cell, deluded, prepares to divide. To the monkey whose kidney may have just lost a few cells, nothing much follows except perhaps the mild discomfort of a chronic kidney infection. But for the new SV40 viruses, released from a dead kidney cell into the full bladder of an infectious but otherwise active monkey, these events are the culmination of a carefully honed plan to reach a jungle full of other — as yet uninfected — monkeys.

In the context of a monkey's kidney cell, the few thousand base pairs of DNA that encode T-antigen have no fewer than five different meanings. First, the sequence itself becomes a double entendre as soon as it is spliced into alternative messenger RNAs. Second, once T-antigen is returned to the nucleus, it finds the regulatory domains of its own gene and, by blocking the "here" sequence in the viral Origin of replication, quickly shuts off the production of its own messenger RNA. T-antigen then obliges the cell to make a new transcript instead, starting again from the Origin and again going halfway around the circle, but in the other direction. This — the third meaning — makes the cell produce millions of empty shells. Fourth, by binding to the viral genome's Origin of DNA replication, T-antigen forces the monkey cell's replication enzymes to make copies of the viral DNA circle, providing new viral genomes for the waiting, empty coats. Fifth, by binding to the cellular proteins that usually block cell division, T-antigen puts the infected kidney cell through a last burst of growth before it dies.

The monkey's infected kidney cell must accept SV40 T-antigen's multiple meanings, even at the cost of its own life. Such an outcome is dramatic, and the death of a monkey cell by SV40 infection may leave one with the sense that the cell was simply mechanically obeying a single set of precise instructions. Such a conclusion would be premature: in a different cellular context, T-antigen's meaning can be equally clear but entirely different. SV40's family name, SV, merely tells us that it is a simian virus; its surname, 40, has a more interesting provenance, which points to the second way a cell can interpret T-antigen. SV40 was the fortieth virus to be found in a wide-ranging search for infectious agents lurking in the cultured cells of monkey kidneys. This was no Nabokovian butterfly hunt; it was a somewhat belated scouring of cell cultures that had been used to grow the polio virus for conversion into vaccines. A small number of those cultured monkey kidney cells would always fill with holes and die, even before they saw any polio virus. These cultures were used anyway — there were no others to turn to — but not before being tested by periodic injection into various laboratory animals: mice, hamsters, and the like.

The search that led to the discovery of SV40 began when an extract of cultured monkey cells injected into a hamster caused a lump to grow under its skin; subsequently, it became clear that the contaminating virus — SV40 — could make tumors in hamsters and mice. Decades later, we can say that the considerable number of people vaccinated for polio with preparations containing SV40 did not come down with tumors any more frequently than those who did not receive any SV40 with their vaccine. This stroke of good fortune has been seen as such by the government agencies that license the sale of pharmaceuticals prepared from the cultured cells of human or primate tissues. All such preparations must now be rigorously tested for the presence of novel viruses well before any new drug or vaccine made from them reaches the market. But all the care in the world cannot guarantee that we will never again discover a latent virus in a pharmaceutical made from cultured primate cells; that is one good reason to welcome the molecular word processor and, with it, the ability to produce vaccines and other recombinant pharmaceuticals in bacterial cells.

Because it could make hamster cells into cancer cells, I took on SV40 as my chosen foe when I enlisted in President Nixon's War on Cancer. I was not a lone soldier; spurred on by the lucky outcome of the vast inadvertent experiment with SV40 that polio vaccination had become, many molecular biologists embraced SV40's ability to cause tumors in mice and hamsters, sure that this very small virus would be — in the jargon typical of the Vietnam era — a good weapon. Its simplicity was its main attraction; such a simple key might well be the best way to unlock the complicated problem of cancer.

Few of us would have predicted then that twenty years later the war would still be fought along pretty much the same lines or that the casualties would be even heavier today. The SV40 key got stuck in the lock back then: when SV40 was first elevated to the status of a model system for cancer, p53, which ultimately provided the explanation for SV40's ability to cause a cell to become a tumor, had not even been discovered. Now that we understand the role of proteins like p53, at least we have a good idea of how the lock works, if not how to slam the door shut again in a cancer cell.

Binding to p53 is the last of the five meanings that T-antigen combines to kill a monkey kidney cell. In a different species of cell — one that can draw from the protein no other meaning except that last one — SV40 T-antigen can mean, not the death of a single cell, but the death of an entire organism. Because monkey and human cells draw all five meanings from SV40 T-antigen, they will both die of the virus, precluding this consequence of a long-term interaction between T-antigen and p53. The species of cells that SV40 virus can transform into cancers are ones in which the virus's T-antigen cannot bring about its own genome's proliferation but can still inactivate the cell's p53: SV40 virus cannot kill, but will transform, the cells of a mouse, a rat, and a hamster with about equal efficiency. Since the other four meanings of T-antigen are played out elsewhere on the viral genome, an isolated gene for SV40 T-antigen will be as effective as the whole virus at transforming cells of these species, and by itself it will also transform monkey cells, even the cells of a monkey kidney. Cells of birds and reptiles have p53 molecules that cannot recognize T-antigen and polymerases that cannot begin to copy SV40 DNA, and so the virus means nothing at all to them.

The capacity of SV40 T-antigen to transform the cells of many different species of mammals suggests that the p53 genes of these species encode versions of p53 that share at least one specific three-dimensional shape or domain — the one that T-antigen can recognize. In fact, the amino acid sequences of a few domains of p53 are almost identical in primates and rodents. This is a clear sign of p53's long history as an important molecule, since it has been at least fifty million years since mice and men — and women — last shared a common ancestor. The conservation of domain structure across so many years explains how T-antigen can form the same tight connection to the p53s of so many species and why in every case the combination subverts p53's ability to keep cells from dividing.

How does SV40 T-antigen make a mouse or hamster cell into the parent of a lethally abnormal growth? Usually, with no explosion of newly made SV40 DNA in the way, a rodent cell exposed to SV40 T-antigen will divide a few times and then, after it digests the irritating pulse of T-antigen and its hapless viral genome, go back to sleep. But every so often the incoming SV40 DNA finds its way into a mouse or hamster nucleus and is recombined into one of the cell's chromosomes. Once this happens, the SV40 genome is no longer vulnerable to the cell's security forces; it is seen by the cell as just another bunch of genes somewhere in its giant genome, genes that will be copied each time the cell's own DNA is replicated.

Unable to make itself fully understood in such a cell, SV40 T-antigen will never have the chance to begin the autonomous duplication of its genome. But its gene can — and will — continue to make T-antigen even after having been incorporated somewhere in the cell's genome, and that T-antigen will force its cell into division in turn. Each time a T-antigen-driven cell divides, the viral gene is copied along with the cell's genome, and as soon as division is complete, both daughter cells are subject to T-antigen and must divide again without delay. The descendants of a cell that has taken T-antigen's gene into its chromosomes can never escape the goad of T-antigen. It stimulates every generation of T-antigen-addled cells to make a new generation of cells in turn. In the body of an adult mouse or hamster, where cell division is very tightly controlled, this is not a healthy situation.*

When a growing nest of unstoppable cells crops up in our body, we call it a tumor. The medical specialty dealing with tumors is called oncology, so a viral gene that converts a normal cell to a tumor cell is called an oncogene, and the

---

* In some tissues, normal cells rarely divide; in others like skin and the lining of the gut, cells divide as a matter of course, but for every cell that is born another dies, shed into the gut or off the body as dandruff. When the obligation to divide is inherited by the descendants of a single cell for many generations, not linked to equivalent cell death, it must produce an ever-larger mass of cells.

process that led to the untoward discovery of SV40 is called oncogenic transformation. Like bacteria in rich broth or primed DNA in a polymerase chain reaction tube, tumor cells grow exponentially. Doubling in about a day, descendants of an SV40-transformed cell will form a visible nodule in a dish in only a few weeks. If a transformed cell is placed in the body of a susceptible mouse or hamster, a tumor appears in about the same time. A million transformed cells — a pinhead clump, too small to feel beneath the skin — will accumulate from one SV40-infected hamster or mouse cell after about twenty doublings, which can take as little as three weeks. Time for another ten doublings — a week and a half — is enough for these million cells each to divide ten times more, producing a billion-celled, pea-size, growing nodule of the sort we are all encouraged to report to our doctors.

T-antigen's inactivation of p53 has taught us that a cancer may begin with the corruption of a single protein of the cell and the subsequent uncalled-for growth of a cluster of cells somewhere in the body. But within that cluster, a selection for the most abnormally vigorous mutant cells goes on constantly: the rest of the brakes on the growth of cells in the body — cell-cell contact, limited energy sources, necessary hormone signals — all select for, and enlarge the fraction of, any rare cell in the initial tumor that may lose sensitivity to these controls by virtue of a second, third, or fourth mutation. In this way, a benign lump or polyp that is constrained from pushing through the layers of tissues that separate the organs of the body will soon harbor within it a more deadly, malignant variant, whose descendants will travel deeper into the body, throwing off tiny microclusters of cells that become secondary tumors throughout the body.

A few hundred growth-controlling genes have been identified as likely targets for mutation in one or another human tumor; cells of malignant colon tumors, for example, are usually mutated in four or more of these genes, and one of them is almost always the p53 gene. Remarkably, a large fraction of tumor-associated human genes — called cellular oncogenes — are closely related to viral oncogenes. It appears that most viruses that cause tumors do so either because in the distant past they captured a mutant form of a cellular oncogene or because — like SV40 — they order a cell to make a protein like T-antigen, which then inactivates one or more of the cell's growth-controlling proteins. Either way, the messages that tumor viruses bring to a cell interrupt the cell's hormonal and genomic dialogue with its neighbors, forcing it to divide and preparing its descendants for the accumulation of further mutations. The oncogenic genes of tumor viruses are intimately related to the growth-controlling proteins of the cell, which explains why cancers can be caused by either viruses or mutagens like cigarette smoke, ultraviolet light, or ionizing radiation: all these agents can change the fate of a cell by bringing on the inherited loss of one or more growth-controlling proteins. *

Once one of our cells has sprung completely loose from the control of proteins like p53 to become a malignant tumor, we have no way today to put its descendants back into a regulated state. Instead, we must remove the initial mass of runaway cancer cells with a knife and try to kill escapees and holdouts with radiation and chemical poisons that damage their DNA. This is a woefully primitive and risky way to deal with the millions of cells in a tumor, and while such treatments may kill most or even all of the tumor's remaining cells, they also may damage the genes for other growth-control proteins in other parts of the body. For the tumors we cannot prevent — the ones that will always occur by random mutation — safe, certain treatment will become available only once we can repair or mimic specific growth-control genes and their proteins in the cancer cells themselves. Until then, we must muddle through as best we can: the best defenses against cancer remain preventive measures such as avoiding mutagens

---

* T-antigen is a member of the family of DNA-binding oncogene proteins. Other oncogenes make counterfeits of cellular proteins that signal the nucleus to begin preparing for cell division. One, for instance, mimics a membrane-bound receptor for a growth-stimulating hormone; a cell that has fake, oncogene-coded receptors on its surface is tricked into acting as if it were bathed in growth-stimulating hormones whether or not any hormones are actually present.

like cigarette smoke and getting checked regularly for small, persistent lumps.

The gene for the T-antigen protein has no single set of meanings; it is an example of molecular polysemy. A mouse cell and a monkey's kidney cell provide the same T-antigen gene with two different contexts, changing T-antigen's meaning in the starkest way. The monkey cell gives the virus a context for self-expression and survival. The moment a monkey cell reads the T-antigen gene of an SV40 genome, it is doomed to convert itself into raw materials for the satisfaction of T-antigen's demands. But if the gene for T-antigen becomes part of the genome of a mouse cell, it is no longer a matter of the cell's being taken over by an unstoppable viral genome but of a cell's being overtaken by its own latent capacity to grow, a body taken over by unstoppable cells. In one context, a cell dies; in the other, it lives and proliferates until its own unnatural vitality threatens to destroy the body of which it had been a part. T-antigen's ability to cause a tumor in a mouse serves its viral genome no purpose; a monkey cell and a mouse cell are like two readers who interpret the meaning of the T-antigen gene in different ways.

Both readings — by the monkey cell ready to die and by the mouse cell ready to be born again as a tumor — are exact, and neither is more nearly correct than the other. Their exactness lies in the three-dimensional shapes of the T-antigen protein's domains. Domains are interdependent contributors to the overall meaning of the molecular sentence that is a protein. Nevertheless, like words in a sentence or the fingers of a hand — recall the handlike DNA polymerase protein — a protein's domains carry their precise meanings separately. Fragments of the T-antigen gene, if addressed properly with the appropriate regulatory sequences, will yield truncated versions of T-antigen carrying some but not all of its domains. When put in a cell, some of these DNA phrases will still be able to carry out one or more of T-antigen's many activities.

As T-antigen comes into intimate contact with different molecules — its own Origin DNA, the monkey or mouse versions of DNA polymerase, p53, RB, and RNA polymerase — each molecule finds different T-antigen domains, and each meets the T-antigen molecule in a special way as the two come together in a complex. What is true for SV40's T-antigen will certainly be true for many human proteins: meanings are added to each protein by the other proteins it joins, and whatever makes the palette of protein interactions different from cell to cell will multiply the contextual meanings of all the proteins in each complex. As the behavior of T-antigen suggests, the ability to understand such layers of meaning will be required of all sophisticated readers of DNA.

∽

Although each domain means one clear thing, there is no rule in the DNA language that prevents two or more domains from saying the same thing: two proteins of different amino acid sequences may fold into almost the same three-dimensional domain. The terrorist's note of a virus like SV40, for example, is written in slightly different ways by different viruses, but they still have the same meaning in the right cell: polyoma is a virus that cannot grow in monkey cells but can do very well in the kidney cell of a mouse. Polyoma makes a T-antigen that does to a mouse's kidney cell precisely what SV40's T-antigen does to a monkey's kidney cell: by commandeering its gene expression and DNA replication, each protein enables its incoming virus to kill a host cell in very short order. Both T-antigens bind to an infected cell's p53 protein: even though the genes and their amino acid sequences are not similar, the three-dimensional shapes of these two T-antigens are similar enough to be recognized by the same p53 proteins.

The capacity of genomes to converge on the same meaning through the evolution of different amino acid sequences that fold into almost identical three-dimensional domains enriches the genomic language's ability to express subtle nuances. Just as a trained scholar may be able to recover the provenance and full meaning of an ancient text by comparing many slightly different drafts done at different times by different people, a comparison of similar domains in proteins that operate in different contexts can show us the domain's range of meaning. There is a striking similarity, for instance, in the way two very different viruses, SV40 and polio, make their outer coats. Both viruses encode a coat protein that folds into a structure resembling a partly opened book standing on its bottom edge. In both cases, five of these open books come together at their spines to form a five-sided dome, and in both cases the five-sided domes assemble into twenty-faceted, roughly spherical coats. SV40 and polio share the domain that folds into a set of hooks and snares that can assemble by fives into domes and then by domes into a hollow shell. Yet SV40 and polio share no base sequence, nor any amino acid sequence, in their coat-protein genes.

Why are the shapes of these domains more similar than their amino acid sequences? When two living things bear a likeness, either both are descended from a common ancestor who shared that characteristic or they have developed it independently in response to similar needs over a long time. In the former case, similarities are said to be homologous, in the latter, analogous. Homologous — but not analogous — similarities allow us to reconstruct evolutionary relationships among today's living things. Are domain similarities homologous or analogous? There is no rule to tell us in advance, but either answer is informative. If many domains turn out to be analogous — the way the separately evolved eyes of a protozoan, a scallop, a squid, a fly, and a person are analogous — that would teach us that the vocabulary of functional domains is a small one, perhaps small enough for us to learn it in its entirety. If we find that the preponderance of domain similarities among proteins are homologous — as we already know many to be — then our ever-growing vocabulary will continue to provide us with the historical context for DNA's current meanings.

One DNA-binding domain critical to the early development of animal embryos has been at work for billions of years. This conserved domain is made from a tight helical cylinder of amino acids that trails a floppy string, with a second cylinder lying crosswise on the first; it looks like one firecracker lying on top of another, tied together by their fuses. The helix-turn-helix domain, as it is called, fits nicely into the wide groove of a DNA molecule. There, specific amino acids recognize specific DNA sequences; when the right DNA sequence is found, the helix-turn-helix domain binds its protein tightly to the

DNA, leaving the other domains of the protein available for interaction with other proteins. Helix-turn-helix domains are so ancient, they are found in proteins that regulate the activity of genes in bacteria and their viruses and in proteins that lay out the futures of cells in very early human embryos. In all cases, from bacterial viruses to the embryos we all once were, the same domain is doing the same thing: helping to turn transcription on or off by binding tightly to the regulatory region of a gene. In animals, the helix-turn-helix domain is so good at what it does, and what it does is so necessary to the formation of an embryo, that the sequences encoding it have been preserved inside a multitude of different genes with only a small amount of mutational variation since the last common ancestor of flies and people grew from a fertilized egg and swam in billion-year-old seas.

Flies, people, and many other multicellular animals have mirror-image right and left sides, with fronts and tops different from backs and bottoms. Bilaterally symmetric animals got that way because as early embryos they were built up, head to tail, from bilaterally symmetric segments; every segment — from the head, thorax, and abdomen of a fly to the head, limbs, and ribs of a person — kept its bilateral symmetry as it developed. All bilaterally symmetric animals use a family of helix-turn-helix proteins to begin this body plan by carving crosswise bands from the mass of early embryonic cells and converting a ball of cells into a Michelin man of stacked segments. The family of genes that causes the head-to-tail segmentation of early embryos was discovered many years ago in the fruit fly as a set of recessive mutations that led to the displacement of organs so that, for instance, a leg might grow from the head in place of an eye. Such massive rearrangements of the body plan are called homeotic, from the Greek for "similarity disease." Each homeotic gene encodes a DNA-binding protein of many domains. Some domains interact with other proteins, others restrict the protein's DNA binding to specific short sequences in the regulatory regions of other genes. But all homeotic genes share one highly conserved DNA sequence encoding the ancient DNA-binding helix-turn-helix domain: the homeobox.

The patterns of transcription of homeobox genes are strikingly similar in the very young embryos of a fly, a frog, and a mouse. In each, families of homeobox genes are sequentially transcribed for short periods of time, starting at the head of the early embryo and sweeping down to its tail. Each family of homeobox genes encodes a set of gene regulators: the earlier, headmost homeotic proteins activate the transcription of later, tailward ones; the tailward ones shut off the synthesis of their activators. Such feedback loops generate pulses of gene transcription, like the pulse of transcription of T-antigen in an infected monkey cell. Rather than leading to cell death in this case, pulses produce bands of cells containing different homeobox proteins, striping the early embryo from front to back. Nuclei in each band, filled with a band-specific set of gene-regulatory proteins, begin different cascades of gene regulation, making their cells differentiate until they become a particular segment of the body. Our brains are made of about a half dozen of these early segments, and a glance at our skeleton tells us that the rest of our bodies are made of segments as well.

Homeobox genes have a special relationship with the chromosomes in which they sit. In the fly's genome and in our own, the genes for each family of homeotic proteins are arrayed on a chromosome in the same order as the positions of the bands they direct the embryo to form. The gene for the earliest, headmost homeotic protein is at one end of a chromosome and is transcribed first, the gene for the tailmost homeotic protein is at the other end of this region of the chromosome and is transcribed last, and all the other homeotic protein genes lie in the order that can be predicted from the sequence and position of their expression in the embryo. These beautiful arrays of genes, their chromosomal positions conveying their intentions even before transcription, stand as a major exception to the general rule that the genome is a lexicon of topics linked only through gene regulation.

As new species of multicellular animals emerged from old, the number of homeotic genes in a family, and even the number of families, has increased. For example, in the fly there is only one family of homeobox genes; in simple vertebrates like the lamprey, two; and in mice and humans there are four.

Tandemly repeated, slightly different genes such as those in the homeobox families accumulate from the slowest but most important kind of DNA movement in the genome: the periodic, accidental duplication of a long stretch of DNA. Rarely, two chromosomes fail to exchange DNA symmetrically during recombination, so one germ cell gets two successive alleles of a gene and the other neither. A sperm or egg with no allele is clearly mutant and likely fatally so, but one with two copies is simply overendowed and usually fertile. In an embryo, the extra copies of genes in a stretch of reduplicated DNA will be redundant, as one allele from each parent takes care of the gene's business.

But redundancy turns out to be a great motor of genomic diversity over time: animals with two versions of a gene on each of their chromosomes will survive despite the accumulation of random mutations in one version as long as the other retains its original, functional sequence. Mutated second genes will usually be of no use, but they expose cells of the body at various times to mutant, variant proteins that need not retain the function of the original. Should this second function be advantageous to the survival of an organism, it will tend to be retained through the generations at the expense of organisms in the same species that lack it. Our color vision, for example, depends on a pigment gene on the X chromosome that duplicated only about thirty-five million years ago, giving us genes for pigments sensitive to red and green light in addition to a gene for blue-sensitive pigment. All descendants of the Old World higher primates, including us, have these three pigment genes; New World monkeys still have only the blue pigment and one other. They see the world the way our common ancestors did long ago, in blues and brownish greens, pretty much the way a color-blind person sees it today.

Because homeobox genes direct the organization of the embryo, each successful duplication has led to a new wrinkle in the basic body plan. The homeobox family expressed in head segments of developing mammalian embryos, for example, has extra, unique genes not found in other animals with backbones, suggesting that an old duplication of segments at the front end of an embryo provided the cellular material for the differentiation of a mammalian brain. There is no reason to think the last gene duplication has occurred; based on the past, it is a safe bet that in the distant future new species will differ from current ones in part because of the novel activity of newly duplicated homeotic genes. Nor are homeotic genes the only ones still being slowly multiplied: duplication of the green-pigment genes happens all the time on the X chromosome, and a few percent of people have four color-pigment genes as a result. In the very long run, their descendants may well see a more colorful world than we do.

~

Homeobox genes, and other genes such as those that encode T-antigen and p53, challenge the ingenuity of prospective readers of the genome. We can fiddle with the sequences of these genes in our molecular word processor, but what good is that if we cannot see the genes in action? These genes have subtle meanings that cannot be fully displayed in a single cell; they require a stage the size of a whole organism and its entire lifetime to play out their roles. Bacteria are not the answer. Inserted into bacterial plasmids, human genes can be grown and harvested or made into simple protein factories, but a human protein cannot completely express itself among a ragtag band of bacterial proteins, few of which will notice it. Nor are cell cultures sufficient; a gene of interest may kill or transform a single cell, but it cannot show what it might have done in an entire embryo. To learn how subtle genes work, we have no choice but to get them into every cell of an embryo and watch their effects over the organism's lifetime.

Genes that begin in the lab and are inserted into a living genome at the earliest possible stage in its development were given a name in 1980 by a biologist at Yale, Frank Ruddle: transgenes. Biologists have been putting genes onstage this way for about twenty years. The easiest to make are plants with transgenes; the genome of a plant cell is far more malleable than any of ours. A skin cell in a dish, for instance, will either grow as a skin cell, transform into a skin tumor, or die, no matter what hormones we present it with. But a cell from the stem or root of a plant, in a dish by itself, can be tricked by simple mixtures of plant hormones into thinking that it is a fertilized egg cell. It will start a plant from scratch out of its own copy of the species' genome, dividing and sending out roots and shoots, leaves and flowers, forming itself into a little plant right in the dish. For uniformity and convenience, most reforestation programs now plant evergreen trees cloned in test tubes from single cells; it is actually easier and cheaper to clone some plants than it is to wait for them to fertilize themselves and provide seed to plant.

With as little effort as it takes to separate plant cells from each other and get the DNA in — this is done by first stripping the cell's wall off, then injecting the DNA or slipping it in by transformation — transgenic plants can be started, planted, and harvested. To begin the cloning sequence, a gene from a molecular word processor is injected into the nucleus of a cultured plant cell before the cell sees any hormones. Then hormones are added, the clonal sprout is cultured in a dish, then in the ground, and soon it becomes a complete, transgenic plant with a copy of the injected gene in every one of its cells. Since the pollen and egg cells of a transgenic plant will carry the transgene, DNA has to be injected only once to begin a bed, or a whole garden, of transgenic plants. Thereafter, they can be bred to one another to make a new strain with whatever feature the transgene confers. Transgenic plants accomplish what natural selection takes much longer to do by gene duplication: they provide a laboratory for the testing of extra, variant copies of plant genes.*

Transgenic plants by the hundreds have been made and grown for their resistance to herbicides. These plants — a mixed message from the molecular word processor — improve crop yields, but they also encourage the use of herbicides to

---

* Some years ago, for instance, scientists discovered how to grow a transgenic plant that could create an antibody. Knowing that an antibody is made of two different proteins that fold into a single active complex, they created two transgenic tobacco plants with DNAs made from the messengers for two proteins. Each made one of the proteins in its leaves; as expected, neither protein had any antibody activity. When the two transgenic plants were crossed, offspring that contained both genes made both proteins, and their leaves filled with active antibodies.

kill competing plants in the field, a practice that has obvious drawbacks. Most important, high doses of herbicide result in the eventual overgrowth of herbicide-resistant weeds by the same logic of natural selection that makes penicillin treatment the cause of penicillin-resistant infections and spraying with DDT a way to generate swamps full of DDT-resistant mosquitoes.

Recently, the Food and Drug Administration decided that transgenic plants could be the source of foods and drugs for general consumption without prior government testing and left the decision of whether to test such plants to their growers. Since many common food plants — potatoes, for instance — contain poisons in parts that are routinely discarded, the government is taking an inexplicably optimistic view about the potential for subtle toxicities in transgenic foodstuffs. Nor is the government requiring that manufacturers and growers label transgenic plants so that consumers would know what they were buying. Like it or not, under current government regulations unlabeled milk, ice cream, and cheese from BST-treated cows and fruit, cereal, and vegetables from transgenic plants will soon be in our stores and on our tables.

~

It doesn't make much sense to put T-antigen, $p53$, or a human homeotic gene into a plant cell. Plants are built up differently from you and me: they have no front or back, differing only from top to bottom. They cannot move around, nor can any but a few of their wooden-walled cells move at all. After every cell division, most plant cells are fixed in place for their lifetime. Like chimneys growing taller by the addition of bricks, the roots and shoots of a plant grow by the division of bands of cells, which are constantly being displaced upward, downward, and outward by the tubes of woody cells they leave behind. Despite their immobility, plant cells communicate with one another as our cells do, by sending proteins and small molecules called plant hormones through hollow tubes filled with fluid. Under the direction of plant hormones, the dividing bands periodically lay down clusters of cells that later undergo meiosis to become the pollen and eggs of a flower. Plants hang their genitals out in the open, and pollen is the one part of a plant that can move; whether by insect, wind, free fall, or fire, a plant must make sure that its pollen gets to an egg cell to start a new plant. Proteins such as T-antigen cannot perform in any sensible way in a plant; the genome of an animal is their only legitimate stage.

There are two ways to generate strains of transgenic animals. The first uses a cancer cell as a vehicle. Mice — and people — sometimes suffer from a rare form of cancer called embryonal carcinoma. Its name conveys the nature of this tumor, which springs from a deranged cell in the tissues that make sperm and egg. Embryonal carcinoma (EC) cells are cancerous; instead of becoming a sperm or egg cell that will contribute to an embryo, they make a horrible kind of tumor, full of differentiating cells that form mockeries of various tissues interleaved with nests of rapidly dividing, undifferentiated EC cells. The undifferentiated cells grow well in a dish, and like many other cultured cells, they can take in a recombinant plasmid and allow its genes to be incorporated into their genome. Unlike almost all other cultured animal cells, though, an EC cell — whose parent cells were about to undergo meiosis — can recombine one of its own genes with a similar sequence that is brought in on a recombinant plasmid. In one more botched attempt at the meiosis it will never get to, an EC cell may eliminate one of its own genes, replacing it with a laboratory version. This noble failure is called site-specific recombination. Through it, a recombinant gene can go directly from the molecular word processor into the EC cell's genome, either knocking out the EC cell's version of the gene or replacing it, giving a newly made variant the perfect stage for a full performance.

Getting the DNA-transformed EC cells into a mouse embryo means interrupting the normal course of mouse development soon after fertilization. Embryos no older than a few hours, and no bigger than a few dozen cells, are dislodged from a recently mated female mouse. Each embryo is a tiny, hollow ball of cells. A transformed EC cell is inserted through a needle into this hollow ball, and the mouse embryo, now bearing a cell that would overwhelm and kill any adult mouse in a few weeks, is returned to the uterus of another mouse. Something amazing happens next: the EC cell starts to divide, but as it does, it ceases to be a cancer cell. Surrounded by the dividing cells of the embryo, the progeny of the EC cell become normal tissue cells, and the mixed ball of cells grows into a mosaic of embryo cells descended both from the fertilized egg and the EC cell. Such a beast — it puts the mythical chimera to shame — has not two but four parents, two of which had conceived the mouse that had carried the embryonal carcinoma in the first place. Tetraparental mice are fertile unless the EC cell's recombinant gene commands otherwise, and so are their descendants. When a son and daughter of a tetraparental mouse are bred, some of their inbred grandchildren will inherit two copies of the recombinant DNA and, if it was initially inserted by site-specific recombination, no normal alleles for that gene will come along.

When a fully recombinant, tetraparental mouse lives a full life, we can conclude with confidence that the injected gene has been given a chance to carry out all the functions and to display all the meanings it encodes, and we can follow these meanings by following the patterns of expression of the gene and its protein. For example, when the regulatory regions of different brain-specific genes are coupled to a marker gene that produces a blue dye, transgenic mice carrying these constructed genes will show streaks of the dye in their brains, mapping exactly where and when each regulatory region is expressed during the development of the mouse. Or we can simply knock a normal gene out of a transgenic mouse by recombining a silent DNA in place of the EC cell's allele to learn whether, and if so where and when, the missing gene is necessary for a normal life.

In one of the earliest experiments along these lines, EC cells had their p53 genes silenced. The prediction was that in the absence of a functional p53 gene, an embryo's cells would go crazy, making a little tumor instead of a mouse. To everyone's surprise, these transgenic mice developed normally, even when they had absolutely no p53 gene activity in any of their cells. They did succumb to a host of tumors in their middle age, confirming the notion that p53 keeps tumors from growing. But by living for months with no apparent problems, these mice forced a fundamental reassessment of p53's meaning. "Knockout" transgenic mice can also display the contribution of a single gene to even the most complex and poorly understood forms of behavior. For example, scientists have found that knocking out one gene encoding a protein that puts phosphorus on a small set of membrane proteins will yield a transgenic mouse that has lost the capacity for long-term memory.

Transgenic mice descended from tetraparental grandparents are exotic, and making and breeding them requires a rare ability to work equally well with cultured tumor cells, recombinant DNA, and colonies of mice. Wouldn't it be simpler just to inject recombinant DNA directly into the nucleus of a fertilized egg cell? Indeed, if the needle is fine enough and the egg is impaled between fertilization and the first cell division, this is the second way to make transgenic strains of mice. It lacks the finesse of an EC cell's specific recombination, because injected DNAs paste themselves at random into the cell's genome. But when site-specific recombination is not needed, direct injection is an easier way to get a gene into every cell of a mouse.

Implanted in the uterus of another female mouse, the injected fertilized egg grows into a many-celled embryo, and the injected DNA is always copied as if it were a cellular gene. Since the new gene has usually integrated in only one chromosome, it is not yet established as a true-breeding mouse gene. As with tetraparental mice, a DNA-injected mouse founds a new strain by mating to an ordinary mouse. Half the litter will carry the injected transgene; when these offspring are mated brother to sister, a fraction of their offspring will have two alleles of the transgene in each cell. Brother-sister mating of the founder's grandchildren will establish the novel strain, each mouse homozygous for the new gene forevermore.

The gene for SV40 T-antigen was one of the first to be inserted into a mouse this way. As expected, if it was provided with a regulatory region that permitted transcription, the protein caused tumors to appear as the transgenic mice grew up. If the molecular word processor was used to link T-antigen's coding region to a regulatory region for a gene active only in one tissue — a liver-specific gene, for instance — the transgenic mouse would come down with tumors of the liver. Even though every one of its cells had the gene, only liver cells could transcribe it and start T-antigen on its malignant way.

A recombinant gene may also be modified prior to injection so that it can be easily rescued from mouse DNA at a later date. One such transgenic strain of mice provides a particularly elegant way to measure the mutagenic effects of chemicals and radiation: the mouse is given a toxic treatment; then the transgene is recovered from its tissues and assayed directly for accumulated mutations. Mice of this strain are for sale; they are called the Big Blue Transgenic Mouse Mutagenesis Assay System, a big but appropriate name for a mouse with an extra bacterial gene that — once recovered and put back into the right bacteria — will turn a bacterial colony blue. It would be fitting to require that Big Blue transgenic mice be used to measure the mutagenic activity of novel herbicides sprayed on the transgenic herbicide-resistant food plants before the fruits and vegetables could be marketed, but that is not likely, at least until the real cost of a new technology is taken into account more carefully than it is today.

A gene intended for integration into a mouse by EC-cell or direct injection does not have to come only from a virus, a bacterium, or a mouse; transgenic mice have been produced with human alleles that function well enough to compensate for damaged or missing mouse alleles. For instance, the transgenic grandpups of fertilized mouse egg cells injected with a human hemoglobin gene produce functional hemoglobin; when the fertilized egg cell comes from an inbred mouse strain suffering an inherited blood disease, the transgene cures the grandpups' symptoms.

The ability of mouse cells to incorporate human genes is very useful in the study of diseases, especially cancer. The potency of new drugs must be tested directly on tumors, and pharmaceutical firms used to inject tumor cells into mice and then add their drugs, a procedure no more reproducible than the constancy of the tumor cells from experiment to experiment. Since 1988 they have been able to turn to a transgenic strain of mice, patented by Harvard University, that has had a human oncogene — called *ras* — inserted in its genome. Licensed by Harvard, the Du Pont Corporation had some success in marketing this strain, called OncoMouse; Du Pont guaranteed that each untreated OncoMouse would develop a lethal tumor within a few months of birth. Cancer labs all over the world began to use the OncoMouse to test possible drug treatments until Du Pont insisted that investigators who developed products with OncoMouse's help had to pay royalties. At that point, many laboratories simply made their own transgenic strains by injecting a human oncogene into a mouse embryo, bypassing the Harvard–Du Pont product.

Big Blue and OncoMouse are not alone: there are HIV mice as well. No ordinary mouse comes down with AIDS, because HIV is so compulsively specific about growing only in one type of human immune-system cell. But an HIV transgenic mouse's immune cells are damaged from within by the HIV genes in every cell; once HIV is bred into the mouse's genome, no further infection is necessary. These mice, tricked from conception by a molecular Trojan horse, offer a model for studying AIDS that develops the disease's symptoms without ever being exposed to the virus itself.

One transgenic mouse strain rich in nuances shows us how wonderfully alike are the homeobox genes of flies and mammals while providing a new way to study a serious birth defect. It has had one of its homeobox genes — called *hox-1.5* — knocked out. The loss of the second copy of *hox-1.5* produces a profoundly damaged mouse, without a thymus or a parathyroid gland and with a number of defects in the formation of the face, the heart, and the head. Two facts about this poor, sick mouse show the power of transgenic technology to explicate the full meaning of a gene and the rigorous preservation of meaning some genes can display even in extraordinarily different contexts. First, these are precisely the sort of defects caused in the fly by mutations of homeobox genes called *Zerknüllt* and *proboscipidia*, whose sequences are strikingly similar to that of the *hox-1.5* gene. The meaning of these mutations is plain: the helix-turn-helix domain and the other interactive domains of *hox-1.5* proteins have affected the development of embryos in the same way for a much longer time than either the fly or mouse has been around, longer than it has been since the last common ancestor of flies and mice was alive. Second, these mutations suggest that people and mice will hardly differ at all in terms of their ways of reading this gene: the birth defects of a *hox-1.5*-deficient mouse are remarkably like those of an infant born with a congenital deficiency called DiGeorge's syndrome. We do not yet know whether the gene that is mutated in DiGeorge's syndrome is the human version of *hox-1.5* or another gene that shares a developmental pathway with it. Either way, the similarity of phenotype in humans and mice suggests that *hox-1.5* knockout mice will be helpful in understanding the human disease.

The *hox-1.5*-deficient mouse is one of an increasing number of transgenic knockout strains that help elucidate inherited diseases of our own, and new medically important transgenic animals are on the way. A strain of transgenic pigs, for instance, may one day replace blood banks. The pigs express a variant of the human gene for hemoglobin. The variant gene — a sequence created in the lab — makes a hemoglobin that will work as a protein without having to be wrapped in a red blood cell. Hemoglobin can be repeatedly harvested from the transgenic pigs and purified for further experimentation. If this line of work is successful, many transfusions of whole blood may no longer be necessary, and emergency operations may be considerably less risky.

Transgenic mice that mimic Alzheimer's disease may also be at hand, although at least two early reports of such models have been retracted after they could not be repeated. In at least one case, though, a form of the disease did develop in a strain of transgenic mice. It was created by introducing a portion of a human gene that is overexpressed in the dying brain cells of an Alzheimer's victim. The transgenic mice are born healthy, but in time their brain cells fill with tangles of threads of this gene's protein as they become demented. The tangles kill brain cells, leaving remnants that pock the parts of the mouse brain responsible for memory, a terrain quite reminiscent of the brains of Alzheimer's disease victims. This cannot be the whole story, though, because while some cases of Alzheimer's disease run in families, most seem to arise spontaneously — or after an injury — and it is unlikely that these instances of dementia could have all stemmed from any single inherited mutant gene.

One clue that might reconcile the complicated patterns of incidence of Alzheimer's disease with the simple results from transgenic mice is the dementia of Down's syndrome: people who inherit three copies of chromosome 21 instead of the usual two become demented at an early age as their brains come to resemble those of Alzheimer's victims. Most neuronal cells in the brain do not normally divide, but injury can stimulate cell division, and with it the possibility of a disordered mitosis that would put a third copy of chromosome 21 in a new neuronal cell. If that were to happen often enough, a person might spontaneously develop a nonfamilial form of Alzheimer's disease late in life due to the overexpression of a neuron-specific gene from three different copies of chromosome 21, as a Down's syndrome person does at an early age. This way of explaining the data makes the prediction — as yet untested — that familial late-onset Alzheimer's would result from inheriting a mutant allele for any of the many genes that contribute to proper chromosome assortment during mitosis.

∼

Though these examples show that we can discover the full meaning of a gene by putting it in a transgenic mouse, transgenic mice will tell us little of what we want to know about the meanings of the human genome. We know there are at least a hundred thousand genes in our genomes, and transgenic mice are not going to be able to tell us about more than a few of them in the next few years, one at a time. Moreover, many traits worthy of study are not the result of one gene's expression but the combined consequence of many genes working together. In principle, we could generate a palette of transgenic strains and then breed them to produce mice that carry any number of different transgenic genes, but this elaborate protocol would go up in cost and complexity very rapidly as the number of human genes involved increased. Besides, a mouse is not as smart as any of us. The parts of our brains that are most interesting, most different, and most obscure to us are assembled and maintained by sets of genes that are not likely to be at work in understandable ways in mice. Some sets of genes, like the ones responsible for the regions of the brain dedicated to language, would probably not even work in transgenic chimpanzees or any other primates, though to a remarkable degree we share genomic coding sequences with them.

Why not transgenic people then? Certainly, there is no technical barrier. The success of in vitro fertilization (IVF) has shown, in passing, that the one-celled human embryo is entirely accessible. IVF is pursued by thousands of couples unable to conceive in the ordinary way; many have had healthy babies by this method. After sperm meets the egg in a dish, the fertilized egg is typically allowed to divide a few times before it is placed in the mother's uterus. For those hours or days, the earliest of human embryos is available for the injection of any DNA sequence one might have made for the purpose. IVF thus presents an undeniable temptation to make a transgenic child.

Most people recoil instinctively from this prospect, since it immediately raises the specter of eugenics and a brave but horrifying new world. But perhaps that is overreaction: what if, for instance, a transgenic child can be born without a congenital disease passed on to her by her parents? Is there a way to use the technology of transgenic development to benefit people and do no harm? In other words, can there be a transgenic medicine consistent with the Hippocratic Oath? The question is neither technical nor conceptual: it is easy to imagine a time when physicians know enough about the genome to say with confidence that one or another sequence would, if properly inserted in a fertilized egg, stop the recurrence of any one of a number of familial diseases. For instance, our medicine already accepts a diagnosis of cystic fibrosis before implantation, and early experiments are under way to replace mutant CFTR protein in the lung cells of cystic fibrosis patients by infecting them with a genetically modified virus carrying a functional copy of the CFTR gene. There is no technical impediment to a combination of these two protocols: inject the CFTR gene into one of the remaining seven cells of an embryo that has been shown to lack a good CFTR allele, and implant the transgenic embryo into a waiting uterus.

The questions that must be answered before such transgenic

medicine — the ultimate in planned parenthood — gets started are social, not scientific. We need to know who is to decide to create the first transgenic embryos. Then — since we can be sure that mistakes will be made — we need to know who is to take responsibility for them. A mistake in this context means, of course, a child born with a defect caused by some step in the experiment. Recently, for example, scientists interested in coloring the hair and eyes of an albino strain of mice transgenically injected the DNA for a missing enzyme that makes black pigment; unexpectedly, they created a strain of transgenic mice whose viscera — heart, stomach, liver, and the like — were all turned around. These mice were unable to live long after birth; careful molecular work showed that the added gene had — while inserting itself in the mouse genome — inadvertently damaged a hitherto unknown gene responsible for maintaining the usual asymmetries of the mouse's internal organs.

Confronting the first, experimental phases of transgenic medicine raises questions that should interest religious leaders, politicians, educators, and parents at least as much as they interest physicians and scientists. The answers we provide — and the nature of the political discourse by which we arrive at them — will determine not so much the medicine of the next century as the manner in which we will live with one another. The issues raised by the potential birth of a failed, experimental, transgenic child are at least as thorny and contentious as the contemporary question of who should decide whether a fetus can be aborted. The passionate and unresolved arguments between "pro-life" advocates, who would forbid abortion as murder, and "pro-choice" defenders, who believe every woman has a right to an abortion on demand, are a foretaste of the disputes that would arise if it were known that any corner of the medical establishment was about to make it possible for a woman to carry a transgenic fetus to term without being able to assure her that the baby would be free of any inadvertent side effects of the DNA injection. Since responsible scientists cannot promise that all experiments will work, I do not see how transgenic medicine can ever be properly undertaken in a democratic society.

Readers of human DNA are not yet at an impasse, but we are surely on the way to one. In a short time we will have transliterated the human genome, played out many parts of it in cells, and gotten some difficult passages translated for us in transgenic animals. Then we will begin to plumb the genome for the passages we want most to know about, the ones that are responsible for our humanity and, if not our souls, then our ability to imagine souls. What we have found about the genome so far suggests that it will be impossible to know ourselves this way through our genomes, but we could easily do great damage to one or more future fellow citizens by trying. As a friend once said to make me think again about performing a particularly seductive experiment, if it isn't worth doing, it isn't worth doing well.

6

~

BETWEEN PHYSICS AND HISTORY:

THE NEW PARADIGM

OF BIOLOGY

TWENTY YEARS AGO the philosopher Thomas Kuhn suggested that a mature science is always guided by a set of theories, standards, and methods, which he called a paradigm. As he explained, this set of tacit or explicit assumptions determines what is seen as important and what is discarded as trivial or unanswerable, focusing a field and often leading to a rapid consolidation of disparate and confusing problems. But as observations accumulate that do not fit the current paradigm, scientists find themselves constrained by what had been a helpful set of standards, one they cannot discard until they find and agree on another, more useful set. As data are accumulated by scientists in a changing field, the same information may be interpreted in different ways, and old, familiar facts may take on new meanings as well. A temporary crisis of meaning occurs when one scientist sees things in a new way while a colleague has not yet come around. Inevitably, scientists who disagree on the meaning of their data will disagree on what to do next until a new paradigm eventually replaces the old and — by agreement of its practitioners — questions that had been marginal become central to the new agenda of a science, and vice versa.

Centuries ago, for example, the intellectual descendants of priests in Europe, Africa, and Asia — the ancestors of today's cosmologists and astronomers — learned to predict the location of planets and stars with considerable accuracy. In order to explain their observations and make accurate predictions while holding to a paradigm that assumed that the earth lay at the center of our solar system and that heavenly bodies traveled only in perfect circles, these early European astronomers were obliged to invent planetary orbits of increasing complexity, intricate circles within circles. A fifteenth-century Polish astronomer — his equivalent of a Nobel Prize was the latinization of his name, from Kopernik to Copernicus — broke the paradigm by reinterpreting available data under the assumption that the sun, not the earth, was at the center of our part of the universe. With that, the extra circlets of planetary motion were no longer necessary; although they were no less efficient at predicting the motion of the planets, they ceased to be of interest. In recent years biomedical science — and especially the sort of science that places the molecular biology of the human genome at its center — has been approaching just such an impasse, one that may herald a new paradigm.

The molecular biology that built its foundations on the presumptions of physics was attended at its birth by a considerable number of physicists. (Francis Crick and Max Delbrück, for instance, were both physicists before turning to biology.) The basic presumption of classical physics — that our cosmos is governed by mathematically precise laws at all scales, from the inside of an atom to the totality of the universe — had undergone its own wrenching reinterpretation with the explication of quantum mechanics. In the 1920s, new data could only be interpreted by using the ideas that the most fundamental atomic phenomena are based on chance and — even more disturbing — that they are not objectively stable but change according to how they are observed. No longer was it possible to imagine that an atom's position and direction could both be known at once; any certainty about the physical world had to be built up from the statistical probabilities and essential ambiguities of quantum mechanics. The deterministic formulas of classical physics still worked for visible objects, which obeyed mathematical laws with precision, but the positions and movements of the invisible atoms that make up all objects were now lost in a probabilistic blur. While the universe remained determinate, the revised mathematical constructs of physics — more accurately reflecting the way atoms behave — could no longer promise completely predictable events and objective, universal knowledge.

With great insight, the earliest molecular biologists extended this new paradigm of physics to biology: living systems, they reasoned, must contain vast numbers of atoms in order to avoid the indeterminacy of small numbers of atoms, and the information that living systems use to construct and replicate themselves must reside in the specific assembly of large molecules from many atoms. Erwin Schrödinger — the inventor of a formula expressing the eerie new reality that atoms and their constituents were neither waves nor particles, but could be conjured as either by the proper choice of detector — was one of the first to use the new physics to address an important question in biology. In *What Is Life?*, published in 1947, he explained why even the smallest living thing had to be made of many atoms. He also called upon statistical mechanics to cut through a thicket of midcentury genetics and correctly predicted that genes would be made of a large, crystalline, but nonrepeating chemical.

In the second half of this century the adopted paradigm of physics has become remarkably fruitful for biology, but it has not converted biology into a branch of physics. Instead, the early ingenuity of physicists who saw the need to study large molecules has brought biology to a stage of certainty — a belief that all answers exist — quite like the one achieved by physics almost a century ago, just before the discovery of quantum mechanics. This faith has survived undimmed for many decades,* but molecular biology now confronts a new and unpredicted uncertainty, a boundary on our ability to know the final meaning of the genes we study. Where once it seemed clear that everything about the living world was intrinsically knowable, we have found — against our expectations — that when sets of genes combine to become the bodies

---

* As Sidney Brenner put it in 1992: "In biology I have said before that in a sense all the answers exist in nature. All we need is the means to look them up, and that's what the techniques [of molecular biology] give us."

and minds of intrinsically unpredictable people, the complete and final meanings of these sets cannot be fully captured. Single genes may one day be totally understood — although that remains to be seen, given the richness of meaning in genes like T-antigen — but the overall meaning of a genome will not be a predictable sum or product of these separate meanings.

The intrinsic incomprehensibility of our own genome cannot be fitted inside the paradigm, derived from physics, that has kept the search for a complete set of time-independent biological mechanisms at the center of molecular biology. For classical physicists, the dust settled when it became clear that tangible objects behaved predictably, although made of unpredictable atoms. For biologists, the challenge will be to come to terms with the discovery that although individual genes may behave predictably, they do not together form a predictable — let alone completely knowable — genome. Experimentation on human genes, no matter how imaginative, will never give a single, complete meaning to the human genome.

Not all biologists have been under the sway of the classical molecular paradigm. Those studying the causes and consequences of natural selection have no hope and no wish for eternal laws: physicists can predict the next solar eclipse, but no one can predict the next species. Trained as scientists but thinking like historians, biologists studying evolution have always embraced the contingent aspects of current and past life and accepted that we will not come this way again. But even though many students of evolution now use the tools of a molecular biologist, their work has for the most part failed to inform the agenda of molecular biology.

This has begun to change. Many molecular biologists are becoming historians in spite of themselves. As they find more examples of the richness of a true historical record — the many-layered, encrypted meanings of an evolved gene — they are beginning to approach the genomes of individuals and species, not as one would approach molecules alone but as one would approach a library of ancient books documenting the history of life on this planet. And as they learn more about ancient gene families that can play similar — but subtly different — roles in the life of a yeast, a fly, and a person, the historical relatedness of all genomes and the intrinsic unpredictability of their futures have slowly but surely amounted to a new way to see molecular biology itself.

The trend is clear: we can expect to find more and more examples of the richness of a real language in our cells. DNA and protein have grammar and syntax, and we have already come upon typographical errors, double meanings, synonyms, and other subtleties. Future studies will build on the fact that the only assembler and preserver of DNA texts until now — natural selection — has generated a matrix of historical, causal relationships so complex that no code linking natural or synthetic DNA sequences to survival of species will be found, and for this reason natural selection will not be reduced to a set of predictable laws.

Once we set aside the futile search for such laws, we will see that genomes like ours, with their networks of interactions and their great multiplicity of meanings, leave us free to use our imagination as we read them. Seen from the vantage point of this new, historical paradigm for biology, genomes that cannot be fully comprehended as the sum of the separate meanings of their genes are nevertheless enormously exciting, while the sort of genome that was believed to be understood as soon as it was transliterated would have left biology a closed science and a servant of its own technology. But imagination is not enough: every pair of people and every pair of living species — whether peach and frog, elephant and dung beetle, *E. coli* and lobster, or chimpanzee and human — have shared a final common ancestor species at some point. To be sure we have access to the texts themselves, we will need to preserve human individuality, despite many temptations to smooth its rough edges, and to understand the historical details of our descent from common ancestors, a history we share with all other creatures, however dissimilar in appearance.

My generation of molecular biologists will likely continue as before: the indeterminacy of the human genome as a whole enlarges the context, but does not reduce the importance, of understanding any allele within it. When a paradigm is supplanted, Kuhn observed, it is the younger members of a field and those just entering it who are quickest to adapt; a real change in direction will come with the next generation. As my future colleagues now in high school and college stake out their own challenges, they will be able to take for granted the central importance of keeping the earth's entire genetic database alive; of establishing the historical record of life's evolution and elucidating the mechanisms of speciation that link all living things by common ancestry; and of uncovering the deep links between our uniquely human use of language and the genomic language used by our genes. Their goals will be, first, to learn the genomic histories of life on Earth, of our species *Homo sapiens,* of our brain's unique capacity for language and thought, and of languages themselves, and then to understand the ways in which these seemingly disparate histories are actually linked and interdependent.

∽

To see these links, it helps to shrink the earth and speed up time by about ten-million-fold each. Now the seven-thousand-mile-diameter earth is about five feet across, not quite as big as our previously magnified SV40 virus. The few-mile-thick layer on the earth's surface that supports all life — from bacteria in the oceans to bacteria in the atmosphere — is a coating no thicker than a dime. Since a billion years of the past collapses into a hundred years of speeded-up time, this miniature earth would have been formed about two thousand years ago. The first living cells would have formed on it almost four hundred years ago; the large creatures with enough bony structure to leave fossils would have lived and died about nine months ago, and the first modern humans — *Homo sapiens* — would have been born about a week ago.

Collapsing perspectives in this way allows us to see that the membrane of living creatures wrapped around our planet is itself a slowly developing, living creature of a sort. Life in this planetary wrapping had a beginning, just as a body begins from a fertilized egg; and from that beginning it has developed as different species — tissues — interact in various ways. Some are shed, others saved; most change, some stay pretty much the same. The growth of cells from a fertilized egg into a living creature is called development; the development of life on

Earth is called evolution. Development and evolution have these things in common, although they work on vastly different dimensional and time scales: they both bring out structures of astounding complexity from the interaction of genes and proteins; they are structured hierarchically; they are time dependent and historically rooted; and, as we are finding out the hard way, neither is totally knowable or predictable.

In some organisms — worms provide a particularly good example — every cell division can be followed and every cell of an adult organism assigned a full genealogy back to the fertilized egg. The totality of genealogies of all cells in an adult organism is called a fate map; the eventual fate of the descendants of every cell in the developing embryo can be read from it. Biologists want a fate map for complex organisms more like ourselves, both to link gene expression to development and to understand more easily the meaning of a given pattern of gene expression in an embryo. We do not have many fate maps yet, but we are confident that they would all look the same in one way: they would all be like a tree, with a trunk from the fertilized egg growing outward through time into many branches and twigs of differentiating tissues and organs.

The fate map of all creatures on Earth looks like the fate map of an embryo. It too begins at some point in time and space — the origin of DNA-and-protein-based life from replicating, catalytic bits of RNA — and grows through almost four billion years (four hundred years in our speeded-up world) into the full complexity of life on Earth today. The fate map of all species alive today is called a phylogenetic tree; it reflects countless specific interactions among species living and dead since life began.

The genomes of all cells in an embryo show a close to perfect resemblance to the genome of their initiating cell, the fertilized egg. Similarly but less perfectly, the genomes of all life on Earth show their descent from a common ancestral sequence. With so much more time for random mutation, DNA movement, and gene duplication, the sequences of species have diverged considerably from one organism to another, but they still show clear signs of their common descent. Proteins, for instance, come in what Ford Doolittle of Dalhousie

University in Canada has called first, second and recent editions. The genes for first-edition proteins are found in all cells; proteins that convert sugars to energy fall in this category. Second-edition proteins are found only in eukaryotes: examples are the histone proteins that wrap DNA for storage in the nucleus and the proteins that confer movement, like actin. Recent editions are found only in plants or in animals but not both: collagen and chlorophyll are examples. There are only about a thousand first-edition genes, each of them very old. Bacteria have one or only a few of each; in their place, the larger chromosomes of cells with nuclei have accumulated extensive families of related descendant genes.

Molecular-genetic fate maps and the phylogenetic tree are hierarchical, because all the branches on each trace back to a single starting point, and because at any level, all twigs on a branch share the attributes of that branch. We can see this in the way we are located on the phylogenetic tree: at the tip of our twiglet we stand alone as a species, *Homo sapiens*. Moving down the twiglet, we come to the twig our twiglet grew from, the genus *Homo*. All other species sharing this genus with us died some tens or hundreds of thousands of years ago. To indicate that the ancestor of all members of the genus *Homo* itself shared an earlier common ancestor with other creatures, we place the ancestor of *Homo* and all its descendant species in the family *hominidae*, the hominids. All other hominids, like all other members of the genus *Homo*, have long since died out. Our closest relatives among the living primates — that is, the ones with whom we share the most recent common ancestor among the extinct primates — are in the superfamily of *hominoidea*, made up of three families: the gibbons, the pongids (orangutans, gorillas, and chimpanzees), and the hominids (us).

We shared an ancestor with the apes, monkeys, and prosimians who did survive, and that shared ancestry puts us with them in the order primates. Primates share body characteristics like live birth, breasts, and hair with a large number of other animals; we indicate this older and broader shared ancestry by placing ourselves in the class *mammalia*, the mammals. Mammals in turn share a backbone with a spinal cord and other anatomical structures, including a common overall body plan, with a host of other animals; these shared characteristics put us in the phylum *chordata*, the chordates. Even earlier, chordates and all other many-celled animals — including the fruit fly, for instance — shared a common many-celled ancestor, and so we and they are all linked in the kingdom metazoa.

Metazoa share nucleated cells with the *metaphyta* or plants, the fungi, and the single-cell protists; creatures in these kingdoms are linked by common origin from the first cell to have a nucleus, which places us on the trunk of the phylogenetic tree in the superkingdom eukaryotes. Finally, we and all other living creatures, whether eukaryotes or prokaryotes without a nucleus, descend from the root of the tree, a common ancestral cell. Although the last of those cells died billions of years ago, we can be confident that the ancestral cell had the attributes that all cells retain to this day: a genome of DNA encoding a set of about a thousand first-edition enzymes to do the work of replication and metabolism, a genetic code, and an RNA-based translation apparatus.

The farther back toward the trunk we go on the phylogenetic tree, the earlier we are in the history of life. Until about six hundred million years ago — when the current phyla diverged — few living things left fossils. Reconstructing earlier chapters in the history of life is strictly a literary enterprise, dependent on the close analysis of conserved DNA sequences. Sequences that are conserved over the widest range of living things are current versions of the most ancient genes. The ribosome genes of our mitochondrial DNA, for example, have been used to confirm the initially controversial hypothesis of Lynn Margulis, of the University of Massachusetts, that symbiogenesis — a series of symbiotic invasions of one primordial cell by another — made possible the evolution of all subsequent eukaryotic life.

According to this hypothesis, more than two billion years ago a primordial purple bacterium set up a stable life inside a primitive eukaryotic cell; in time this bacteria and its descendants lost their freedom to live anywhere but inside another cell, thereby becoming the symbiotic ancestors of the mitochondria inside almost all eukaryotic cells alive today.* A subsequent seduction of eukaryotic cells by bacteria — this time blue-green ones, which could turn sunlight into sugars — gave the ancestor of today's green plants the beginnings of what would become chloroplasts. We can recover signs of these long-term symbiotic events — palimpsests like the Old Testament phrase in the line from James — because chloroplasts and mitochondria still retain genomic circles of DNA from the days when their ancestors were free-living bacteria, and these genomes still carry genes for their own ribosomes. Once the sequences of these genes could be compared with the sequences of ribosomal genes from the cells themselves and from various strains of bacteria, it quickly became evident that ribosomes of chloroplasts and mitochondria are not similar to the genes of any eukaryotic ribosomes. Rather, they most closely resemble the genes of certain bacteria that grow in hot, sulfurous springs, an environment evocative of one of life's more auspicious homes a few billion years ago.

The efforts to construct molecular-genetic fate maps — the trees of gene-regulatory pathways that accompany differentiation and development in a single plant or animal — and to recreate the phylogenetic tree of life on Earth are related in a simple way. Disparities of size and duration — individual organisms are smaller than the planet; individual lifetimes are shorter than the lifetimes of the species — have until recently kept these two fields from informing each other's efforts, but to obtain the fullest possible meaning of the individual genes they study, molecular biologists will have to know a gene's history and the roles played by homologous genes in other organisms. The Harvard geneticist Richard Lewontin caught the cusp of this in 1982, just as the tools of the molecular word processor were in their earliest stages of development: "The great evolutionist Theodosius Dobzhansky wrote that 'nothing in biology makes sense except in the light of evolution.' But

---

* An exception worth mentioning is the intestinal parasite *Giardia lamblia*, which has no mitochondria at all. Its nuclear genome diverges from all other eukaryotic genomes; *Giardia lamblia* is perhaps the sole descendant of a eukaryotic cell line that lived before the mitochondrial invasion.

we must add that 'nothing in human evolution makes sense except in the light of history.'"

A new, historical approach has already made itself felt in molecular biology: every newly sequenced piece of a genome is "looked up" by computer programs that use the fact of common descent to search for sequence homologies in a growing data bank of hundreds of millions of base pairs from hundreds of species. Coding sequences that have no homology with any known gene are increasingly rare, and it is possible that we may learn the vocabulary of regulatory domains before too long. In filling out these time-dependent, historical maps — the DNA and protein sequence analysis of homologies among DNAs, the phylogenetic reconstruction of relationships among all living creatures, and the molecular biology of development — some molecular biologists are already contributing to a more complete, historically informed biology.

At the same time, the mechanistic lines of inquiry that until recently defined molecular biology have increasingly become dependent on their utility and profitability rather than their intrinsic interest. While laboratories isolating genes associated with human disease or crop development remain magnetic attractors of private and government funds, the five hundredth such human gene hardly generates the buzz that heralded the first five. In place of the simple cloning and sequencing of a human gene, critical experiments now revolve around the use of transgenic mice to reveal the fullest possible meaning of the gene in the richest available context, and the centrality of the recovered gene itself has begun to be displaced by the possibility of creating — writing — a new version of it in our word processor, and then drawing out our own version's meaning in the transgenic context.

~

To see the world as a sphere covered in a thin skin of tissue called life, with a particular history that will not happen again, is to bring the variable of time to molecular biology and thus allow genomes, their encoded proteins, and the networks of regulation that bring these proteins into the world to be seen as natural creations sharing two properties with literature, art, and science itself: knowable pasts and unknowable futures. In the case of our own genome, time and evolution have led to the unbounded and unpredictable attributes of consciousness and language. Historically based molecular biology will want to understand the genomic contribution to these two uniquely human attributes. Acquiring this knowledge begins with a fuller understanding of the origin and history of our species, so let us return to the phylogenetic tree to see how we compare with our nearest neighbors.

The first hallmarks of a future that would include us are in ancestral mammals who lived at least two hundred million years ago. From that stock, mammals diversified — sometimes slowly, sometimes quickly, especially after the cataclysmic death of the dinosaurs sixty-five million years ago — into a set of about four thousand living species, different enough from each other to be placed in no fewer than fifteen different orders, including our own, primates. Recall that among primates, we share the most characteristics with other members of the hominoid superfamily of gibbons, orangutans, gorillas, and chimps. Our genomes and those of the great apes — particularly the African forms — are very similar, with more than 98 percent sequence homology between the genomes of chimp and human and not much less between human and gorilla or chimp and gorilla.

The last common ancestor of the living hominoids died off no later than ten million years ago, and for much of that time none of the hominoids were particularly human. About eight million years later — two million years ago — the first *Homo* species whose fossils we have found, *Homo habilis*, appeared and lived among other, smaller-brained cousins, the Australopithecenes. *Homo habilis* made tools, was about three feet high, and had a brain volume of about twenty-three ounces. In rather short order a bigger species, *Homo erectus*, appeared in Africa, in time supplanting *Homo habilis*, and spread to parts of Europe and Asia, living from about 1.8 million years ago until about four hundred thousand years ago. By then various strains of *Homo erectus* had grown to about six feet tall and had up to thirty-three-ounce brains.

The pace of change was accelerating: about three hundred thousand years ago, even the biggest and brainiest *H. erectus* had died off, and in their place we find the fossils of the first of our own species, archaic *Homo sapiens*. These early humans, with brains at least as large as ours at forty-five to fifty ounces, left a cultural heritage that includes the wonderful grave at Shanidar in Iran, in which an archaic *Homo sapiens* of the Neanderthal type was lovingly buried with flowers. Anatomically modern *Homo sapiens* first appeared in eastern Africa about a hundred thousand to a hundred and twenty-five thousand years ago and began migrating soon thereafter. Europe, Asia, and Africa saw many millennia of joint habitation by archaic and modern humans, but the Neanderthal people of Europe died off about forty thousand years ago, and we have been the lone members of the genus *Homo* ever since.

The molecular biological investigation that would help us understand many of the open questions in this history has only just begun. We do not know, for example, whether modern and archaic *Homo sapiens* ever interbred, nor in particular whether current Europeans carry any DNA sequences inherited from the Neanderthals. There is evidence, however, that modern *Homo sapiens* lived for some time in Africa before migrating north, west, and east to every continent beginning about a hundred and fifty thousand years ago, quickly establishing all races of humankind in the process. For example, certain stretches of mitochondrial DNA are more diverse in Africans than in people of any other continent, suggesting that their ancestors — who might have lived in Africa for some time before their great migration — had more time to accumulate allelic variations than did the small groups of migrating African ancestors who became today's Asians and Europeans. But the evidence is not conclusive, and some paleontological evidence supports the possibility that Europe and Asia — both possibly populated for a million or more years by descendants of the early migration of *Homo erectus* from Africa — were also the home of their own versions of archaic *Homo sapiens* before the second migration from Africa took place. In that case, some scientists have argued, the modern peoples of Europe and Asia might be the descendants, not only of the exodus of African *Homo sapiens*, but of separate, locally evolved versions of *Homo sapiens* as well. Molecular homologies fall on the side of the hypothesis that we are all the descendants of the second, more recent African exodus, but only barely, and much more work needs to be done to reconcile molecular with paleontological data.

Over the sweep of the thousand centuries since we began to establish ourselves on all the continents, modern *Homo sapiens* has been a remarkably promiscuous species. Many of our genes may exist in any of a number of different but functional alleles, and almost all normal alleles can be found — at various frequencies — in human chromosomes all over the planet. We have only begun to characterize the incidence of various alleles in genomes from representatives of the thousands of ethnic groups, but even this earliest work reveals that the genomes of today's Europeans are a hybrid intermediate between Asian and African ancestors. This could not be so unless mating occurred frequently among the ancestors of currently isolated groups of people. The genetic diversity between any two ethnic groups — quantified by measuring allelic frequencies — is usually small, relative to the diversity between individuals in one group. The result is clear: when it comes to our species, you really can't judge a genetic book by its cover. Molecular-historical biology has therefore already told us something important about our behavior as a species: despite our tendency to live or die by the dream that it might be so, none of us has come from a pure ethnic or racial stock.*

◇

In his private notebooks Darwin wrote, "Why is thought — being a secretion of the brain — more wonderful than gravity a property of matter[?] It is our arrogance, our admiration of ourselves." Perhaps, but this secretion has made it possible for a DNA-based life form to understand that it is constructed by a text written in an ancient language, and surely there is nothing more appropriate for students of DNA to learn than where in the genome the ability to comprehend any language resides.

---

* In any case, race is a cultural, not a biological, term when it is applied to our species. For instance, as a consequence of the period when African people were bought, sold, and bred as property, "white" people in the southern United States today have a higher frequency of alleles associated with people from Africa than do "white" Northerners or "white" Canadians.

Languages, tribes, and races are all relatively recent developments in our forty thousand years of uncontested survival as
the only hominid. Because the phylogenetic tree allows us to
use comparative anatomy to tell us about our past, we can see
how our survival may have depended on a new use of the lungs
and larynx for speech. The mouth of all primates feeds into
two tubes: one — which is joined by a path through the nose
— goes to the lungs; the other goes to the stomach. In other
primates, the epiglottis keeps the nose-lung pipe open while
directing the contents of the mouth to the stomach, allowing
them to eat and breathe at the same time. In humans, the
position and large size of the larynx — essential for speech —
prevent the epiglottis from separating the two pipes, so we can
choke if we eat and breathe at the same time. Fossil evidence
suggests that archaic *Homo sapiens* had the usual primate
epiglottis; it appears unlikely that the throat of a Neanderthal
could form a complex string of sounds. Our larynx is uniquely
placed to intervene in the flow of air from the lungs. Apparently the risk of choking was overridden by the benefits of
language when we shared the continents with archaic *Homo
sapiens*.

What in our genomes gives us language? When phylogenetic
relatedness is assessed by form, the degree of similarity between individuals or fossils can be measured by counting the
number of shared attributes, usually called characters. Molecular biology has had little to contribute to the notion of
characters; they may have a wide range of molecular complexity. A single base-pair difference may count as a character in
one study, whereas another study will consider the difference
between chimps who lack spoken language and humans who
have it to be one character. Since about four tenths of all the
messenger RNAs made from the human genome are made
only in the human brain, it is possible that a character such as
the ability to form languages has the molecular complexity of
tens of thousands of genes.

At least some of the human genes involved in creating language must be active in the assembly and operations of a small
sector of the human brain named for the scientist Paul Broca;
structures in this region are closely associated with the capacity to speak and understand a language and next to structures

involved in repetitive motions of the arms and fingers. Since we know that complex stone tools of the Achulean type were manufactured by *Homo erectus* as early as 1.4 million years ago, an appealing model for the origin of languages is pre-adaptive; that is, our facility for language may be the result of an evolved use of neural circuits selected in *Homo erectus* or its ancestors for their role in repetitive motions with tools.

Languages, as MIT's professor of linguistics Noam Chomsky was the first to show, are organized hierarchically, and comparative studies of the brains and behaviors of living primates support the notion that the Broca region of our last common ancestor directed complex, hierarchical manipulations of objects, a function it still serves in chimpanzees and in humans until about age two. Patricia Greenfield of the University of California has connected Chomsky's observation with data drawn from observing primate behavior to suggest that the function of the primate Broca region has always been to assemble hierarchies: first, hierarchies of manipulation for the body's hands; later, and only secondarily, hierarchies of linguistic structures for the organs of speech and hearing.

Most primates besides ourselves and the Old World apes have Broca regions that function like those of a one-year-old human child. In mature humans, chimps, and gorillas, the nerve cells of the Broca region are connected to areas of the brain that drive the hands, mouth, and tongue, permitting adult chimps and gorillas to make and use single tools. The Broca region in our brain is bigger than a chimp's, and it also makes connections to regions at the front of our brain that are lacking in chimps and other primates. From age two on, human brains develop neural circuits in and around the Broca region that confer the ability to assemble both complex languages and complex combinations of objects; chimpanzees lack this second cycle of postnatal development. Grown chimps, with Broca regions most like ours, can make a simple subassembly by combining two tools into a third. But only humans use tools to make a new tool and then use that in another assembly, in ever-deepening hierarchies of complexity. And while other primates have a rich vocabulary of purposeful sounds, only human languages organize words hierarchically, and only humans assemble words hierarchically to make a language, using words to make clauses, clauses to make sentences, and sentences to make arguments.

Persons unable to make full use of the human capacity for spoken language can use their Broca regions, their capacity for language, and their hands to communicate in the rich language of Sign. Deaf children raised by parents who use Sign develop their language skills through a formative period of the hand equivalent of babbling, and when Sign is used by a grown person, the Broca region — as well as the regions normally given over to hand movements — is activated in the brain. Small lesions in the human Broca region, though, can cause the loss of both hierarchical capacities: a man with such a lesion can assemble strings of words but no clauses or sentences; he will be able to put blocks in a row, but not to assemble structures from them.

Even as we begin to understand the biology of thought and language, we must acknowledge how little we know about the genomic contribution to consciousness. The frontal regions of our brain, in which abstract notions are processed and which through their connections to the Broca region drive our language skills, develop from a segment laid down in early embryonic development by a member of a family of genes containing homeoboxes. But which homeobox genes are most closely associated with the assembly of the frontal regions of the brain in humans? And did the duplication of a homeobox gene at the "head" of a family of genes, in an ancestral primate a few million years ago, set a primate line on the path to language, knowledge, and thought? Which genes are activated in the Broca region of the human brain, and the regions it feeds, as a two-year-old acquires grammatical language skills? We don't know the answers to any of these questions; it will be the task of a new generation of molecular neurobiologists, versed in the historical context of hominid evolution and the comparative anatomy and genetics of the primates, to search them out.

≈

A developing connection between genetics and linguistics gives rise to another, if less likely, series of questions for the new biology. Our myriad languages divide us, even as our capacity for language defines our common humanity. From the global vantage point we are a fractured species, separated by language into hundreds of groups. On every continent many — although not all — languages are wrapped in flags to signify that they have been elevated to the formal autonomy of nationhood. Given the shared power of language, why has our species chosen to separate itself into mutually uncomprehending tribes, states, nations, kingdoms, and empires? How did languages develop among us, separating us this way? Have languages affected our genomes? These hardly seem like questions for classical molecular biology, but if we want to know the history and the full meaning of the many alleles spread among our species, we will very likely need to know the history of the development of our languages from their beginnings. To begin, we might ask: why should the genomes of people speaking different languages be different?

The words of a particular language are arbitrary; it is only necessary that all who speak it agree on their meanings. Let us assume that all living people are the descendants of ancestors who lived in Africa for some long period and that these ancestors used the anatomical and mental capacities of *Homo sapiens* to speak a language. As these ancestors migrated outward to populate Turkey, the Middle East, Europe, Asia, and later Polynesia, Australia, and the Americas, physical separation would have allowed "speciation" of languages: the language spoken in each newly reached, isolated part of the world would have been free to change in ways that might easily render it incomprehensible to the people occupying a different range or continent. Dispersion and lack of contact with other people would therefore be accompanied by the evolution of different languages. In their search for the hypothetical tree of ancestry for languages, linguists who analyze the degree of homology of two languages by comparison of phonemes, words, and grammars have already found evidence for the evolution of languages from common ancestors. As with the phylogenetic tree, however, the further back the splitting, the more difficult to reconstruct the ancestral tongue.

The languages of Europe have been particularly carefully analyzed, and the results suggest that the people of Europe continued to fragment and refragment into noncommunicat-

ing groups well after the hunter-gatherer tribes that first populated the continent were supplanted by farmers. English, for
example, is one of about a hundred languages that have split
from the language — called Proto-Indo-European — spoken by
the first modern humans to arrive on the European continent.
As Proto-Europeans spread west about eight thousand years
ago from what is now Turkey to Greece, then north to what
are now the Slavic and German-speaking lands, then west and
south again to what are now the Latin countries, their language split into mutually incomprehensible dialects over and
over again.

The first offspring languages are — like the progenitors of
phylogenetic orders — long since dead: Anatolian, Aryano-
Greco-Armenian, Celto-Italo-Tocharian, and Balto-Slavo-Ger-
manic. Each became the parent of many languages. Balto-
Slavo-Germanic, for instance, was replaced in various parts of
northern Europe by Balto-Slavic, Northern Germanic, and
Western Germanic, three dead languages that kept the ancient
peoples of northern Europe divided into mutually uncomprehending regions. More recently, the territory of Western Germanic speakers divided further, into regions speaking English,
Flemish, Dutch, Low German, and High German; one of these
regions later acquired the trappings of a nation-state. In two of
the most recent bifurcations, High German and Yiddish split
about a thousand years ago, Dutch and Afrikaans about three
hundred years ago. In all these examples, and in all the other
cases we might examine anywhere on the planet, the appearance of new languages signaled the separation of a group of
people into mutually uncomprehending subgroups, a process
that has gone on since our emergence as a species.

Proto-Indo-European is just one branch — and not even a
major one — on the tree of languages. Just as our genomes
contain many genes with domains derived from a small number of ancient, first-edition genes whose initial functions were
too important ever to be lost by any living cell, so can some of
our words still be traced back to the speakers of our species'
first language, called Proto-World. In both cases the principle
of conservation is the same: the sequences — genes, domains,
or words — that are most widely distributed among today's
species or languages are the ones likely to have existed at the

earliest stages in the formation of the evolutionary tree. For example, the words *haku* and *hita* in Proto-World changed hardly at all to *haku* and *-ita* in Nostratic, the precursor of Proto-Indo-European, then became *hakw* and *hed* in Proto-Indo-European, *aqua* and *edere* in Latin, *wazzan* and *ezzan* in Old German, and "water" and "eat" in English. At the same time but in another part of the world, in Amerind — the root language of many indigenous North and South American peoples — the words again hardly changed from Proto-World, becoming *hakw* and *hit-*.

Once groups of early people separated completely from one another by migration through continents devoid of other humans, neither their languages nor their alleles could be exchanged, so allele frequencies as well as languages were likely to diverge. When Luigi Cavalli-Sforza of Stanford University examined the amino acid and base-pair sequence differences for a set of proteins in representatives of human cultures from all over the planet, he found that people whose languages are known to have separated more recently from a common ancestral language have fewer sequence differences in their alleles than people whose languages have been apart for a very long time.

The initial appearance of separate languages can be explained as the result of the physical isolation of separate migrating bands of hunters and farmers, but why did languages and genomes continue to diverge once people began to share the same territories? When a group of people live in the same region and intermarry over a long period, they will share the same allele frequencies for multi-allelic genes; this sharing is called gene flow. When different allele frequencies appear in a population — whether by random drift or, as with sickle-cell anemia, in an adaptive response to a local change in the environment — they can be maintained only if gene flow is very limited. The link between our languages and our genomes turns out to be simple: language differences are a powerful constraint on the selection of a spouse and therefore a barrier to gene flow.

Because languages keep groups of people in genetic isolation from one another, separate languages preserve local concentrations of alleles that contribute to differences in appearance.

Once this occurs, language and appearance mutually reinforce a positive feedback loop that drives our species into an ever larger number of groups of ever more different-looking people. Not even nations, with all their powers to set boundaries and wage war, are as effective at keeping people apart as languages; nationalism based on language is therefore a particularly powerful way to enforce isolation, even though xenophobia may be a common consequence.

Robert Sokal, at the State University of New York in Stony Brook, has shown how efficient languages are at preserving differences in alleles. He examined the genomes of people from all over Europe, measuring the frequencies of 63 alleles of 19 genes at more than three thousand locales. He discovered that in 33 places in Europe, allele frequencies changed very sharply across short distances, which he called boundaries. Some 22 boundaries were mapped onto barriers that might be expected to keep gene flow down by simple physical isolation: 18 were oceanic and 4 were mountainous. But the most striking barrier was neither rock nor water but language: 9 allele boundaries overlaid no physical boundary but only a linguistic one, 31 of the 33 boundaries separated linguistic families or dialects, and 27 were zones of contact of ethnic groups that had originated far from one another. For example, an allelic boundary in Iceland traveled along terrain separating the regions of Iceland settled by immigrants from Norway and Ireland, a migration that ended a thousand years ago. Unlike the preservation of the sickle-cell allele in malarial regions, such allelic boundaries cannot be the result of adaptation to a specific environment. Instead, they provide strong evidence for the inherent capacity of language differences to preserve and widen genetic differences by inhibiting gene flow.

Studies on languages and alleles have brought us full circle: the human capacity for many languages has had consequences for the genome that confers it. The future development of studies on the genomic contribution to the capacity for language, and the linguistic contribution to genomic differences, will make this branch of molecular biology into a behavioral science. But at the same time, molecular techniques have given us the capacity to be far more intrusive than any other branch of behavioral science: we also have the capacity to change alleles in human DNA by direct intervention, adding a fateful, prognostic voice to the language-intensive but otherwise free choice of two people to have a child.

∾

The years that end and begin millennia are notable numbers, deep reminders of our temporary place in the long passage of time. They make us take notice of where we are, the way we do when all the little wheels on our car's odometer turn, as 19,999 becomes 20,000 miles. At the end of the last millennium, the world that kept measure by a Christian calendar awaited apocalypse and the end of days. As this millennium draws to a close on a planet of many religions but — from convenience if not faith — one calendar, a sense of foreboding has reappeared at a critical time in the study of three of the planet's most interesting histories — of life, of *Homo sapiens*, and of language. Since their basic texts are genomic, all three histories will remain obscure until molecular biologists develop their skills at genomic analysis. But as we approach the third millennium, it is apparent that our species, fragmented among nations, has done serious, long-term damage to the earth's capacity to support life itself, so portions of the basic texts carrying these three histories are at risk of being lost before we have even opened them.

As Edward O. Wilson of Harvard details in *The Diversity of Life*, the loss of tropical rain forest in the 1980s has meant the loss of about 1 in 200 species every year. Though precise estimates are difficult to get, it seems clear that each day — as about a quarter of a million new humans join the five billion of us already here — at least a hundred of Earth's five million to fifty million species disappear.* In the last decades of this millennium, a political movement to halt and reverse ecologi-

---

* The broad range in estimates of the number of different species tells us how much work remains to be done before we can claim to have even the outlines of a record of life's diversity. While forms visible to the eye have been catalogued for centuries, new species still remain to be discovered in remote areas, and the terrain of microscopic life remains largely unmapped: a spadeful of soil taken anywhere is almost certain to contain unreported species of microbes.

cal degradation and the loss of species has developed in response to these facts, as people in many countries of the world — speaking many languages, governed in many ways, and worshiping many gods — begin to see the need to think and act as members of one among many species in order not to ruin our common planetary home.

To sectors of this environmental movement, all science is at best a mixed blessing. In their terms, the planet's troubles arose in the first place as one branch of science after another lost sight of its supposed reason for being — the careful elucidation of nature's ways — to serve instead a perverse variant of Jeremy Bentham's utilitarianism, the production of greater piles of goods for greater numbers of people. The result of one final century of belching smokestacks and burgeoning populations, they argue, is a planet that shows signs of serious discomfort with us: a burned-out ozone layer, a blanket of warming carbon dioxide changing our climate, poisonous metals and bits of our Styrofoam coffee cups in the deepest oceans, and so forth. This view of the future can be carried too far, until it becomes a modern version of the blood and soil romanticism of the last century, a fundamentalist revulsion with science and technology that portrays our planet as a single, living organism so glutted and clogged with the outpourings of our technology as to be infected, rather than populated, by us. But environmental activists who have taken the trouble to study the sciences of ecology and evolution and who have at least an acquaintance with their biological, geological, and chemical underpinnings see that while we humans are a problem for the planet, all of us (even the scientists) belong here too. These environmentalists know that our species is but one of many, with no more right to a place on the planet than any other, but certainly no less; and they call on scientists to protect our common and only home in the ways each of us knows best.

The classic molecular biology that studies the mechanisms of the action of specific genes and proteins will not cease — nor will it necessarily be overrun or supplanted — because some molecular biologists see in the richness of DNA texts a new reason to speak out in defense of the preservation of species diversity. But the longer molecular biology clings to its paradigm of physics and keeps itself aloof from matters of history, the more likely it will be that the loss of genetic variation — in food crops, in wild animals, in the millions of unrecorded species, and in our own species — will degrade and destroy just those undiscovered DNA sequences that might have led to a more complete comprehension of our own genes and genomes.

The loss of species by deforestation and other human activities is as pivotal a threat to new molecular biology as the pillaging of Alexandria's library or the burning of books by Hitler's university students were to the enterprise of history itself. As we enter the next millennium, historically grounded molecular biology and scientifically informed environmentalism will find their common ground — if both are alert and flexible enough to grasp the opportunity — in a shared view of the world as a single home for us all and of us all as part of a single human family.

⁓

Once molecular biologists accept the central importance of preserving and studying the diversity of genomes — some because they are interested in the new questions to be asked of these historical texts; others because human genomes are the only source of nature's experiments on human genes — they will see the need to stem the loss of indigenous peoples and languages. Whether an indigenous people become victims of war or economic casualties or they themselves choose to join a larger society, once they are lost, a portion of the human genome's complete library of drafts — some novel assortments of alleles, perhaps even some novel alleles as well — can never be recovered. While the Human Genome Project labors to harvest a single allelic sequence for one consensus human genome, others are more interested in the diversity of our species' genomes than in acquiring any one version of it. Luigi Cavalli-Sforza, Kenneth Kidd of Yale, and the late Alan Wilson of the University of California informally began what they call the Human Genomes Project a few years ago, a far-flung effort to collect blood samples and DNA from members of vanishing indigenous peoples around the world. Their work has cost very little and gained hardly any of the visibility of the Human

Genome Project, but in time their archive will be appreciated as the first international attempt to preserve our genomic inheritance.

The genomic archive at Yale is just the beginning: a new generation of molecular historians will see the attraction of collaborating with environmentalists in the establishment of a fundamental database, a planetary encyclopedia of genomes. This encyclopedia would be a collection of genomes — prepared as DNA libraries, referenced by PCR — of representative members of the diverse species that live above, on, and in the earth's continents and oceans. Many countries already have museums of natural history, private and public institutions charged with assembling and maintaining collections of creatures great and small. With PCR as a magnifier of bits and pieces of DNA, and with homology between living and dead species as a guide to the synthesis of proper primers, museum collections also offer us a chance to recover portions of genomes from extinct species. DNA sequences have been recovered from the feathers and skin and seeds of dried, pickled, and stuffed specimens of now-extinct species, but PCR — which can amplify short stretches of mitochondrial DNA from insects trapped in fossilized amber a hundred million years ago — has barely been brought to most collections.

While the bodies and tissues of specimens often cannot be easily moved from one museum to another, DNA libraries are as portable as CDs, and transliterated sequences are as light as bytes. Molecular biology makes its home today in universities, medical centers, government laboratories, and private companies. As museums change the way they gather, maintain, characterize, and share their collections, they will join with and perhaps one day regain their preeminence among the venues for the humane but scientific study of life.

∾

What lies ahead for molecular biology? It would be paradoxical to have argued that the biological future is not predictable, only to predict the future of biology. But extrapolations from current research can serve to sharpen the issues that all of us — not just scientists, but also citizens, voters, parents, and children — will have to face. Molecular biology, like any other science, has been guided by little more than the tastes and drives of its practitioners. A new, broader context will take hold only if the best of today's scientists see the historical paradigm as a source of new questions worthy of their attention. But in this period of adjustment — between paradigms, as it were — molecular biologists have a rare chance to think again of the possible consequences of their work before they go too far up an expensive blind alley or down a road that leaves the rest of us facing a mess we neither asked for nor know how to control.

Consider, for instance, the kind of information that might come out of a merger of DNA analysis with twin studies. Scientists who compare identical with fraternal twins have shown that the inherited component of any complicated human difference — in height, say, or musical ability, or sexual preference, or intelligence — is usually the consequence of allelic differences in many genes. Until recently, it was impractical to untangle such complex patterns of inheritance. But with the power of PCR and with increasingly facile computer programs, it will soon be possible to identify and analyze the particular alleles that all members of a family carry for hundreds of different genes and DNA marker sequences. As researchers apply the techniques of DNA analysis to the genomes of identical twins and their families, we have reason to expect they will extend the work of scientists like Dean Hamer to discover sets of DNA sequences that correlate with just the attributes listed above.

Recall that Craig Venter has obtained thousands of partial sequences from messenger RNAs expressed specifically by portions of our brains. Venter's many sequences make excellent and appropriate probes for these studies, and no technological barrier would prevent them from eventually being applied in IVF preimplantation analysis as well. Here is how Nick Martin, a scientist engaged in these studies in Brisbane, Australia, sees the immediate future, in a recent interview in *Science* magazine:

Martin believes the same approach could be used with genes for IQ and personality. "I can't wait to get into it," he says.

And although a practical application for such research is now a "pie in the sky," says Martin, it is exactly the kind of work that could lead to such *Brave New World* activities as measuring the precise genetic makeup of children so that the teaching environment could be tailored to shape their development efficiently.

By the light of such Panglossian eagerness, the importance of the new paradigm in biology is apparent: seeing all the living world's DNA as a set of historically related texts is less hazardous — as well as more accurate — than seeing it as a vastly complicated set of molecules from which laws may be derived, personality traits decoded, or new ways found to "measure the precise genetic makeup of children." No serious historian expects the historical record to yield rules that predict the behavior of a person or the course of history, but biology has all too often provided scientific cover for those who would write such rules into laws governing our behavior, even though every claim to have found such laws in science has turned out to be premature, and some have also provided excuses for terrible, lethal behavior.

My generation of molecular biologists has already come upon the temptations and risks of molecular eugenics, embodied by the development of technologies for intervention in human reproduction on a mass scale. Here, for example, is a description of one component of the procedures used in a 1989 study published in the prestigious British medical journal *Lancet*, "Biopsy of Human Preimplantation Embryos and Sexing by DNA Amplification":

> After approval of the project by the ethics committee of the Royal Postgraduate Medical School and the Voluntary Licensing Authority for Human in Vitro Fertilization and Embryology, patients were approached at least one month before proposed IVF for tubal infertility to ascertain whether they would consider donating "surplus" embryos, if available as a consequence of their treatment, for studies aimed at better diagnosis of genetic disease.

That is, women waiting for IVF were asked to give over extra eggs for experimental fertilization, and the resulting embryos were then used to establish that PCR could differentiate male from female embryos. This study was "aimed at better diagnosis of genetic disease," only because the authors intended to use their procedure to identify — not implant — the IVF boys of mothers carrying X-linked mutations.

As this example suggests, we are only just beginning to see what may lie ahead: the direct, eugenic selection permitted by IVF (whether negative selection through assay for problematic alleles or positive selection through transgenic IVF); the development of a molecular pharmacology for controlling human sexuality; or the allelic fingerprinting of everyone at birth for purposes related to bearing or raising children. All these procedures will undoubtedly be proposed with great enthusiasm in the coming years, but once they are seen in the light of the human genome's global impenetrability, these dead ends of an old paradigm will appear as wrong, and as dangerous, and as the establishment of separate culture vessels for alphas and betas in the *Brave New World* of Huxley or the numbering of people by a tattoo on their arms in the real world of German concentration camps.

The genome's indeterminacy provides us with an appealing alternative: to see DNA as literature. One of the best definitions of literature comes from the Italian novelist Italo Calvino; in his *Six Memos for the Next Millennium*, Calvino tried to characterize the essence of great literature. His prescription for the literature of the twenty-first century included five qualities: lightness, quickness, exactitude, visibility, and multiplicity. As it happens, the genome of a person has all of these qualities in abundance. It is light because it is as small as the rigors of natural selection permit. It is quick because it must be: the life of a cell is short, and the entire text of the genome must be copied in a few hours; in the case of an embryo, the genomic text must make a person ready for the world — starting from a single cell — in only a few months. It is exact because its base sequences and the proteins they encode create the specificity of surfaces that gives living things their distinctive complexity and efficiency in a disordered universe. It is visible because cells, the genome's readers, assemble into a living thing from its instructions. But above all, the human genome is multiple. We are different from one another, and this allows the DNA texts within us to carry the infinite multiplicity of possibility in human character and, most especially, in the hopes we have for our children.

Calvino himself saw a necessary connection between science and literature. As he wrote in *Six Memos*:

> Only if poets and writers set themselves tasks that no one else dares imagine will literature continue to have a function. Since science has begun to distrust general explanations and solutions that are not sectorial and specialized, the grand challenge for literature is to be capable of weaving together the various branches of knowledge, the various "codes," into a manifold and multifaceted vision of the world.

In DNA, nature has created a manifest and multifaceted text. Once we finally see that all genomes are a form of literature, we will be able to approach them properly, as a library of the most ancient, precious, and deeply important books. Only then can the new biology be born.

CONCLUSION

LESS THAN A DECADE after the ashes of the Second World War had cooled, James Watson and Francis Crick were making tin and paper models of DNA and uncovering the set of laws that govern all inheritance. Since then we have come to understand that DNA is a chemical text that instructs our bodies in all their operations while copying itself so faithfully that these instructions can be passed from generation to generation, enabling life to persist on our planet. These discoveries have revolutionized biology, and the study of genetics is now so complex and ambitious that it has spilled beyond the boundaries of science: human chromosomes, and the information carried by their DNA, will increasingly guide and perhaps even direct our politics as well as our research in the next century. Meanwhile, some of the deepest assumptions of a free society — each of us is an individual; each of us has a private life; we are all equal under the law — have once again been called into question by the work of biologists. The risks posed by investigations into the workings of the human genome come from nineteenth-century notions of eternal progress through science, this time linked to a new and extraordinary power to change inheritance through the reordering of DNA.

Earlier in this century, physicists were lucky enough to have two decades in which to recast the paradigm of their field and then pursue their discoveries while still inside a cocoon of ostensibly pure, objective science, above human frailty, beyond petty politics, motivated by curiosity and intellectual adventure alone. Though the context of their work changed, they managed to preserve the context of their profession. That they ultimately did not live up to their own professional standards of distance and objectivity — the atomic bomb was as much the work of American physicists as were the theories that allowed them to design it; the expedient anti-Semitism of physicists in Germany canceled the lead German physics had enjoyed in the decades before the war — did not keep them from passing those standards on to us. The idea that scientists ought to work at a remove from the concerns of common humanity remains powerful indeed.

Molecular biologists ought not to repeat their mistake. Somehow, by a grace I do not understand, we have not thrown the switch of nuclear war a second time in the past half century. In this period of grace we have developed the capacity to read, to edit, to rewrite, and perhaps to begin to understand our DNA texts. If we can give ourselves the time, our genomes will together teach us that we are all profoundly related, that we are all one human family. Abandoning hope of final closure on the language meaning of the human genome, future molecular biologists will be free to be critics and historians, expert at multiple interpretations, even able to go back and forth between the white lab coat and the jacket of a critical scholar or the blue suit of a public servant. My colleagues have never had a better opportunity to become engaged in the political, economic, and social consequences of our science, setting a new example by taking responsibility for the larger results of our research, along with credit for the results themselves.

∾

But time is short. Biomedical science is about to change whether or not scientists choose to help steer a new course. The fundamental premise of molecular biology — that any question about a living thing can be answered, any disease understood and eradicated, by learning the detailed interactions of appropriate DNAs, RNAs, and proteins — has grown from an optimistic research strategy to the dominant agenda of a multibillion-dollar research juggernaut. Preventive medicine, public health, and universal education about the workings of the human body have all been overshadowed by the dream that cures for all diseases would flow from an understanding of their molecular mechanisms. The conquests of molecular biology have been many, but in their frothy wake, many implicit promises have gone unmet. Newborn children die in the United States more frequently than they do in more than a dozen other countries, including many that spend far less per person on health care than we do; cancer is not diminishing as a cause of death; and after a decade and billions of dollars, the fact that HIV is more clearly understood as a molecular entity than any other animal virus is small solace to the million Americans who are infected with it or the many millions more who have lost a friend or relative to AIDS.

Molecular biologists have two choices. They can continue working out the meanings of individual genes, going into business for themselves with the discoveries they have made in tax-supported laboratories, shortcutting peer review using news conferences and patent secrecy, taking tax money from their forty million fellow Americans who cannot afford any health insurance at all, and ignoring any potential eugenic uses of their work. Or they can begin to rethink what it is they do and why they do it. An agenda for the next stage of molecular biology is going to be assembled before this century is out, in any event, because the various groups who can pay for basic research — government agencies, agribusiness and pharmaceutical firms, the military, the criminal justice apparatus, would-be eugenicists — need one in order to make their own plans.

These groups will set the future of molecular biology to suit their purposes unless the scientists who would find themselves constrained to carry it out choose to join the debate. The dream of pure and unfettered research is ultimately dangerous; despite the hopes of some of its brightest practitioners, the path of a science — or at least of the science I know — is not self-correcting. Only by openly sharing concerns with others and asking for the broadest possible audience to help set its agenda can science meet its responsibilities to the society that supports it.

∾

I am not sophisticated about music, but when I find something that speaks to me, I listen to it over and over again. Once, as this book was reaching its final state, I heard in Beethoven's Triple Concerto an argument I had been struggling to formulate in words. Beginning with the few genes that are transcribed in the very first cells of an embryo, our bodies play their genomes as if they were instruments playing a concerto or a symphony. Like the Triple Concerto, these melodies of transcription and translation start quietly and simply, then build, interweave, and modulate one another until with a great thumping there is just silence. It follows that since few scientists are Beethovens, the rest of us had best be careful not to bring discord into the wonderfully rich scores that play in each of us every moment of our lives.

The fear of fateful discordances runs deep in our literature. In Part Two of *Faust*, Goethe shows the devil Mephistopheles as a creative if difficult scientist whose research includes a line of experimentation with in vitro homunculi that should by now be startlingly familiar: "Much have I seen, in wandering to and fro, Including crystallized humanity." After being led through many fine experiments by Mephistopheles, Dr. Faust dies a blind fool, thinking he is directing his technicians to produce new crops when in fact he is among zombies who dig his grave. But even as he dies, Faust is busy imagining the culmination of his research plans, sure that if he could make them work, his reputation as a scientist would be secure.

On the other hand, Goethe himself, in conversations recorded by his friend Eckermann, tells us the importance and value of our inability to completely understand his *Faust* and, by extension, why we should not expect to completely understand our genomes: "In such compositions what really matters is that the single masses should be clear and significant, while the whole remains incommensurable; and by that very reason, like an unsolved problem, draws mankind to study it again and again." The issue we face today is whether molecular biology will accept the insights of Goethe or continue to imitate his creations, Mephistopheles and Dr. Faust.

Dr. Faust was only one of a long line of talented but dangerous scientists brought to life in fiction over the years. Many think of Mary Shelley's Dr. Frankenstein — who assembled the parts of corpses into a failed human — as the worst of them and consider his monster the ultimate vision of biomedical science gone awry. But H. G. Wells, a scientifically well-informed writer of the next generation, created in *The Island of Dr. Moreau* a far more chilling and believable vision of the molecular biologist at home in a horrible world of his own making.

Isolated on his island, Dr. Moreau has no wish to touch another person, dead or alive. Instead, he cuts and tweaks the bodies and minds of beasts until they become semihuman. They worship and fear him as their Creator; he modestly accepts this as fitting. But in his experiments on transspecies tissue differentiation the animal sometimes prevails, and once it does, the reverted beasts destroy the doctor, his laboratory, and all else but Prendick, the surviving witness left to tell the tale. Here is how Dr. Moreau explains himself to Prendick:

> "You see, I went on with this research just the way it led me. That is the only way I ever heard of research going. I asked a question, devised some method of getting an answer, and got — a fresh question. Was this possible, or that possible? You cannot imagine what this means to an investigator, what an intellectual passion grows upon him. You cannot imagine the strange colorless delight of these intellectual desires. The thing before you is no longer an animal, a fellow creature, but a problem . . ."
>
> "But," said I, "the thing is an abomination — "
>
> "To this day I have never troubled about the ethics of the matter. The study of Nature makes man at last as remorseless as Nature . . . Each time I dip a living creature into the bath of burning pain, I say, This time I will burn out all the animal, this time I will make a rational creature of my own. After all, what is ten years? Man has been a hundred thousand in the making."

Beyond H. G. Wells and Dr. Moreau, there is of course Aldous Huxley, whose *Brave New World* casts such long shadows over the future of molecular biology. Huxley revisited that book's terrain twenty years after it appeared — soon after the structure of DNA was discovered — and came to this conclusion:

An education for freedom (and for love and intelligence which are at once the conditions and the results of freedom) must be, among other things, an education in the proper uses of language. . . . [This education should teach] the value, first of all, of individual freedom, based on the facts of human diversity and genetic uniqueness; the value of charity and compassion, based on the old familiar fact, lately rediscovered by psychiatry, the fact that, whatever their mental and physical diversity, love is as necessary to human beings as food or shelter; and finally, the value of intelligence, without which love is impotent and freedom unattainable.

Perhaps the first task of the education that Huxley describes is to teach all of us that to be born mortal with a mind that can imagine perfection or immortality is a cruel joke of nature. My colleagues and I can outwit this devil of our imagination, not by serving it, but by understanding that despite their imperfections our children — the world's children — are the only immortality we are allowed. As characters in the literature of DNA, we must work to preserve their futures while we can.

FURTHER READING

The following four lists of references should make it easy to learn more about the subjects and issues of this book. The first is a selection of general textbooks and reviews; the second a collection of books I found particularly helpful while writing this book; the third, four lists covering the main topics of this book; and the last, a collection of important, primary references from scientific journals arranged by chapter.

GENERAL REFERENCES

After fifteen years, the best book for the general reader on the history of molecular biology is still Judson's *Eighth Day of Creation*. For a closer and more recent — but dryer — look at the subject, I recommend Darnell's hefty textbook, *Molecular Cell Biology*. Revised every few years, this single volume captures the excitement of a fast-moving science through its lucid descriptions and colorful illustrations.

The other biology textbooks — Alberts, de Duve, Holtzman, Miklos, and Watson — are each somewhat more specialized than Darnell, but all are easy to find and worth the effort to read. While all biology texts discuss evolution, it is the central theme in Gould, King, Lewontin, Strickberger, and Tattersall. Likewise, Kandel and Gregory are good sources of detailed science concerning the mind and brain, and Miller is an excellent source of information on language. The beautiful pictures in Pauling and Morrison nicely complement the sometimes dense prose of any textbook.

Alberts, B., et al., 1990. *Molecular biology of the cell*, 2d ed. New York: Garland.

Darnell, J., et al., 1990. *Molecular cell biology*, 2d ed. New York: W. H. Freeman.

de Duve, C., 1984. *A guided tour of the living cell*. San Francisco: Freeman.

Gould, S. J., 1977. *Ontogeny and phylogeny*. Cambridge: Belknap Press of Harvard University Press.

Gregory, R. L., ed., 1987. *The Oxford companion to the mind*. New York: Oxford University Press.

Holtzman, E., and A. Novikoff, 1984. *Cells & organelles*, 3d ed. Philadelphia: Saunders.

Judson, H. F., 1979. *The eighth day of creation*. New York: Simon and Schuster.

Kandel, E., and J. Schwartz, 1981. *Principles of neural science*. New York: Elsevier.

King, J. C., 1981. *The biology of race*. Los Angeles: University of California Press.

Lewontin, R., 1982. *Human diversity*. New York: Scientific American Books, W. H. Freeman.

Miklos, D., and G. Freyer, 1990. *DNA science: A first course in recombinant DNA technology*. Cold Spring Harbor, N.Y.: Cold Spring Harbor Laboratory Press.

Miller, G., 1991. *The science of words*. New York: Freeman–Scientific American.

Morrison, P., P. Morrison, and the Office of C. Eames, 1982. *Powers of ten*. San Francisco: Scientific American Press of W. H. Freeman.

Pauling, L., and R. Hayward, 1964. *The architecture of molecules*. San Francisco: W. H. Freeman.

Strickberger, M., 1989. *Evolution*. Boston: Jones and Bartlett.

Tattersall, I., et al., 1986. *Encyclopedia of human evolution and prehistory*. New York: Garland.

Watson, J. D., et al., 1987. *Molecular biology of the gene*. Menlo Park, Calif.: Benjamin/Cummings.

BOOKS TO READ

These are the books from which I have drawn some of my arguments. Many — Dante, Darwin, Gamow, Goethe, Huxley, Koestler, Kuhn, Orwell, Solzhenitsyn, Schrödinger, Watson, Wells — are classics, either of the general culture or of science. The more recent remainder — Calvino, Chatwin, Crick, Edelman, Gore, Gould, Jacob, Rosenfield, Thomas, and Wilson — are likely to be of equally lasting importance.

Calvino, I., 1988. *Six memos for the next millennium.* Cambridge: Harvard University Press.

Chatwin, B., 1988. *The songlines.* New York: Penguin.

Crick, F. R. C., 1988. *What mad pursuit.* New York: Basic Books.

Dante Alighieri, 1954. *The inferno.* Translated by J. Ciardi, reprinted 1982. New York: Signet.

Darwin, Charles, 1859. *The origin of species.* London: John Murray. Reprint, New York: Penguin Classics, 1984.

Edelman, G., 1992. *Bright air, brilliant fire.* New York: Basic Books.

Gamow, G., 1947. *One, two, three . . . infinity.* New York: Viking Press.

Goethe, J., 1975. *Faust.* Translated by Philip Wayne. London: Penguin.

Gore, A., 1992. *Earth in the balance.* Boston: Houghton Mifflin.

Gould, S. J., 1981. *The mismeasure of man.* New York: Norton.

Huxley, A., 1932. *Brave new world.* Reprinted 1989. New York: Harper & Row.

———, 1958. *Brave new world revisited.* Reprinted 1989. New York: Harper & Row.

Jacob, F., 1982. *The logic of life.* New York: Random House.

Koestler, A., 1941. *Darkness at noon.* New York: Macmillan.

Kuhn, T., 1962. *The structure of scientific revolutions.* International Encyclopedia of Unified Science 2, reprinted 1970. Chicago: University of Chicago Press.

Orwell, G., 1949. *1984.* London: Martin Secker and Warburg.

Rosenfield, I., 1992. *The strange, familiar and forgotten.* New York: Knopf.

Schrödinger, E., 1944. *What is life?* Cambridge, Eng.: Cambridge University Press. Reprint, Cambridge, Eng.: Cambridge University Press, 1988.

Snow, C. P., 1959. *The two cultures and the scientific revolution.* Cambridge, Eng.: Cambridge University Press.

Solzhenitsyn, A., 1968. *The first circle.* New York: Harper & Row.

Thomas, L., 1974. *Lives of a cell.* New York: Viking.

———, 1983. *The youngest science.* New York: Viking.

Watson, J. D., 1968. *The double helix.* New York: Atheneum. Reprint, New York: Norton Critical Edition, ed. G. Stent, 1980.

Wells, H. G., 1984 (reprint). *The island of Dr. Moreau.* New York: Signet.

Wilson, E. O., 1992. *The diversity of life.* Cambridge: Harvard University Press.

SPECIALIZED BACKGROUND BOOKS

These four sets of books each delve into specifics of one of the four major topics of this book: molecular biology and genetics, evolution and the history of life on earth, the nature and history of language, and the politics of medicine and science. The politics — or, to the fastidious, the ethics — of medical science is a booming subject in its own right; by far the greatest number of books in these lists are ones that attempt to map the boundaries of this branch of science.

Molecular Biology and Genetics

Alberts, B., ed., 1988. *Mapping and sequencing the human genome.* Washington, D.C.: National Research Council, National Academy of Sciences.

Bonner, J. T., 1974. *On development.* Cambridge: Harvard University Press.

Brandon, L., 1991. *Introduction to protein structure.* New York: Garland Press.

Buchsbaum, R., 1948. *Animals without backbones.* Chicago: University of Chicago Press.

de Pomerai, D., 1985. *From gene to animal.* Cambridge, Eng.: Cambridge University Press.

Gierasch, L., and J. King, eds., 1990. *Protein folding.* Washington, D.C.: AAAS.

Keller, E., 1983. *A feeling for the organism.* New York: W. H. Freeman.

Krimsky, S., 1983. *Genetic alchemy.* Cambridge: MIT Press.

Levine, A. J., ed., 1992. *Tumor suppressor genes, the cell cycle and cancer.* Cold Spring Harbor, N.Y.: Cold Spring Harbor Laboratory Press.

National Research Council, 1992. *DNA technology in forensic science.* National Academy of Sciences Press.

Office of Technology Assessment, 1988. *Mapping our genes: Genome projects, how big, how fast?* Baltimore: Johns Hopkins University Press.

Office of Technology Assessment, 1992. *A new technological era for American agriculture.* Washington, D.C.: U.S. Congress.

Office of Technology Assessment, 1992. *Cystic fibrosis and DNA tests: Implications of carrier screening.* Washington, D.C.: U.S. Congress.

Pollack, R., 1981. *Readings in mammalian cell culture,* 2d ed. Cold Spring Harbor, N.Y.: Cold Spring Harbor Press.

Tooze, J., ed., 1980. *Molecular biology of tumor viruses.* Cold Spring Harbor, N.Y.: Cold Spring Harbor Press.

Evolution and the History of the Earth

Albritton, C. C., Jr., 1980. *The abyss of time.* San Francisco: Freeman, Cooper. Reprint, Los Angeles: Tarcher, 1986.

Clapham, W., 1981. *Human ecosystems.* New York: Macmillan.

Dawkins, R., 1976. *The selfish gene.* New York: Oxford.

Ereshevsky, M., 1992. *The units of evolution: Essays on the nature of species.* Cambridge: MIT Press.

Lewontin, R., 1974. *The genetic basis of evolutionary change.* New York: Columbia University Press.

Li, W.-H., and D. Graur, 1991. *Fundamentals of molecular evolution.* Sunderland, Mass.: Sinauer.

Margulis, L., and K. Schwartz, 1982. *Five kingdoms, An illustrated guide to the phyla of life on Earth.* New York: W. H. Freeman.

———, and L. Olendzenski, eds., 1992. *Environmental evolution.* Cambridge: MIT Press.

Mayr, E., 1988. *Toward a new philosophy of biology.* Cambridge: Harvard University Press.

Selander, R., A. Clark, and T. Whittam, 1991. *Evolution at the molecular level.* Sunderland, Mass.: Sinauer.

Origins and Mechanisms of Language

Bruner, J., 1990. *Acts of meaning.* Cambridge: Harvard University Press.

Delbrück, M., 1975. *Mind from matter?* Palo Alto: Blackwell.

Johnson, G., 1992. *In the palaces of memory.* New York: Vintage.

Klima, E., and U. Bellugi, 1978. *The signs of language.* Cambridge: Harvard University Press.

Landau, M., 1991. *Narratives of evolution.* New Haven: Yale University Press.

Politics of Science and Medicine

Angier, N., 1988. *Natural obsessions.* Boston: Houghton Mifflin.

Annas, G., 1992. *Gene mapping: Using law and ethics as guides.* New York: Oxford University Press.

Bankowski, Z., and A. Capron, eds., 1991. *Genetics, ethics and human values: Human genome mapping, genetic screening and gene therapy.* World Health Organization.

Bulger, R., E. Heitman, and S. J. Reiser, 1993. *The ethical dimensions of the biological sciences.* New York: Cambridge University Press.

Davis, B., ed., 1992. *The genetic revolution: Scientific prospects and public perception.* Baltimore: Johns Hopkins University Press.

de Solla Price, D. J., 1963. *Little science, big science.* New York: Columbia University Press.

Dubos, R., 1961. *The dreams of reason.* New York: Columbia University Press.

Ginzberg, E., 1990. *The medical triangle.* Cambridge: Harvard University Press.

Hall, S., 1992. *Mapping the next millennium: The discovery of the new geographics.* New York: Random House.

Holtzman, N., 1989. *Proceed with caution: Predicting genetic risks in the recombinant DNA era.* Baltimore: Johns Hopkins.

Kevles, D., and L. Hood, eds., 1992. *The code of codes: Scientific and social issues in the human genome project.* Cambridge: Harvard University Press.

Kevles, D. J., 1985. *In the name of eugenics.* New York: Knopf.

Lange, J., et al., 1940. *Erbpathologie.* Vol. 1 of *Menschliche erblehre und rassenhygiene.* Munich: Lehmanns.

Lappe, M., 1984. *Broken code: The exploitation of DNA.* San Francisco: Sierra Club Books.

Lee, Thomas, 1992. *Human genome project: Quest for the code of life.* New York: Plenum.

Lifton, R., 1986. *The Nazi doctors.* New York: Basic Books.

Müller-Hill, B., 1988. *Murderous science.* New York: Oxford University Press.

Nelkin, D., and L. Tancredi, 1989. *Dangerous diagnostics.* New York: Basic Books.

Nichols, E. K., 1988. *Human gene therapy.* Cambridge: Harvard University Press.

Pollack, R., et al., 1973. *Biohazards in biological research.* Cold Spring Harbor, N.Y.: Cold Spring Harbor Press.

Proctor, R., 1988. *Racial hygiene.* Cambridge: Harvard University Press.

Rainger, R., 1992. *An agenda for antiquity.* University of Alabama Press.

Suzuki, D., and P. Knudtson, 1989. *Genethics: The clash between the new genetics and human value.* Cambridge: Harvard University Press.

Weatherall, D., 1991. *The new genetics and clinical practice.* New York: Oxford University Press.

Wingerson, L., 1990. *Mapping our genes.* New York: Plume.

JOURNAL ARTICLES

These lists would not be complete without a sampling, by chapter, of information written by one scientist for another. I drew many of my examples of DNA as a language from this primary scientific literature. These papers are for the most part also good examples of the style by which — in fits and starts — the molecular biology of our species advances.

Chapter 1

Watson, J. D., and F.H.C. Crick, 1953. A structure for deoxyribose nucleic acid. *Nature,* April 25: 737–38.
———. Genetical implications of the structure of deoxyribonucleic acid. *Nature,* May 30: 964–67.

Chapter 2

Charlesworth, B., 1991. The evolution of sex chromosomes. *Science* 251: 1030–33.
Clark, L., et al., 1992. Defective epithelial chloride transport in a gene-targeted mouse model of cystic fibrosis. *Science* 257: 1125–30.
Diamond, J., 1991. Curse and blessing of the ghetto. *Discover,* March 1991: 60–65.
Gusella, J., et al., 1983. A polymorphic DNA marker genetically linked to Huntington's disease. *Nature* 306: 234–38.
Hamer, D., et al., 1993. A linkage between DNA markers on the X chromosome and male sexual orientation. *Science* 261: 5119–22.
Harley, V., et al., 1992. DNA binding activity of recombinant SRY from normal males and XY females. *Science* 255: 453–56.
Merz, B., 1987. Matchmaking scheme solves Tay-Sachs problem. *J. Amer. Med. Assoc.* 258: 2636–37.
News item, 1968. Logic of biology. *Nature* 220: 429–30.
Potter, H., 1991. Review and hypothesis: Alzheimer disease and Down syndrome: Chromosome 21 nondisjunction

may underlie both disorders. *Am. J. Human Genetics* 48: 1192–1200.

Rommens, J. M., et al., 1989. Identification of the cystic fibrosis gene: Chromosome walking and jumping. *Science* 245: 1059–80.

Chapter 3

Aggarwal, A., et al., 1988. Recognition of a DNA operator by the repressor of phage 434: A view at high resolution. *Science* 242: 899–906.

Benner, M., et al., 1989. Modern metabolism as a palimpsest of the RNA world. *Proc. Nat. Acad. Sci.* 86: 7054.

Brendel, V., et al., 1986. Linguistics of nucleotide sequences: Morphology and comparison of vocabularies. *J. Biomolecular Structure and Dynamics* 4: 11–21.

Darnell, J., 1982. Variety in the level of gene control in eukaryotic cells. *Nature* 297: 499–506.

De Duve, C., et al., 1988. The second genetic code. *Nature* 333: 117–18.

Dombroski, B., et al., 1991. Isolation of an active human transposable element. *Science* 254: 1805–7.

Ealick, S., et al., 1991. Three-dimensional structure of recombinant human interferon-γ. *Science* 252: 698–702.

Francklyn, E., et al., 1992. Overlapping nucleotide determinants for specific aminoacylation of RNA microhelices. *Science* 255: 1121–25.

Fu, Y.-H., et al., 1992. An unstable triplet repeat in a gene related to myotonic muscular dystrophy. *Science* 255: 1256–58.

Gething, M., and J. Sambrook, 1992. Protein folding in the cell. *Nature* 355: 33–45.

Gogos, J., et al., 1992. Sequence discrimination by alternatively spliced isoforms of a DNA binding zinc finger domain. *Science* 257: 1951–55.

Hanscombe, O., et al., 1991. Importance of globin gene order for correct developmental expression. *Genes & Development* 5: 1387–94.

Hard, T., et al., 1990. Solution structure of the glucocorticoid receptor DNA-binding domain. *Science* 249: 157–60.

Helfman, D., et al., 1988. Alternative splicing of tropomyosin pre-mRNAs in vitro and in vivo. *Genes & Development* 2: 1627–38.

Jurka, J., 1990. Novel families of interspersed repetitive elements from the human genome. *Nucleic Acids Research* 18: 137–41.

Koch, C., et al., 1991. SH2 and SH3 domains: Elements that control interactions of cytoplasmic signalling proteins. *Science* 252: 668–74.

Kuhl, P., et al., 1992. Linguistic experience alters phonetic perception in infants by 6 months of age. *Science* 252: 606–8.

McClintock, B., 1984. The significance of responses of the genome to challenge. *Science* 226: 792–801.

Nathans, J., et al., 1989. Molecular genetics of human blue cone monochromacy. *Science* 245: 831–38.

Piatigorsky, J., and G. Wistow, 1991. The recruitment of crystallins: New functions precede gene duplication. *Science* 252: 1078–79.

Ptashne, M., and A. Gann, 1990. Activators and targets. *Nature* 346: 329–31.

Reilly, J., et al., 1990. Once more with feeling: Affect and language in atypical populations. *Development and Psychopathology* 2: 367–91.

Schulman, L., and H. Pelka, 1989. The Anticodon contains a major element of the identity of Arginine Transfer RNAs. *Science* 246: 1595–97.

Shih, M.-C., et al., 1988. Intron existence predated the divergence of eukaryotes and prokaryotes. *Science* 242: 1164–66.

Spector, D., 1990. Higher order nuclear organization: Three dimensional distribution of small nuclear ribonucleoprotein particles. *Proc. Nat. Acad. Sci.* 87: 147–51.

Stanfield, R., et al., 1990. Crystal structures of an antibody to a peptide and its complex with peptide antigen at 2.8 Å. *Science* 248: 712–19.

Thal, D., et al., 1989. Language and cognition in two children with William's syndrome. *J. Speech and Hearing Res.* 32: 489–500.

Thibodeau, S., et al., 1993. Microsatellite instability of cancer of the proximal colon. *Science* 260: 816–22.

Treisman, J., et al., 1989. A single amino acid can determine the DNA binding specificity of homeodomain proteins. *Cell* 59: 553–62.

Vinson, C., et al., 1989. Scissors-grip model for DNA recognition by a family of leucine zipper proteins. *Science* 246: 911–16.

Zahler, A., et al., 1993. Distinct functions of SR proteins in alternative pre-mRNA splicing. *Science* 360: 219–22.

Chapter 4

Blaese, M., 1993. Development of gene therapy for immunodeficiency: Adenosine deaminase deficiency. *Pediatric Research* 33 (suppl.): S49–S55.

Brosius, J., 1991. Retroposons — seeds of evolution. *Science* 251: 753–54.

Cantor, C., 1990. Orchestrating the human genome project. *Science* 248: 49–51.

Chakraborty, R., and K. Kidd, 1991. The utility of DNA typing in forensic work. *Science* 254: 1735–39.

Davis, B., et al., 1990. The human genome and other initiatives. *Science* 342–43.

Engelhardt, J., et al., 1993. Direct gene transfer of human CFTR into human bronchial epithelia of xenografts with E1-deleted adenoviruses. *Nature Genetics* 4: 27–34.

Erlich, H., 1991. Recent advances in the Polymerase Chain Reaction. *Science* 252: 1643–50.

Jeskevich, J., and C. Guyer, 1990. Bovine growth hormone: Human food safety evaluation. *Science* 249: 875–84.

Kieleczawa, J., et al., 1992. DNA sequencing by primer walking with strings of contiguous hexamers. *Science* 258: 1787–91.

Le Gal La Salle, G., et al., 1993. An adenovirus vector for gene transfer into neurons and glia in the brain. *Science* 259: 988–90.

Lewontin, R., and D. Hartl, 1991. Population genetics in forensic DNA typing. *Science* 254: 1745–50.

Li, H., et al., 1988. Amplification and analysis of DNA sequences in single human sperm and diploid cells. *Nature* 335: 414–17.

Lusher, J., et al., 1993. Recombinant factor VIII for the treatment of previously untreated patients with hemophilia A. *New England J. Medicine* 328: 453–59.

NIH/CEPH Collaborative Mapping Group, 1992. A comprehensive genetic linkage map of the human genome. *Science* 258: 67–86; appendix, 148–62.

Olson, M., et al., 1989. A common language for physical mapping of the human genome. *Science* 245: 1434–35.

Patterson, A., et al., 1988. Resolution of quantitative traits into Mendelian factors by using a complete linkage map of restriction fragment length polymorphisms. *Nature* 335: 721.

Radmacher, M., et al., 1992. From molecules to cells: Imaging soft samples with the atomic force microscope. *Science* 257: 1900–05.

Reilly, P., 1992. ASHG statement on genetics and privacy: Testimony to United States Congress. *Am. J. Human Genetics* 50: 640–42.

Risch, N., and B. Devlin, 1992. On the probability of matching DNA fingerprints. *Science* 255: 717–20.

Vasil, I., 1990. The realities and challenges of plant biotechnology. *Bio/technology* 8: 296–301.

Watson, J. D., 1990. The human genome project: Past, present and future. *Science* 248: 44–48.

Weissenbach, J., et al., 1992. A second-generation linkage map of the human genome. *Nature* 359: 794–801.

Chapter 5

Aaltonen, L., et al., 1993. Clues to the pathogenesis of familial colorectal cancer. *Science* 260: 812–16.

Aldous, P., 1993. European biotech: Thumbs down for cattle hormone. *Science* 261: 418.

Anderson, C., 1993. Researchers win decision on knockout mouse pricing. *Science* 260: 23–24.

Behringer, R., et al., 1989. Synthesis of functional human hemoglobin in transgenic mice. *Science* 245: 971–73.

Borowiec, J., et al., 1990. Binding and unwinding: How T antigen engages the SV40 origin of DNA replication. *Cell* 60: 181–84.

Chisaka, O., and M. Capecchi, 1991. Regionally restricted developmental defects resulting from targeted disruption of the mouse homeobox gene *hox-1.5*. *Nature* 350: 473–79.

Daubert, William, et al., petitioners, v. Merrell Dow Pharmaceuticals, Inc. Supreme Court decision 92–102, decided June 28, 1993. *United States Law Week* 6-29-93: 4805–11.

DePamphilis, M., and M. Bradley, 1986. SV40. Chapter 3 in *The papovaviridae*, vol. I. New York: Plenum.

Dyson, N., et al., 1990. Large T antigens of many polyoma viruses are able to form complexes with the retinoblastoma protein. *J. Virol.* 64: 1353–56.

Frebourg, T., et al., 1992. Germ-line mutations of p53 suppressor gene in patients with high risk for cancer inactivate the p53 protein. *Proc. Nat. Acad. Sci.* 89: 6413–17.

Galton, D., 1988. Molecular genetics of coronary heart disease. *Euro. J. Clin. Invest.* 18: 219–25.

Grant, S., et al., 1992. Impaired long-term potentiation, spatial learning, and hippocampal development in fyn mutant mice. *Science* 258: 1903–10.

Handyside, A., et al., 1992. Birth of a normal girl after in vitro fertilization and pre-implantation testing for cystic fibrosis. *New England J. Medicine* 327: 905–9.

Hiatt, A., et al., 1989. Production of antibodies in transgenic plants. *Nature* 342: 76–78.

Jaenisch, R., 1988. Transgenic animals. *Science* 240: 1468–74.

Kawabata, S., et al., 1991. Amyloid plaques, neurofibrillary tangles and neuronal loss in brains of transgenic mice overexpressing a C-terminal fragment of human amyloid precursor protein. *Nature* 354: 476–78.

———, 1992. Alzheimer's retraction. *Nature* 356: 23.

Kessel, M., and P. Gruss, 1990. Murine developmental control genes. *Science* 249: 374–79.

Kuerbitz, S., et al., 1992. Wild-type p53 is a cell cycle checkpoint determinant following irradiation. *Proc. Nat. Acad. Sci.* 89: 7491–95.

Leonard, J. M., et al., 1988. Development of disease and virus recovery in transgenic mice containing HIV proviral DNA. *Science* 242: 1665–70.

Levine, A., et al., 1991. The p53 tumour suppressor gene. *Nature* 351: 453–56.

Loeber, G., et al., 1989. The zinc finger region of SV40 large T antigen. *J. Virology* 63: 94–100.

Mason, H., et al., 1992. Expression of hepatitis B surface antigen in transgenic plants. *Proc. Nat. Acad. Sci.* 89: 11745–49.

McVey, D., et al., 1989. Properties of the DNA-binding domain of the SV40 large T antigen. *Mol. Cell. Biol.* 9: 5525–36.

Padgette, S., et al., 1989. Selective herbicide tolerance through protein engineering. *Cell Cult. Somatic Cell Gen. Plants* 6: 441–76.

Paszkowski, J., et al., 1988. Gene targeting in plants. *EMBO J.* 7: 4021–26.

Peltomaki, P., et al., 1993. Genetic mapping of a locus predisposing to human colorectal cancer. *Science* 260: 810–12.

Qian, Y., et al., 1989. The structure of the Antennapedia homeo domain determined by NMR spectroscopy: Comparison with prokaryotic repressors. *Cell* 59: 573–80.

Ratcliff, R., et al., 1993. Production of severe cystic fibrosis mutation in mice by gene targeting. *Nature Genetics* 4: 35–41.

Sepulveda, A., et al., 1989. Development of a transgenic mouse system for the analysis of stages of liver carcinogenesis using tissue-specific expression of SV40 Large T-antigen controlled by regulatory elements of the human α-1-antitrypsin gene. *Cancer Research* 49: 6108–17.

Vogelstein, B., and K. Kinzler, 1992. p53 function and dysfunction. *Cell* 70: 523–26.

Walsh, C., and C. Cepko, 1992. Widespread dispersion of neuronal clones across functional regions of the cerebral cortex. *Science* 255: 434–40.

Yokoyama, T., et al., 1993. Reversal of left-right asymmetry: A sinus inversus mutation. *Science* 260: 679–82.

Chapter 6

Abelson, J., 1990. Directed evolution of nucleic acids by independent replication and selection. *Science* 249: 488–89.

Aldhous, P., 1992. The promise and pitfalls of molecular genetics. *Science* 257: 164–65.

Asfaw, B., et al., 1992. The earliest Acheulean from Konso-Gardula. *Nature* 330: 732–35.

Ayala, F., 1986. On the virtues and pitfalls of the molecular evolutionary clock. *J. Heredity* 77: 226–35.

Bailey, J., et al., 1993. Heritable factors influence sexual orientation in women. *Arch. Gen. Psychiatry* 50: 217–23.

Barbujani, G., and R. Sokal, 1990. Zones of sharp genetic change in Europe are also linguistic boundaries. *Proc. Nat. Acad. Sci.* 87: 1816–19.

Begun, D., 1992. Miocene fossil hominids and the chimp-human clade. *Science* 257: 1929–32.

Bouchard, T., et al., 1990. Sources of human psychological differences: The Minnesota study of twins reared apart. *Science* 250: 223–28.

Caldeira, K., et al., 1992. The life span of the biosphere revisited. *Nature* 360: 721–23.

Cann, R., et al., 1987. Mitochondrial DNA and human evolution. *Nature* 325:31–36.

Cavalli-Sforza, L., 1990. How can one study individual variation for 3 billion nucleotides of the human genome? *Am. J. Human Genetics* 46: 649–51.

———, et al., 1988. Reconstruction of human evolution: Bringing together genetic, archaeological and linguistic data. *Proc. Nat. Acad. Sci.* 85: 6002–6.

———, 1993. Demic expansions and human evolution. *Science* 259: 639–46.

Churchland, P., and T. Sejnowski, 1988. Perspectives on cognitive neuroscience. *Science* 242: 741–45.

Corina, D., et al., 1992. The linguistic basis of left hemisphere specialization. *Science* 255: 1258–60.

Coyne, J., 1992. Genetics and speciation. *Nature* 355: 511–15.

Deacon, T., 1990. Rethinking mammalian brain evolution. *Amer. Zool.* 30: 629–705.

DeSalle, R., et al., 1992. DNA sequences from a fossil termite in Oligo-Miocene amber and their phylogenetic implications. *Science* 257: 1933–37.

Gazzaniga, M., 1989. The organization of the human brain. *Science* 245: 947–52.

Gingerich, P., 1985. Species in the fossil record: Concepts, trends and transitions. *Paleobiology* 11: 27–41.

Goodman, M., 1989. Emerging alliance of phylogenetic systematics and molecular biology: A new age of exploration. *The hierarchy of life*, eds. B. Fernholm et al., ch. 4: 43–61. New York: Elsevier.

Green, P., et al., 1993. Ancient conserved regions in new gene sequences and the protein databases. *Science* 259: 1711–16.

Hall, S., 1992. How technique is changing science. *Science* 257: 344–49.

Han, T.-M., et al., 1992. Megascopic eukaryotic algae from the 2.1-billion-year-old Negaunee iron-formation, Michigan. *Science* 257: 232–35.

Handyside, A., et al., 1989. Biopsy of human preimplantation embryos and sexing by DNA amplification. *Lancet* Feb. 18: 347–49.

Knoll, A., 1992. The early evolution of eukaryotes: A geological perspective. *Science* 256: 622–27.

Lake, J., 1990. Origin of the metazoa. *Proc. Nat. Acad. Sci.* 87: 763–66.

Lander, E., and D. Botstein, 1989. Mapping mendelian factors underlying quantitative traits using RFLP linkage maps. *Genetics* 121: 185.

Lightman, A., and O. Gingerich, 1991. When do anomalies begin? *Science* 255: 690–95.

May, R., 1988. How many species are there on Earth? *Science* 241: 1441–49.

Morton, N., et al., 1993. Kinship bioassay on hypervariable loci in Blacks and Caucasians. *Proc. Nat. Acad. Sci.* 90: 1892–96.

Murtha, M., et al., 1991. Detection of homeobox genes in development and evolution. *Proc. Nat. Acad. Sci.* 88: 10711–15.

Novacek, M., 1992. Mammalian phylogeny: Shaking the tree. *Nature* 356: 121–25.

Pimm, S., and J. Gittleman, 1992. Biological diversity: Where is it? *Science* 255: 940.

Pinker, S., and P. Bloom, 1990. Natural language and natural selection. *Behav. and Brain Sci.* 13: 707–84.

Plomin, R., 1990. The role of inheritance in behavior. *Science* 248: 183–88.

Poinar, G., et al., 1993. Terrestrial soft-bodied protists and other microorganisms in Triassic amber. *Science* 259: 222–24.

Risch, N., 1992. Genetic linkage: Interpreting Lod scores. *Science* 255: 803–4.

Schopf, W., 1993. Microfossils of the early Archean Apex Chert: New evidence for the antiquity of life. *Science* 260: 640–46.

Sleep, N., et al., 1989. Annihilation of ecosystems by large asteroid impacts on the early Earth. *Nature* 342: 139–42.

Smouse, P., et al., 1982. Multiple-locus allocation of individuals to groups as a function of the genetic variation within and differences among human populations. *Amer. Nat.* 119: 445–63.

Sokal, R., et al., 1990. Genetics and language in European populations. *Amer. Nat.* 135: 157–75.

Tianyuan, L., and D. Etler, 1992. New middle Pleistocene hominid crania from Yunxian in China. *Nature* 357: 404–7.

van den Bergh, S., 1992. The age and size of the universe. *Science* 258: 421–23.

Vigilant, L., et al., 1991. African populations and the evolution of human mitochondrial DNA. *Science* 253: 1503–7.

Wood, B. 1992. Origin and evolution of the genus *Homo*. *Nature* 355: 783–90.

Yoon, C., 1993. Counting creatures great and small. *Science* 260: 620–22.

Conclusion

Brown, G., 1992. Rational science, irrational reality: A congressional perspective on basic research and society. *Science* 258: 200–01.

Glass, B., 1971. Science: Endless horizons or golden age? *Science* 171: 23–29.

Lederman, L., 1992. The advancement of science. *Science* 256: 1119–24.

•

INDEX